Predicting and changing
health behaviour

Predicting and changing health behaviour

Research and Practice with Social Cognition Models

Third edition

Edited by
Mark Conner and Paul Norman

McGraw Hill Education Open University Press

Open University Press
McGraw-Hill Education
McGraw-Hill House
Shoppenhangers Road
Maidenhead
Berkshire
England
SL6 2QL

email: enquiries@openup.co.uk
world wide web: www.openup.co.uk

and Two Penn Plaza, New York, NY 10121-2289, USA

First published 1995
Second edition published 2005
First published in this third edition 2015

A catalogue record of this book is available from the British Library

ISBN-13: 978-0-335-26378-3
ISBN-10: 0-335-26378-X
eISBN: 978-0-335-26379-0

Library of Congress Cataloging-in-Publication Data
CIP data applied for

Typeset by Aptara, Inc.

Fictitious names of companies, products, people, characters and/or data that may be used herein (in case studies or in examples) are not intended to represent any real individual, company, product or event.

Praise for this book

John Muir (1838–1914)

Contents

List of tables

List of figures

Contributors

Charles Abraham is Professor of Psychology at Peninsular Medical School, University of Exeter, Exeter, UK.

Henk Boer is Associate Professor in Health Psychology and Programme Leader of Psychology at the University of Twente, Enschede, The Netherlands.

Nikos L.D. Chatzisarantis is Professor of Psychology with the Health Psychology and Behavioural Medicine Research Group in the School of Psychology and Speech Pathology, Curtin University, Perth, WA, Australia.

Mark Conner is Professor of Applied Social Psychology at the School of Psychology, University of Leeds, Leeds, UK.

Stephanie D. Finneran is a PhD student in health-social psychology at the University of Connecticut, Storrs, CT, USA.

Meg Gerrard is Research Professor of Psychology at the University of Connecticut, USA.

Rick Gibbons is Professor of Psychology at the University of Connecticut, Storrs, CT, USA.

Peter M. Gollwitzer is Professor of Social Psychology and Motivation at the University of Konstanz, Germany and Psychology Department, New York University, New York, USA.

Martin S. Hagger is John Curtin Distinguished Professor with the Health Psychology and Behavioural Medicine Research Group in the School of Psychology and Speech Pathology, Curtin University, Perth, WA, Australia.

Aleksandra Luszczynska is Professor of Psychology at the University of Social Sciences and Humanities, Poland, and Associate Research Professor at the Trauma, Health, and Hazards Center, University of Colorado, Colorado Springs, CO, USA.

Susan Michie is Professor of Health Psychology and Director of the Centre for Behaviour Change at University College London, London, UK.

Barbara Mullan is Associate Professor with the Health Psychology and Behavioural Medicine Research Group in the School of Psychology and Speech Pathology, Curtin University, Perth, WA, Australia.

Paul Norman is Professor of Health Psychology at the Department of Psychology, University of Sheffield, Sheffield, UK.

Andrew Prestwich is Senior Lecturer in Health and Social Psychology at the School of Psychology, University of Leeds, Leeds, UK.

Ralf Schwarzer is Research Professor of Psychology at the Institute of Positive Psychology and Education, Australian Catholic University, Sydney, NSW, Australia, Professor of Psychology at the University of Social Sciences and Humanities, Poland, and Emeritus Professor at the Institut für Psychologie, Freie Universität Berlin, Berlin, Germany.

Erwin R. Seydel was, until 2012, Professor of Organizational and Health Communication at the Department of Communication Studies, University of Twente, Enschede, The Netherlands.

Paschal Sheeran is Professor of Psychology at the Department of Psychology, University of North Carolina at Chapel Hill, Chapel Hill, NC, USA.

Paul Sparks is Senior Lecturer at the Department of Psychology, University of Sussex, Brighton, UK.

Michelle L. Stock is Associate Professor of Psychology at The George Washington University, Washington, DC, USA.

Stephen Sutton is Professor of Psychology at the University of Cambridge, Institute of Public Health, Cambridge, UK.

Thomas L. Webb is Reader in Social Psychology at the Department of Psychology, University of Sheffield, Sheffield, UK.

Caroline E. Wood is Senior Research Associate in the Department of Clinical, Educational and Health Psychology at University College London and Assistant Director of the UCL Centre for Behaviour Change, London, UK.

Preface

The study of behaviours that influence health, the factors that determine which individuals perform these behaviours, and how to change them is a key area of research within health psychology. As the third edition of this book testifies, there is a considerable and impressive body of research in this area. The purpose of this book is to provide in a single source an overview of current research and practical details of how to apply the most widely used social cognition models to the prediction of the performance of health behaviours and to use them to change such behaviours. Social cognition models start from the assumption that an individual's behaviour is best understood in terms of his or her perceptions of the social environment. Such an approach has been widely and successfully used by psychologists to help understand a range of human behaviours, and by health psychologists to understand health behaviours in particular.

The chapters in this book bring together detailed reviews and descriptions of the most common social cognition models and their application to understanding and changing health behaviours. It is hoped that this will provide a useful resource to those interested in work in this area, and make the described approaches to understanding and changing health behaviours more accessible and more appropriately applied. Moreover, by bringing together these models, similarities and differences between approaches can be examined and the whole approach critically evaluated.

The introductory chapter examines the concept of health behaviour and briefly reviews epidemiological work on the variation in who performs the different health behaviours. It then outlines the general social cognitive approach taken to understanding and predicting health behaviour. The key features of the social cognition models described in the subsequent chapters are then outlined. Similarities, differences, and the potential for integration among these models are then discussed. Finally, the potential for using social cognition models to change health behaviours are outlined.

Following the introductory chapter are nine individual chapters describing the most widely applied social cognition models: the health belief model, protection motivation theory, self-determination theory, the theory of planned behaviour, the prototype/willingness model, social cognitive theory, the health action process approach, stage models (transtheoretical model, precaution adoption process model), and implementation intentions. Each of these 'model' chapters has been produced by prominent researchers in the area and, in general, follows a common structure. Section 1 outlines the background to and origins of the model. This is followed, in Section 2, by a description of the model, including full details of each of its components. Section 3 contains a summary of research using the model and the findings with a range of health behaviours. Section 4 examines recent developments and expansions to the model. Section 5 provides a detailed consideration of the procedures for developing appropriate measures for each component of the model. Section 6 reviews intervention studies that have been conducted using the model to change health behaviours. The final section reviews potential future directions for research with the model.

The penultimate chapter focuses on the techniques that can be used to change health behaviours, often by targeting variables outlined in the main social cognition models. As a result, this chapter follows a slightly different structure to those focusing on individual models. The final chapter considers some of the major unresolved issues relating to predicting and changing health behaviour that are common to the social cognitive approach.

The book is not intended to be a 'cookbook' of how to apply social cognition models to predict and change health behaviours. Rather, the intention is to introduce readers to the general social cognitive approach to the understanding of such behaviours, to describe the most commonly used social cognition models, to consider their differences and similarities as well as their advantages and disadvantages, and to enable researchers to apply each model appropriately to predict and change health behaviour within their own area of interest. Useful directions for future research within this paradigm are described both in the model chapters and final chapter of the book.

We would like to thank the authors of the chapters for all their hard work in producing such clear descriptions of these models and extensive reviews of the relevant literature. We would also like to thank Open University Press for its help and encouragement during the preparation of the third edition of this book.

Mark Conner and Paul Norman

Abbreviations

A	attitude towards behaviour
AIDS	acquired immune deficiency syndrome
BB	behavioural beliefs
BCT	behaviour change technique
BCTTv1	Behaviour Change Technique Taxonomy version 1
BCW	Behaviour Change Wheel
BI	behavioural intention
BSE	breast self-examination
CB	control beliefs
CDT	cognitive dissonance theory
CHD	coronary heart disease
ELM	elaboration likelihood model
EVP	expectancy-value perspective
FOBT	foecal occult blood test
GNAT	Go/NoGo Task
HAPA	health action process approach
HBCC	Health Behaviour Change Competency Framework
HBM	health belief model
HIV	human immunodeficiency virus
IAT	Implicit Association Test
MAP	model of action phases
MOST	Multiphase Optimization Strategy
MRI	magnetic resonance imaging
NB	normal beliefs
PAPM	precaution adoption process model
PBC	perceived behavioural control
PED	performance-enhancing drug
PHM	preventive health model
PMT	protection motivation theory
PWM	prototype/willingness model
RCT	randomized controlled trial
RIM	reflective–impulsive model
RPM	relapse prevention model
SAM	self-affirmation manipulation
SCM	social cognition model
SCT	social cognitive theory
SDT	self-determination theory
SES	socio-economic status

SET	self-efficacy theory
SEU	subjective expected utility
SN	subjective norm
SRBAI	self-report behavioural automaticity index
SRHI	self-report habit index
STD	sexually transmitted disease
TCS	Theory Coding Scheme
TDF	Theoretical Domains Framework
TIB	theory of interpersonal behaviour
TPB	theory of planned behaviour
TRA	theory of reasoned action
TSE	testicular self-examination
TST	temporal self-regulation theory
TTM	transtheoretical model

Chapter 1

Predicting and changing health behaviour: a social cognition approach

Mark Conner and Paul Norman

1 Introduction

A considerable body of research has examined the role of social cognitive factors in predicting health behaviour (see Conner and Norman 1995, 2005; Norman *et al.* 2000). This chapter overviews the social cognition approach to understanding health behaviours; introduces key theories employed; compares theories; considers theory integration; and, finally, examines the value of the approach for changing health behaviour.

Justification for the study of health behaviours is based on two assumptions: that in industrialized countries a substantial proportion of the mortality from the leading causes of death is due to particular behaviour patterns, and that these behaviour patterns are modifiable. It is now recognized that individuals can make contributions to their own health and well-being through adopting particular health-enhancing behaviours (e.g. exercise) and avoiding other health-compromising behaviours (e.g. smoking). The identification of the factors that underlie such 'health behaviours' has become a focus of research in psychology and other health-related disciplines since the mid 1980s (e.g. Winett 1985; Adler and Matthews 1994; Conner and Norman 1995, 2005; Baum and Posluszny 1999; Norman *et al.* 2000). The importance of behaviour change to this research should not be underestimated. Although gaining an understanding of the reasons why individuals perform a variety of behaviours has often been the focus of research, this should be seen as a first step in designing better interventions to change the prevalence of health behaviours and so produce improvements in individuals' and populations' health.

The health behaviours focused on have been extremely varied, from health-enhancing behaviours such as exercise participation and healthy eating, through health-protective behaviours such as health screening clinic attendance, vaccination against disease, and condom use in response to the threat of AIDS, to avoidance of health-harming behaviours such as smoking and excessive alcohol consumption, and sick-role behaviours such as compliance with medical regimens. A unifying theme has been that they each have immediate or long-term effects on the individual's health and are at least partially within the individual's control. Epidemiological studies have revealed considerable variation in who performs these behaviours. Approaches taken to understanding factors underlying this variation have been many and varied. A broad distinction can be made between factors intrinsic to the individual (e.g. socio-demographic factors, personality, social support, cognitions) and factors extrinsic to the individual, which can be further divided into incentive structures (e.g. taxing tobacco and alcohol, subsidizing sporting facilities) and legal restrictions (e.g. banning dangerous substances, fining individuals for not wearing seatbelts). Of the two, intrinsic factors have received most attention from psychologists, of which cognitive factors have been considered the most important proximal determinants. Models of how such cognitive factors produce various 'social' behaviours are commonly referred to as social cognition models (SCMs) and have been widely used by health psychologists. They are considered to have provided a contribution to the greater understanding of who performs health behaviours (Marteau 1989) and to explaining how extrinsic factors may produce behaviour change (e.g. Rutter *et al.* 1993). The justifications for focusing on social cognitive determinants in SCMs are twofold. First, these 'health cognitions' are assumed to be important causes of behaviour that mediate the effects of other determinants (e.g. social class). Second, they are assumed to be more open to change than other factors (e.g. personality). These justifications imply that effective interventions could usefully be based on manipulations of cognitive factors shown to determine health behaviours.

2 Health behaviours

Health behaviours have been defined as 'Any activity undertaken by a person believing himself to be healthy for the purpose of preventing disease or detecting it at an asymptomatic stage' (Kasl and Cobb 1966: 246). There are limitations to this conception, including the omission of lay or self-defined health behaviours and the exclusion of activities carried out by people with recognized illnesses that are directed at self-management, delaying disease progression or improving general well-being. In contrast, in the *Handbook of Health Behavior Research*, Gochman defines health behaviours as '... overt behavioral patterns, actions and habits that relate to health maintenance, to health restoration and to health improvement' (1997: 3). A useful broad definition would include any activity undertaken for the purpose of preventing or detecting disease or for improving health and well-being (Conner and Norman 1995, 2005). A variety of behaviours fall within such a definition, including medical service usage (e.g. physician visits, vaccinations, screening), adherence to medical regimens (e.g. dietary, diabetic, anti-hypertensive regimens), and self-directed health behaviours (e.g. diet, exercise, smoking). This section looks at the role of such behaviours in health outcomes, what is known about who performs these behaviours, ways of classifying these behaviours, and the broad range of factors that are predictive of the performance of such behaviours.

2.1 The role of health behaviours in health outcomes

Studies of the relationship between the performance of health behaviours and a variety of health outcomes have been conducted for more than 40 years (e.g. Belloc and Breslow 1972; Whitehead

1988; Blaxter 1990). For example, studies in Alameda County, California identified seven features of lifestyle – not smoking, moderate alcohol intake, sleeping 7–8 hours per night, exercising regularly, maintaining a desirable body weight, avoiding snacks, and eating breakfast regularly – that together were associated with lower morbidity and higher subsequent long-term survival (Belloc and Breslow 1972; Belloc 1973; Breslow and Enstrom 1980). There now exists a considerable body of research demonstrating the importance of a variety of health behaviours for both morbidity and mortality. For example, research into the major causes of premature death in the Western world (e.g. cardiovascular diseases and cancer) has emphasized the importance of behaviours such as smoking, alcohol consumption, dietary choice, sexual behaviours, and physical exercise (e.g. Smith and Jacobson 1988), together with gaps in primary prevention and screening uptake (Amler and Eddins 1987). In addition, several authors have pointed out that health behaviours may have a positive impact on quality of life via delaying the onset of chronic disease and extending active lifespan (e.g. Conner and Norman 1995, 2005).

Baum and Posluszny (1999) note three basic ways in which behaviour exerts its influence on health: (1) by producing direct biological changes; (2) by conveying health risks or protecting against them; or (3) by leading to the early detection or treatment of disease. So, for example, smoking may lead to changes in the cells of the lungs that predispose an individual to lung cancer; using condoms may protect against the transmission of HIV or other sexually transmitted infections; and breast or testicular self-examination can lead to detection of lumps and the early treatment of abnormalities.

2.2 Who performs health behaviours?

Given the impact of a range of health behaviours on health outcomes, one might expect there to be detailed information available on who performs what health behaviours and how this varies across different segments of the population. Unfortunately, although there is a growing body of research that details variations in health behaviours across the population, there is also considerable unevenness in the data and its availability. A lot more is known about the distribution of behaviours such as smoking than say testicular or breast self-examination. There is also considerable variation across countries. In the USA, for example, the Centers for Diseases Control collects and produces regular summaries for health behaviours such as smoking, alcohol consumption, physical activity, and sleep (CDC 2013). Similarly, the UK Data Service (www.ukdataservice.ac.uk) provides access to a number of key surveys that provide overview data for a range of health behaviours across the UK population as a whole (e.g. General Lifestyle Survey), together with more detailed information on specific cohorts often followed at regular intervals (e.g. Longitudinal Study of Young People in England). The data collected and made publicly available for other countries is much more varied and in many cases more limited, particularly for Third World countries. A single, publicly available source bringing together the most recent data from different nations on who performs various health behaviours would be an invaluable resource to researchers working in this area. Such data would allow researchers to make better comparisons across countries or points in time, as well as explore more specific information on differences by type of behaviour, and to explore variations by demographic variables such as gender, age, ethnic group, education, and socio-economic status.

Data for the USA (CDC 2013) reveals complex variations by behaviour and demographics. In relation to risky behaviours, the CDC report revealed that about 25% of US adults had five or more alcoholic drinks in one day at least once in the past year, 20% of adults were current cigarette smokers, about 33% of adults were completely inactive in terms of leisure-time aerobic activity, and nearly 75% of adults never did muscle-strengthening activity. Based on demographic differences in the performance of risky behaviours, men were more likely than women to smoke cigarettes and to engage in at-risk drinking but less likely than women to be physically inactive in terms of both aerobic and muscle-strengthening activities. Adults aged 65 and over were the least likely (of all the age groups) to be current smokers or to have had five or more alcoholic drinks in one day at least once in the past year, but were the most likely to be physically inactive in their leisure time. Asian adults had significantly lower rates of at-risk drinking than white, black, American Indian or Alaska Native adults. Adults with higher levels of education were less likely than those with fewer years of education to be current smokers, and to be physically inactive in leisure time. Adults with higher family income had lower rates of cigarette smoking, physical inactivity in leisure time, and insufficient sleep, but higher rates of at-risk drinking. Married adults had lower prevalence of current cigarette smoking than all other marital status groups.

In relation to healthy behaviours, about 60% of adults had never smoked cigarettes, about 50% of adults met guidelines for aerobic physical activity, and about 25% of adults met the guidelines for muscle-strengthening activity. Based on demographic differences in the performance of healthy behaviours, men were more likely than women to meet physical activity guidelines (both aerobic and muscle-strengthening) through leisure-time activities, but women were more likely than men to be lifetime non-smokers and to be at a healthy weight. Adults aged 18–24 years had the highest prevalence for all healthy behaviours. Black adults and Asian adults were more likely than white adults to have never smoked cigarettes. White adults and Asian adults were more likely than black adults to meet guidelines for aerobic physical activity. White adults were more likely than black adults or Asian adults to meet guidelines for muscle-strengthening activity. Those with higher levels of education were more likely than those with less education to have never smoked cigarettes, and to have met the physical activity guidelines. Adults in the highest income groups were more likely than low-income adults to have never smoked, and to have met the physical activity guidelines (both aerobic and muscle-strengthening). Never-married and married adults were more likely than adults in the other marital status groups to have never smoked cigarettes.

There were also trends across time. For example, the percentage of adults who had five or more alcoholic drinks in one day at least once in the past year increased from 20.5% (2005–2007) to 23.6% (2008–2010), although adult smoking prevalence remained unchanged between 2005–2007 (20.4%) and 2008–2010 (20.2%). The percentage of adults who were completely aerobically inactive declined from 39.7% (2005–2007) to 33.9% (2008–2010).

Variations in who performs different health behaviours is of particular interest here given that the focus of the present volume is on examining the factors that might explain such variations. For example, variations across social class groups in who smokes might be fully or partially explained (or mediated) by differences across such groups in terms of attitudes, norms or intentions in relation to smoking. In addition, the importance of factors that explain differences in who performs health behaviours might vary across social class groups. Such moderation effects can be important in directing interventions more appropriately. For example, Conner *et al.* (2013) showed intentions to be better predictors of a number of health behaviours among those from higher versus lower social class groups.

2.3 Classifying health behaviours

The majority of the research in this volume focuses on behaviour-specific cognitions. This means that, for example, intentions to quit smoking are thought to be relevant to predicting quitting smoking but not relevant to other health behaviours. Work on health behaviour change similarly often focuses on single behaviours. However, this raises the issue of the extent to which we can generalize across health behaviours. For example, the social cognitive predictors of smoking behaviour might be different from the social cognitive predictors of fruit and vegetable consumption. Similarly, intervention techniques that help an individual quit smoking might not be useful or relevant for increasing fruit and vegetable consumption. In part, the answer to this point may depend on how similar different health behaviours are. In this section, a number of classifications of health behaviours that might inform such issues are overviewed.

One approach to classifying health behaviours has been to empirically examine which behaviours are performed together. This is sometimes known as the *frequency of engagement* approach and has identified either a single dimension (e.g. Jessor *et al.* 1998) or multiple dimensions (e.g. Roysamb *et al.* 1997), although the nature and number of dimensions identified appears to be a function of the behaviours examined. An alternative approach has been the *functional approach*, whereby health behaviours are grouped according to their function. The most common distinction in this area is between behaviours that enhance (i.e. approach) or impair (i.e. avoidance) health. Health-impairing behaviours have harmful effects on health or otherwise predispose individuals to disease, and include smoking, excessive alcohol consumption, and high dietary fat consumption. In contrast, health-enhancing behaviours convey health benefits or otherwise protect individuals from disease, and include physical activity and exercise, fruit and vegetable consumption, and condom use in response to the threat of sexually transmitted diseases. Various other sub-divisions of these two categories have been suggested. For example, Rothman and Salovey (1997) highlight the distinction between preventive health behaviours (those that aim to prevent the onset of ill health), detective health behaviours (those that aim to detect potential problems), and curative health behaviours (those that aim to cure or treat a health problem). These three categories have also been described as primary, secondary, and tertiary prevention respectively.

A different approach to classifying behaviours is based on their *key characteristics*. McEachan *et al.* (2010) noted that some studies have classified health behaviours by familiarity (i.e. degree of experience the individual has with the behaviour; Notani 1998), habitualness (based on frequency of opportunity to perform and stability of context in which the behaviour is performed; Ouellette and Wood 1998) or volitional control (i.e. degree to which the behaviour requires other resources to perform it, or is simply based on decision to act; Ajzen 1991). McEachan *et al.* (2010) measured perceptions of a number of health behaviours along a range of dimensions and identified three dimensions along which they consistently varied: (1) 'easy immediate pay-offs' vs. 'effortful long-term pay-offs'; (2) 'private and un-problematic vs. public and problematic'; and (3) 'important routines vs. unimportant one-offs'. For example, risk behaviours were clearly differentiated by being perceived as 'easy immediate pay-offs' and 'public and problematic', whereas approach behaviours such as physical activity behaviours were perceived as 'effortful long-term pay-offs'.

These different ways of classifying health behaviours clearly provide some insights into similarities and differences between health behaviours. However, to date it is unclear whether any single classification system can provide a sound basis for generalizing from one health behaviour to another in relation to the key factors that predict or change these behaviours. Indeed, a classification system that attempted to classify health behaviours according to similarity of key determinants (e.g. intention-based behaviours) or the most effective means of changing behaviour (e.g. self-efficacy is key to change these behaviours) might be the most useful approach in this regard.

2.4 Predicting the performance of health behaviours

Can we understand and predict who performs health behaviours? This would contribute to our understanding of the variation in the distribution of health across society. It might also indicate targets for interventions designed to change health behaviours. As one might expect, a variety of factors account for individual differences in the propensity to undertake health behaviours, including demographic factors, social factors, emotional factors, perceived symptoms, factors relating to access to medical care, personality factors, and cognitive factors (Rosenstock 1974; Taylor 1991; Adler and Matthews 1994; Baum and Posluszny 1999).

In addition to demographic variables such as age, gender, ethnicity, and socio-economic status (see Section 2.2), social factors such as parental models are important in instilling health behaviours early in life. The influence of peers is also important, such as in starting smoking (e.g. McNeil *et al.* 1988). Cultural values are also influential, for instance in determining the number of women exercising in a particular culture (e.g. Wardle and Steptoe 1991). Emotional factors play a role in the practise of some health habits, for example overeating is linked to stress in some obese people (e.g. Greeno and Wing 1994). Self-esteem also plays a role in influencing the practise of health behaviours by some (e.g. Royal College of Physicians 1992). Perceived symptoms will control health habits when, for example, a smoker regulates his or her smoking on the basis of sensations in the throat. Finally, the accessibility of medical care services has been found to influence the use of those health services (e.g. Whitehead 1988).

Personality theory proposes that traits or combinations of traits are fundamental determinants of behaviour and there is considerable evidence linking personality and behaviour (for a general review, see Hampson 2012). Personality factors have been either positively (e.g. conscientiousness) or negatively (e.g. negative affectivity) associated with the practise of health behaviours (Adler and Matthews 1994; Steptoe *et al.* 1994; for a discussion, see Norman and Conner, Chapter 12 this volume).

Finally, cognitive factors also determine whether or not an individual practises health behaviours. For example, knowledge about links between behaviour and health (i.e. risk awareness) is an essential factor in an informed choice concerning a healthy lifestyle. The reduction of smoking over the past 20–30 years in the Western world can be attributed to a growing awareness of the serious health risks posed by tobacco use brought about by widespread publicity. A variety of other cognitive variables have been studied. These factors include perceptions of health risk, potential efficacy of behaviours in reducing this risk, perceived social pressures to perform the behaviour, and control over performance of the behaviour.

A wide range of variables, from several models, has been related to the performance of health behaviours (for reviews, see Cummings *et al.* 1980; Becker and Maiman 1983; Mullen *et al.* 1987; Weinstein 1993). For example, Cummings *et al.* (1980) had experts sort 109 variables derived from 14 different health behaviour models. On the basis of non-metric multidimensional scaling, six distinct factors were derived:

1. Accessibility of health care services
2. Attitudes to health care (beliefs about quality and benefits of treatment)
3. Perceptions of disease threat
4. Knowledge about disease
5. Social network characteristics
6. Demographic factors.

Factors 2–5 represent social cognitive factors (beliefs, attitudes, knowledge). Such factors have been central to a number of models of the determinants of health behaviours for several reasons. These factors are enduring characteristics of the individual that shape behaviour and are acquired through socialization processes. They differentiate between individuals from the same background in terms of their propensity to perform health behaviours. They are also open to change and hence represent one route to intervening to change health behaviours. Cognitive factors represent an important area of study in health promotion because they may mediate the effects of many of the other factors discussed earlier and because they are believed to be a good focus of attention in interventions to change health behaviours. These cognitive factors constitute the content of a small number of widely used models of health behaviour. Such models have been labelled 'social cognition models' because of their use of a number of cognitive variables in researching individual social (including health) behaviours.

3 Social cognition approach to health behaviour

Social cognition is concerned with how individuals make sense of social situations. The approach focuses on individual cognitions or thoughts as processes that intervene between observable stimuli and responses in specific real-world situations (Fiske and Taylor 1991, 2013). A significant proportion of social psychology over the last 35 years has started from this assumption that social behaviour is best understood as a function of people's perceptions of reality, rather than as a function of an objective description of the stimulus environment. The question of which cognitions are important in predicting behaviour has been the focus of a great deal of research. This 'social cognitive' approach to the person as a thinking organism has been dominant in social psychology for the past two decades or more (Schneider 1991). The vast majority of work in social cognition can be broadly split into how people make sense of others (person perception) and themselves (self-regulation) (Fiske and Taylor 1991: 14). The focus in this volume is on self-regulation processes and how various social cognitive processes relate to health behaviour.

Self-regulation processes can be defined as those '... mental and behavioral processes by which people enact their self-conceptions, revise their behavior, or alter the environment so as to bring about outcomes in it in line with their self-perceptions and personal goals' (Fiske and Taylor 1991: 181). As such, self-regulation can be seen as emerging from a clinical tradition in psychology that sees the individual as engaging in behaviour change efforts designed to eliminate dysfunctional patterns of thinking or behaviour (Turk and Salovey 1986). Models of the cognitive determinants of health behaviour are part of this tradition. Self-regulation involves the setting of goals, cognitive preparations, and the ongoing monitoring and evaluation of goal-directed activities. Two phases are commonly distinguished: motivational and volitional (model of action phases; Gollwitzer 1993). The motivational phase involves the deliberation of incentives and expectations in order to choose between goals and implied actions. This phase ends with a decision concerning the goal to be pursued. The second, volitional phase involves planning and action towards achieving the set goal. Research concerned with developing models that explain the role of cognitive variables in the motivational phase still dominates the area, although increasingly researchers have sought to redress this balance by developing models of the role of cognitive variables in the volitional phase (e.g. Kuhl 1984; Kuhl and Beckmann 1985, 1994; Weinstein 1988; Heckhausen 1991; Bagozzi 1992, 1993; Gollwitzer 1993) with increasing applications to health behaviours (e.g. Schwarzer 1992; Schwarzer and Luszczynska, Chapter 8 this volume; Sutton, Chapter 9 this volume; Prestwich *et al.*, Chapter 10 this volume).

Social cognition models (SCMs) describing the key cognitions and their inter-relationships in the regulation of behaviour have been developed and widely applied to the understanding of health behaviours. Two broad types of SCMs have been applied in health psychology, predominantly to explain health-related behaviours and response to health threats (Conner 1993).

The first type involves attribution models concerned with individuals' causal explanations of health-related events (e.g. King 1982). However, most research within this tradition has focused on how people respond to a range of serious illnesses, including cancer (Taylor *et al.* 1984), coronary heart disease (Affleck *et al.* 1987), diabetes (Tennen *et al.* 1984), and end-stage renal failure (Witenberg *et al.* 1983) rather than the health-enhancing and compromising behaviours of otherwise healthy individuals. More recent work on illness representations (Petrie and Weinman 1997; Moss-Morris *et al.* 2002; Hagger and Orbell 2003), based on Leventhal's self-regulation model (Leventhal *et al.* 1984), also falls into this category. This work seeks to examine individuals' reactions to a disease (or disease threat). In particular, the model delineates three stages. In the first stage, the individual forms an illness representation along five core dimensions: disease identity (i.e. the symptoms experienced as part of the condition), consequences (i.e. the perceived range and severity of the consequences of the disease), causes (i.e. the perceived causes of the disease), timeline (i.e. the extent to which the disease is perceived to be acute or chronic in nature), and control/cure (i.e. the extent to which the patient and others can manage the disease). In the second stage, the illness representation is used to guide the choice of coping efforts, while in the third stage the outcomes of coping efforts are appraised and used to adjust the illness representation. Thus in this model, individuals' perceptions of their illness are seen to have a central role in determining coping efforts and subsequent adaptation. However, a meta-analysis conducted by Hagger and Orbell (2003) of studies on illness representations only revealed evidence for a weak correlation between the control/cure dimension and specific problem-focused coping efforts (e.g. medication adherence). In contrast, stronger correlations were found between illness representations and various measures of physical and psychological well-being.

The second type of SCM examines various aspects of an individual's cognitions in order to predict future health-related behaviours and outcomes. The SCMs commonly used to predict health behaviours include: the health belief model (e.g. Becker 1974; Janz and Becker 1984; Abraham and Sheeran, Chapter 2 this volume); protection motivation theory (e.g. Maddux and Rogers 1983; Van der Velde and Van der Pligt 1991; Norman *et al.*, Chapter 3 this volume); self-determination theory (e.g. Deci and Ryan 2002; Hagger and Chatzisarantis, Chapter 4 this volume); the theory of reasoned action/theory of planned behaviour (e.g. Ajzen 1991; Fishbein and Ajzen 2010; Conner and Sparks, Chapter 5 this volume); the prototype-willingness model (Gibbons *et al.* 2003; Gibbons *et al.*, Chapter 6 this volume); social cognitive theory (e.g. Bandura 1982, 2000; Schwarzer 1992; Luszczynska and Schwarzer, Chapter 7 this volume); and the health action process approach (e.g. Schwarzer 2008; Schwarzer and Luszczynska, Chapter 8 this volume). Another set of models focuses on the idea that behaviour change occurs through a series of qualitatively different stages. These so-called 'stage' models (Sutton, Chapter 9 this volume) include the transtheoretical model of change (Prochaska and DiClemente 1984) and the precaution-adoption process (Weinstein 1988). Finally, some recent work examining health behaviours has focused on specific volitional variables (e.g. Kuhl 1984; Gollwitzer 1993, 1999; Abraham *et al.* 1999). In particular, implementation intentions (Gollwitzer 1993) have emerged as a useful technique for changing health behaviours (Prestwich *et al.*, Chapter 10 this volume).

These SCMs provide a basis for understanding the determinants of behaviour and behaviour change. They also provide a list of important targets that interventions designed to change behaviour might focus upon if they are to be successful. Each of these models emphasizes the rationality of human behaviour. Thus, the health behaviours to be predicted are considered to be the end result of a rational decision-making process based upon deliberative, systematic processing of the available information. Most assume that behaviour and decisions are based upon an elaborate, but subjective, cost–benefit analysis of the likely outcomes of differing courses of action. As such they have roots going back to expectancy-value theory (Peak 1955) and subjective expected utility theory (Edwards 1954). It is assumed that individuals generally aim to maximize utility and so prefer behaviours that are associated with the highest expected utility.

The overall utility or desirability of a behaviour is assumed to be based upon the summed products of the probability (expectancy) and utility (value) of specific, salient outcomes or consequences. This can be represented as:

$$\text{SEU}_j = \sum_{i=1}^{i=m} \text{P}_{ij} \cdot \text{U}_{ij},$$

where SEU_j is the subjective expected utility of behaviour j, P_{ij} is the perceived probability of outcome i of action j, U_{ij} is the subjective utility or value of outcome i of action j, and m is the number of salient outcomes. Different behaviours may have differing subjective expected utilities because of the value of the different outcomes associated with each behaviour, and the probability of each behaviour being associated with each outcome. While such a model allows for subjective assessments of both probability and utility, it is assumed that these assessments are combined in a rational, consistent way. Outcome expectancies can be usefully classified along a limited number of key dimensions. For example, Bandura (2000) distinguishes between outcome expectancies as physical, social or self-evaluative, while Ajzen and Fishbein (1980) distinguish between social outcomes and other outcomes. More recently, Rhodes and Conner (2010) distinguished outcome expectancies in terms of positive-negative, immediate-distal, and instrumental-affective dimensions. The relative importance of different types of outcome expectancies has been a recent focus of attention (e.g. Lawton *et al.* 2007).

Such judgements underlie many of the widely used SCMs, including the health belief model, protection motivation theory, theory of reasoned action/planned behaviour, and social cognitive theory (Weinstein 1993, 2000; Van der Pligt 1994). While such considerations may well provide good predictions of health behaviours, several authors have noted that they do not provide an adequate description of the way in which individuals make decisions (e.g. Jonas 1993; Frisch and Clemen 1994). For example, except for the most important decisions, it is unlikely that individuals integrate information in this way (Van der Pligt *et al.* 2000).

4 Overview of commonly used social cognition models

In this section, we outline the different SCMs that form the focus of this volume. We briefly describe how each model conceptualizes the social cognitive variables or health cognitions important in determining behaviour, and the way in which these variables are combined to predict behaviour (see other chapters in this volume for a detailed review of each SCM).

4.1 Health belief model

The health belief model (HBM) is perhaps the oldest and most widely used social cognition model in health psychology (Rosenstock 1966; Becker 1974; Abraham and Sheeran, Chapter 2 this volume). Rather than a formal model, the HBM has been considered more a loose association of variables that have been found to predict behaviour (Conner 1993).

The HBM uses two aspects of individuals' representations of health behaviour in response to threat of illness: perceptions of illness threat and evaluation of behaviours to counteract this threat. Threat perceptions are seen to depend upon two beliefs: the perceived susceptibility to the illness and the perceived severity of the consequences of the illness. Together these two variables are believed to determine the likelihood of the individual following a health-related action, although their effect is modified by individual differences in demographic variables, social pressures, and personality. It is thought that the particular action taken is determined by an evaluation of the available alternatives, focusing on the benefits or efficacy of the health behaviour and the perceived costs or barriers to performing the behaviour. Thus, individuals are likely to follow a particular health action if they believe themselves to be susceptible to a particular condition that they also consider to be serious, and believe that the benefits of the action taken to counteract the health threat outweigh the costs.

Two other variables commonly included in the model are cues to action and health motivation. Cues to action are assumed to include a diverse range of triggers to the individual taking action, which may be internal (e.g. physical symptom) or external (e.g. mass media campaign, advice from others) to the individual (Janz and Becker 1984). Furthermore, as Becker (1974) has argued, certain individuals may be predisposed to respond to such cues because of the value they place on their health (i.e. health motivation).

4.2 Protection motivation theory

Protection motivation theory (PMT; Rogers 1975) was originally proposed to provide conceptual clarity to the understanding of fear appeals. The theory has been revised on a number of occasions (Norman *et al.*, Chapter 3 this volume). As typically applied (Maddux and Rogers 1983; Rogers 1983), PMT describes adaptive and maladaptive responses to a health threat as the result of two appraisal processes: threat appraisal and coping appraisal. *Threat appraisal* is based upon a consideration of perceptions of susceptibility to, and severity of, a health threat. *Coping appraisal* involves the process of assessing the behavioural alternatives that might diminish the threat. This process is assumed to be based on the individual's expectancy that performing a certain behaviour can remove the threat (response efficacy) and a belief in one's capability to successfully execute the recommended courses of action (self-efficacy).

Together, these two appraisal processes result in the intention to perform adaptive (protection motivation) or maladaptive responses. *Adaptive responses* are held to be more likely if the individual perceives him or herself to be facing a severe health threat to which he or she is susceptible. Adaptive responses are also more likely if the individual perceives such responses to be effective in reducing the threat and believes that he or she can successfully perform the adaptive response. These two cognitive appraisals feed into *protection motivation*, an intervening variable that arouses, sustains, and directs activity to protect the self from danger. Protection motivation is typically operationalized as intention to perform the health-protective behaviour or avoid the health-compromising behaviour. Actual behaviour is assumed to be a function of intentions.

The revised theory (Maddux and Rogers 1983), described here, can be seen as a hybrid theory (Prentice-Dunn and Rogers 1986) with susceptibility, severity, response-efficacy, and response costs (i.e. perceived barriers) components, all originating from the health belief model, and self-efficacy originating from Bandura's social cognitive theory (Bandura 1982).

4.3 Self-determination theory

Self-determination theory (SDT; Deci and Ryan 1985; Ryan and Deci 2000; Hagger and Chatzisarantis, Chapter 4 this volume) represents a somewhat different approach to the prediction of health behaviour. A key focus of the theory is that motivation to participate in behaviour is driven by the extent to which the behaviour is perceived to satisfy three basic psychological needs: the needs for autonomy (Deci 1975), competence (Harter 1978), and relatedness (Baumeister and Leary 1995). The extent to which these needs are considered satisfied determines the type of quality of motivation experienced by the individual with respect to the behaviour.

Self-determination theory makes an important distinction between different types of motivation. These are placed along a continuum according to the degree to which the motivation to perform a behaviour is perceived to emanate from the self (i.e. is self-determined or autonomous). At one end of the continuum is amotivation, a state that reflects a lack of intention to act. Amotivation is seen to result from an individual not valuing the target activity, not feeling competent to perform the activity, and not expecting that the activity will lead to a desired outcome. At the other end of the continuum is intrinsic motivation, which is highly autonomous and represents the prototypical case of self-determination. Behaviour that is regulated by intrinsic motivation is performed for its own sake – that is, for the inherent enjoyment of performing the behaviour.

Between amotivation and intrinsic motivation lies extrinsic motivation, which reflects that the behaviour is performed to obtain some outcome, other than the inherent satisfaction or enjoyment of performing the behaviour. Self-determination theory proposes that behaviours that are extrinsically motivated vary according to their relative autonomy and outlines four regulatory styles that can be used to guide such behaviours. The first is *external regulation*, where behaviour is performed to satisfy an external demand or reward contingency. Second, behaviours that are guided by *introjected regulation* are performed to avoid negative feelings such as guilt or shame. Behaviours guided by these first two regulatory styles are clearly intended, in that individuals will feel competent to perform the behaviours and believe that they will lead to certain outcomes, but they cannot be said to be autonomous given that the value and regulation of the behaviour have not been internalized and integrated into the self. Third, behaviours guided by *identified regulation* are seen to be more autonomous and self-determined in nature. Such behaviours are experienced by individuals as being important for functioning effectively in the social world. Fourth, and the most autonomous form of extrinsic motivation, is *integrated regulation*, which occurs when the value and regulation of the behaviour are fully assimilated by the self. In other words, performance of the behaviour is consistent with the individual's other values and needs. Behaviours guided by these last two regulatory styles share many qualities with those regulated by intrinsic motivation but they are still considered to be the result of extrinsic motivation as they are performed to obtain outcomes other than the inherent enjoyment of performing the behaviour. In many SDT studies, integrated and intrinsic motivation are combined to form an 'autonomous motivation' measure that can be contrasted with more 'controlled' or extrinsic motivation. Most important, for the prediction of health behaviour, behaviours that are perceived as autonomously motivated, and satisfying of psychological needs, are more likely to be engaged in, and persisted with, in the absence of any discernible extrinsic contingency. This means that autonomously motivated individuals are more likely to be effective in self-regulating their behaviour without the need for external prompts.

Self-determination theory has been integrated with other theories, such as the theory of planned behaviour (Ajzen, 1991), to provide a broader model of the determinants of health behaviours (see Hagger and Chatzisarantis, Chapter 4 this volume).

4.4 Theory of planned behaviour

Developed by social psychologists, the theory of planned behaviour (TPB) has been widely applied to the understanding of a variety of behaviours (Ajzen 1991; Armitage and Conner 2001; Conner and Sparks, Chapter 5 this volume). The TPB outlines the factors that determine an individual's decision to follow a particular behaviour. This theory is itself an extension of the widely applied theory of reasoned action (Fishbein and Ajzen 1975; Ajzen and Fishbein 1980; for an integration of these models, see Fishbein and Ajzen 2010).

The TPB proposes that the proximal determinants of behaviour are intention to engage in that behaviour and perceptions of control over that behaviour. Intentions represent a person's motivation in the sense of his or her conscious plan or decision to exert effort to perform the behaviour. Perceived behavioural control is a person's expectancy that performance of the behaviour is within his or her control. This concept is similar to Bandura's (1982) concept of self-efficacy (see Trafimow *et al.* 2002). Control is seen as a continuum with easily executed behaviours at one end and behavioural goals demanding resources, opportunities, and specialized skills at the other.

Intention is itself determined by three sets of factors: (1) attitudes, which are the overall evaluations of the behaviour by the individual; (2) subjective norms, which consist of a person's beliefs about whether significant others think he or she should engage in the behaviour; and (3) perceived behavioural control, which is the individual's perception of the extent to which performance of the behaviour is easy or difficult. Each of these three components is also held to have prior determinants. *Attitudes* are a function of beliefs about the perceived consequences of the behaviour based upon two perceptions: the likelihood of an outcome occurring as a result of performing the behaviour and the evaluation of that outcome. *Subjective norms* are a function of normative beliefs, which represent perceptions of specific significant others' preferences about whether one should or should not engage in a behaviour. This is quantified as the subjective likelihood that specific salient groups or individuals (referents) think the person should perform the behaviour, multiplied by the person's motivation to comply with that referent's expectation. Judgements of *perceived behavioural control* are influenced by beliefs concerning whether one has access to the necessary resources and opportunities to perform the behaviour successfully, weighted by the perceived power of each factor to facilitate or inhibit the execution of the behaviour. These factors include both internal control factors (information, personal deficiencies, skills, abilities, emotions) and external control factors (opportunities, dependence on others, barriers).

4.5 Prototype-willingness model

The prototype-willingness model (PWM; Gibbons *et al.* 2003; Gibbons *et al.*, Chapter 6 this volume) was developed out of the theory of reasoned action/theory of planned behaviour (TRA/TPB) in order to take account of less reasoned pathways that might influence behaviour. Gibbons *et al.* (2003) argue that models like the TRA/TPB may provide relatively poor predictions of health-impairing or health-risk behaviours such as unprotected sex, particularly among young people. Gibbons and Gerrard (1995, 1997) argue that young people are likely to experience opportunities to engage in health-risk behaviours. In such situations, they may be 'willing' to engage in the behaviour given the opportunity to do so. Thus, their behaviour reflects a reaction to the social situation rather than a premeditated intention to engage in a health-risk behaviour. The PWM was developed to provide an account of such health-risk behaviour among adolescents and young people.

The PWM outlines two 'pathways' to health-risk behaviour among adolescents and young adults. The first is a 'reasoned pathway' reflecting the operation of more or less rational decision-making processes as outlined in the major SCMs. In this pathway, health-risk behaviour is based on a consideration of the risks of performing the behaviour. Thus, behavioural intention is seen to be the proximal predictor of health-risk behaviour in this pathway. The second pathway to health-risk behaviour is a 'social reaction pathway' that forms the cornerstone of the PWM. This pathway includes four factors that impact on individuals' willingness to engage in health-risk behaviours when they encounter risk-conducive situations. First are *subjective norms*, which focus on perceptions of whether important others engage in the behaviour and whether they are likely to approve or disapprove of the individual performing the behaviour. In this way, Gibbons and Gerrard (1995, 1997) highlight the importance of both descriptive and injunctive social norms (Cialdini *et al.* 1991). Second are *attitudes*, which are primarily concerned with the perceived likelihood of negative outcomes (e.g. perceived vulnerability). In particular, a willingness to perform a health-risk behaviour in a risk-conducive situation may be associated with a downplaying of the risks associated with the behaviour. Third is *past behaviour*. The fourth factor in the PWM is the *prototype* associated with the health-risk behaviour – that is, the image that people have of the type of person who engages in a particular behaviour (e.g. the 'typical ecstasy user'). According to the PWM, prototype favourability (i.e. the extent to which the image is positively evaluated) and prototype similarity (i.e. the perceived similarity between the image and one's self) interact to impact on individuals' willingness to engage in a health-risk behaviour. The four factors identified in the 'social reaction pathway' are seen to exert their influence through *behavioural willingness*. Gibbons and Gerrard (1995, 1997) argue that the willingness to engage in a health-risk behaviour in a risk-conducive situation provides a better prediction of subsequent behaviour than does behavioural intention, as it reflects the social reactive nature of many of the health-risk behaviours performed by young people.

4.6 Social cognitive theory

Social cognitive theory (Bandura 1982; Luszczynsha and Schwarzer, Chapter 7 this volume) forms the basis of a further model of the determinants of health behaviour. In this approach, goals and action are assumed based on two types of expectancy (action-outcome, self-efficacy) in addition to socio-structural factors. *Action-outcome expectancy* is the belief that a given behaviour will or will not lead to a given outcome. For example, the belief that quitting smoking will lead to a reduced risk of lung cancer would represent an action-outcome expectancy. *Self-efficacy expectancy* is the belief that an individual is confident about performing a particular behaviour. *Socio-structural factors* represent aspects of the environment that facilitate or impede performance of the behaviour. Goals represent plans or intentions to perform the behaviour. Self-efficacy is the key component of the model, as reflected in the largest number of paths to behaviour.

There is also a clear causal ordering among these different influences. Action-outcome expectancies are assumed to impact upon behaviour directly or via their influence upon goals or intentions to engage in the behaviour. Self-efficacy expectancies are assumed to have a direct impact on behaviour and indirect effects via their influence on goals/intentions, action-outcome expectancies, and socio-structural factors. The direct link is attributable to the fact that optimistic self-beliefs predict actual behavioural performance through greater effort and persistence. The first indirect link reflects the fact that individuals typically intend to perform (or form goals towards) behaviours they perceive to be within their control. The second indirect link reflects the fact that individuals with high self-efficacy tend to expect more positive outcomes to follow from the behaviour. The third indirect link reflects the fact that individuals high in self-efficacy try harder to overcome impediments in the environment or are better at drawing on socio-structural facilitators (Schwarzer 1992; Bandura 2000; Luszczynska and Schwarzer, Chapter 7 this volume).

4.7 Health action process approach

The health action process approach (HAPA; Schwarzer 1992; Schwarzer and Luszczynska, Chapter 8 this volume) assumes that although behaviour change can be described as a continuous process, it can also be described in terms of qualitative stages or phases. It can be considered to be a hybrid model that includes elements from social cognitive theory and the theory of planned behaviour as well as stages from models such as the transtheoretical model (see Section 4.8). The three stages distinguished are pre-intenders, intenders, and actors. Respectively, these refer to the influences on deciding whether to change one's behaviour, the influences on deciding how to act in support of the decision to change, and the influences on acting and continuing to act. Like social cognitive theory, *pre-intenders* see outcome expectancies and (action) self-efficacy as key determinants of intentions with the added predictor of risk perceptions. Here risk perceptions refer to the likely outcomes of not changing the current behaviour. *Intenders* see action and coping planning along with coping self-efficacy as key to turning intention into action, while *actors* distinguish between action initiation and maintenance to differentiate between issues linked to starting a behaviour versus continuing it over a prolonged period. Coping self-efficacy and action control are seen as key to progress in this stage and recovery self-efficacy is seen as key to dealing with setbacks or lapses in the performance of the behaviour. A growing body of literature has used the HAPA to explore predictors of engaging in various health behaviours, and to inform the design of interventions to change such behaviours (Schwarzer and Luszczynska, Chapter 8 this volume). In relation to the latter, the HAPA differs from models such as social cognitive theory in suggesting that different interventions may be appropriate depending on what stage or phase the individual is currently in.

4.8 Stage models of health behaviour

A number of researchers have suggested that there may be qualitatively different stages in the initiation and maintenance of a health behaviour, and that to obtain a full understanding of the determinants of health behaviour it is necessary to conduct a detailed analysis of the nature of these stages (see Sutton, Chapter 9 in this volume, for a review). From a social cognitive perspective, an important implication of this position is that different cognitions may be important at different stages in promoting health behaviour, and that different interventions may be appropriate for individuals in different stages.

One of the first stage models was the transtheoretical model (TTM) proposed by Prochaska and DiClemente (1984). Their model has been widely applied to analyse the process of change in alcoholism treatment (DiClemente and Hughes 1990) and smoking cessation (DiClemente *et al.* 1991). In one recent form, DiClemente *et al.* (1991) identify five stages of change: pre-contemplation, contemplation, preparation, action, and maintenance. Individuals are seen to progress through each stage to achieve successful maintenance of a new behaviour. Taking the example of smoking cessation, it is argued that in the *pre-contemplation stage* the smoker is unaware that his or her behaviour constitutes a problem and has no intention to quit. In the *contemplation stage*, the smoker starts to think about changing his or her behaviour, but is not committed to try to quit. In the *preparation stage*, the smoker has an intention to quit and starts to make plans about how to quit. The *action stage* is characterized by active attempts to quit, and after six months of successful abstinence the individual moves into the *maintenance stage*, characterized by attempts to prevent relapse and to consolidate the newly acquired non-smoking status. The TTM also includes variables assumed to predict stage change and processes that determine change (see Sutton, Chapter 9 this volume).

Another important stage model is the precaution-adoption process (Weinstein 1988, Weinstein and Sandman 1992; Sutton, Chapter 9 this volume). This includes seven stages: unaware of issue, unengaged by issue, deciding about acting, decided not to act, decided to act, acting, and maintenance. These seven stages show a number of parallels with, and also differences from, the five stages included of the TTM. A range of evidence in support or against such stage models has accumulated; opinion is divided on the added value of such an approach (Sutton, Chapter 9 this volume).

4.9 Implementation intentions

The main social cognition models of health behaviour can be seen to be primarily concerned with people's motivations to perform a health behaviour (the health action process approach is an exception) and, as such, can be considered to provide strong predictions of behavioural intentions (i.e. the end of a motivational phase). However, strong intentions do not always lead to corresponding actions. In his meta-analysis of meta-analyses, Sheeran (2002) reported an average intention–behaviour correlation of 0.53. However, the major social cognition models do not directly address the issue of how intentions are translated into action. A construct that appears important to the translation of intentions into actions is implementation intentions (Gollwitzer 1993, 1999; for a review in relation to health behaviours, see Prestwich *et al.*, Chapter 10 this volume).

Gollwitzer (1993) made the distinction between goal intentions and implementation intentions. While the former is concerned with intentions to perform a behaviour or achieve a goal (i.e. 'I intend to achieve X'), the latter is concerned with plans as to when, where, and how the goal intention is to be translated into behaviour (i.e. 'I intend to initiate the goal-directed behaviour X when situation Y is encountered'). The important point about implementation intentions is that they commit the individual to a specific course of action when certain environmental conditions are met and, in so doing, they help translate goal intentions into action. Take the example of going swimming: an individual may have the goal intention to go swimming, but this may not be translated into behaviour if he or she does not have an implementation intention that specifies when, where, and how he or she will go swimming. Gollwitzer (1993) argues that by making implementation intentions, individuals pass control over to the environment. The environment therefore acts as a cue to action, such that when certain conditions are met, the performance of the intended behaviour follows relatively automatically. Factors promoting the effectiveness of implementation intentions in relation to health behaviour change are an important focus of research attention.

Prestwich *et al.* (Chapter 10 this volume) provide an in-depth review of both basic and applied research with implementation intentions. In particular, implementation intentions are shown to increase the performance of a range of behaviours with, on average, a medium effect size.

5 Comparison and integration of key social cognition models

5.1 Empirical comparisons

Despite the substantial volume of empirical work using the main social cognition models to predict a range of health behaviours, comparatively little empirical work has directly compared the predictive power of the different models (Noar and Zimmerman 2005; Glanz and Bishop 2010). As Weinstein (1993) notes, the lack of comparison studies means there is little consensus on whether some variables are more influential than others and whether some models of health behaviour are more predictive than others. While this criticism of research with social cognition models is clearly valid, it is also evident that those studies that have attempted to compare different models have provided insights. This section overviews a number of these comparison studies for the key SCMs (see also Bagozzi 1992; Bagozzi and Kimmel 1995; Hunter *et al.* 2003) and then examines the evidence from meta-analytic reviews of the power of individual variables to predict behaviour.

Several early studies compared the health belief model (HBM; i.e. susceptibility, severity, benefits, barriers, health motivation) with the theory of reasoned action (TRA; i.e. attitude, subjective norm). For example, Hill *et al.* (1985) found the two models to explain similar amounts of variance in women's intentions to perform breast self-examination (17–20% of variance) and to have a Pap test/cervical smear (26–32% of variance). Mullen *et al.* (1987) found the HBM and TRA to provide similar levels of prediction for changes in a range of health behaviours over an eight-month period. Although these two studies reported the HBM to predict slightly more variance than the TRA, Oliver and Berger (1979) found the TRA to be a better predictor of inoculation behaviour, as did Rutter (1989) in relation to AIDS-prevention behaviour. In other early studies, Conner and Norman (1994) examined the determinants of attendance at a health check and found the models to predict intentions and behaviour to a similar degree, while Bakker *et al.* (1994) found the theory of planned behaviour (TPB) to be more predictive of condom use among heterosexuals. More recent studies have also reported the TPB to have greater predictive power than the HBM for behaviours such as uptake of human papillomavirus vaccine (Gerend and Shepherd 2012), bicycle helmet use (Lajunen and Rasanen 2004), seat belt use (Simsekoglu and Lajunen 2008), and condom use behaviour (Montanaro and Bryan 2014). Montanaro and Bryan (2014) also used an intervention targeted at changing components of the HBM and TPB to study effects on later behaviour. The intervention successfully changed perceived susceptibility, perceived benefits, and attitudes towards condom use. However, only attitudes and self-efficacy were associated with intentions, the only predictor of behaviour change.

Two comparison studies have focused on self-efficacy in relation to the main SCMs. Seydel *et al.* (1990) compared the HBM (i.e. susceptibility, severity, outcome expectancies) with protection motivation theory (PMT; i.e. susceptibility, severity, outcome expectancies, self-efficacy) and reported outcome expectancies and self-efficacy to be the most important predictors of cancer-related preventive intentions and behaviour. Dzewaltowski (1989) compared the TRA with social cognitive theory (SCT) in relation to exercise behaviour using a prospective design. The SCT provided stronger predictions of exercise behaviour than the TRA, with self-efficacy emerging as the most important single predictor.

Other comparison studies have generally reported similar levels of predictive power for the SCMs examined. For example, Boer and Mashamba (2005) reported that the TPB and PMT performed similarly in explaining intentions to use condoms among adolescents in South Africa. Blanchard *et al.* (2011) concluded that the TPB, PMT, and SCT were similarly useful in predicting physical activity among those engaged in home-based cardiac rehabilitation. Plotnikov *et al.* (2014) used the same three theories in relation to physical activity in adults with type 2 diabetes. Each explained similar, but small, amounts of variance in both objective and self-reported physical activity. Matterne *et al.* (2011) compared the TPB, prototype-willingness model (PWM), and the health action process approach (HAPA) in a sample with occupational skin disease and reported that they provided similar levels of prediction of skin protection behaviour. In another study, Orbell *et al.* (2006) reported the TPB to be better than self-regulation theory (Leventhal *et al.* 1984) for predicting adherence to treatment following cervical cancer screening.

Although further comparison studies would be informative, in general, the studies reported to date have shown that many of the main SCMs are similarly able to predict intentions and behaviour. In contrast, meta-analytic reviews of the power of individual variables to predict intentions and behaviour (Table 1.1) provide clearer support for some health cognitions over others. Cohen (1992) suggests that correlations of 0.5 equate to large effect sizes (d_+), 0.3 to medium effect sizes, and 0.1 to small effect sizes. Meta-analyses indicate self-efficacy, attitudes, outcome expectancies, norms, and response costs have medium-to-large effects on intentions, while response efficacy, prototypes, susceptibility, and severity have small-to-medium effects on intentions. In contrast, intentions, willingness, self-efficacy, planning, perceived barriers, outcome expectancies, and attitudes have medium-to-large effects on behaviour, while perceived benefits, response costs, norms, and severity have small-to-medium effects on behaviour, and susceptibility has a very small effect on behaviour.

Meta-analytic reviews have also attempted to identify the causal role of health cognitions in changing intentions and behaviour. These reviews included studies that reported changes

Table 1.1 Summary of meta-analyses of the power of different health cognitions to predict intentions and behaviour

Construct	Theory	Effect size (r_+)	
		Intention	Behaviour
Behavioural intention/protection motivation/goals	TPB, PMT, SCT, HAPA, PWM	—	0.42
Behavioural willingness	PWM	—	0.44
Planning	HAPA	—	0.34
Susceptibility/vulnerability/risk perception	HBM, PMT, HAPA	0.13	0.05
Severity	HBM, PMT	0.10	0.15
Perceived benefits	HBM	—	0.27
Perceived barriers	HBM	—	0.30
Response efficacy	PMT	0.29	0.09
Response costs	PMT	−0.34	−0.25
Self-efficacy/perceived behavioural control	PMT, TPB, SCT, HAPA, PWM	0.60	0.38
Outcome expectancies	SCT, TPB, HAPA	0.40	0.30
Attitudes	TPB, PWM	0.45	0.30
Norms	TPB, PWM	0.35	0.18
Prototypes	PWM	0.26	—

Note: Data taken from meta-analyses focusing on prospective tests on health behaviours, and data from reviews with larger numbers of studies or averages across reviews. See relevant theory chapter in this volume for further details. r_+ = sample weighted average correlations.

to a health cognition and the consequent impact on intentions and/or behaviour. For example, Webb and Sheeran (2006) reviewed studies that significantly changed intentions ($d_+ = 0.66$) and reported that these studies had medium-sized effects on behaviour ($d_+ = 0.36$). Sheeran *et al.* (submitted) examined the impacts of changing attitudes/outcome expectancies, norms, and self-efficacy/perceived behavioural control on intentions and behaviour. Changes in attitudes, norms, and self-efficacy were associated with medium-sized changes in intentions ($d_+ = 0.50$; $d_+ = 0.41$; $d_+ = 0.50$ respectively) and small-to-medium sized changes in behaviour ($d_+ = 0.37$; $d_+ = 0.20$; $d_+ = 0.46$ respectively) (for further discussion, see Norman and Conner, Chapter 12 this volume).

This meta-analytic evidence provides support for self-efficacy, attitudes, outcome expectancies, norms, and response costs as important predictors of intentions (although the number of studies testing response costs is more limited). It also suggests intentions, willingness, self-efficacy, planning, perceived barriers, outcome expectancies, and attitudes are important predictors of behaviour (although the number of studies testing willingness, planning, and perceived barriers is more limited).

5.2 Theoretical comparisons

A number of authors have commented on the considerable overlap between constructs contained in the main social cognition models of health behaviour (Kirscht 1982; Armitage and

Conner 2000; Gebhardt and Maes 2001; Norman and Conner, Chapter 12 this volume). Moreover, as Cummings *et al.* (1980) note, where differences do appear they tend to represent differences in labelling rather than differences in underlying constructs. This suggests that there might be some benefit in developing integrated social cognition models of health behaviour. This section considers some of the main constructs outlined in social cognition models of health behaviour and the extent to which they may overlap. Seven main areas of overlap are identified.

First, models that have been developed specifically to predict health behaviour (i.e. health action process approach, health belief model, protection motivation theory) focus on the notion of threat as measured by perceived susceptibility/vulnerability and perceived severity. In addition, social cognitive theory (SCT) focuses on expectancies about environmental cues (i.e. risk perception; Rosenstock *et al.* 1988). In contrast, the theory of planned behaviour (TPB) does not explicitly cater for emotional or arousal variables, leading some authors to suggest that the TPB may be limited to the rational part of a health decision (Oliver and Berger 1979). Weinstein (1993) argues against this view, pointing out that perceptions of severity may be tapped indirectly by the evaluation component of behavioural beliefs, while perceptions of susceptibility may be tapped by belief strength. For example, a behavioural belief may focus on the perceived likelihood that continued smoking might lead to lung cancer (i.e. perceived susceptibility) and an evaluation of this consequence (i.e. perceived severity). However, while perceptions of susceptibility and severity may be tapped by a consideration of behavioural beliefs, it may be advantageous to maintain the distinction between threat perception and behavioural beliefs (see Norman *et al.* 1999).

Second, most social cognition models of health behaviour focus on the perceived consequences of performing a health behaviour (Rosenstock *et al.* 1988; Weinstein 1993; Conner and Norman 1994; Van der Pligt 1994). For example, in the TPB and prototype-willingness model (PWM), the focus is on behavioural beliefs, in the health belief model (HBM) it is on the benefits and costs of performing a health behaviour, in SCT and the health action process approach (HAPA) it is on outcome expectancies, and in protection motivation theory (PMT) it is on response-efficacy and response costs.

Third, there is considerable overlap between the perceived behavioural control component of the TPB and self-efficacy (Ajzen 1991). A number of the models also focus on specific control issues or barriers to the performance of health behaviour. Thus, a similarity can be noted between control beliefs in the TPB, the perceived barriers dimension of the HBM, and response costs in the PMT (Conner and Norman 1994; Van der Pligt 1994). Rosenstock *et al.* (1988) have further considered the overlap between the perceived barriers dimension of the HBM and self-efficacy. They consider the perceived barriers dimension to be a 'catch-all' term for all the potential barriers to action, both internal and external. As a result, they argue for the inclusion of self-efficacy as a separate construct within the HBM, highlighting two important consequences: first, it would help delimit the scope of the barriers dimension, and second, it would add to the predictive power of the HBM.

Fourth, social cognition models of health behaviour do not explicitly cover normative influences on behaviour (Conner and Norman 1994), with the exception of the TPB, which includes the subjective norm construct and underlying normative beliefs, and the PWM, which also includes the prototype construct. In the HBM, normative influences are simply listed as one of many potential cues to action. In SCT, normative influences may be covered by outcome expectancies that focus on the perceived social consequences of behaviour. However, Schwarzer (1992) has questioned the extent to which it is necessary to differentiate between social outcome expectancies and other expectancies in SCT (see Bandura 2000). Weinstein (1993) has put forward a similar argument in relation to normative beliefs and behavioural beliefs in the TPB. Nevertheless, there may be some merit in limiting the scope of outcome expectancies or behavioural beliefs so that the independent influence of normative influences can be considered in more detail (Trafimow and Fishbein 1995).

Fifth, nearly all models include an intervening variable that is seen to mediate the relationship between other social cognitive variables and behaviour (Weinstein 1993). In the majority of models this variable is behavioural intention, while in PMT it is labelled protection motivation, although Prentice-Dunn and Rogers (1986) state that protection motivation is most appropriately assessed by behavioural intention measures. The PWM includes measures of behavioural intention and behavioural willingness, while SDT includes different types of motivation (i.e. amotivation through to intrinsic motivation). In contrast, the HBM does not include a measure of behavioural intention, although a number of researchers have called for its addition to act as a mediating variable between the HBM variables and behaviour (e.g. Becker *et al.* 1977; King 1982; Calnan 1984).

Sixth, the TPB, SCT, and HAPA all postulate a direct relationship between self-efficacy (or perceived behavioural control) and behaviour in addition to the one between intention and behaviour. This is important because it highlights that not all influences on behaviour are fully mediated by intentions. Models such as the PWM also include behavioural willingness as an additional direct predictor of behaviour, while SCT includes outcome expectancies as direct predictors and HAPA includes planning as a mediator between intentions and behaviour.

Finally, there are a number of similarities in more recent models (e.g. HAPA) that have sought to outline the variables that are important in the volitional phase of health behaviour (e.g. Weinstein 1988; Heckhausen 1991; Bagozzi 1992; Schwarzer 1992; Gollwitzer 1993; Kuhl and Beckmann 1994). In particular, these models emphasize the need for individuals to deploy a range of self-regulatory skills and strategies to ensure that strong intentions are translated into behaviour. For example, Kuhl (1984) details a wide range of action control processes that can be used to strengthen and protect intentions from alternative action tendencies, whereas both the HAPA (Schwarzer 1992) and implementation intentions (Gollwitzer 1993) emphasize the importance of formulating action plans specifying where, when, and how an intended behaviour is to be performed.

Five main conclusions can be drawn from the above comparisons. First, there is considerable overlap between the constructs included in the models. For example, most focus on outcome expectancies or the consequences of performing a behaviour. Second, some of the models may usefully be expanded to consider normative influences and perceived threat. Third, there is a strong case for including self-efficacy in all models of health behaviour. Fourth, behavioural intention should be included in all models as a mediating variable between other social cognitive variables and behaviour. Not only does intention typically emerge as the strongest predictor of behaviour but it also marks the end of a motivational phase of decision-making that many SCMs focus upon. Fifth, models need to consider post-intentional influences on behaviour.

5.3 Integration

Given the considerable overlap between constructs, it is not surprising that some researchers have attempted to produce integrated social cognition models of health behaviour (Norman and Conner 1995; Armitage and Conner 2000; Fishbein *et al.* 2001; Fishbein and Ajzen 2010).

Most prominent among these attempts is the work of a number of major theorists who attended a workshop organized by the National Institute of Mental Health in response to the need to promote HIV-preventive behaviours. At the workshop were Bandura (social cognitive theory), Becker (health belief model), Fishbein (theory of reasoned action), Kanfer (self-regulation), and Triandis (theory of interpersonal behaviour; see Norman and Conner, Chapter 12 this volume), who sought to 'identify a finite set of variables to be considered in any behavioral analysis' (Fishbein *et al.* 2001: 3). They identified eight variables, which, they argued, should account for most of the variance in any (deliberative) behaviour (Figure 1.1). These were organized into two sets. The first set were those variables that they viewed as necessary and sufficient determinants of behaviour. Thus, for behaviour to occur, an individual must (i) have a strong intention, (ii) have the necessary skills to perform the behaviour, and (ii) experience an absence of environmental constraints that could prevent behaviour. The variables in the second set were primarily seen to influence intention, although it was noted that some of the variables may also have a direct effect on behaviour. Thus, a strong intention is likely to occur when an individual (iv) perceives the advantages (or benefits) of performing the behaviour to outweigh the perceived disadvantages (or costs), (v) perceives the social (normative) pressure to perform the behaviour to be greater than that not to perform the behaviour, (vi) believes that the behaviour is consistent with his or her self-image, (vii) anticipates the emotional reaction to performing the behaviour to be more positive than negative, and (viii) has high levels of self-efficacy.

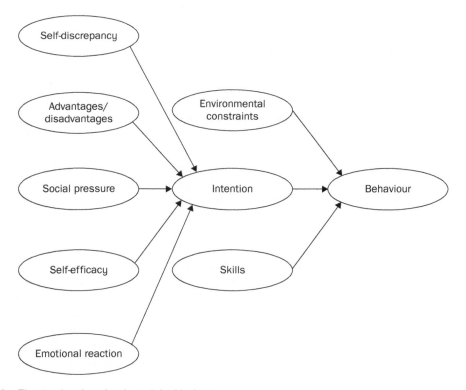

Figure 1.1 The 'major theorists' model of behaviour

This 'major theorists' model has a number of positive features. In particular, it is both logical and parsimonious and incorporates many of the key constructs included in the main social cognition models. Nonetheless, there are a number of observations that can be made about this model. First, it includes a number of constructs that do not feature in the main social cognition models. For example, although some researchers have suggested that self-identity should be included as an additional predictor in the theory of planned behaviour (e.g. Charng et al. 1988), subsequent research has shown that it explains little additional variance (Conner and Armitage 1998). Similarly, anticipated affect has also been put forward as an additional predictor (e.g. Conner and Armitage 1998), although Ajzen and Fishbein (2005) have argued that anticipated emotions should be considered as a subset of behavioural beliefs. Second, it is noteworthy that the integrated model fails to include perceptions of susceptibility and severity, which are key constructs in the health belief model and protection motivation theory. Third, the model lacks detail regarding the relationships between its constructs. In fact, Fishbein et al. (2001) noted that the major theorists were unable to agree on the likely nature of these relationships. Fourth, no empirical test of the model has been conducted to date (see Fishbein and Ajzen 2010). Finally, the model is fairly mute on the post-intentional (i.e. volitional) phase of health behaviour, simply stating that in addition to a strong intention, an individual must also possess the necessary skills to perform the behaviour and not encounter any environmental constraints that could prevent performance of the behaviour. However, recently developed volitional models identify a wide range of variables that might be important in translating intentions into action (e.g. Weinstein 1988; Heckhausen 1991; Bagozzi 1992; Schwarzer 1992; Gollwitzer 1993; Kuhl and Beckmann 1994).

6 Using social cognition models to change health behaviour

One important development in recent years has been the increased use of social cognition models to develop interventions to change health behaviours (e.g. Rutter and Quine 2002; Michie and Wood, Chapter 11 this volume). The chapters in this volume provide reviews of applications of the major SCMs to health behaviour change: the health belief model (Abraham and Sheeran, Chapter 2 this volume), protection motivation theory (Norman et al., Chapter 3 this volume), self-determination theory (Hagger and Chatzisarantis, Chapter 4 this volume), the theory of planned behaviour (Conner and Sparks, Chapter 5 this volume), the prototype-willingness model (Gibbons et al., Chapter 6 this volume), social cognitive theory (Luszczynska and Schwarzer, Chapter 7 this volume), the health action process approach (Schwarzer and Luszczynska, Chapter 8 this voume), stage models (Sutton, Chapter 9 this volume), and implementation intentions (Prestwich et al., Chapter 10 this volume). Michie and Wood (Chapter 11 this volume) provide a broader review of work on health behaviour change. Importantly, Michie and Wood overview the way in which theory can inform intervention design, present a methodology for specifying interventions in terms of their component behaviour change techniques (BCTs), overview attempts to develop a taxonomy of BCTs, and report on a methodology for investigating the effectiveness of individual BCTs and combinations of BCTs in changing behaviour. Finally, Norman and Conner (Chapter 12 in this volume) consider a number of general issues relating to use of social cognition models to develop interventions to change health behaviours.

The focus on behaviour change is welcome for several reasons. First, appropriate intervention studies can provide strong tests of SCMs. In particular, where interventions appropriately target and successfully manipulate components of an SCM, they can provide good tests of the proposed causal relationships within the SCM. Second, if a key justification for the SCM approach to health behaviours is their ability to produce more effective interventions, then this assumption needs to be tested. Third, interest in health behaviours is at least partly based on the impact these behaviours have on health outcomes such as morbidity and mortality. Demonstrating that research on predicting and changing health behaviours can improve such outcomes is the cornerstone to the utility of the social cognition approach.

7 Conclusions: using social cognition models in predicting and changing health behaviours

This chapter has set out the rationale for the interest in understanding health behaviours, particularly as a basis for attempting to change their occurrence in order to increase both length and quality of life. Social cognition models provide an important and widely used approach to understanding health behaviour in describing the important social cognitive variables predicting such behaviours. As such, these models provide an important basis for achieving the aim of changing health behaviour by providing a means for identifying appropriate targets for intervention work. Intervention work is now proceeding to test the causal role of these variables, as identified in SCMs, as a means to change health behaviour and promote health outcomes. Other work has focused on a broader set of behaviour change techniques (BCTs) that might be usefully employed in changing different health behaviours (Michie and Wood, Chapter 11 this volume). A closer integration of these parallel strands of work is needed to further the science of behaviour change. For example, work on SCMs can provide useful insights into the process of behaviour change by examining the impact of BCTs (that successfully change behaviour) on mediating social cognitions.

References

Abraham, C., Sheeran, P., Norman, P., Conner, M., De Vries, N. and Otten, W. (1999) When good intentions are not enough: modeling postdecisional cognitive correlates of condom use, *Journal of Applied Social Psychology*, 29, 2591–612.

Adler, N. and Matthews, K. (1994) Health psychology: why do some people get sick and some stay well? *Annual Review of Psychology*, 45, 229–59.

Affleck, G., Tennen, H., Croog, S. and Levine, S. (1987) Causal attribution, perceived control, and recovery from a heart attack, *Journal of Social and Clinical Psychology*, 5, 356–64.

Ajzen, I. (1991) The theory of planned behavior, *Organizational Behavior and Human Decision Processes*, 50, 179–211.

Ajzen, I. and Fishbein, M. (1980) *Understanding Attitudes and Predicting Social Behavior*. Englewood Cliffs, NJ: Prentice-Hall.

Ajzen, I. and Fishbein, M. (2005) The influence of attitudes on behavior, in D. Albarracin, B.T. Johnson and M.P. Zanna (eds.) *Handbook of Attitudes and Attitude Change: Basic Principles* (pp. 173–221). Mahwah, NJ: Erlbaum.

Amler, R.W. and Eddins, D.L. (1987) Cross-sectional analysis: precursors of premature death in the U.S., in R.W. Amler and H.B. Dull (eds.) *Closing the Gap* (pp. 54–87). New York: Oxford University Press.

Armitage, C.J. and Conner, M. (2000) Social cognition models and health behaviour: a structured review, *Psychology and Health*, 15, 173–89.

Armitage, C.J. and Conner, M. (2001) Efficacy of the theory of planned behaviour: a meta-analytic review, *British Journal of Social Psychology*, 40, 471–99.

Bagozzi, R.P. (1992) The self-regulation of attitudes, intentions and behavior, *Social Psychology Quarterly*, 55, 178–204.

Bagozzi, R.P. (1993) On the neglect of volition in consumer research: a critique and proposal, *Psychology and Marketing*, 10, 215–37.

Bagozzi, R.P. and Kimmel, S.K. (1995) A comparison of leading theories for the prediction of goal-directed behaviours, *British Journal of Social Psychology*, 34, 437–61.

Bakker, A.B., Buunk, A.P. and Siero, F.W. (1994) Condom use of heterosexuals: a comparison of the theory of planned behavior, the health belief model and protection motivation theory. Unpublished manuscript.

Bandura, A. (1982) Self-efficacy mechanism in human agency, *American Psychologist*, 37, 122–47.

Bandura, A. (2000) Health promotion from the perspective of social cognitive theory, in P. Norman, C. Abraham and M. Conner (eds.) *Understanding and Changing Health Behaviour: From Health Beliefs to Self-regulation* (pp. 229–42). Amsterdam: Harwood Academic.

Baum, A. and Posluszny, D.M. (1999) Health psychology: mapping biobehavioral contributions to health and illness, *Annual Review of Psychology*, 50, 137–63.

Baumeister, R. and Leary, M.R. (1995) The need to belong: desire for interpersonal attachments as a fundamental human motivation, *Psychological Bulletin*, 117, 497–529.

Becker, M.H. (1974) The health belief model and sick role behavior, *Health Education Monographs*, 2, 409–19.

Becker, M.H., Haefner, D.P., Kasl, S.V., Kirscht, J.P., Maiman, L.A. and Rosenstock, I.M. (1977) Selected psychosocial models and correlates of individual health-related behaviors, *Medical Care*, 15, 27–46.

Becker, M.H. and Maiman, L.A. (1983) Models of health-related behavior, in D. Mechanic (ed.) *Handbook of Health, Health Care and the Health Professions* (pp. 539–68). New York: Free Press.

Belloc, N.B. (1973) Relationship of health practices to mortality, *Preventive Medicine*, 2, 67–81.

Belloc, N.B. and Breslow, L. (1972) Relationship of physical health status and health practices, *Preventive Medicine*, 9, 409–21.

Blanchard, C.M., Reid, R.D., Morrin, L.I., McDonnell, L., McGannon, K., Rhodes, R.E. *et al.* (2011) Understanding physical activity during home-based cardiac rehabilitation from multiple theoretical perspectives, *Journal of Cardipulmonary Rehabilitation and Prevention*, 31, 173–80.

Blaxter, M. (1990) *Health and Lifestyles*. London: Tavistock.

Boer, H. and Mashamba, M.T. (2005) Psychosocial correlates of HIV protection motivation among black adolescents in Venda, South Africa, *AIDS Education and Prevention*, 17, 590–602.

Breslow, L. and Enstrom, J.E. (1980) Persistence of health habits and their relationship to mortality, *Preventive Medicine*, 9, 469–83.

Calnan, M. (1984) The health belief model and participation in programmes for the early detection of breast cancer, *Social Science and Medicine*, 19, 823–30.

Centers for Diseases Control (CDC) (2013) *Health Behaviors of Adults: United States, 2008–2010*. Washington, DC: USDHHS.

Charng, H.-W., Piliavin, J.A. and Callero, P.L. (1988) Role identity and reasoned action in the prediction of repeated behavior, *Social Psychology Quarterly*, 51, 303–17.

Cialdini, R.B., Kallgren, C.A. and Reno, R.R. (1991) A focus theory of normative conduct: a theoretical refinement and re-evaluation of the role of norms in human behaviour, in M.P. Zanna (ed.) *Advances in Experimental Social Psychology* (Vol. 24, pp. 201–34). San Diego, CA: Academic Press.

Cohen, J. (1992) A power primer, *Psychological Bulletin*, 112, 155–9.

Conner, M.T. (1993) Pros and cons of social cognition models in health behaviour, *Health Psychology Update*, 14, 24–31.

Conner, M. and Armitage, C.J. (1998) Extending the theory of planned behavior: a review and avenues for further research, *Journal of Applied Social Psychology*, 28, 1430–64.

Conner, M. and Norman, P. (1994) Comparing the health belief model and the theory of planned behaviour in health screening, in D.R. Rutter and L. Quine (eds.) *Social Psychology and Health: European Perspectives* (pp. 1–24). Aldershot: Avebury.

Conner, M. and Norman, P. (eds.) (1995) *Predicting Health Behaviour: Research and Practice with Social Cognition Models*. Buckingham: Open University Press.

Conner, M. and Norman, P. (eds.) (2005) *Predicting Health Behaviour: Research and Practice with Social Cognition Models* (2nd edn.). Maidenhead: Open University Press.

Conner, M., McEachan, R., Jackson, C., McMillan, B., Woolridge, M. and Lawton, R. (2013) Moderating effect of socioeconomic status on the relationship between health cognitions and behaviors, *Annals of Behavioral Medicine*, 46, 19–30.

Cummings, M.K., Becker, M.H. and Maile, M.C. (1980) Bringing models together: an empirical approach to combining variables used to explain health actions, *Journal of Behavioral Medicine*, 3, 123–45.

Deci, E.L. (1975) *Intrinsic Motivation*. New York: Plenum Press.

Deci, E.L. and Ryan, R.M. (1985) *Intrinsic Motivation and Self-determination in Human Behavior*. New York: Plenum Press.

Deci, E.L. and Ryan, R.M. (2002) An overview of self-determination theory: an organismic-dialectical perspective, in E.L. Deci and R.M. Ryan (eds.) *Handbook of Self-determination Research* (pp. 3–33). New York: University of Rochester Press.

DiClemente, C.C. and Hughes, S.O. (1990) Stages of change profiles in outpatient alcoholism treatment, *Journal of Substance Abuse*, 2, 217–35.

DiClemente, C.C., Prochaska, J.O., Fairhurst, S.K., Velicer, W.F., Velasquez, M.M. and Rossi, J.S. (1991) The process of smoking cessation: an analysis of precontemplation, contemplation, and preparation stages of change, *Journal of Consulting and Clinical Psychology*, 59, 295–304.

Dzewaltowski, D.A. (1989) Toward a model of exercise motivation, *Journal of Sport and Exercise Psychology*, 32, 11–28.

Edwards, W. (1954) The theory of decision making, *Psychological Bulletin*, 51, 380–417.

Fishbein, M. and Ajzen, I. (1975) *Belief, Attitude, Intention, and Behavior*. New York: Wiley.

Fishbein, M. and Ajzen, I. (2010) *Predicting and Changing Behavior: The Reasoned Action Approach*. New York: Psychology Press.

Fishbein, M., Triandis, H.C., Kanfer, F.H., Becker, M., Middlestadt, S.E. and Eichler, A. (2001) Factors influencing behavior and behavior change, in A. Baum, T.A. Revenson and J.E. Singer (eds.) *Handbook of Health Psychology* (pp. 3–17). Mahwah, NJ: Erlbaum.

Fiske, S.T. and Taylor, S.E. (1991) *Social Cognition*. New York: McGraw-Hill.

Fiske, S.T. and Taylor, S.E. (2013) *Social Cognition: From Brains to Culture* (2nd edn.). Los Angeles, CA: Sage.

Frisch, D. and Clemen, R.T. (1994) Beyond expected utility: rethinking behavioral decision making, *Psychological Bulletin*, 116, 46–54.

Gebhardt, W.A. and Maes, S. (2001) Integrating social-psychological frameworks for health behaviour research, *American Journal of Health Behavior*, 25, 528–36.

Gerend, M.A. and Shepherd, J.E. (2012) Predicting human papillomavirus vaccine uptake in young adult women: comparing the health belief model and theory of planned behavior, *Annals of Behavioral Medicine*, 44, 171–80.

Gibbons, F.X. and Gerrard, M. (1995) Predicting young adults' health risk behavior, *Journal of Personality and Social Psychology*, 69, 505–17.

Gibbons, F.X. and Gerrard, M. (1997) Health images and their effects on health behaviour, in B.P. Buunk and F.X. Gibbons (eds.) *Health, Coping and Well-being: Perspectives from Social Comparison Theory* (pp. 63–94). Hillsdale, NJ: Erlbaum.

Gibbons, F.X., Gerrard, M. and Lane, D.J. (2003) A social-reaction model of adolescent health risk, in J.M. Suls and K.A. Wallston (eds.) *Social Psychological Foundations of Health and Illness* (pp. 107–36). Oxford: Blackwell.

Glanz, K. and Bishop, D.B. (2010) The role of behavioral science theory in the development and implementation of public health interventions, *Annual Review of Public Health*, 31, 399–418.

Gochman, D.S. (ed.) (1997) *Handbook of Health Behavior Research* (Vol. 1). New York: Plenum Press.

Gollwitzer, P.M. (1993) Goal achievement: the role of intentions, *European Review of Social Psychology*, 4, 142–85.

Gollwitzer, P.M. (1999) Implementation intentions: strong effects of simple plans, *American Psychologist*, 54, 493–503.

Greeno, C.G. and Wing, R.R. (1994) Stress-induced eating, *Psychological Bulletin*, 115, 444–64.

Hagger, M. and Orbell, S. (2003) A meta-analytic review of the common-sense model of illness representations, *Psychology and Health*, 18, 141–84.

Hampson, S.E. (2012) Personality processes: mechanisms by which personality traits 'get outside the skin', *Annual Review of Psychology*, 63, 315–39.

Harter, S. (1978) Effectance motivation reconsidered: toward a developmental model, *Human Development*, 1, 661–9.

Heckhausen, H. (1991) *Motivation and Action*. Berlin: Springer.

Hill, D., Gardner, G. and Rassaby, J. (1985) Factors predisposing women to take precautions against breast and cervix cancer, *Journal of Applied Social Psychology*, 15, 59–79.

Hunter, M.S., Grunfeld, E.A. and Ramirez, A.J. (2003) Help-seeking intentions for breast-cancer symptoms: a comparison of the self-regulation model and the theory of planned behaviour, *British Journal of Health Psychology*, 8, 319–33.

Janz, N.K. and Becker, M.H. (1984) The health belief model: a decade later, *Health Education Quarterly*, 11, 1–47.

Jessor, R., Turbin, M.S. and Costa, F.M. (1998) Protective factors in adolescent health behaviour, *Journal of Personality and Social Psychology*, 75, 788–800.

Jonas, K. (1993) Expectancy-value models of health behaviour: an analysis by conjoint measurement, *European Journal of Social Psychology*, 23, 167–83.

Kasl, S.V. and Cobb, S. (1966) Health behavior, illness behavior and sick role behavior, *Archives of Environmental Health*, 12, 246–66.

King, J. (1982) The impact of patients' perceptions of high blood pressure on attendance at screening, *Social Science and Medicine*, 16, 1079–91.

Kirscht, J.P. (1982) Preventive health behaviour: a review of research and issues, *Health Psychology*, 2, 277–301.

Kuhl, J. (1984) Volitional aspects of achievement motivation and learned helplessness: toward a comprehensive theory of action control, *Progress in Experimental Personality Research*, 13, 99–171.

Kuhl, J. and Beckmann, J. (eds.) (1985) *Action Control: From Cognition to Behavior*. Berlin: Springer.

Kuhl, J. and Beckmann, J. (eds.) (1994) *Volition and Personality: Action Versus State Orientation*. Göttingen: Springer.

Lajunen, T. and Rasanen, M. (2004) Can social psychological models be used to promote bicycle helmet use among teenagers? A comparison of the health belief model, theory of planned behavior and the locus of control, *Journal of Safety Research*, 35, 115–23.

Lawton, R., Conner, M. and Parker, D. (2007) Beyond cognition: predicting health risk behaviors from instrumental and affective beliefs, *Health Psychology*, 26, 259–67.

Leventhal, H., Nerenz, D.R. and Steele, D.F. (1984) Illness representations and coping with health threats, in A. Baum and J. Singer (eds.) *A Handbook of Psychology and Health* (pp. 219–52). Hillsdale, NJ: Erlbaum.

Maddux, J.E. and Rogers, R.W. (1983) Protection motivation and self-efficacy: a revised theory of fear appeals and attitude change, *Journal of Experimental Social Psychology*, 19, 469–79.

Marteau, T.M. (1989) Health beliefs and attributions, in A.K. Broome (ed.) *Health Psychology: Processes and Applications* (pp. 1–23). London: Chapman & Hall.

Matterne, U., Diepgen, T.L. and Weisshaar, E. (2011) A longitudinal application of three health behaviour models in the context of skin protection behaviour in individuals with occupational skin disease, *Psychology and Health*, 26, 1188–1207.

McEachan, R.R.C., Lawton, R.J. and Conner, M. (2010) Classifying health-related behaviours: exploring similarities and differences amongst behaviours, *British Journal of Health Psychology*, 15, 347–66.

McNeil, A.D., Jarvis, M.J., Stapleton, J.A., Russell, M.A.H., Eiser, J.R., Gammage, P. *et al.* (1988) Prospective study of factors predicting uptake of smoking in adolescents, *Journal of Epidemiology and Community Health*, 43, 72–8.

Montanaro, E.A. and Bryan, A.D. (2014) Comparing theory-based condom interventions: health belief model versus theory of planned behavior, *Health Psychology*, 33, 1251–60.

Moss-Morris, R., Weinman, J., Petrie, K.J., Horne, R., Cameron, L.D. and Buick, D. (2002) The revised Illness Perception Questionnaire (IPQ-R), *Psychology and Health*, 17, 1–16.

Mullen, P.D., Hersey, J.C. and Iverson, D.C. (1987) Health behaviour models compared, *Social Science and Medicine*, 24, 973–81.

Noar, S.M. and Zimmerman, R.S (2005) Health behavior theory and cumulative knowledge regarding health behaviors: are we moving in the right direction? *Health Education Research*, 20, 275–90.

Norman, P., Abraham, C. and Conner, M. (2000) *Understanding and Changing Health Behaviour: From Health Beliefs to Self-regulation*. Amsterdam: Harwood Academic.

Norman, P. and Conner, M. (1995) The role of social cognition models in predicting health behaviours: future directions, in M. Conner and P. Norman (eds.) *Predicting Health Behaviour: Research and Practice with Social Cognition Models* (pp. 197–225). Buckingham: Open University Press.

Norman, P., Conner, M. and Bell, R. (1999) The theory of planned behavior and smoking cessation, *Health Psychology*, 18, 89–94.

Notani, A.S. (1998) Moderators of perceived behavioural control's predictiveness in the Theory of Planned Behaviour: a meta-analysis, *Journal of Consumer Psychology*, 7, 247–71.

Oliver, R.L. and Berger, P.K. (1979) A path analysis of preventive health care decision models, *Journal of Consumer Research*, 6, 113–22.

Orbell, S., Hagger, M., Brown, V. and Tidy, J. (2006) Comparing two theories of health behavior: a prospective study of noncompletion of treatment following cervical cancer screening, *Health Psychology*, 25, 604–15.

Ouelette, J.A. and Wood, W. (1998) Habit and intention in everyday life: the multiple processes by which past behavior predicts future behavior, *Psychological Bulletin*, 124, 54–74.

Peak, H. (1955) Attitude and motivation, in M.R. Jones (ed.) *Nebraska Symposium on Motivation* (Vol. 3, pp. 149–88). Lincoln, NB: University of Nebraska Press.

Petrie, K.J. and Weinman, J. (1997) *Perceptions of Health and Illness: Current Research and Applications*. Amsterdam: Harwood Academic.

Plotnikov, R.C., Lubans, D.R., Penfold, C.M. and Courneya, K.S. (2014) Testing the utility of three social-cognitive models for predicting objective and self-report physical activity in adults with type 2 diabetes, *British Journal of Health Psychology*, 19, 329–46.

Prentice-Dunn, S. and Rogers, R.W. (1986) Protection motivation theory and preventive health: beyond the health belief model, *Health Education Research*, 1, 153–61.

Prochaska, J.O. and DiClemente, C.C. (1984) *The Transtheoretical Approach: Crossing Traditional Boundaries of Therapy*. Homewood, IL: Dow Jones Irwin.

Rhodes, R. and Conner, M. (2010) Comparison of behavioral belief structures in the physical activity domain, *Journal of Applied Social Psychology*, 40, 2105–20.

Rogers, R.W. (1975) A protection motivation theory of fear appeals and attitude change, *Journal of Psychology*, 91, 93–114.

Rogers, R.W. (1983) Cognitive and physiological processes in fear appeals and attitude change: a revised theory of protection motivation, in J.T. Cacioppo and R.E. Petty (eds.) *Social Psychophysiology: A Source Book* (pp. 153–76). New York: Guilford Press.

Rosenstock, I.M. (1966) Why people use health services, *Milbank Memorial Fund Quarterly*, 44, 94–124.

Rosenstock, I.M. (1974) Historical origins of the health belief model, *Health Education Monographs*, 2, 1–8.

Rosenstock, I.M., Strecher, V.J. and Becker, M.H. (1988) Social learning theory and the health belief model, *Health Education Quarterly*, 15, 175–83.

Rothman, A.J. and Salovey, P. (1997) Shaping perceptions to motivate healthy behaviour: the role of message framing, *Psychological Bulletin*, 121, 3–19.

Royal College of Physicians (RCP) (1992) *Smoking and the Young*. Sudbury, UK: Lavenham Press.

Roysamb, E., Rise, J. and Kraft, P. (1997) On the structure and dimensionality of health-related behaviour in adolescents, *Psychology and Health*, 12, 437–52.

Rutter, D.R. (1989) Models of belief–behaviour relationships in health, *Health Psychology Update*, November, pp. 8–10.

Rutter, D.R. and Quine, L. (eds.) (2002) *Changing Health Behaviour*. Buckingham: Open University Press.

Rutter, D.R., Quine, L. and Chesham, D.J. (1993) *Social Psychological Approaches to Health*. London: Harvester-Wheatsheaf.

Ryan, R.M. and Deci, E.L. (2000) Self-determination theory and the facilitation of intrinsic motivation, social development, and well-being, *American Psychologist*, 55, 68–78.

Schneider, D.J. (1991) Social cognition, *Annual Review of Psychology*, 42, 527–61.

Schwarzer, R. (1992) Self-efficacy in the adoption and maintenance of health behaviors: theoretical approaches and a new model, in R. Schwarzer (ed.) *Self-efficacy: Thought Control of Action* (pp. 217–43). London: Hemisphere.

Schwarzer, R. (2008) Modeling health behavior change: how to predict and modify the adoption and maintenance of health behaviors, *Applied Psychology: An International Review*, 57, 1–29.

Seydel, E., Taal, E. and Wiegman, O. (1990) Risk-appraisal, outcome and self-efficacy expectancies: cognitive factors in preventive behavior related to cancer, *Psychology and Health*, 4, 99–109.

Sheeran, P. (2002) Intention–behavior relations: a conceptual and empirical review, in W. Strobe and M. Hewstone (eds.) *European Review of Social Psychology* (Vol. 12, pp. 1–30). Chichester: Wiley.

Sheeran, P., Maki, A., Montanaro, E., Bryan, A., Klein, W.M.P., Miles, E. *et al.* (submitted) The impact of changing attitudes, norms, and self-efficacy on health-related intentions and behavior: a meta-analysis.

Simsekoglu, O. and Lajunen, T. (2008) Social psychology of seat belt use: a comparison of theory of planned behavior and health belief model, *Transportation Research Part F: Traffic Psychology and Behaviour*, 11, 181–91.

Smith, A. and Jacobson, B. (1988) *The Nation's Health: A Strategy for the 1990s*. London: Kings Fund.

Steptoe, A., Wardle, J., Vinck, J., Tuomisto, M., Holte, A. and Wichstrom, L. (1994) Personality and attitudinal correlates of healthy and unhealthy lifestyles in young adults, *Psychology and Health*, 9, 331–43.

Taylor, S. (1991) *Health Psychology*. New York: McGraw-Hill.

Taylor, S., Lichtman, R.R. and Wood, J.V. (1984) Attributions, beliefs about control and adjustment to breast cancer, *Journal of Personality and Social Psychology*, 46, 489–502.

Tennen, H., Affleck, G., Allen, D.A., McGrade, B.J. and Ratzan, S. (1984) Causal attributions and coping with insulin-dependent diabetes, *Basic and Applied Social Psychology*, 5, 131–42.

Trafimow, D. and Fishbein, M. (1995) Do people really distinguish between behavioural and normative beliefs? *British Journal of Social Psychology*, 34, 257–66.

Trafimow, D., Sheeran, P., Conner, M. and Finlay, K.A. (2002) Evidence that perceived behavioral control is a multidimensional construct: perceived control and perceived difficulty, *British Journal of Social Psychology*, 41, 101–21.

Turk, D.C. and Salovey, P. (1986) Clinical information processing: bias inoculation, in R.E. Ingham (ed.) *Information Processing Approaches to Clinical Psychology* (pp. 305–23). New York: Academic Press.

Van der Pligt, J. (1994) Risk appraisal and health behaviour, in D.R. Rutter and L. Quine (eds.) *Social Psychology and Health: European Perspectives* (pp. 131–52). Aldershot: Avebury.

Van der Pligt, J., de Vries, N.K., Manstead, A.S.R. and Van Harreveld, F. (2000) The importance of being selective: weighting the role of attribute importance in attitudinal judgment, *Advances in Experimental Social Psychology*, 32, 135–200.

Van der Velde, W. and Van der Pligt, J. (1991) AIDS-related behavior: coping, protection motivation, and previous behavior, *Journal of Behavioral Medicine*, 14, 429–51.

Wardle, J. and Steptoe, A. (1991) The European Health and Behaviour Survey: rationale, methods and initial results from the United Kingdom, *Social Science and Medicine*, 33, 925–36.

Webb, T.L. and Sheeran, P. (2006) Does changing behavioral intentions engender behavior change? A meta-analysis of the experimental evidence, *Psychological Bulletin*, 132, 249–68.

Weinstein, N.D. and Sandman, P.M. (1992) The precaution adoption process model, in K. Glanz, B.K. Rimer and F.M. Lewis (eds.) *Health Behavior and Health Education: Theory, Research, and Practice* (3rd edn., pp. 121–43). San Francisco, CA: Jossey-Bass.

Weinstein, W.D. (1988) The precaution adoption process, *Health Psychology*, 7, 355–86.

Weinstein, W.D. (1993) Testing four competing theories of health-protective behavior, *Health Psychology*, 12, 324–33.

Weinstein, W.D. (2000) Perceived probability, perceived severity, and health-protective behavior, *Health Psychology*, 19, 65–74.

Whitehead, M. (1988) The health divide, in *Inequalities in Health: The Black Report and the Health Divide* (pp. 217–356). London: Penguin.

Winett, R.A. (1985) Ecobehavioral assessment in health life-styles: concepts and methods, in P. Karoly (ed.) *Measurement Strategies in Health Psychology* (pp. 147–81). Chichester: Wiley.

Witenberg, S.H., Blanchard, E.B., Suls, J., Tennen, H., McCoy, G. and McGoldrick, M.D. (1983) Perceptions of control and causality as predictors of compliance with hemodialysis, *Basic and Applied Social Psychology*, 1, 319–36.

Chapter 2

The health belief model

Charles Abraham and Paschal Sheeran

1 General background

In the 1950s, US public health researchers began developing psychological models designed to enhance the effectiveness of health education programmes (Hochbaum 1958; Rosenstock 1966). Demographic characteristics such as socio-economic status, gender, ethnicity, and age were known to be associated with preventive health-related behaviour patterns (i.e. patterns of behaviour predictive of differences in morbidity and mortality) as well as differential use of health services (Rosenstock 1974). Even when services were publicly financed, socio-economic status was associated with health-related behaviour patterns. Demographic and socio-economic characteristics could not be modified through health education but it was hypothesized that other potentially modifiable individual characteristics associated with health-related behaviour patterns could be changed through educational interventions, and thus shift health behaviour patterns at population levels.

Beliefs provide a crucial link between socialization and behaviour. Beliefs are enduring individual characteristics that shape behaviour and can be acquired through primary socialization. Beliefs are also modifiable and can differentiate between individuals from the same background. If persuasive techniques can be used to change behaviour-related beliefs and such interventions result in behaviour change, this provides a theoretical and practical basis for evidence-based health education.

The relationship between health beliefs and behaviours was conceptualized primarily in terms of Lewin's (1951) idea of 'valence'. Particular beliefs were thought to make behaviours more or less attractive. This resulted in an expectancy-value model of belief–behaviour relationships in which events believed to be more or less likely were positively or negatively evaluated by individuals. In particular, the likelihood of experiencing a health problem, the severity of the consequences of that problem, and the perceived benefits of a preventive behaviour, in combination with its potential costs, were seen as key beliefs that shaped health-related behaviour patterns. Early research found that these health beliefs were indeed correlated with differ-ences in health-related behaviour patterns (referred to below as 'health behaviours' or 'health behaviour patterns') and so could be used to differentiate between those who did and did not undertake such behaviours. The model was initially applied to preventive behaviours but later successfully extended to identify the correlates of health service usage and adherence to medi-cal advice (Becker *et al.* 1977b).

Rosenstock (1974) attributed the first health belief model (HBM) research to Hochbaum's (1958) studies of the uptake of tuberculosis X-ray screening. Hochbaum found that perceived sus-ceptibility to tuberculosis and the belief that people with the disease could be asymptomatic (mak-ing screening beneficial) distinguished between those who had and had not attended for chest X-rays. Similarly, a prospective study by Kegeles (1963) showed that perceived susceptibility to the worst imaginable dental problems and awareness that visits to the dentist might prevent these problems were useful predictors of the frequency of dental visits over the next three years. Haefner and Kirscht (1970) took this research further by demonstrating that an HBM-based health educa-tion intervention designed to increase participants' perceived susceptibility, perceived severity, and anticipated benefits resulted in a greater number of check-up visits to the doctor compared with no intervention over an eight-month follow-up. Thus, by the early 1970s a series of studies suggested that the HBM specified a series of key health beliefs that provided a useful framework for understanding individual differences in health behaviour patterns and for designing behaviour change interventions.

The HBM had the advantage of specifying a discrete set of common-sense beliefs that appear to explain, or mediate, the effects of demographic variables on health behaviour pat-terns and are amenable to change through educational intervention. The model could be applied to a range of health behaviours and so provided a framework for shaping behaviour patterns relevant to public health as well as training health care professionals to work from their patients' subjective perceptions of illness and treatment. Consensus regarding the utility of the HBM was important for public health research and, simultaneously, placed cognition modelling at the centre of health service research.

The HBM was consolidated when Becker *et al.* (1977b) published a consensus statement from the Carnegie Grant Subcommittee on Modification of Patient Behavior for Health Mainte-nance and Disease Control. This paper considered a range of alternative approaches to under-standing the social psychological determinants of health and illness behaviour and endorsed the HBM framework. The components of the model were defined and further research on the relationships between individual beliefs and health behaviours was called for.

2 Description of the model

The HBM focused on two aspects of individuals' representations of health and health behav-iour: threat perception and behavioural evaluation. Threat perception was construed as two key beliefs: perceived susceptibility to illness or health problems, and anticipated severity of the consequences of illnesses. Behavioural evaluation also consisted of two distinct sets of beliefs: those concerning the benefits or efficacy of a recommended health behaviour, and those con-cerning the costs of, or barriers to, enacting the behaviour. In addition, the model proposed that cues to action can activate health behaviour when appropriate beliefs are held. These 'cues'

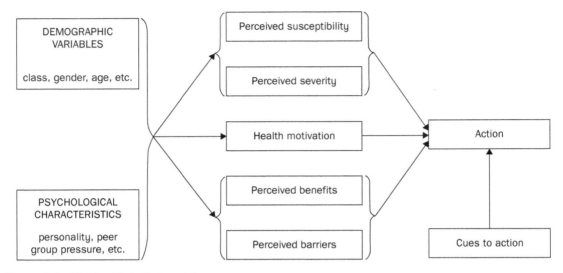

Figure 2.1 The health belief model

included a diverse range of triggers, including individual perceptions of symptoms, social influence, and health education campaigns. Finally, an individual's general health motivation, or 'readiness to be concerned about health matters', was included in later versions of the model (e.g. Becker *et al.* 1977b). There were therefore six distinct constructs specified by the HBM.

As Figure 2.1 indicates, there were no clear guidelines on how to operationalize the links between perceived susceptibility, severity, and overall threat perception. Similarly, although it was suggested that perceived benefits were 'weighted against' perceived barriers (Becker *et al.* 1977b), no formula for creating an overall behavioural evaluation measure was developed. Consequently, the model has usually been operationalized as a series of up to six separate independent variables that potentially account for variance in health behaviours. Even the definition of these six constructs was left open to debate. Rosenstock (1974) and Becker and Maiman (1975) illustrated how various researchers used somewhat different operationalizations of these constructs and, in a meta-analysis of predictive applications of the HBM, Harrison *et al.* (1992) concluded that this lack of operational homogeneity weakens the HBM's status as a coherent psychological model of the prerequisites of health behaviour. Nevertheless, a series of studies has shown that these various operationalizations allowed identification of beliefs correlated with health behaviours (e.g. Janz and Becker 1984).

3 Summary of research

3.1 Overview of HBM applications and research strategies

The HBM has been applied to the prediction of an impressively broad range of health behaviours among a wide range of populations. Table 2.1 illustrates the range of behaviours that have been examined. Three broad areas can be identified: (1) preventive health behaviours, which include health-promoting (e.g. diet, exercise) and health-risk (e.g. smoking) behaviours as well as vaccination and

Table 2.1 Illustrative applications of the HBM

Behaviour	Researchers
Preventive behaviours	
Screening	
• genetic	Tay-Sachs trait: Becker *et al.* (1975); faecal occult blood: Hoogewerf *et al.* (1990)
• health	Hypertension: King (1984); cervical cancer: Orbell *et al.* (1995); colorectal cancer: Rawl *et al.* (2001), Hay *et al.* (2003); mammography: Aiken *et al.* (1994a, 1994b); STI test: Simon and Das (1984); HIV test: Dorr *et al.* (1999)
Risk behaviours	
• smoking	Penderson *et al.* (1982), Gianetti *et al.* (1985), Mullen *et al.* (1987), Stacy and Lloyd (1990)
	Exposure to environmental tobacco smoke: Li *et al.* (2003)
• alcohol	Portnoy (1980), Beck (1981), Gottlieb and Baker (1986)
• eating meat	Weitkunat *et al.* (2003)
Influenza vaccination	Cummings *et al.* (1979), Oliver and Berger (1979), Rundall and Wheeler (1979), Larson *et al.* (1982)
Breast self-examination	Champion (1984), Calnan (1985), Owens *et al.* (1987), Ronis and Harel (1989), Umeh and Rogan-Gibson (2001), Norman and Brain (2005)
Contraceptive use (including condom use)	Eisen *et al.* (1985), Hester and Macrina (1985), Lowe and Radius (1987) Abraham *et al.* (1992, 1996), Lollis *et al.* (1997), Adih and Alexander (1999), Volk and Koopman (2001), Drayton *et al.* (2002), Winfield and Whaley (2002)
Diet and exercise	Langlie (1977), Aho (1979a)
	In relation to osteoporosis prevention: Silver Wallace (2002)
Dental behaviours	
• dental visits	Kegeles (1963), Chen and Land (1986)
• brushing/flossing	Chen and Tatsuoka (1984)
Others	Cholera prevention: Ogionwo (1973); coronary heart disease prevention: Ali (2002); osteoporosis prevention: Schmiege *et al.* (2007); safety helmet use: Quine *et al.* (1998)
Sick role/adherence behaviours	
Anti-hypertensive regimens	Kirscht and Rosenstock (1977), Nelson *et al.* (1978), Taylor (1979), Hershey *et al.* (1980)
Diabetic regimens	Harris and Lynn (1985), Bradley *et al.* (1987), Brownlee-Duffeck *et al.* (1987), Wdowik *et al.* (2001)
Renal disease regimens	Heinzelmann (1962), Hartman and Becker (1978), Cummings *et al.* (1982)
Psychiatric regimens	Kelly *et al.* (1987), Smith *et al.* (1999), Perkins (2002)
Parental adherence to children's regimens	Obesity: Becker *et al.* (1977b); rheumatic fever: Gordis *et al.* (1969); otitis medea: Charney *et al.* (1967), Becker *et al.* (1972); asthma: Becker *et al.* (1978)

(Continued)

Table 2.1 *Continued*

Behaviour	Researchers
Others	Regimen for urinary tract infection: Reid and Christensen (1988); malaria prophylaxis regimens: Abraham *et al.* (1999a), Farquharson *et al.* (2004)
Clinic use	
Physician visits	
• preventive	Kirscht *et al.* (1976), Leavitt (1979), Berkanovich *et al.* (1981), Norman and Conner (1993)
• parent and child	Becker *et al.* (1972, 1977a), Kirscht *et al.* (1978)
• psychiatric	Connelly *et al.* (1982), Connelly (1984), Rees (1986), Pan and Tantam (1989)

contraceptive practices; (2) sick role behaviours, particularly adherence to recommended medical regimens; and (3) clinic use, which includes physician visits for a variety of reasons.

Early HBM studies focused on prediction of preventive health behaviours. One of the first reviews of research (Becker *et al.* 1977a) examined 20 studies, 13 of which were investigations of preventive actions. These 13 studies examined seven distinct behaviours (X-ray screening for TB, polio vaccination, influenza vaccination, use of safety gloves, pap test, preventive dental visits, and screening for Tay-Sachs trait). In contrast, six of the remaining seven studies of sick role behaviours concerned adherence to penicillin prescriptions. When Janz and Becker reviewed the HBM literature in 1984, smoking, alcohol use, dieting, exercise, and attendance at blood pressure screening had been added to the list of preventive behaviours examined from an HBM perspective. Studies of sick role behaviours also increased to include adherence to regimens for hypertension, insulin-dependent and non-insulin-dependent diabetes, end-stage renal disease, obesity, and asthma. Studies often examined a range of outcomes relevant to a particular regimen. For example, Cummings and colleagues' (1982) study of end-stage renal disease patients included measures of serum phosphorus and potassium levels, fluid intake, weight gain, and patients' self-reports of diet and medication. Subsequent research has extended the range of behaviours examined to include contraceptive use, including condom use, and personal dental behaviours such as teeth brushing and flossing, as well as screening for faecal occult blood, colorectal cancer, and sexually transmitted diseases.

Many HBM predictive studies have employed cross-sectional designs, although Janz and Becker's (1984) review found that 40% ($n = 18$) of identified HBM studies were prospective. Prospective studies are important because simultaneous measurement of health beliefs and (especially self-reported) behaviour may be subject to memory and social desirability biases and do not permit causal inferences (Field 2000). Most studies also have used self-report measures of behaviour but some have used physiological measures (e.g. Bradley *et al.* 1987), behavioural observations (e.g. Alagna and Reddy 1984; Dorr *et al.* 1999; Hay *et al.* 2003) or medical records (e.g. Orbell *et al.* 1995; Drayton *et al.* 2002) as outcome measures. While the majority of measures of health beliefs employ self-completion questionnaires, structured face-to-face (e.g. Cummings *et al.* 1982; Volk and Koopman 2001) and telephone (e.g. Grady *et al.* 1983) interviews have also been employed. The use of random sampling techniques is commonplace and specific representation of low-income and minority groups is also evident (e.g. Becker *et al.* 1974; Mullen *et al.* 1987; Ronis and Harel 1989; Winfield and Whaley 2002).

Findings from research studies employing the HBM are reviewed below. We first examine evidence for the predictive utility of the model's four major constructs: susceptibility, severity, benefits, and barriers. Second, we consider findings relating to cues to action and health motivation, which have received more limited empirical attention. Third, we examine the issue of combining health beliefs and the potential importance of interactions among beliefs. Finally, we discuss the extent to which health beliefs have been successful in mediating the effects of social structural variables and past behaviour.

3.2 Utility of perceived susceptibility, severity, benefit, and barrier constructs

Three quantitative reviews of research using the HBM with adults have been published (Janz and Becker 1984; Harrison *et al.* 1992; Carpenter 2010). These reviews adopted different strategies in quantifying findings from primary research studies. There is also a substantial literature reporting applications of the HBM to children's behaviour, which we do not discuss below (see, for example, Gochman and Parcel 1982).

In their review, Janz and Becker (1984) employed a vote count procedure (see Cooper 1986: 36). A significance ratio was calculated 'wherein the number of positive and statistically significant findings for an HBM dimension are divided by the total number of studies which reported significance levels for that dimension'. Janz and Becker's significance ratios show the percentage of times each HBM construct was statistically significant in the predicted direction across 46 studies. Across all studies, the significance ratios are very supportive of HBM predictions. Susceptibility was significant in 81% (30/37) of studies, severity in 65% (24/37), benefits in 78% (29/37), and barriers in 89% (25/28). When prospective studies only ($n = 18$) were examined, findings appeared to confirm a predictive role for these health beliefs. The ratios were 82%, 65%, 81%, and 100% for susceptibility, severity, benefits, and barriers based on 17, 17, 16, and 11 studies, respectively. Results show that barriers are the most reliable predictor of behaviour, followed by susceptibility and benefits, and finally severity.

Figure 2.2 presents significance ratios separately for preventive, sick role, and clinic utilization behaviours based in each case on the number of studies examined by Janz and Becker.[1] Across 24 studies of preventive behaviours, barriers were significant predictors in 93% of hypotheses, susceptibility in 86%, benefits in 74%, and severity in 50%. Barriers were also the most frequent predictor in 19 studies of sick role behaviours (92%), with severity second (88%) followed by benefits (80%) and susceptibility (77%). Janz and Becker only included three clinic use studies in their review. Benefits were significant in all studies, susceptibility was significant in two of three, and severity was significant in one of three. Barriers were significant in one of the two studies of clinic use that examined this component. It is interesting to note that while severity has only a moderate effect upon preventive behaviour or clinic utilization, it is the second most powerful predictor of sick role behaviour. Janz and Becker suggest that these differences might be due to respondents' difficulty in conceptualizing this component when they are asymptomatic or when the effects of the health threat are unfamiliar or only occur in the long term.

Janz and Becker's findings appear to provide strong support for the HBM across a range of behaviours, although limitations of the vote count procedure suggest caution in interpreting these results. The significance ratios only reveal how often HBM components were significantly associated with behaviour, not how large the effects of HBM measures were on outcomes (e.g. behaviour). Moreover, significance ratios give equal weighting to findings from studies with

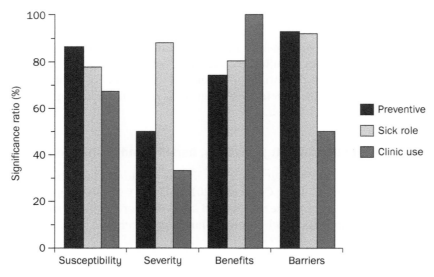

Figure 2.2 Significance ratios for HBM constructs for preventive, sick role and clinic use behaviours (after Janz and Becker 1984)

large and small numbers of participants, and do not differentiate between bivariate relationships between an HBM construct and behaviour and multivariate associations. In addition, Janz and Becker's analysis did not properly control for multiple behavioural outcomes.

Harrison and colleagues' (1992) meta-analytic review of the HBM addressed these methodological issues. Harrison *et al.* originally identified 234 published empirical tests of the HBM. Of these, only 16 studies (6.8%) measured all four major components and included reliability checks. This clearly demonstrates the extent to which operationalizations of the HBM have failed to measure all constructs or provide psychometric tests of measures (see Conner 1993). The meta-analysis involved converting associations between HBM constructs and behaviour measures, in each study, into a common effect size, namely Pearson's *r*. A weighted average of these effect sizes was then computed for each component (see Rosenthal 1984). Figure 2.3 shows that, across all studies, the average correlations between HBM components and behaviour were 0.15, 0.08, 0.13, and 0.21 for susceptibility, severity, benefits, and barriers, respectively. While these correlations are statistically significant they are all small, with individual constructs accounting for between just 0.5% and 4% of the variance in behaviour across studies. Unlike Janz and Becker (1984), Harrison *et al.* found that HBM components had different associations in cross-sectional versus longitudinal designs. Both benefits and barriers had significantly larger effect sizes in prospective than in retrospective studies, whereas in the case of severity, the effect size was significantly larger in retrospective studies.

Updating Harrison and colleagues' work, Carpenter (2010) conducted a meta-analysis of 18 studies in which HBM measures had been used to prospectively predict health behaviours, including 12 studies published after Harrison *et al.* (1992) and involving 2702 respondents. The studies reviewed focused on a range of health behaviours, including screening attendance, dental care, condom use, smoking cessation, and diet and exercise; the predictive period ranged between 2 and 365 days. As can be seen from Table 2.2, apart from perceived susceptibility,

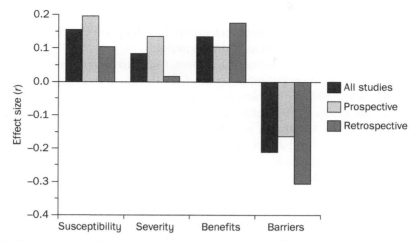

Figure 2.3 Effect sizes for HBM constructs for prospective and retrospective studies (after Harrison *et al.* 1992)

Carpenter found somewhat higher average correlations between health beliefs and measures of behaviour than did Harrison *et al.* (0.05, 0.15, 0.27, and 0.30, respectively), suggesting that associations between benefits and barriers and health-related behaviours may be stronger than indicated by Harrison *et al.* Carpenter also noted that these correlations were higher when the time interval between belief and behavioural measurement was shorter, and that correlations varied across health behaviours. Overall, all three of the reviews considered here confirm a consistent pattern of small, significant correlations between HBM-specified beliefs and measures of health-related behaviours varying across behavioural measures and follow-up periods.

Table 2.2 Average correlations between HBM-specified beliefs and health behaviours

Review	Susceptibility	Severity	Benefits	Barriers
Harrison *et al.* (1992)	0.15	0.08	0.13	0.21
Carpenter (2010)	0.05	0.15	0.27	0.30

3.3 Utility of cues to action and health motivation constructs

Cues to action and health motivation have been relatively neglected in empirical tests of the HBM. Janz and Becker (1984), Harrison *et al.* (1992), and Carpenter (2010) did not include these components in their reviews because of the paucity of studies including these measures. One reason for researchers' failure to measure these components may be the lack of clear construct definitions. Unlike the four key health beliefs included in the HBM, 'cues to action' can include a wide range of experiences and contexts and so have been operationalized differently by different researchers. For example, Grady *et al.* (1983) found significant associations between the numbers of family members with breast and other cancers and participation in a breast self-examination teaching programme. These authors did not, however, refer to these measures as 'cues to action', while an almost identical measure in Keesling and Friedman's (1987) study of skin cancer prevention was categorized as a 'cue to action'.

Physicians' advice or recommendations have been found to be successful cues to action in the contexts of smoking cessation (Weinberger *et al.* 1981; Stacy and Lloyd 1990) and flu vaccination (Cummings *et al.* 1979). Postcard reminders have also been successful (e.g. Larson *et al.* 1982; Norman and Conner 1993), although the effect of other media cues to action is less clear. While Ogionwo (1973) found that a radio, film, and poster campaign was successful in attempts to prevent cholera, Bardsley and Beckman (1988) reported a negative effect of an advert for alcoholism treatment. Mullen *et al.* (1987) found no effect for memory of a mass media campaign upon smoking, while Li *et al.* (2003) found that reported exposure to anti-smoking campaigns on radio, TV, and billboards was not associated with young people's exposure to tobacco smoke. Knowing someone who is HIV positive or has AIDS has not been predictive of behavioural change among gay men (e.g. McCuskar *et al.* 1989; Wolcott *et al.* 1990), and Winfield and Whaley (2002) found that a multi-item scale, including assessment of knowledge of others with HIV/AIDS, previous discussion of HIV/AIDS, and exposure to HIV/AIDS campaigns, was not significantly correlated with condom use among African American college students. Similarly, Umeh and Rogan-Gibson (2001) found that a multi-item cues-to-action scale that included social pressure, recommendations from health care professionals, family experiences, and physical symptoms was not associated with reported breast self-examination. However, Aho (1979b) found that knowing someone who had experienced negative side-effects from influenza vaccination was negatively related to inoculation behaviour. Perhaps unsurprisingly, measures of 'internal' cues to action, namely the presence or intensity of symptoms, have also been generally predictive of behaviour (King 1984; Harris and Lynn 1985; Kelly *et al.* 1987).

Measures of 'health motivation' have generally been single questionnaire items, usually expressing general 'concern' about health, although a few researchers have developed psychometric scales (e.g. Maiman *et al.* 1977; Champion 1984; Umeh and Rogan-Gibson 2001). Bivariate relationships between health motivation and health behaviour are generally small but statistically significant (e.g. Ogionwo 1973; Berkanovich *et al.* 1981; Champion 1984; Casey *et al.* 1985; Ali 2002), with some non-significant exceptions (e.g. Harris and Guten 1979; Rayant and Sheiham 1980; Umeh and Rogan-Gibson 2001). Findings from multivariate analyses are mixed, with some studies finding positive relationships (e.g. Portnoy 1980; Thompson *et al.* 1986; Ali 2002) and others finding no association (e.g. King 1982; Wagner and Curran 1984). Health motivation has also been used as an outcome in predictive studies using the HBM when HBM measures are used to predict intentions (e.g. Petosa and Kirby 1991). Overall, however, the primary challenge in operationalizing 'cues to action' and 'health motivation' either as explanatory measures or intervention targets is that their broad definitions may mean that they can refer to quite different modifiable psychological factors across different populations, behaviour patterns, and contexts.

3.4 Combining HBM components

Failures to operationalize the HBM in its entirety may be partly due to the early suggestion that susceptibility and severity could be combined under a single construct, that is 'threat', and similarly, that benefits and barriers should be subtracted from one another rather than treated as separate constructs (Becker and Maiman 1975). Some researchers have used a threat index rather than measure susceptibility and severity separately (e.g. Kirscht *et al.* 1976). This appears to violate the expectancy-value structure of the HBM and so can be seen as an inferior, and perhaps incorrect, operationalization of the model (see Feather 1982).

While most HBM studies measure benefits and barriers, some researchers have also combined benefits and barriers in a single index (e.g. Oliver and Berger 1979; Gianetti *et al.* 1985). This practice raises theoretical and empirical issues. At a theoretical level, Weinstein (1988) suggests that there is a qualitative difference between benefits and barriers, at least in hazardous situations, which means that they should be treated as distinct constructs. For example, while barriers relating to taking exercise or giving up salt are certain and concrete (e.g. time and effort, loss of pleasure), the benefits in terms of avoiding hypertension are more hypothetical. At an empirical level, the benefits construct may comprise distinct components, namely the efficacy of the behaviour in achieving an outcome (response efficacy) as well as possible psychosocial benefits such as social approval. Similarly, the barriers construct may comprise both physical limitations on performing a behaviour (e.g. expense) and psychological costs associated with its performance (e.g. distress). It is unlikely that a single index could adequately represent these different outcome expectancies. An empirical approach to resolving this issue is to employ factor and reliability analyses to assess whether, and which, benefits and barriers can be legitimately combined, from a psychometric perspective (e.g. Abraham *et al.* 1992).

A separate issue concerns whether susceptibility and severity scores should combine additively or multiplicatively as the HBM's expectancy-value structure would suggest. Rogers and Mewborn (1976) have investigated this issue experimentally from a protection motivation theory perspective. These researchers found no support for the predicted susceptibility × severity interaction (see also Weinstein 1982; Maddux and Rogers 1983; Rogers 1983; Ronis and Harel 1989). In a rare HBM study addressing this question, Lewis (1994) noted that the severity manipulation check in Rogers and Mewborn's study was not successful, so their data did not represent a useful test of the interaction hypothesis. Lewis's data found no support for the interaction hypothesis using parametric and non-parametric statistical tests on retrospective data. However, in a prospective study employing a small sample, the susceptibility × severity interaction contributed a significant proportion of unique variance ($sr^2 = 0.12$, $p < 0.05$). Lewis suggests that the equation

$$\text{threat} = \text{susceptibility} + (\text{susceptibility} \times \text{severity})$$

may better represent the effects of the severity component, at least for some health behaviours, than a simple additive model. Kruglanski and Klar (1985) and Weinstein (1988) concur, suggesting that severity must reach a certain magnitude to figure in health decisions, but once that magnitude has been reached, decisions are based solely on perceived susceptibility. The relatively poor findings for the severity component in quantitative reviews appear to support these interpretations, although further research on this issue is required.

3.5 Utility of HBM components in mediating the impact of past experience or social structural position

In a useful review of literature on the impact of past experience of a behaviour upon its future performance, Sutton (1994) points out that almost all health behaviours are capable of being repeated. Janz and Becker (1984: 44) acknowledge that 'some behaviours (e.g. cigarette smoking, tooth-brushing) have a substantial habitual component obviating any ongoing psychosocial decision-making process', but do not address the question of whether health beliefs might have a role in breaking unhealthy habits. While the issue of whether cognitions mediate the effects of past experience has been a central concern of researchers using the theory of reasoned action (see Bentler and Speckart 1979), few HBM studies measure past behaviour.

Some researchers using HBM have explicitly addressed this mediation hypothesis. In a prospective study, Cummings *et al.* (1979) found both direct and indirect effects for 'past experience with flu shots' upon subsequent inoculation behaviour. Perceived efficacy of vaccination (a benefit) and the behavioural intention construct of the theory of reasoned action (Fishbein and Ajzen 1975) were both partial mediators of the effects of experience. Similarly, Norman and Brain (2005) found that perceived susceptibility and barriers both partially mediated the effects of past behaviour on subsequent breast self-examination. Two studies by Otten and van der Pligt (1992) tested whether perceived susceptibility mediated the relationship between past and future preventive health behaviours. While past behaviour was predictive of susceptibility assessments and a proxy measure of future behaviour (behavioural expectation; Warshaw and Davis 1985), susceptibility was negatively associated with expectation and did not mediate the effects of past behaviour. Otten and van der Pligt's (1992) studies underline the need for further longitudinal research on this issue.

Another important, and neglected, issue concerns the ability of HBM components to mediate the effects of social structural position upon health behaviour. Cummings *et al.* (1979) found that socio-economic status (SES) was not related to health beliefs, although both SES and beliefs were significantly related to inoculation behaviour in bivariate analyses. Orbell *et al.* (1995), on the other hand, found that perceived susceptibility and barriers entirely mediated the effects of social class upon uptake of cervical screening. Direct effects were, however, obtained for both marital status and sexual experience. Salloway *et al.* (1978) obtained both direct and indirect effects of occupational status, sex, and income and an indirect effect of education upon appointment-keeping at an inner-city hypertension clinic (see also Chen and Land 1990; Sullivan *et al.* 2004).

Salloway *et al.* (1978) are critical of Rosenstock's (1974) contention that the HBM may be more applicable to middle-class samples because of their orientation towards the future, deliberate planning, and deferment of immediate gratification. Salloway *et al.* (1978: 113) point out that working-class people 'are subject to real structural barriers and constrained by real differences in social network structure which are not present in middle-class populations'. Further research is needed to determine the impact of SES upon health beliefs and their relationship to behaviour, and to discriminate between the effects of cognitions and the effects of factors such as financial constraints, culture of poverty/network effects, and health system/provider barriers upon the likelihood of health behaviours (Rundall and Wheeler 1979).

4 Developments

Recognizing limitations of the HBM, Rosenstock (1974) suggested that a more comprehensive model of cognitive antecedents could reveal how health beliefs are related to other psychological stages in decision-making and action. King (1982) demonstrated how this might be achieved by 'extending' the HBM in a study of screening for hypertension. She included measures of individuals' causal understanding of high blood pressure derived from 'attribution theory'

(Kelley 1967), which she theorized as determinants of health beliefs, which, in turn, prompted intention formation (Fishbein and Ajzen 1975), a more immediate cognitive antecedent of action. Using a prospective design, King found that eight measures, including intention, could correctly classify 82% of respondents as either attenders or non-attenders. She also reported that four measures (perceived severity, two measures of perceived benefits, and the extent to which respondents identified one or many causes of high blood pressure) accounted for 18% of the variance in behavioural intention, which was the best single predictor of attendance. This study is noteworthy because it combined constructs from a number of theories (attribution theory, the HBM, and the theory of reasoned action) and created a new model that simultaneously explored the cognitive foundations of health beliefs and sketched a mechanism by which they might generate action. King's research is a good example of how pathways between cognition measures may be empirically examined to provide evidence relating to psychological processes rather than static belief strengths and valences. Unfortunately, studies of this kind are rare in HBM research (but see Quine *et al.* 1998; Abraham *et al.* 1999a). This failure to extend the model has distanced it from theoretical advances in social cognition research, and later attempts to situate health beliefs in more comprehensive models of the cognitive antecedents of action have tended to abandon the HBM structure in favour of new conceptual frameworks (e.g. protection motivation theory; Prentice-Dunn and Rogers 1986).

By 1980, work on 'locus of control' by Rotter (1966) and Wallston and Wallston (1982) and, more importantly, 'perceived self-efficacy' by Bandura (1977) had established perceived control as an important determinant of health behaviour. King (1982) included a measure of perceived control derived from attribution theory, which was found to predict attendance. Later, Janz and Becker (1984) also recognized the importance of perceived control but speculated that it might be thought of as a component of perceived barriers rather than an additional theoretical construct. Consequently, the HBM remained unmodified, whereas Ajzen added perceived behavioural control to the theory of reasoned action to re-launch it as the theory of planned behaviour (TPB; Ajzen and Madden 1986; Ajzen 1998). Two years later, Rosenstock *et al.* (1988) acknowledged that Janz and Becker (1984) underestimated the importance of self-efficacy and proposed that it be added to the HBM. Subsequent studies have tested the predictive utility of an extended HBM, including self-efficacy, and generally confirmed that self-efficacy is a useful additional predictor (e.g. Silver Wallace 2002; Wallace 2002; Hay *et al.* 2003; Norman and Brain 2005; Schmiege *et al.* 2007). When floor or ceiling effects are observed, such as when participants are uniformly confident that they can take action, self-efficacy may not provide additional discrimination (e.g. Weitkunat *et al.* 2003) between those who act and those who do not. Often, however, self-efficacy is a useful additional predictor, partly because it reflects individuals' views of the behaviour being predicted rather perceived health risk. For example, Schmiege *et al.* (2007) found that health beliefs about current preventive behaviours, including perceived barriers and self-efficacy, were more powerful predictors of calcium consumption and weight-bearing exercise, at six months follow-up, than beliefs about potential negative health outcomes.

Unfortunately, unlike King (1982), Rosenstock *et al.* (1988) offered no new theoretical formulation for considering self-efficacy. They suggested that self-efficacy could be added to the other HBM constructs without elaboration of the model's theoretical structure. This may have been short-sighted because subsequent research indicated that key HBM constructs have indirect effects on behaviour as a result of their effect on perceived control and intention, which may, therefore, be regarded as more proximal determinants of action (Schwarzer 1992; Abraham *et al.* 1999a). For example, Schmiege *et al.* (2007) found that intention measures entirely mediated the effects of health beliefs on behaviour.

A number of researchers have included HBM-specified health beliefs in more comprehensive models of the cognitive antecedents of action. For example, Schwarzer's (1992) 'health action process approach' combines constructs from the HBM with those from other social cognitive models (see Schwarzer and Luszczynska, Chapter 8 this volume). Susceptibility and severity beliefs are construed as antecedents of outcome expectancies and intention, and intention and self-efficacy are identified as more proximal antecedents of action. Abraham *et al.* (1999a) found that including health beliefs (concerning perceived susceptibility and perceived side-effects) in a TPB model helped identify key cognitive antecedents of the intention to adhere to malaria prophylaxis after returning from a malarious region. Like King, Abraham *et al.* found that specific health beliefs enhanced the prediction of intention and that intention was the strongest predictor of adherence. Intention mediated the effects of most cognitions on behaviour, although among a sample taking a drug known to have serious side-effects, perceived side-effects added to the variance explained in adherence, after controlling for the effects of intention. Jones *et al.* (2001) found that an HBM-derived measure of perceived threat contributed to the prediction of intention to use sunscreen in a model that also included measures of knowledge, norms, importance of short-term negative consequences, and self-efficacy. Such research suggests that health beliefs may be more usefully construed as cognitive antecedents of self-efficacy and intention, rather than direct antecedents of action. However, in certain circumstances, particularly salient beliefs about a procedure or medication (e.g. beliefs about perceived side-effects) may enhance the prediction of behaviour, controlling for the effects of intention and self-efficacy.

Correspondence between social cognition models has been recognized for some time. For example, Kirscht (1983: 287) noted that HBM constructs could be 'mapped onto' the theory of reasoned action. Prompted by efforts to promote HIV-preventive behaviours, leading theorists held a workshop in 1991 to 'identify a finite set of variables to be considered in any behavioural analysis' (Fishbein *et al.* 2001: 3). Theorists included Fishbein (theory of planned behaviour; e.g. Fishbein and Ajzen 1975), Bandura (social cognitive theory and self-efficacy; e.g. Bandura 1977), and Becker (health belief model; e.g. Becker *et al.* 1977a, 1977b). They identified eight core variables important to explaining behaviour and promoting behaviour change. Three variables were regarded as necessary and sufficient prerequisites, namely a strong intention, the necessary skills, and the absence of environmental constraints that prevent the specified actions. In addition, five further antecedents were identified as determinants of intention strength: self-efficacy, the belief that advantages (e.g. benefits) outweigh disadvantages (e.g. costs), the perception of greater social (normative) pressure to perform the behaviour than not to perform the behaviour, the belief that the action is consistent with the person's self-image, and anticipation of a more positive than negative emotional reaction to undertaking the specified action(s). This framework maps the main constructs from the HBM onto the more general attitude and normative constructs included in the theory of reasoned action. Beliefs about the seriousness of a health threat, personal susceptibility to the threat, efficacy of medication, and side-effects of medication are all construed as perceived advantages and disadvantages of action, which are, in turn, determinants of strength of intention. This produces a logical and parsimonious framework that incorporates the two-stage model of decision-making and action inherent in the theory of reasoned action (Fishbein and Ajzen 1975) – that is, intention predicts behaviour and is predicted by a series of other cognitive antecedents. This amalgamation of predictive models is a helpful development for researchers wishing to apply social cognition models. However, researchers should continue to explore and measure health beliefs because research has shown that such beliefs can explain additional variance in intention beyond that engendered by general measures of attitude (e.g. semantic differential measures; Fishbein *et al.* 2001: 11). Overall, however, with some exceptions, it may be prudent to regard many HBM-specified beliefs as antecedents of intention, rather than predictors of behaviour.

5 Operationalization of the model

Below we outline the steps involved in developing an HBM questionnaire. We briefly review available instruments and analyse a study by Champion (1984) in which she developed health belief scales to investigate the frequency of breast self-examination. Determination of reliability and validity of scales is addressed in some depth. Finally, we identify some conceptual difficulties with HBM components and briefly address problems of response bias.

5.1 Developing an HBM questionnaire

Formulating hypotheses or research questions clearly so that they translate into relationships between variables, defining an appropriate sample, gaining access to that sample, and deciding the mode of data collection (e.g. pencil-and-paper test or telephone interview) are generally prerequisites of instrument development. There are two ways to determine the content of the items of the questionnaire. The first is to conduct a literature search for previous HBM studies in the area and determine whether previous instruments are published or available from authors. Scales should be checked to determine whether internal reliability is satisfactory and whether the scale has face validity (respondents believe that the scale measures what it says it does). A scale obtained in this way might be used in its entirety but may require modification if it is to be used with a different sample.

The HBM scales from the Standardized Compliance Questionnaire (Sackett *et al.* 1974) have been modified for use in a variety of settings (e.g. Cerkoney and Hart 1980; Bollin and Hart 1982; Connelly 1984) but this instrument may be difficult to obtain and other scales have also been employed. For example, Calnan (1984) and Hallal (1982) employed measures derived from Stillman's (1977) research on breast cancer. Fincham and Wertheimer (1985) used items derived from Leavitt (1979) in their study of uptake of prescriptions, while Hoogewerf *et al.* (1990) examined compliance with genetic screening using items from Halper *et al.* (1980). There are also published HBM scales in the areas of compliance with hypertension regimens (Abraham and Williams 1991), children's obesity regimens (Maiman *et al.* 1977), breast self-examination (Champion 1984), and other behaviours.

If no appropriate, previously developed HBM measures are available, researchers must develop their own (for a general guide to scale development, see DeVellis 1991). A useful example of this process is provided by Champion's (1984) study of breast self-examination The first step involves generating items that purport to measure HBM components (the item pool). Again, previous HBM studies can be used as a guide. It is good practice, however, for researchers to conduct semi-structured interviews with 20 or 30 potential respondents in order to determine respondents' perceptions of the health threat and beliefs about the behaviour in an open-ended manner. This process will ensure that questionnaire items are salient to the population of interest and will provide guidance on how well respondents will understand medical terminology and other terms. Identification of sample relevant benefits, barriers, and cues to action is likely to provide better behavioural predictors than researcher-imposed conceptualizations. Relevant experts can also be used to develop and select items.

Champion initially developed 20–24 items for each HBM component (excluding cues to action) but then retained only those items that at least six of eight judges (faculty and doctoral students knowledgeable about the HBM) agreed represented the constructs in question. Random presentation of items to judges allowed assessment of the content (or face) validity of each scale – that is, the extent to which the items accurately and adequately reflected the content of HBM constructs.

The next step in developing the instrument is the pilot study. While a small number of studies in the literature report pilots of the instruments employed in the main study (e.g. Eisen *et al.* 1985; Orbell *et al.* 1995), these, unfortunately, are exceptions rather than the rule, and this lack of piloting may help to explain some of the difficulties with previous research using the HBM. Champion's pilot questionnaires included the items judged to have good content validity (10–12 items for each construct) and employed a 5-point Likert scale for responses (where 5 = 'strongly agree' and 1 = 'strongly disagree'). The questionnaires were posted to a convenience sample of women together with a prepaid return envelope. Three hundred and one women participated.

Reliability and validity analyses constitute the final step in determining scale items. When a scale has high reliability, random measurement error is low and the items can be viewed as indices of one underlying construct. Scale reliability can be assessed using Cronbach's alpha coefficient (Cortina 1993) or the Spearman–Brown formula (Rust and Golombok 1990). One can determine error over time by correlating scores on the same scale at different time points, for example, two weeks apart. Champion determined alpha coefficients for each HBM component, dropping items that reduced the reliability of the scale. While coefficients for three constructs exceeded the generally accepted level of 0.70 (susceptibility = 0.78, severity = 0.78, and barriers = 0.76), the reliabilities for benefits and health motivation were weaker (0.62 and 0.61, respectively). Two weeks after the original questionnaires were distributed, these revised scales were sent to a subsample that had agreed to take part in a further study. Correlations were computed between scores on the scales at these two time-points. These test–retest correlations were satisfactory (> 0.70) for four of the five components (susceptibility = 0.86, severity = 0.76, benefits = 0.47, barriers = 0.76, health motivation = 0.81).

The construct validity of the scales (the extent to which scales measure what they are designed to measure) was next determined by factor analysing all of the item scores. This statistical procedure sorts individual items into groupings or factors on the basis of correlations between items. Factor analysis showed that, with one exception, items all loaded on the factors (HBM constructs) they were originally assigned to, demonstrating satisfactory construct validity. Criterion validity was also determined by demonstrating that the HBM measures were significantly related to previous practice of breast self-examination. Table 2.3 presents the items used to measure the susceptibility, severity, benefits and barriers constructs, following the reliability and validity checks.

Table 2.3 Items representing susceptibility, severity, benefits, and barriers components in a study of breast self-examination (Champion 1984)

HBM constructs, items, and reliability

Susceptibility
1. My chances of getting breast cancer are great.
2. My physical health makes it more likely that I will get breast cancer.
3. I feel that my chances of getting breast cancer in the future are good.
4. There is a good possibility that I will get breast cancer.
5. I worry a lot about getting breast cancer.
6. Within the next year I will get breast cancer.

Cronbach's alpha = 0.78

Severity
1. The thought of breast cancer scares me.
2. When I think about breast cancer I feel nauseous.
3. If I had breast cancer, my career would be endangered.
4. When I think about breast cancer, my heart beats faster.
5. Breast cancer would endanger my marriage (or a significant relationship).
6. Breast cancer is a hopeless disease.
7. My feelings about myself would change if I got breast cancer.
8. I am afraid to even think about breast cancer.
9. My financial security would be endangered if I got breast cancer.
10. Problems I would experience from breast cancer would last a long time.
11. If I got breast cancer, it would be more serious than other diseases.
12. If I had breast cancer, my whole life would change.

Cronbach's alpha = 0.70

Benefits
1. Doing self-breast exams prevents future problems for me.
2. I have a lot to gain by doing self-breast exams.
3. Self-breast exams can help me find lumps in my breast.
4. If I do monthly breast exams, I may find a lump before it is discovered by regular health exams.
5. I would not be so anxious about breast cancer if I did monthly exams.

Cronbach's alpha = 0.61

Barriers
1. It is embarrassing for me to do monthly breast exams.
2. In order for me to do monthly breast exams, I have to give up quite a bit.
3. Self-breast exams can be painful.
4. Self-breast exams are time-consuming.
5. My family would make fun of me if I did self-breast exams.
6. The practice of self-breast exams interferes with my activities.
7. Doing self-breast exams would require starting a new habit, which is difficult.
8. I am afraid I would not be able to do self-breast exams.

Cronbach's alpha = 0.76

Although there were some difficulties with Champion's (1984) analyses, this paper provides an example of good practice in the design of a study applying the HBM. Champion rightly contrasts her own study with previous research, pointing out that the validity and reliability of HBM measures has rarely been tested, that multiple-item measures are not routinely employed, that operational definitions vary across studies, and that the use of response options that generate nominal or ordinal (as opposed to interval) data limits statistical exploration of relationships between measures.

5.2 Problems of operationalization: conceptual difficulties with HBM components

Champion (1984) describes regression of a measure of breast self-examination practice on HBM components as evidence for construct validity. We would argue that these data are indicative of criterion validity. There is also some difficulty with interpretation of the factor analysis in that a three-factor solution for the perceived severity component was not pursued. An item relating to having 'relatives and friends with breast cancer' (p. 83) was not interpreted as a cue to action, so this component of the HBM was ignored in Champion's analysis. Finally, further item development on the benefits component should properly have been conducted to improve its poor reliability. Both the methodological problems revealed by consideration of Champion's (1984) paper and the heterogeneity of effect sizes obtained by Harrison *et al.* (1992) and Carpenter (2010) highlight difficulties with the conceptual definition of HBM constructs. A variety of theorists have drawn attention to problematic assumptions inherent in the HBM, including the assumption that HBM constructs are unidimensional and that relationships between HBM constructs and behaviour are fixed and linear. In this sub-section, we briefly review theoretical issues relevant to the conceptualization of each of the HBM constructs.

5.2.1 Susceptibility

Becker and Maiman (1975: 20) acknowledge the wide variety of operationalizations of susceptibility:

> Hochbaum's questions apparently emphasized the concept of perceived *possibility* of contracting the disease; Kegeles' questions were directed at the *probability* of becoming ill; Heinzelmann requested estimates of likelihood of *recurrence*, while Elling *et al.* asked for similar *re-susceptibility* estimates from the mother concerning her child; and Rosenstock introduced '*self-reference*' versus '*reference to men (women) your age*' (as well as 'fixed-alternative' versus 'open-ended' items). [original emphasis]

Tversky and Kahneman (1981) showed that even quite small changes in the wording of risk choices have significant and predictable effects upon responses. Thus, considerable care needs to be taken in the phrasing of items measuring perceived susceptibility, and multi-item measures are essential.

People may employ cognitive heuristics in their susceptibility judgements. Slovic *et al.* (1977) pointed out that, in general, people seem to overestimate the frequency of rare causes of death and underestimate common causes of death. In particular, events that are dramatic or personally relevant, and therefore easy to imagine or recall, tend to be overestimated. There is also a tendency for people to underestimate the extent to which they are personally vulnerable to health and life-threatening problems. Weinstein (1980) has termed this phenomenon 'unrealistic optimism'. This sense of unique invulnerability has been demonstrated in the context of both relative risk comparisons of self to others (e.g. Weinstein 1984) and subjective versus objective risk appraisals (Gerrard and Warner 1991). Cognitive factors, including perceptions of control, egocentric bias, personal experience, and stereotypical beliefs, have been posited as explanations for this tendency, as well as motivational factors, including self-esteem maintenance and defensive coping (see Van der Pligt *et al.* 1993). The impact of these cognitive and motivational processes on risk estimation may help to explain the small effect sizes obtained for associations between perceived susceptibility and health-protective behaviours (Harrison *et al.* 1992).

Weinstein (1988) has also drawn attention to other difficulties with the HBM conceptualization of susceptibility. He suggests that beliefs about susceptibility should be characterized in terms of three stages. The first stage involves the awareness that the health threat exists. The second stage involves determining how dangerous the threat is and how many people are likely to be affected. This is inevitably an ambiguous question and many people will display unrealistic optimism at this stage. Only in the final stage, when the threat has been personalized, will personal susceptibility be acknowledged. This processual account of risk perception implies that susceptibility levels are likely to change over time as populations are influenced by health education and that, consequently, the point at which susceptibility is measured may determine the strength of its association with subsequent health behaviour.

The interpretation of correlations between perceived susceptibility and health behaviour may also be problematic in cross-sectional studies because both positive and negative associations between risk and behaviour are easily interpreted. For example, suppose someone believes he or she is at risk of HIV infection and therefore decides that he or she will use a condom during sex. In this case, high susceptibility leads to safer behaviour and so the correlation is positive. The same person, having adopted consistent condom use, however, may now estimate his or her risk of infection as low. In this case, protective behaviour leads to lowered susceptibility, resulting in a negative correlation. Cross-sectional data do not allow determination of the causal relationships between beliefs and behaviour and vice versa. In a review of this issue, Weinstein and Nicolich (1993: 244) concluded that: 'the correlation between perceived personal risk and simultaneous preventive behaviors should not be used to assess the effects of perceptions on behavior. It is an indicator of risk perception accuracy.' Gerrard *et al.* (1996) supported this conclusion by examining four prospective studies that measured perceived susceptibility to HIV infection and subsequent safer sexual behaviour. They found no evidence that perceived susceptibility predicts behaviour when the effects of past behaviour were controlled. By contrast, they found a small but significant average weighted association ($r_+ = -0.11$) between past risk behaviour and perceived HIV susceptibility across 26 cross-sectional studies. Gerrard *et al.* point out that sexual behaviour is social and complex and that the impact of perceived susceptibility may be reduced for these reasons. Nonetheless, these findings underline the need for longitudinal studies and analyses that control for the effects of past behaviour in modelling the impact of perceived susceptibility (and other cognitions) on future behaviour. Such findings also suggest that, when evaluating the impact of belief-changing interventions, it is important to assess cognitions immediately after risk information has been received – that is, before participants have had an opportunity to change their behaviour.

Finally, individual differences may moderate the relationship between past risk behaviour and perceived susceptibility. For example, Gerrard *et al.* found that this relationship was strongest among older respondents, women (vs. men), gay (vs. straight) men, and college (vs. clinic) samples. Smith *et al.* (1997) found that self-esteem moderated the effect of past behaviour on perceived susceptibility, and Gladis *et al.* (1992) found that although for most participants previous risk behaviour was positively related to perceived susceptibility, this relationship was reversed among pupils classed as 'repressors'. Myers (2000) further highlighted the importance of this personality trait in studies of health beliefs and cognitions. There is also evidence that personality differences moderate the relationship between perceived risk and subsequent behaviour. For example, Hampson *et al.* (2000) found that perceived risk was associated with a reduction in cigarettes smoked indoors but only for those high in conscientiousness.

5.2.2 Severity

Severity has been conceptualized as a multidimensional construct involving both the medical severity of a disease (pain, complications, etc.) and its psychosocial severity (e.g. the extent to which illness might interfere with valued social roles). Unfortunately, as Haefner (1974: 96) noted: 'examining the literature, one becomes aware of the variation in the selection of particular dimensions of seriousness to be studied'. For example, in a study of osteoporosis prevention, Smith Klohn and Rogers (1991) used essays to manipulate three severity dimensions: visibility of disablement (high vs. low), time of onset (near vs. distant future), and rate of onset (gradual vs. sudden). These researchers obtained a significant main effect for visibility and a significant interaction between visibility and time of onset on post-test intention measures. The more visibly disabling descriptions of the effects of osteoporosis were, the stronger were intentions to take preventive action. In addition, low visibility consequences in the distant future were associated with weaker intentions than high visibility consequences with either time of onset. These findings underline the importance of pilot work in identifying salient dimensions of severity, including beliefs about visibility and how quickly consequences are likely to occur.

Ronis and Harel (1989) combined elements of the HBM and subjective expected utility (SEU) theory in a study of breast examination behaviours. Since breast examination leads to early detection and treatment, these researchers divided the severity component into severity following action (severity of breast cancer if treated promptly) and severity following inaction (severity of breast cancer if treated late). They found support for this distinction using confirmatory factor analysis. Path analysis showed that severity dimensions did not directly affect behaviour. Rather, the benefits constructs entirely mediated the effects of severity. This study offered an interesting reconceptualization of the threat component of the HBM. Instead of directly influencing behaviour, threat appraisal is thought to contribute to the subjective utility of taking action versus not taking action. This is reflected in Schwarzer's (1992) health action process approach, in which perceived threat is construed as a determinant of outcome expectancies and intention. Further research comparing direct effects (Janz and Becker 1984), interactions (e.g. Lewis 1994), and mediational (Ronis and Harel 1989) models of severity would be informative.

5.2.3 Benefits, barriers, cues to action, and health motivation

The remaining HBM constructs have also raised problems of multidimensionality in operationalizations of the model. As we have noted, the benefits construct comprises both medical and psychosocial benefits of engaging in health-promoting behaviours. Similarly, the barriers component comprises practical barriers to performing the behaviour (e.g. time, expense, availability, transport, waiting time), as well as psychological costs associated with performing the behaviour (pain, embarrassment, threat to well-being or lifestyle and livelihood). Later HBM formulations (Rosenstock *et al.* 1988) included psychological barriers to performing the behaviour. While self-efficacy has received considerable attention (Bandura 1986, 1997), other specific psychological barriers might include poor understanding of complex recommendations (e.g. by a learning disabled person with diabetes) or a lack of social skills (e.g. to negotiate condom use successfully). Indeed, later work has indicated that social skills prerequisite to interpersonal negotiation may be more important predictors of safer sexual behaviour than the beliefs specified by the HBM (Bandura 1992; Abraham and Sheeran 1993, 1994).

As we have seen, the cues to action construct can encompass a variety of influences upon behaviour, ranging from awareness and memory of mass media campaigns, through leaflets and reminder letters, to perceived descriptive and injunctive normative influence exerted by health care professionals and significant others. Thus the coherence of this construct has been questioned by a number of researchers. For example, Weinstein (1988) argued that the construct does not fit easily alongside the rational expectancy-value structure of the model's major constructs. Mattson (1999) suggested that 'cues to action' could include all persuasive experiences, including interpersonal communication, exposure to mass media, and internal responses to threat. Conceptualized in this way, cues to action are causally prior to beliefs and the effect of cues on beliefs depends on the content of the persuasive communications (e.g. fear appeals vs. self-efficacy enhancing communication). Schwarzer (1992) suggested that actual and perceived cues should be distinguished and that cues to action might be more appropriately construed as antecedents of intention formation and action (once other beliefs were established). Arguably, operationalizations of cues to action could ask respondents about the presence or absence of cues and also ask them to indicate the extent to which cues were available and influenced their decisions (see Bagozzi 1986). Such measures may more closely represent the original conception of 'cues'. The challenge facing researchers is to define this construct so that it can be translated into clearly defined measures that have both theoretical and psychometric coherence or, alternatively, to divide the construct into a series of clearly defined behavioural prompts.

Multi-item measures of health motivation have included a variety of items. For example, Chen and Land's (1986) measure included items relating to control over health and perceived health status, while Umeh and Rogan-Gibson (2001) included measures of past performance of a range of health behaviours. This underlines problems with the discriminant validity of the health motivation construct. If health motivation is to be used as a distinct measure, further research is needed to clarify the relationship between this construct and related constructs, including past behaviour, health locus of control (Wallston and Wallston 1982), health value (Kristiansen 1985), and intention, as specified in the theories of reasoned action and planned behaviour (Fishbein and Ajzen 1975).

5.3 Problems of operationalization: response bias

A final problem, common to all social cognition models, concerns social desirability. Respondents may be aware of the purposes of interviews and questionnaires and so may be motivated to exaggerate both the desirability of their beliefs and behaviours and the consistency between the two. Unfortunately, this issue has received little attention. Prospective studies and objective outcome measures help to reduce bias, and individual difference measures of social desirability may also identify participants most likely to shape their responses to present a socially desirable picture of themselves. Sheeran and Orbell (1995) found that responses to HBM measures may also be subject to bias when questionnaire items are not randomized and can easily be 'read' by respondents.

6 Intervention studies

We have examined the utility of the HBM as a model of modifiable cognitive determinants of health-related behaviour and reviewed studies evaluating its utility as a predictive model of behaviour. This is foundational because accurate prediction is an indicator of veridical explanation. As Sutton (1998: 1317) observed, 'models that do not enable us to predict behaviour are unlikely to be useful as explanatory models'. Explanatory models are useful to behaviour change intervention designers to the extent that they identify modifiable intrapersonal factors that underpin the regulation of behaviours that health care professionals wish to promote or discourage. Thus, if HBM-specified beliefs can be changed and such changes result in changes in health behaviour patterns, such as increasing the prevalence of consistent condom use among sexually active adolescents (e.g. Abraham *et al.* 1992; Abraham and Sheeran 1994; Sheeran *et al.* 1999), then the model provides a useful resource for behaviour change intervention designers.

The HBM specifies a series of potentially modifiable cognitions. Perceived susceptibility and severity represent perceived illness threat, and while these beliefs may be prerequisite to preventive motivation, they may be less strongly associated with behaviour than beliefs about the specific behaviour, such as benefits, barriers, and self-efficacy (Sullivan *et al.* 2004). Other cognition models, such as the theory of planned behaviour (Ajzen 1991, 1998) and the health action process approach (Schwarzer 1992, 2008), have conceptualized all HBM cognitions as determinants of the strength and stability of motivation to change behaviour, with self-efficacy also having effects on the translation of motivation into action. However, the impact of changing any cognition on subsequent behaviour depends on the target audience and the behaviour. For example, even when self-efficacy is a strong correlate of a specified preventive behaviour pattern in a particular population, changing self-efficacy is only likely to promote behaviour change among those with low behaviour-specific self-efficacy beliefs. The selection of cognition targets for intervention design must be group specific.

Once modifiable cognitions are identified, intervention designers need to identify particular change techniques known to effectively change those cognitions (Abraham and Michie 2008). For example, an intervention may use the technique of 'communicating group-specific disease incidence' in order to increase perceived susceptibility. However, even when one or more evidence-based change techniques are identified, many design and implementation choices remain. Disease incidence may be communicated in different ways using different media. Abraham (2012) discusses how health care professionals can use identified change targets and techniques to develop text-based change techniques in paper or electronic media (see also Abraham *et al.* [2002] and Abraham *et al.* [2007] for analyses of how identified change targets have, in practice, been translated into text-based communication in nationally available, European leaflets intended to promote condom use and reduce excessive alcohol use, respectively).

Alternatively, rather than text-based communication, an intervention designer might find evidence suggesting that a drama-based approach to incidence communication would be more effective than a text-based intervention. For example, in the 'handshake transmission activity' (e.g. Stephenson *et al.* 2004), students are instructed to shake hands with other students (or not) and then later asked to stand depending on status. The handshake can represent sexual intercourse and standing can represent being infected with a specific sexually transmitted infection. Some standing students represent initially infected individuals, others those who become infected during the encounter, while those who remain sitting represent those who avoided infection because they used condoms or avoided having sex (by not shaking hands). This mode of delivery is more resource intensive than provision of a text-based leaflet or website but may be more effective in changing perceived susceptibility than other delivery formats. The Intervention Mapping framework (Bartholomew *et al.* 2011) guides intervention designers through such decisions (for a discussion of the contextualization and use of intervention mapping in behaviour change intervention design, evaluation, and implementation, see Denford *et al.* 2015).

It is important to remember that interventions differ across multiple dimensions when attributing differences in effectiveness to particular characteristics of behaviour change interventions. For example, one HBM-based intervention targeting perceived susceptibility may be effective while another, also targeting perceived susceptibility, may be ineffective because the particular change techniques or mode of delivery differ and/or the implementation of the intervention was more or less well suited to the recipients and context. Moreover, de Bruin *et al.* (2010) demonstrated that the content of active control conditions, such as 'usual care', can determine the effectiveness of interventions. If an intervention is compared with optimal usual care as opposed to poor usual care, it is less likely to appear effective. Thus investigation of associations between targeted cognitions and intervention effectiveness can provide helpful guidance to intervention designers (for an insightful illustration, see Albarracín *et al.* 2005). However, all such advice should be considered in the context of the multiple dimensions along which intervention designs and evaluations differ.

Below we consider behaviour change intervention evaluations in which the HBM was identified as the theoretical or 'logic' model identifying potentially modifiable beliefs. Table 2.4 lists 19 HBM-based, behaviour change intervention evaluations that illustrate the diversity of this literature. We have not included intervention evaluations that used knowledge and health beliefs as outcome measures (e.g. Booth *et al.* 1999; Out and Lafreniere 2001; Aoun *et al.* 2002).

Among this small sample of intervention studies, there is evidence of selectivity in the choice of health behaviours targeted for intervention: Some behaviours were targeted several times (e.g. mammogram screening), whereas other behaviours were not targeted at all. Some interventions were derived directly from the HBM (e.g. Carmel *et al.* 1996; Toro-Alfonso *et al.* 2002; Anderson *et al.* 2011), whereas others drew upon HBM and other social cognition models in order to target a broader range of cognitions (e.g. Strecher *et al.* 1994; Lu 2001). Some interventions took the form of educational presentations to groups in classes or workshops (e.g. Ford *et al.* 1996; Abood *et al.* 2003; Shariatjafari *et al.* 2012) and/or involved the distribution of leaflets or booklets (e.g. Carmel *et al.* 1996; Hawe *et al.* 1998), whereas others were delivered at an individual level (referred to variously as 'educational' or 'counselling' interventions) and often involved assessment of the recipient's current beliefs before new information and persuasive arguments were presented (e.g. Cummings *et al.* 1981; Jones *et al.* 1988a, 1988b; Hegel *et al.* 1992; Champion 1994; Anderson *et al.* 2011). Such interventions are tailored to the individual's cognitions. Computer-generated, individually tailored letters have also been used (Strecher *et al.* 1994). All of these interventions relied on information provision and verbal persuasion as means to change HBM-specified beliefs.

Table 2.4 Evaluations of behaviour change interventions based on the HBM

Behaviour	Target group	Investigators/effectiveness	Intervention
Screening behaviours			
Stroke-risk screening	Adults with stroke risk	**Anderson et al. (2011)**	Motivational telephone call
Preventive behaviours			
Smoking cessation	Adult patients	**Strecher et al. (1994)**	Tailored letters
	Women with cardiac risk	Schmitz et al. (1999)	Individual educational programme
Breast self-examination	Female adolescents	**Ludwick and Gaczkowski (2001)**	Teaching with video role model
	Taiwanese beauticians	**Lu (2001)**	Instruction, practice, and follow-up
Mammogram screening	Elderly minority women	**Fox et al. (2001)**	Postal advice on cost
	Women (40–48 years)	**Champion (1994)**	Home interview
	Women (35+ years)	**Champion (1995)**	Home interview
	Women (50–85 years)	**Champion et al. (2003)**	Various (five interventions)
Safer sexual practices	Men who have sex with men	**Toro-Alfonso et al. (2002)**	Workshop
Condom use	Low-cost sex workers	**Ford et al. (1996)**	Outreach group educational programmes
Teenage contraception	Adolescents	Eisen et al. (1992)	HBM-based sex education
Healthy diet	University employees	**Abood et al. (2003)**	Eight-week worksite intervention
	Healthy women	**Shariatjafari et al. (2012)**	Three-session group education and cooking instruction
Sun exposure protection	Elderly kibbutz members	**Carmel et al. (1996)**	Multi-component intervention
Measles vaccination	Parents (pre-vaccination)	**Hawe et al. (1998)**	Modified postal reminder card
Adherence behaviours			
Time in treatment	Alcohol clinic patients	Rees (1986)	Weekly group meeting
Fluid restrictions	Male haemodialysis patients	Hegel et al. (1992)	HBM-based counselling
Keeping appointments	Emergency room patients (11 problems)	**Jones et al. (1988b)**	HBM-promoting interviews

Note: Studies highlighted in bold found evidence of behaviour change following the HBM-based intervention.

Fifteen of these 19 evaluations (79%), highlighted in bold in Table 2.4, found evidence of behaviour change following HBM-based interventions. This is very encouraging, suggesting that HBM-specified cognitions can provide an important basis for behaviour change intervention design. However, because these evaluations were not systematically selected or assessed for methodological rigour, conclusions regarding effectiveness should be examined on a study-by-study basis. For example, some evaluations did not include a control group (e.g. Carmel *et al.* 1996), and weaknesses inherent in before-and-after designs mean that observed changes in such evaluations cannot be confidently assigned to the intervention. Other evaluations employed randomized controlled trials (RCTs) and some investigated moderator effects (see Baron and Kenny 1986). For example, Strecher *et al.* (1994) found that their computer-tailored letters were effective for moderate but not heavy smokers in two studies using random assignment to an intervention or control group. Some evaluations also report intervention effects on hypothesized cognitive mediators (e.g. changes in targeted health beliefs). We will highlight methodological and theoretical issues emerging from this literature by considering four of these 19 intervention evaluations in greater detail.

Ludwick and Gaczkowski (2001) used a pre-/post-test design without a control group to evaluate an HBM-based intervention to increase breast self-examination (BSE) among ninety-three 14- to 18-year-old US teenagers. The intervention was a school-based, multi-stage teaching session delivered by an undergraduate nursing student. Fibrocystic changes and risks of contracting breast cancer were explained to classes in order to increase knowledge of perceived susceptibility and severity. Cards that could be placed in showers were distributed as cues to action. Classes also watched a video that explained breast anatomy, showed teenagers performing BSE, and demonstrated mammography. In addition, classes watched a demonstration of BSE on a breast model and practised BSE on breast models under supervision. The intervention was evaluated by questionnaire one month after the teaching session. Self-reported BSE increased significantly. For example, the proportion that had never performed BSE fell from 64% to 32%. The HBM components were measured using multi-item scales but the authors do not report pre-/post-test comparisons of HBM measures. It is, therefore, unclear whether the observed self-report behaviour change could be explained by changes in the target HBM cognitions. Although the increase in reported BSE initiation is substantial, this evaluation is weak because no control group was included and the follow-up was short-term. Thus, for example, the results do not clarify whether the completion of BSE-related questionnaires on its own might have prompted increased BSE (without the class), or what proportion of these teenagers were still performing BSE at three months or a year post-intervention.

Lu (2001) assessed the effectiveness of a work-site intervention designed to promote BSE among women who scored highly on a measure of perceived barriers to BSE. High scoring women were allocated by place of work to a control group ($n = 40$) or intervention group ($n = 30$). The educational programme was based on the HBM, the theory of reasoned action, and Bandura's (1977) social cognitive theory. A brief description indicates that the intervention included BSE instructions and practice using breast models as well as discussion of individual barriers to BSE performance. In addition, participants received a monthly reminder telephone call. The intervention was evaluated using self-report questionnaires three months later. The HBM constructs were measured using multi-item scales derived from Champion's work (see, for example, Table 2.3). Significant differences between the intervention and control group were found for reported BSE, BSE accuracy, perceived susceptibility, perceived benefits and barriers, perceived competency, perceived normative influence, and intention, but not for perceived seriousness at three-month follow-up. However, these analyses did not control for pre-intervention scores (e.g. using analysis of covariance) and no mediation analysis is reported. Consequently, it is unclear whether differences between the intervention and control group on HBM-specified beliefs accounted for differences in reported BSE. Multiple regression analyses indicated that perceived competency and normative influence were significant predictors of BSE frequency (with perceived competency accounting for 13% of the variance in BSE frequency) but that HBM-specified beliefs did not add to the variance explained in BSE. This implies that HBM-specified beliefs may not be the most important cognitive targets for BSE-promoting interventions.

The intervention evaluations reported by Lu (2001) and Ludwick and Gaczkowski (2001) suggest that educational programmes, including BSE instruction, practice with breast models, and follow-up reminders, are likely to promote BSE (see also Champion 1995). However, more sophisticated intervention evaluation designs, such as RCTs, with longer-term follow-up, are required before conclusions can be reached about evidence-based practice for health educators in this field. Although these interventions were, at least partially, inspired by the HBM, it is unclear whether their apparent effectiveness depended on promotion of HBM-specified beliefs. It is possible, for example, that enhanced self-efficacy, rather than changes in HBM-specified beliefs, is crucial to the effectiveness of such BSE educational programmes.

Champion (1994) reported a more robust evaluation of an intervention designed to promote mammography attendance in women over 35 years. An RCT was used to compare four conditions: a no-intervention control group, an information-giving intervention, an individual counselling intervention designed to change HBM-specified beliefs, and a combined intervention designed both to provide information and change health beliefs. Self-reported adherence to mammography attendance guidelines was assessed for 301 women one year later. Controlling for pre-intervention compliance, the results indicated that only the combination intervention had a significantly greater post-intervention adherence rate than the control group, with this group being almost four times more likely to adhere. Thus, this evaluation establishes that both information provision and belief-change interventions are required to maximize mammography adherence (see also Champion and Huster 1995; Mandelblatt and Yabroff 1999). The belief-change interventions resulted in greater perceived seriousness, greater benefits, and reduced barriers but did not increase perceived susceptibility. However, no mediation analysis was reported and, since knowledge and perceived control were also enhanced, the findings do not demonstrate conclusively that HBM-specified belief changes were critical to intervention effectiveness.

Jones *et al.* (1988b) report an RCT of an intervention designed to persuade patients using hospital emergency services to make and keep follow-up appointments with their own doctor. The sample comprised 842 patients with 11 presenting problems (chest pain, hypertension, asthma, otitis media, diabetes, urinary tract infection, headache, urethritis [men], vaginitis [women], low back pain, and rash) that did not require hospitalization. An intervention for individual patients was developed. This involved assessment of patients' HBM-specified beliefs and delivery of protocol-based, condition-specific educational messages to target beliefs that were not accepted by recipients. The intervention was designed to increase the patients' perceived susceptibility to illness complications, perceived seriousness of the complications, and benefits of a follow-up referral appointment in terms of avoiding further complications. It was delivered by a research nurse during necessary nursing care. Four intervention conditions were tested: (1) a routine care, control group; (2) an individual, nurse-delivered hospital intervention; (3) the hospital intervention combined with a follow-up telephone call; and (4) a follow-up telephone call without the hospital intervention. Only 33% of the control group patients scheduled a follow-up appointment, whereas 76% of the hospital intervention group, 85% of the telephone intervention group, and 85% of the combined intervention group did so. Twenty-four per cent of the control group kept a follow-up appointment compared with 59% in the hospital intervention group, 59% in the telephone intervention group, and 68% in the combination group. Thus, the combination intervention worked most effectively. Jones *et al.* did not conduct a cost-effectiveness analysis but noted that the telephone intervention alone might be the most effective practical intervention when costs such as staff training and staff time are taken into account.

Jones *et al.* (1988b) found that presenting problem had a moderating effect on the impact of the intervention – that is, there were no significant differences between conditions in relation to keeping a follow-up appointment for four of the 11 illness groups (i.e. diabetes, headache, urethritis, and vaginitis). The results of this study were also reported separately for asthmatic patients (Jones *et al.* 1987a), hypertensive patients (Jones *et al.* 1987b), low back pain patients (Jones *et al.* 1988a), urinary tract patients (Jones *et al.* 1991a), and chronic versus acute patients (Jones *et al.* 1991b). Mediation analysis was conducted. The researchers found that among those patients who had scheduled a follow-up appointment, the interventions did not have an effect on keeping an appointment. This suggests that the interventions were effective because they prompted appointment scheduling. The availability of childcare and being older than 30 years also made keeping a scheduled appointment more likely. These mediation and moderation analyses help clarify how the intervention(s) work and for whom. However, the researchers did not report analyses testing whether differences in pre- and post-intervention HBM-specified beliefs could account for the effect of the intervention on scheduling follow-up appointments. Nonetheless, these studies indicate that a HBM-based intervention worked for a variety of patients and that the model of delivery could enhance effectiveness.

These illustrative evaluation studies demonstrate that the HBM has inspired effective behaviour change interventions across a range of health behaviours. However, these studies also highlight six key shortcomings in studies evaluating HBM-inspired interventions. First, some evaluation designs are limited due to the lack of appropriate control groups, lack of randomization to condition, samples that do not support generalization or short-term follow-up. Second, the variety of behaviours targeted and the multidimensionality of HBM constructs means that the nature of persuasive messages may differ across behaviours and thereby undermine the validity of cross-behaviour cognition and technique comparisons. For example, one intervention may attempt to reduce perceived barriers by informing patients of available financial support (e.g. Fox *et al.* 2001), while another attempts to reduce barriers by enhancing communication about risk and precautions in sexual relationships (e.g. Toro-Alfonso *et al.* 2002). The HBM-specified change process is the same (perceived barriers to behaviour change) but the content of the intervention is quite different. Third, the HBM, like other social cognition models, does not describe *how* to change beliefs. It is possible to combine models like the HBM with cognition change theories such as the elaboration likelihood model (ELM; Petty and Cacioppo 1986; for an empirical example, see Quine *et al.* 2001) or cognitive dissonance theory (CDT; Festinger 1957; for an empirical example, see Stone *et al.* 1994) but this approach is not typical of HBM based interventions. Consequently, the selection of change techniques is often not, or not explicitly, theory based. Fourth, interventions usually comprise a variety of change techniques, making it unclear which particular technique (or combinations of techniques) is/are crucial to effectiveness. For example, in considering the BSE-promoting interventions by Ludwick and Gaczkowski (2001) and Lu (2001), we might ask whether practice examination of breast models is crucial to effectiveness or whether reminders are necessary to ensure maintenance. To identify the contribution of specific change techniques, evaluations need to test effects on changing specified cognitions (e.g. perceived barriers) and behaviours of single techniques and combinations of techniques. Fifth, to establish whether an intervention generates behaviour change because it alters target beliefs, it is necessary both to measure cognition and behaviour pre- and post-intervention and to relate the former to the latter including mediation analyses (Baron and Kenny 1986). However, mediation analysis is rarely reported in HBM-based intervention evaluations. Consequently, even when these interventions are effective in changing behaviour, it is unclear whether such effects are due to changes in HBM-specified beliefs. Sixth, once an effective technique is identified, it is important to explore moderating effects such as patient type and mode of delivery to establish for whom (and how) the intervention is most likely to be effective.

To date, only two meta-analyses have been conducted that provide useful insights into the utility of the HBM as a model to inform the design of health behaviour change interventions. Jones *et al.* (2013) conducted a systematic review of evaluations of HBM-based interventions designed to increase adherence to medical regimens as measured by behaviour change. Eighteen intervention evaluations were included. Fourteen targeted adults and 9 targeted patients' adherence behaviours across a range of illnesses including alcoholism, asthma, diabetes, and obstructive sleep apnoea. Sixteen used RCTs to evaluate the intervention with follow-up periods ranging from one to twelve months. Overall, 14 of the 18 studies (77%) reported significant improvements in adherence behaviours following an HBM-based behaviour change intervention. Effect sizes varied from small to large (Cohen's d ranged from 0.2 to 1.0), with six studies (33%) reporting moderate to large effect sizes ($d > 0.5$). As Jones *et al.* note, the HBM was originally developed to guide public health interventions, and all three studies reporting large ($d > 0.8$) significant effects on adherence behaviours were aimed at primary prevention of disease. Moreover, two of these three studies used objective measures of patient attendance. Jones *et al.* noted that the interventions used a variety of behaviour change techniques but were unable to map change techniques onto specific HBM beliefs, or to relate changes in HBM beliefs to changes in adherence behaviour. Jones *et al.* (2013) found that interventions varied in the HBM beliefs that were targeted, with 16 targeting perceived benefits, 15 targeting perceived susceptibility, 14 targeting perceived barriers, 11 targeting perceived severity, 7 targeting cues to action, and 4 targeting self-efficacy. The authors did not include health motivation in their conceptualization of the HBM. Overall, despite the small sample of studies included, this review suggests that HBM-based behaviour change interventions can effectively promote adherence behaviours and, in certain cases, are surprisingly effective (e.g. achieving d values of 0.8 and above).

Meta-analyses of correlational data (e.g. Harrison *et al.* 1992; Carpenter 2010) and meta-analyses focusing on changes in outcome behaviours (e.g. Jones *et al.* 2013) cannot assess the extent to which beliefs specified by the HBM have a causal impact on health-related behaviours (see our fifth shortcoming above). A recent meta-analysis explored this issue by selecting studies that (1) randomly assigned participants to intervention versus control conditions, (2) observed a significant increase in perceived susceptibility or perceived severity due to the intervention, and (3) compared subsequent behaviour for treatment versus control participants (Sheeran *et al.* 2014). Findings showed that interventions that increased perceptions of susceptibility or severity led to significant changes in behaviour in the predicted direction (mean $d = 0.25$ and 0.34, respectively).

There was also evidence that heightening perceptions of *both* susceptibility and severity led to greater changes in behaviour compared with heightening either susceptibility or severity on its own. Interventions that increased perceptions of susceptibility also had larger effects on behaviour when perceived benefits (response efficacy) or self-efficacy were simultaneously enhanced. The largest effect on behaviour was observed when interventions were successful in increasing perceived susceptibility, response efficacy, *and* self-efficacy (average $d = 0.52$). These results indicate that successfully changing beliefs specified by the original HBM and by an extended HBM effectively promote health behaviour change. Overall, then, the HBM, which has been used to guide health behaviour change interventions since 1970 (e.g. Haefner and Kirscht 1970), appears to have considerable potential as a basis for health behaviour change intervention design, despite its relatively poor predictive utility. They key to effectiveness may be identification of predictive beliefs that are missing and amenable to change within particular populations.

7 Future directions

The HBM has provided a useful theoretical framework for the identification of modifiable beliefs predictive of health-related behaviours for more than 50 years (Rosenstock 1974). The model's common-sense constructs are easy for non-psychologists to assimilate and can be readily and inexpensively operationalized in self-report questionnaires. The HBM has focused researchers' and health care professionals' attention on modifiable psychological prerequisites of behaviour and provided a basis for practical interventions across a range of behaviours. Research has, however, predominantly employed cross-sectional correlational designs, and further experimental studies are required to clarify the causal impact of changing beliefs specified by the HBM on a range of health behaviours (e.g. Sheeran *et al.* 2014). The proposed mediation of socio-economic influences on health behaviour by health beliefs also remains unclear. Research identifying which beliefs or cognitions mediate the effects of socio-economic status in relation to particular health behaviours (e.g. Orbell *et al.* 1995) would be especially valuable.

The common-sense, expectancy-value framework of the HBM simplifies health-related representational processes. Further elaboration of HBM constructs, as seen in Weinstein's (1988) precaution adoption process, may therefore be necessary. The model also excludes cognitions that have been shown to be powerful predictors of behaviour. In contrast to the theory of reasoned action, it fails to highlight the importance of intention formation or the influence that others' approval may have upon our behaviour. It portrays individuals as asocial, economic decision-makers and consequently fails to account for behaviour under social and affective control. This is evident in applications to sexual behaviour, where, despite initial optimism, it has failed to distinguish between 'safer' and 'unsafe' behaviour patterns. The model is also limited because it does not articulate hierarchical or temporal relationships between cognitions. Despite King's (1982, 1984) innovative extension, the model has not distinguished between proximal and distal antecedents of behaviour. More recent models, such as the theory of planned behaviour (Ajzen and Madden 1986) and protection motivation theory (Prentice-Dunn and Rogers 1986), propose direct and indirect cognitive influences on behaviour. This facilitates a more powerful analysis of data and a clearer indication of how interventions might exert their effects. For example, if a certain level of perceived severity must be reached before perceived susceptibility becomes dominant in guiding behaviour, this would explain why severity generally has weak associations with behaviour and suggest that this variable should be regarded as a more distal cognitive antecedent (Schwarzer 1992). Intentions and perceived self-efficacy may mediate the effects of health beliefs on behaviour (Cummings *et al.* 1979; Warwick *et al.* 1993), confirming Rosenstock's (1974) suggestion that HBM constructs could be seen as 'the setting for...subsequent responses at other stages in the decision process' leading to action. More recent research has focused upon specifying cognitions that distinguish between people who intend and subsequently undertake behaviours and people with equivalent intentions who do not act (Abraham *et al.* 1999b; Gollwitzer 1999; Sheeran 2002; Sheeran and Abraham 2003). Health beliefs may, therefore, be seen as distant from action facilitation and self-regulation processes. Nonetheless, even if other models specify stronger predictors of behaviour, in certain instances, beliefs about susceptibility, benefits of precautions or treatments or barriers to performing health behaviours may remain potentially important if variability in these beliefs is key to motivation to act.

Further systematic examination of evaluations of HBM-inspired interventions could clarify patterns of effectiveness across this literature. However, given the heterogeneity of evaluation designs, intervention techniques, target behaviours, and populations, it is likely that reviews focusing on interventions designed to change particular behaviours for particular populations will be most informative (e.g. Kelley *et al.* 2001). For example, in a review of 63 interventions designed to increase mammography use, Yabroff and Mandelblatt (1999) found that four theory-based interventions drawing upon the HBM (see Aiken *et al.* 1994a, 1994b; Champion 1994) increased mammography utilization, on average, by an impressive 23% compared with usual care. The review also indicated that theory-based cognitive interventions that did not involve interpersonal interaction (e.g. those distributing letters or videos) were not effective. Meta-analyses of this kind can identify types of intervention and modes of intervention delivery that are effective in changing specified health behaviours. This information could then be used to design experimental studies that isolate particular techniques and combinations of techniques and measure potential mediators, including pre- and post-intervention beliefs. Such findings would permit identification of techniques that are effective in changing certain beliefs that are important to particular health behaviours and allow these techniques to be tested against one another (see, for example, Hegel *et al.* 1992). Much remains to be done but, overall, evaluation studies and meta-analyses highlight the ongoing usefulness of the HBM as a basis for behaviour change intervention design and evaluation.

Note

1. The number of hypotheses examined for each HBM component varies across behaviour types. The relevant numbers for vulnerability, severity, benefits, and barriers in the case of preventive behaviours are 21, 18, 19, and 14 respectively. In the case of sick role behaviours, the numbers of hypotheses are 13, 16, 15, and 12 respectively.

References

Abood, D.A., Black, D.R. and Feral, D. (2003) Smoking cessation in women with cardiac risk: a comparative study of two theoretically based therapies, *Journal of Nutrition Education and Behavior*, 35, 260–7.

Abraham, C. (2012) Mapping change mechanisms and behaviour change techniques: a systematic approach to promoting behaviour change through text, in C. Abraham and M. Kools (eds.) *Writing Health Communication: An Evidence-Based Guide* (pp. 83–98). London: Sage.

Abraham, C. and Michie, S (2008) A taxonomy of behavior change techniques used in interventions, *Health Psychology*, 27, 379–87.

Abraham, C. and Sheeran, P. (1993) In search of a psychology of safer-sex promotion: beyond beliefs and texts, *Health Education Research: Theory and Practice*, 8, 245–54.

Abraham, C. and Sheeran, P. (1994) Modelling and modifying young heterosexuals' HIV-preventive behaviour: a review of theories, findings and educational implications, *Patient Education and Counselling*, 23, 173–86.

Abraham, C. and Sheeran, P. (2003) Implications of goal theories for the theories of reasoned action and planned behaviour, *Current Psychology*, 22, 264–80.

Abraham, C., Clift, S. and Grabowski, P. (1999a) Cognitive predictors of adherence to malaria prophylaxis regimens on return from a malarious region: a prospective study, *Social Science and Medicine*, 48, 1641–54.

Abraham, C., Krahé, B., Dominic, R. and Fritsche, I. (2002) Do health promotion messages target cognitive and behavioural correlates of condom use? A content analysis of safer-sex promotion leaflets in two countries, *British Journal of Health Psychology*, 7, 227–46.

Abraham, C., Sheeran, P., Abrams, D. and Spears, R. (1996) Health beliefs and teenage condom use: a prospective study, *Psychology and Health*, 11, 641–55.

Abraham, C., Sheeran, P., Norman, P., Conner, M., de Vries, N. and Otten, W. (1999b) When good intentions are not enough: modeling post-intention cognitive correlates of condom use, *Journal of Applied Social Psychology*, 29, 2591–612.

Abraham, C., Sheeran, P., Spears, R. and Abrams, D. (1992) Health beliefs and the promotion of HIV-preventive intentions amongst teenagers: a Scottish perspective, *Health Psychology*, 11, 363–70.

Abraham, C., Southby, L., Quandte, S., Krahé, B. and van der Sluijs, W. (2007), What's in a leaflet? Identifying research-based persuasive messages in European alcohol-education leaflets, *Psychology and Health*, 22, 31–60.

Abraham, I.L. and Williams, B.M. (1991) Hypertensive elders' perception and management of their disease: health beliefs or health decisions? *Journal of Applied Gerontology*, 10, 444–54.

Adih, W.H. and Alexander, C.S. (1999) Determinants of condom use to prevent HIV infection among youth in Ghana, *Journal of Adolescent Health*, 24, 63–72.

Aho, W.R. (1979a) Smoking, dieting and exercise: age differences in attitudes and behaviour relevant to selected health belief model variables, *Rhode Island Medical Journal*, 62, 95–102.

Aho, W.R. (1979b) Participation of senior citizens in the Swine Flu inoculation programme: an analysis of health belief model variables in preventive health behaviour, *Journal of Gerontology*, 34, 201–8.

Aiken, L.S., West, S.G., Woodward, C.K. and Reno, R.R. (1994a) Health beliefs and compliance with mammography-screening: recommendations in asymptomatic women, *Health Psychology*, 13, 122–9.

Aiken, L.S., West, S.G., Woodward, C.K., Reno, R.R. and Reynolds, K.D. (1994b) Increasing screening mammography in asymptomatic women: evaluation of a second generation theory-based program, *Health Psychology*, 13, 526–38.

Ajzen, I. (1991) The theory of planned behavior, *Organizational Behavior and Human Decision Processes*, 50, 179–211.

Ajzen, I. (1998) Models of human social behaviour and their application to health psychology, *Psychology and Health*, 13, 735–9.

Ajzen, I. and Madden, T.J. (1986) Prediction of goal-directed behaviour: attitudes, intentions and perceived behavioral control, *Journal of Experimental Social Psychology*, 22, 453–74.

Alagna, S.W. and Reddy, D.M. (1984) Predictors of proficient technique and successful lesion detention in breast self-examination, *Health Psychology*, 3, 113–27.

Albarracín, D., Gillete, J.C., Earl, A.N., Glasman, L.R. and Durantini, M.R. (2005) A test of major assumptions about behavior change: a comprehensive look at the effects of passive and active HIV-prevention interventions since the beginning of the epidemic, *Psychological Bulletin*, 131, 856–97.

Ali, N.S. (2002) Prediction of coronary heart disease preventive behaviors in women: a test of the Health Belief Model, *Women and Health*, 35, 83–96.

Anderson, R.T., Camacho, F., Iaconi, A.I., Tegeler, C.H. and Balkrishnan, R. (2011) Enhancing the effectiveness of community stroke risk screening: a randomised controlled trial, *Journal of Stroke and Cerebrovascular Diseases*, 20, 330–5.

Aoun, S., Donovan, R.J., Johnson, L. and Egger, G. (2002) Preventive care in the context of men's health, *Journal of Health Psychology*, 7, 243–52.

Bagozzi, R.P. (1986) Attitude formation under the theory of reasoned action and a purposeful behaviour reformulation, *British Journal of Social Psychology*, 25, 95–107.

Bandura, A. (1977) Self-efficacy: towards a unifying theory of behavioural change, *Psychological Review*, 84, 191–215.

Bandura, A. (1986) *Social Foundations of Thought and Action*. Englewood Cliffs, NJ: Erlbaum.

Bandura, A. (1992) Exercise of personal agency through the self-efficacy mechanism, in R. Schwarzer (ed.) *Self-Efficacy: Thought Control of Action* (pp. 3–38). Washington, DC: Hemisphere.

Bandura, A. (1997) *Self-Efficacy: The Exercise of Control*. New York: Freeman.

Bardsley, P.E. and Beckman, L.J. (1988) The health belief model and entry into alcoholism treatment, *International Journal of the Addictions*, 23, 19–28.

Baron, R. and Kenny, D.A. (1986) The moderator–mediator variable distinction in social psychological research: conceptual, strategic, and statistical considerations, *Journal of Personality and Social Psychology*, 51, 1173–82.

Bartholomew, L.K., Parcel, G.S., Kok, G., Gottlieb, N.H. and Fernández, M.E. (2011) *Planning Health Promotion Programs: An Intervention Mapping Approach*. San Francisco, CA: Jossey-Bass.

Beck, K.H. (1981) Driving while under the influence of alcohol: relationship to attitudes and beliefs in a college sample, *American Journal of Drug and Alcohol Abuse*, 8, 377–88.

Becker, M.H. and Maiman, L.A. (1975) Sociobehavioural determinants of compliance with health and medical care recommendations, *Medical Care*, 13, 10–24.

Becker, M.H., Drachman, R.H. and Kirscht, J.P. (1972) Predicting mothers' compliance with pediatric medical regimens, *Journal of Pediatrics*, 81, 843–54.

Becker, M.H., Drachman, R.H. and Kirscht, J.P. (1974) A new approach to explaining sick-role behaviour in low income populations, *American Journal of Public Health*, 64, 205–16.

Becker, M.H., Haefner, D.P. and Maiman, L.A. (1977b) The health belief model in the prediction of dietary compliance: a field experiment, *Journal of Health and Social Behaviour*, 18, 348–66.

Becker, M.H., Radius, S.M. and Rosenstock, I.M. (1978) Compliance with a medical regimen for asthma: a test of the health belief model, *Public Health Reports*, 93, 268–77.

Becker, M.H., Haefner D.P., Kasl, S.V., Kirscht, J.P., Maiman, L.A. and Rosenstock, I.M. (1977a) Selected psychosocial models and correlates of individual health-related behaviors, *Medical Care*, 15, 27–46.

Becker, M.H., Kaback, M.M., Rosenstock, I.R. and Ruth, M. (1975) Some influences of public participation in a genetic screening program, *Journal of Community Health*, 1, 3–14.

Bentler, P.M. and Speckart, G. (1979) Models of attitude–behaviour relations, *Psychological Review*, 86, 452–64.

Berkanovich, E., Telesky, C. and Reeder, S. (1981) Structural and social psychological factors on the decision to seek medical care for symptoms, *Medical Care*, 19, 693–709.

Bollin, N.W. and Hart, L.K. (1982) The relationship of health belief motivations, health focus of control and health valuing to dietary compliance of haemodialysis patients, *American Association of Nephrology Nurses and Technicians Journal*, 9, 41–7.

Booth, R.E., Zhang, Y. and Kwiatkowski, C.F. (1999) The challenge of changing drug and sex risk behaviors of runaway and homeless adolescents, *Child Abuse and Neglect*, 23, 1295–306.

Bradley, C., Gamsu, D.S. and Moses, S.L. (1987) The use of diabetes-specific perceived control and health belief measures to predict treatment choice and efficacy in a feasibility study of continuous subcutaneous insulin infusion pumps, *Psychology and Health*, 1, 133–46.

Brownlee-Duffeck, M., Peterson, L. and Simonds, J.F. (1987) The role of health beliefs in the regimen adherence and metabolic control of adolescents and adults with diabetes mellitus, *Journal of Consulting and Clinical Psychology*, 55, 139–44.

Calnan, M. (1984) The health belief model and participation in programmes for the early detection of breast cancer: a comparative analysis, *Social Science and Medicine*, 19, 823–30.

Calnan, M. (1985) An evaluation of the effectiveness of a class teaching breast self-examination, *British Journal of Medical Psychology*, 53, 317–29.

Carmel, S., Shani, E. and Rosenberg, L. (1996) Skin cancer protective behaviors among the elderly: explaining their response to a health education program using the health belief model, *Educational Gerontology*, 22, 651–68.

Carpenter, C.J. (2010) A meta-analysis of the effectiveness of health belief model variables in predicting behaviour, *Health Communication*, 25, 661–9.

Casey, R., Rosen, B., Glowasky, A. and Ludwig, S. (1985) An intervention to improve follow-up of patients with otitis media, *Clinical Pediatrics*, 24, 149–52.

Cerkoney, K.A. and Hart, K.L. (1980) The relationship between the health belief model and compliance of persons with diabetic regimens, *Diabetes Care*, 3, 594–8.

Champion, V.L. (1984) Instrument development for health belief model constructs, *Advances in Nursing Science*, 6, 73–85.

Champion, V.L. (1994) Strategies to increase mammography utilization, *Medical Care*, 32, 118–29.

Champion, V.L. (1995) Results of a nurse-delivered intervention on proficiency and nodule detection with BSE, *Oncology Nursing Forum*, 22, 819–24.

Champion, V. and Huster, G. (1995) Effect of interventions on stage of mammography adoption, *Journal of Behavioral Medicine*, 18, 169–87.

Champion, V., Maraj, M., Hui, S., Perkins, A.J., Tierney, W., Menon, U. *et al.* (2003) Comparison of tailored interventions to increase mammography screening in nonadherent older women, *Preventive Medicine*, 36, 150–8.

Charney, E., Bynum, R., Eldridge, D., Frank, D., MacWhinney, J.B., McNabb, N. *et al.* (1967) How well do patients take oral penicillin? A collaborative study in private practice, *Journal of Pediatrics*, 40, 188–95.

Chen, M. and Land, K.C. (1986) Testing the Health Belief Model: Lisrel analysis of alternative models of causal relationships between health beliefs and preventive dental behaviour, *Social Psychology Quarterly*, 49, 45–60.

Chen, M. and Land, K.C. (1990) Socioeconomic status (SES) and the health belief model: LISREL analysis of unidimensional versus multidimensional formulations, *Journal of Social Behaviour and Personality*, 5, 263–84.

Chen, M. and Tatsuoka, M. (1984) The relationship between American women's preventive dental behaviour and dental health beliefs, *Social Science and Medicine*, 19, 971–8.

Connelly, C.E. (1984) Compliance with outpatient lithium therapy, *Perspectives in Psychiatric Care*, 22, 44–50.

Connelly, C.E., Davenport, Y.B. and Nurnberger, J.I. (1982) Adherence to treatment regimen in a lithium carbonate clinic, *Archives of General Psychiatry*, 39, 585–8.

Conner, M. (1993) Pros and cons of social cognition models in health behaviour, *Health Psychology Update*, 14, 24–30.

Cooper, H.M. (1986) *Integrating Research: A Guide for Literature Reviews*. London: Sage.

Cortina, J.M. (1993) What is coefficient alpha? An examination of theory and applications, *Journal of Applied Psychology*, 78, 98–104.

Cummings, K.M., Becker, M.H. and Kirscht, J.P. (1982) Psychosocial factors affecting adherence to medical regimens in a group of haemodialysis patients, *Medical Care*, 20, 567–79.

Cummings, K.M., Becker, M.H., Kirscht, J.P. and Levin, N.W. (1981) Intervention strategies to promote compliance with medical regimens by ambulatory haemodialysis patients, *Journal of Behavioral Medicine*, 4, 111–27.

Cummings, K.M., Jette, A.M. and Brock, B.M. (1979) Psychological determinants of immunization behaviour in a swine influenza campaign, *Medical Care*, 17, 639–49.

De Bruin, M., Viechtbauer, W., Schaalma, H.P., Kok, H., Abraham, C. and Hospers, H.J. (2010) Standard care impact on effects of highly active antiretroviral therapy adherence interventions: A meta-analysis of randomized controlled trials, *Archives of Internal Medicine*, 170, 240–50.

Denford, S., Abraham, C., Smith, J., Lloyd, J.J., White, M., Tarrant, M. *et al.* (2015) Designing and evaluating behavior change interventions to promote health, in K.J. Reynolds and N.R. Branscombe (eds.) *The Psychology of Change: Life Contexts, Experiences, and Identities*. New York: Psychology Press.

DeVellis, R.F. (1991) *Scale Development: Theory and Applications*. Newbury Park, CA: Sage.

Dorr, N., Krueckeberg, S., Strathman, A. and Wood, M.D. (1999) Psychosocial correlates of voluntary HIV antibody testing in college students, *AIDS Education and Prevention*, 11, 14–27.

Drayton, V.L.C., Montgomery, S.B., Modeste, N.N. and Frye-Anderson, B.A. (2002) The Health Belief Model as a predictor of repeat pregnancies among Jamaican teenage mothers, *International Quarterly of Community Health Education*, 21, 67–81.

Eisen, M., Zellman, G.L. and McAlister, A.L. (1985) A health belief model approach to adolescents fertility control: some pilot program findings, *Health Education Quarterly*, 12, 185–210.

Eisen, M., Zellman, G.L. and McAlister, A.L. (1992) A health belief model–social learning theory approach to adolescents' fertility control: findings from a controlled field trial, *Health Education Quarterly*, 19, 249–62.

Farquharson, L., Noble, L., Barker, C. and Behrens, R.H. (2004) Health beliefs and communication in the travel clinic as predictors to adherence to malaria chemoprophylaxis, *British Journal of Health Psychology*, 9, 201–17.

Feather, N.T. (1982) *Expectations and Actions: Expectancy-value Models in Psychology*. Hillsdale, NJ: Erlbaum.

Festinger, L. (1957) *A Theory of Cognitive Dissonance*. Stanford, CA: Stanford University Press.

Field, A. (2000) *Discovering Statistics: Using SPSS for Windows*. London: Sage.

Fincham, J.E. and Wertheimer, A.L. (1985) Using the health belief model to predict initial drug therapy defaulting, *Journal of Psychology*, 118, 101–5.

Fishbein, M. and Ajzen, I. (1975) *Belief, Attitude, Intention and Behavior: An Introduction to Theory and Research*. Reading, MA: Addison-Wesley.

Fishbein, M., Triandis, H.C., Kanfer, F.H., Becker, M., Middlestadt, S.E. and Eichler, A. (2001) Factors influencing behaviour and behaviour change, in A. Baum, T.A. Revenson and J.E. Singer (eds.) *Handbook of Health Psychology* (pp. 3–17). Mahwah, NJ: Erlbaum.

Ford, K., Wirawan, D.N., Fajans, P., Meliawan, P., MacDonald, K. and Thorpe, L. (1996) Behavioural interventions for reduction of sexually transmitted disease/HIV transmission among female commercial sex workers and clients in Bali, Indonesia, *AIDS*, 10, 213–22.

Fox, S.A., Stein, J.A., Sockloskie, R.J. and Ory, M.G. (2001) Targeted mailed materials and the Medicare beneficiary: increasing mammogram screening among the elderly, *American Journal of Public Health*, 91, 55–61.

Gerrard, M. and Warner, T.D. (1991) Antecedents of pregnancy among women marines, *Journal of the Washington Academy of Sciences*, 80, 1015.

Gerrard, M., Gibbons, F.X. and Bushman, B.J. (1996) Relation between perceived vulnerability to HIV and precautionary sexual behaviour, *Psychological Bulletin*, 119, 390–409.

Gianetti, V.J., Reynolds, J. and Rihen, T. (1985) Factors which differentiate smokers from ex-smokers among cardiovascular patients: a discriminant analysis, *Social Science and Medicine*, 20, 241–5.

Gladis, M.M., Michela, J.L., Walter, H.J. and Vaughan, R.D. (1992) High school students' perceptions of AIDS risk: realistic appraisal or motivated denial? *Health Psychology*, 11, 307–16.

Gochman, D.S. and Parcel, G.S. (eds.) (1982) Children's health beliefs and health behaviours, Special Issue of *Health Education Quarterly*, 9, 104–270.

Gollwitzer, P.M. (1999) Implementation intentions: strong effects of simple plans, *American Psychologist*, 54, 493–503.

Gordis, L., Markowitz, M. and Lilienfeld, A.M. (1969) Why patients don't follow medical advice: a study of children on long-term antistreptococcal prophylaxis, *Journal of Pediatrics*, 75, 957–68.

Gottlieb, N.H. and Baker, J.A. (1986) The relative influence of health beliefs, parental and peer behaviours and exercise program participation on smoking, alcohol use and physical activity, *Social Science and Medicine*, 22, 915–27.

Grady, K.E., Kegeles, S.S., Lund, A.K., Wolk, C.H. and Farber, N.J. (1983) Who volunteers for a breast self-examination program? Evaluating the bases for self-selection, *Health Education Quarterly*, 10, 79–94.

Haefner, D.P. (1974) The health belief model and preventive dental behavior, in M.H. Becker (ed.) *The Health Belief Model and Personal Health Behavior* (pp. 93–105). Thorofare, NJ: Slack.

Haefner, D.P. and Kirscht, J.P. (1970) Motivational and behavioural effects of modifying health beliefs, *Public Health Reports*, 85, 478–84.

Hallal, J.C. (1982) The relationship of health beliefs, health locus of control, and self-concept to the practice of breast self-examination in adult women, *Journal of Nursing Research*, 31, 127–42.

Halper, M., Winawer, S. and Body, R. (1980) Issues of patient compliance, in S. Winawer, D. Schottenfeld and P. Sherlock (eds.) *Colorectal Cancer: Prevention, Epidemiology and Screening* (pp. 299–310). New York: Raven Press.

Hampson, S.E., Andrews, J.A., Barckley, M., Lichenstein, E. and Lee, M.E. (2000) Conscientiousness, perceived risk and risk reduction behaviors: a preliminary study, *Health Psychology*, 19, 496–500.

Harris, D.M. and Guten, S. (1979) Health protective behaviour: an exploratory study, *Journal of Health and Social Behaviour*, 20, 17–29.

Harris, R. and Lynn, M.W. (1985) Health beliefs, compliance and control of diabetes mellitus, *Southern Medical Journal*, 2, 162–6.

Harrison, J.A., Mullen, P.D. and Green, L.W. (1992) A meta-analysis of studies of the health belief model with adults, *Health Education Research*, 7, 107–16.

Hartman, P.E. and Becker, M.H. (1978) Non-compliance with prescribed regimen among chronic haemodialysis patients, *Journal of Dialysis and Transplantation*, 7, 978–86.

Hawe, P., McKenzie, N. and Scurry, R. (1998) Randomised controlled trial of the use of a modified postal reminder card in the uptake of measles vaccination, *Archives of Disease in Childhood*, 79, 136–40.

Hay, J.L., Ford, J.S., Klein, D., Primavera, L.H., Buckley, T.R. Stein, T.R. *et al.* (2003) Adherence to colorectal cancer screening in mammography-adherent older women, *Journal of Behavioral Medicine*, 26, 553–76.

Hegel, M.T., Ayllon, T., Thiel, G. and Oulton, B. (1992) Improving adherence to fluid restrictions in male hemodialysis patients: a comparison of cognitive and behavioural approaches, *Health Psychology*, 11, 324–30.

Heinzelmann, F. (1962) Factors in prophylaxis behaviour in treating rheumatoid fever: an exploratory study, *Journal of Health and Human Behaviour*, 3, 73.

Hershey, J.C., Morton, B.G., Davis, J.R. and Reichgolt, M.J. (1980) Patient compliance with antihypertensive medication, *American Journal of Public Health*, 70, 1081–9.

Hester, N.R. and Macrina, D.M. (1985) The health belief model and the contraceptive behaviour of college women: implications for health education, *Journal of American College Health*, 33, 245–52.

Hochbaum, G.M. (1958) *Public Participation in Medical Screening Programs: A Socio-Psychological Study*. Public Health Service Publication #572. Washington, DC: US Government Printing Office.

Hoogewerf, P.E., Hislop, T.G., Morrison, B.J., Burns, S.D. and Sitzo, R. (1990) Health belief and compliance with screening for faecal occult blood, *Social Science and Medicine*, 30, 721–6.

Janz, N. and Becker, M.H. (1984) The health belief model: a decade later, *Health Education Quarterly*, 11, 1–47.

Jones, C.J., Smith, H. and Llewellyn, C. (2013) Evaluating the effectiveness of health belief model interventions in improving adherence: a systematic review, *Health Psychology Review*, 8, 253–69.

Jones, F., Abraham, C., Harris, P., Schulz, J. and Chrispin, C. (2001) From knowledge to action regulation: modeling the cognitive prerequisites of sunscreen use in Australian and UK samples, *Psychology and Health*, 16, 191–206.

Jones, P.K., Jones, S.L. and Katz, J. (1987a) Improving compliance for asthmatic patients visiting the emergency department using a health belief model intervention, *Journal of Asthma*, 24, 199–206.

Jones, P.K., Jones, S.L. and Katz, J. (1987b) Improving follow-up among hypertensive patients using a health belief model intervention, *Archives of Internal Medicine*, 147, 1557–60.

Jones, S.L., Jones, P.K. and Katz, J. (1988a) Compliance for low-back pain patients in the emergency department: a randomized trail, *Spine*, 13, 553–6.

Jones, S.L., Jones, P.K. and Katz, J. (1988b) Health belief model intervention to increase compliance with emergency department patients, *Medical Care*, 26, 1172–84.

Jones, S.L., Jones, P.K. and Katz, J. (1991a) A randomized trial to improve compliance in urinary tract patients in the emergency department, *Annals of Emergency Medicine*, 19, 16–20.

Jones, S.L., Jones, P.K. and Katz, J. (1991b) Compliance in acute and chronic patients receiving a health belief model intervention in the emergency department, *Social Science and Medicine*, 32, 1183–9.

Keesling, B. and Friedman, H.S. (1987) Psychological factors in sunbathing and sunscreen use, *Health Psychology*, 6, 477–93.

Kegeles, S.S. (1963) Why people seek dental care: a test of a conceptual formulation, *Journal of Health and Human Behaviour*, 4, 166–73.

Kelley, H.H. (1967) Attribution theory in social psychology, in D. Levine (ed.) *Nebraska Symposium on Motivation* (pp. 192–241). Lincoln, NB: University of Nebraska Press.

Kelley, K., Bond, R. and Abraham, C. (2001) Effective approaches to persuading pregnant women to quit smoking: a meta-analysis of intervention evaluation studies, *British Journal of Health Psychology*, 6, 207–28.

Kelly, G.R., Mamon, J.A. and Scott, J.E. (1987) Utility of the health belief model in examining medication compliance among psychiatric outpatients, *Social Science and Medicine*, 25, 1205–11.

King, J.B. (1982) The impact of patients' perceptions of high blood pressure on attendance at screening: an extension of the health belief model, *Social Science and Medicine*, 16, 1079–91.

King, J.B. (1984) Illness attributions and the health belief model, *Health Education Quarterly*, 10, 287–312.

Kirscht, J.P. (1983) Preventive health behaviour: a review of research and issues, *Health Psychology*, 2, 277–301.

Kirscht, J.P. and Rosenstock, I.M. (1977) Patient adherence of antihypertensive medical regimens, *Journal of Community Health*, 3, 115–24.

Kirscht, J.P., Becker, M.H. and Eveland, P. (1976) Psychological and social factors as predictors of medical behaviour, *Journal of Medical Care*, 14, 422–31.

Kirscht, J.P., Becker, M.H., Haefner, D.P. and Maiman, L.A. (1978) Effects of threatening communications and mothers' health beliefs on weight change in obese children, *Journal of Behavioural Medicine*, 1, 147–57.

Kristiansen, C.M. (1985) Value correlates of preventive health behaviour, *Journal of Personality and Social Psychology*, 49, 748–58.

Kruglanski, A.W. and Klar, Y. (1985) Knowing what to do: on the epistemology of actions, in J. Kuhl and J. Beckmann (eds.) *Action Control: From Cognition to Behaviour* (pp. 41–60). Berlin: Springer.

Langlie, J.K. (1977) Social networks, health beliefs and preventive health behaviour, *Journal of Health and Social Behaviour*, 18, 244–60.

Larson, E.B., Bergman, J. and Heidrich, F. (1982) Do postcard reminders improve influenza vaccination compliance? *Journal of Medical Care*, 20, 639–48.

Leavitt, F. (1979) The health belief model and utilization of ambulatory care services, *Social Science and Medicine*, 13, 105–12.

Lewin, R.W. (1951) *Field Theory in Social Science*. New York: Harper.

Lewis, K.S. (1994) An examination of the health belief model when applied to diabetes mellitus. Unpublished doctoral dissertation, University of Sheffield.

Li, C., Unger, J.B., Schuster, D., Rohrbach, L.A., Howard-Pitney, B. and Norman, G. (2003) Youths' exposure to environmental tobacco smoke (ETS): associations with health beliefs and social pressure, *Addictive Behaviors*, 28, 39–53.

Lollis, C.M., Johnson, E.H. and Antoni, M.H. (1997) The efficacy of the health belief model for predicting condom usage and risky sexual practices in university students, *AIDS Education and Prevention*, 9, 551–63.

Lowe, C.S. and Radius, S.M. (1987) Young adults' contraceptive practices: an investigation of influences, *Adolescence*, 22, 291–304.

Lu, Z.J. (2001) Effectiveness of breast self-examination nursing interventions for Taiwanese community target groups, *Journal of Advanced Nursing*, 34, 163–70.

Ludwick, R. and Gaczkowski, T. (2001) Breast self-exams by teenagers: outcome of a teaching program, *Cancer Nursing*, 24, 315–19.

Maddux, J.E. and Rogers, R.W. (1983) Protection motivation and self-efficacy: a revised theory of fear appeals and attitude change, *Journal of Experimental Social Psychology*, 19, 469–79.

Maiman, L.A., Becker, M.H., Kirscht, J.P., Haefner, D.P. and Drachman, R.H. (1977) Scales for measuring health belief model dimensions: a test of predictive value, internal consistency and relationships among beliefs, *Health Education Quarterly*, 4, 215–31.

Mandelblatt, J.S and Yabroff, K.R. (1999) Effectiveness of interventions designed to increase mammography use: a meta-analysis of provider-targeted strategies, *Cancer Epidemiology, Biomarkers and Prevention*, 8, 759–67.

Mattson, M. (1999) Towards a reconceptualization of communication cues to action in the health belief model: HIV test counselling, *Communication Monographs*, 66, 240–65.

McCuskar, J., Stoddard, A.M., Zapka, J.G., Zorn, M. and Mayer, K.H. (1989) Predictors of AIDS-preventive behaviour among homosexually active men: a longitudinal analysis, *AIDS*, 3, 443–8.

Mullen, P.D., Hersey, J.C. and Iversen, D.C. (1987) Health behaviour compared, *Social Science and Medicine*, 24, 973–81.

Myers, L.B. (2000) Identifying repressors: a methodological issue for health psychology, *Psychology and Health*, 15, 205–14.

Nelson, E.C., Stason, W.B. and Neutra, R.R. (1978) Impact of patients' perceptions on compliance with treatment for hypertension, *Journal of Medical Care*, 16, 893–906.

Norman, P. and Brain, K. (2005) An application of the extended health belief model to the prediction of breast self-examination among women with a family history of breast cancer, *British Journal of Health Psychology*, 10, 1–16.

Norman, P. and Conner, M. (1993) The role of social cognition models in predicting attendance at health checks, *Psychology and Health*, 8, 447–62.

Ogionwo, W. (1973) Socio-psychological factors in health behaviour: an experimental study of methods and attitude change, *International Journal of Health Education*, 16 (suppl.), 1–14.

Oliver, R.L. and Berger, P.K. (1979) A path analysis of preventive care decision models, *Journal of Consumer Research*, 6, 113–22.

Orbell, S., Crombie, I. and Johnston, G. (1995) Social cognition and social structure in the prediction of cervical screening uptake, *British Journal of Health Psychology*, 1, 35–50.

Otten, W. and van der Pligt, J. (1992) Risk and behaviour: the mediating role of risk appraisal, *Acta Psychologia*, 80, 325–46.

Out, J.W. and Lafreniere, K. (2001) Baby think it over: using role play to prevent teen pregnancy, *Adolescence*, 36, 571–82.

Owens, R.G., Daly, J., Heron, K. and Lemster, S.J. (1987) Psychological and social characteristics of attenders for breast screening, *Psychology and Health*, 1, 303–13.

Pan, P. and Tantam, D. (1989) Clinical characteristics, health beliefs and compliance with maintenance treatment: a comparison between regular and irregular attenders at a depot clinic, *Acta Psychiatrica Scandinavica*, 79, 564–70.

Penderson, L.L., Wanklin, J.M. and Baskerville, J.C. (1982) Multivariate statistical models for predicting change in smoking behaviour following physician advice to stop smoking, *Journal of Preventive Medicine*, 11, 536–49.

Perkins, D.O. (2002) Predictors of noncompliance in patients with schizophrenia, *Journal of Clinical Psychiatry*, 63, 1121–8.

Petosa, R. and Kirby, J. (1991). Using the health belief model to predict safer sex intentions among adolescents, *Health Education Quarterly*, 18, 463–76.

Petty, R.E. and Cacioppo, J.T. (1986) The elaboration likelihood model of persuasion, in L. Berkowitz (ed.) *Advances in Experimental Social Psychology* (Vol. 19, pp. 123–205). New York: Academic Press.

Portnoy, B. (1980) Effects of a controlled-usage alcohol education program based on the health belief model, *Journal of Drug Education*, 10, 181–95.

Prentice-Dunn, S. and Rogers, R.W. (1986) Protection motivation theory and preventive health: beyond the health belief model, *Health Education Research: Theory and Practice*, 3, 153–61.

Quine, L., Rutter, D.R. and Arnold, L. (1998) Predicting and understanding safety helmet use among schoolboy cyclists: a comparison of the theory of planned behaviour and the health belief model, *Psychology and Health*, 13, 251–69.

Quine, L., Rutter, D.R. and Arnold, L. (2001) Persuading school-age cyclists to use safety helmets: effectiveness of an intervention based on the theory of planned behaviour, *British Journal of Health Psychology*, 6, 327–45.

Rawl, S., Champion, V., Menon, U., Loehrer, P.J., Vance, G.H. and Skinner, C.S. (2001) Validation of scales to measure benefits of and barriers to colorectal cancer screening, *Journal of Psychosocial Oncology*, 19, 47–63.

Rayant, G.A. and Sheiham, A. (1980) An analysis of factors affecting compliance with tooth-cleaning recommendations, *Journal of Clinical Periodontology*, 7, 289–99.

Rees, D.W. (1986) Changing patients' health beliefs to improve compliance with alcohol treatment: a controlled trial, *Journal of Studies on Alcoholism*, 47, 436–9.

Reid, L.D. and Christensen, D.B. (1988) A psychosocial perspective in the explanation of patients' drug-taking behaviour, *Social Science and Medicine*, 27, 277–85.

Rogers, R.W. (1983) Cognitive and physiological processes in fear appeals and attitude change: a revised theory of protection motivation, in J. Cacioppo and R. Petty (eds.) *Social Psychophysiology* (pp. 153–76). New York: Guilford Press.

Rogers, R.W. and Mewborn, C.R. (1976) Fear appeals and attitude change: effects of a threat's noxiousness, probability of occurrence and the efficacy of coping responses, *Journal of Personality and Social Psychology*, 34, 54–61.

Ronis, D.L. and Harel, Y. (1989) Health beliefs and breast examination behaviours: analysis of linear structural relations, *Journal of Psychology and Health*, 3, 259–85.

Rosenstock, I.M. (1966) Why people use health services, *Milbank Memorial Fund Quarterly*, 44, 94–124.

Rosenstock, I.M. (1974) Historical origins of the health belief model, *Health Education Monographs*, 2, 328–335.

Rosenstock, I.M., Strecher, V.J. and Becker, M.H. (1988) Social learning theory and the health belief model, *Health Education Quarterly*, 15, 175–83.

Rosenthal, R. (1984) *Meta-analysis Procedures for Social Research*. Beverly Hills, CA: Sage.

Rotter, J.B. (1966) Generalized expectancies for internal versus external control of reinforcement, *Psychological Monographs*, 80 (whole no. 609), 1–28.

Rundall, T.G. and Wheeler, J.R. (1979) The effect of income on use of preventive care: an evaluation of alternative explanations, *Journal of Health and Social Behaviour*, 20, 397–406.

Rust, J. and Golombok, S. (1990) *Modern Psychometrics*. London: Routledge.

Sackett, D.L., Becker, M.H. and MacPherson, A.S. (1974) *The Standardized Compliance Questionnaire*. Hamilton, Ontario: McMaster University.

Salloway, J.C., Pletcher, W.R. and Collins, J.J. (1978) Sociological and social psychological models of compliance with prescribed regimen: in search of a synthesis, *Sociological Symposium*, 23, 100–21.

Schmiege, S.J., Aiken, L.S., Sander, J.L. and Gerend, M.A. (2007) Osteoporosis prevention among young women: psychological models of calcium consumption and weight bearing exercise, *Health Psychology*, 26, 577–87.

Schmitz, J.M., Spiga, R., Rhoades, H.M., Fuentes, F. and Grabowski, J. (1999) Nutrition education worksite intervention for university staff: application of the health belief model, *Nicotine and Tobacco Research*, 1, 87–94.

Schwarzer, R. (1992) Self-efficacy in the adoption and maintenance of health behaviours: theoretical approaches and a new model, in R. Schwarzer (ed.) *Self-Efficacy: Thought Control of Action* (pp. 217–42). Washington, DC: Hemisphere.

Schwarzer, R. (2008) Modeling health behavior change: how to predict and modify the adoption and maintenance of health behaviors, *Applied Psychology*, 57, 1–29.

Shariatjafari, S., Omidvar, N., Shakibazadeh, E., Majdzadeh, R., Minaei, M. and Gholamzade, M. (2012) Effectiveness of community-based intervention to promote Iran's food-based dietary guidelines. *International Journal of Preventive Medicine*, 4, 249–61.

Sheeran, P. (2002) Intention–behavior relations: a conceptual and empirical review, in W. Stroebe and M. Hewstone (eds.) *European Review of Social Psychology* (Vol. 12, pp. 1–36). Chichester: Wiley.

Sheeran, P. and Abraham, C. (2003) The importance of temporal stability of intention relative to other moderators of the intention–behavior relation, *Personality and Social Psychology Bulletin*, 29, 205–15.

Sheeran, P. and Orbell, S. (1995) How confidently can we infer health beliefs from questionnaire responses? *Psychology and Health*, 11, 273–90.

Sheeran, P., Abraham, C. and Orbell, S. (1999) Psychosocial correlates of condom use: a meta-analysis, *Psychological Bulletin*, 125, 90–132.

Sheeran, P., Harris, P. and Epton, T. (2014) Does heightening risk appraisals change people's intentions and behavior? A meta-analytic review of the experimental evidence, *Psychological Bulletin*, 140, 511–43.

Silver Wallace, L. (2002) Osteoporosis prevention in college women: application of the expanded health belief model, *American Journal of Health Behavior*, 26, 163–72.

Simon, K.J. and Das, A. (1984) An application of the health belief model toward educational diagnosis for VD education, *Health Education Quarterly*, 11, 403–18.

Slovic, P., Fischoff, B. and Lichtenstein, S. (1977) Behavioral decision theory, *Annual Review of Psychology*, 28, 1–39.

Smith, G.E., Gerrard, M. and Gibbons, F.X. (1997) Self-esteem and the relation between risk behaviour and perceptions of vulnerability to unplanned pregnancy in college women, *Health Psychology*, 16, 137–46.

Smith, J.A., Hughes, I.C.T. and Budd, R.J. (1999) Non-compliance with anti-psychotic medication: users' views on advantages and disadvantages, *Journal of Mental Health*, 8, 287–96.

Smith Klohn, L. and Rogers, R.W. (1991) Dimensions of severity of health threat: the persuasive effects of visibility, time of onset and rate of onset on young women's intentions to prevent osteoporosis, *Health Psychology*, 10, 323–9.

Stacy, R.D. and Lloyd, B.H. (1990) An investigation of beliefs about smoking among diabetes patients: information for improving cessation efforts, *Journal of Patient Education and Counselling*, 15, 181–9.

Stephenson, J.M., Strange, V., Forrest, S., Oakley, A., Copas, A., Allen, E. *et al.* (2004) Pupil-led sex education in England (RIPPLE study): cluster-randomised intervention trial, *Lancet*, 364, 338–46.

Stillman, M. (1977) Women's health beliefs about breast cancer and breast self-examination, *Nursing Research*, 26, 121–7.

Stone, J., Aronson, E., Crain, A.L., Winslow, M.P. and Fried, C.B. (1994) Inducing hypocrisy as a means of encouraging young adults to use condoms, *Personality and Social Psychology Bulletin*, 20, 116–28.

Strecher, V.J., Kreuter, M., DenBoer, D.J., Kobrin, S., Hospers, H.J. and Skinner, C.S. (1994) The effects of computer-tailored smoking cessation messages in family practice settings, *Journal of Family Practice*, 39, 262–70.

Sullivan, K., Pasch, L.A., Cornelius, T. and Cirigliano, E. (2004) Predicting participation in premarital prevention programs: the health belief model and social norms, *Family Process*, 43, 175–93.

Sutton, S. (1998) Predicting and explaining intentions and behavior: how well are we doing? *Journal of Applied Social Psychology*, 15, 1317–38.

Sutton, S.R. (1994) The past predicts the future: interpreting behaviour–behaviour relationships in social-psychological models of health behaviours, in D.R. Rutter and L. Quine (eds.) *Social Psychology and Health: European Perspectives* (pp. 71–88). Aldershot: Avebury Press.

Taylor, D.W. (1979) A test of the health belief model in hypertension, in R.B. Haynes, D.W. Taylor and K.L. Sackett (eds.) *Compliance in Health Care* (pp. 103–9). Baltimore, MD: Johns Hopkins University Press.

Thompson, R.S., Michnich, M.E., Gray, J., Friedlander, L. and Gilson, B. (1986) Maximizing compliance with hemoccult screening for colon cancer in clinical practice, *Medical Care*, 24, 904–14.

Toro-Alfonso, J., Varas-Dias, N. and Andujar-Bello, I. (2002) Evaluation of an HIV/AIDS prevention intervention targeting latino gay men and men who have sex with men in Puerto Rico, *AIDS Education and Prevention*, 14, 445–56.

Tversky, A. and Kahneman, D. (1981) The framing of decisions and the psychology of choice, *Science*, 211, 453–8.

Umeh, K. and Rogan-Gibson, J. (2001) Perceptions of threat, benefits, and barriers in breast self-examination amongst young asymptomatic women, *British Journal of Health Psychology*, 6, 361–72.

Van der Pligt, J., Otten, W., Richard, R. and Van der Velde, F. (1993) Perceived risk of AIDS: unrealistic optimism and self-protective action, in J.B. Prio and G.D. Reeder (eds.) *The Social Psychology of HIV Infection* (pp. 39–58). Hillsdale, NJ: Erlbaum.

Volk, J.E. and Koopman, C. (2001) Factors associated with condom use in Kenya: a test of the health belief model, *AIDS Education and Prevention*, 13, 495–508.

Wagner, P.J. and Curran, P. (1984) Health beliefs and physician identified 'worried well', *Health Psychology*, 3, 459–74.

Wallace, L.S. (2002) Osteoporosis prevention in college women: application of the expanded health belief model, *American Journal of Health Behavior*, 26, 163–72.

Wallston, K.A. and Wallston, B.S. (1982) Who is responsible for your health? The construct of health locus of control, in G.S. Sanders and J. Suls (eds.) *The Social Psychology of Health and Illness* (pp. 65–95). Hillsdale, NJ: Erlbaum.

Warshaw, P.R. and Davis, F.D. (1985) Disentangling behavioral intention and behavioral expectation, *Journal of Experimental Social Psychology*, 21, 213–28.

Warwick, P., Terry, D. and Gallois, C. (1993) Extending the theory of reasoned action: the role of health beliefs, in D.J. Terry, C. Gallois and M. McCamish (eds.) *The Theory of Reasoned Action: Its Application to AIDS-Preventive Behaviour* (pp. 117–34). Oxford: Pergamon Press.

Wdowik, M.J., Kendall, P.A., Harris, M.A. and Auld, G. (2001) Expanded health belief model predicts diabetes self-management in college students, *Journal of Nutrition Education*, 33, 17–23.

Weinberger, M., Green, J.Y. and Mandin, J.J. (1981) Health beliefs and smoking behaviour, *American Journal of Public Health*, 71, 1253–5.

Weinstein, N.D. (1980) Unrealistic optimism about future life events, *Journal of Personality and Social Psychology*, 39, 806–20.

Weinstein, N.D. (1982) Unrealistic optimism about susceptibility to health problems, *Journal of Behavioral Medicine*, 5, 441–60.

Weinstein, N.D. (1984) Why it won't happen to me: perceptions of risk factors and illness susceptibility, *Health Psychology*, 3, 431–57.

Weinstein, N.D. (1988) The precaution adoption process, *Health Psychology*, 7, 355–86.

Weinstein, N.D. and Nicolich, M. (1993) Correct and incorrect interpretations of correlations between risk perceptions and risk behaviours, *Health Psychology*, 12, 235–45.

Weitkunat, R., Pottgiesser, C., Meyer, N., Crispin, A., Fischer, R., Schotten, K. *et al.* (2003) Perceived risk of bovine spongiform encephalopathy and dietary behaviour, *Journal of Health Psychology*, 8, 373–81.

Winfield, E.B. and Whaley, A.L. (2002) A comprehensive test of the health belief model in the prediction of condom use among African American college students, *Journal of Black Psychology*, 28, 330–46.

Wolcott, D.L., Sullivan, G. and Klein, D. (1990) Longitudinal change in HIV transmission risk behaviours by gay male physicians, *Journal of Psychosomatics*, 31, 159–67.

Yabroff, K.R. and Mandelblatt, J.S. (1999) Interventions targeted towards patients to increase mammography use, *Cancer Epidemiology, Biomarkers and Prevention*, 8, 749–57.

Chapter 3

Protection motivation theory

Paul Norman, Henk Boer, Erwin R. Seydel and Barbara Mullan

1 General background

Rogers (1975) developed protection motivation theory (PMT) as a framework for understanding the impact of fear appeals. A revision of PMT (Rogers 1983) extended the theory to provide a more general account of the impact of persuasive communications, with an emphasis on the cognitive processes that mediate behaviour change. Subsequent research has typically taken two forms: first, PMT has been used as a framework to develop and evaluate persuasive communications; and second, PMT has been used as a model to predict health behaviour.

The origins of PMT lie in early work on the persuasive impact of fear appeals that focused on the conditions under which fear appeals may influence attitudes and behaviour. Central to this work was whether fear appeals could, in themselves, influence attitudes and behaviour, or whether their effects were more indirect. The Yale Program of Research on Communication and Attitude Change (Hovland *et al.* 1953) provided a systematic study of the ways and conditions under which fear appeals may change attitudes and behaviour. The research was based on the fear-drive model, which proposed that fear acts as a driving force that motivates trial-and-error behaviour. If a communication evokes fear, then the recipient will be motivated to reduce this unpleasant emotional state. If the communication also contains behavioural advice, then following this advice may reduce the threat. If following the behavioural advice leads to a reduction of fear, then the behavioural response will be reinforced and the probability of performing the behaviour in the future is enhanced. However, if following the behavioural advice does not lead to fear reduction, or if the communication does not contain behavioural advice, alternative maladaptive coping responses, such as avoidance or denial, may be used to reduce fear.

The fear-drive model proposed a non-monotonic relationship between fear arousal and the probability of following recommended advice (i.e. acceptance). In particular, Janis (1967) argued that as well as motivating the recipient to find ways to reduce the danger (i.e. facilitation), fear may also lead to a more critical evaluation of the recommended advice (i.e. interference). As fear increases (from nil), facilitation is assumed to increase at a faster rate than interference. However, above a certain (optimal) level, the interfering effects of fear are assumed to increase faster than the facilitating effects. As a result, an inverted U-shaped relationship is predicted between fear arousal and acceptance of a recommended action. However, little evidence has been found for this inverted U-shaped relationship (Leventhal 1970; Rogers and Deckner 1975). Instead, a review of early studies (between 1953 and 1980) concluded that there was stronger evidence for a positive linear relationship (Sutton 1982).

Protection motivation theory was developed to provide conceptual clarity to work on fear appeals. In particular, Rogers (1975) sought to identify the key variables in fear appeals as well as their cognitive mediational effects. Protection motivation theory was based on the work of Hovland *et al.* (1953), who proposed that there are three main stimulus variables in a fear appeal: (1) the magnitude of noxiousness or severity of an event; (2) the probability of the event occurring if no protective behaviour is adopted or existing behaviour modified; and (3) the efficacy of a recommended coping response to reduce or eliminate the noxious event. Rogers (1975) included these variables in the original formulation of PMT and further proposed that each stimulus variable initiates a corresponding cognitive mediational process. Thus, the magnitude of noxiousness of an event initiates perceptions of severity, the probability that the event will occur initiates perceptions of vulnerability, and the availability of an effective coping response initiates perceptions of response efficacy. In other words, the impact of the stimulus variables in a fear appeal is mediated by perceived severity, vulnerability, and response efficacy. These perceptions, in turn, influence protection motivation (i.e. intention to follow the behavioural advice). Protection motivation is seen to be the proximal determinant of protective behaviour, as it 'arouses, sustains, and directs activity' (Rogers 1975: 94).

Rogers (1983) subsequently revised PMT to provide a more general theory of persuasive communication and underlying cognitive mediating processes. In particular, the revised version included a broader range of factors that initiate cognitive processes in addition to persuasive communications. These included observational learning, past experience, and personality. The theory was also expanded to incorporate additional cognitive mediating processes, including perceptions of the rewards of maladaptive responses, self-efficacy, and response costs, organized into two independent cognitive mediating processes: threat appraisal and coping appraisal.

Protection motivation theory has similarities with Leventhal's (1970) parallel response model, which distinguishes between two independent control processes that are initiated by a fear appeal. The first, fear control, focuses on attempts to reduce the emotional threat (e.g. avoidance), while the second, danger control, focuses on attempts to reduce the threatened danger (e.g. following behavioural advice). The parallel response model is important in that it proposes that protection motivation results from danger control processes (i.e. cognitive responses) rather than from fear control processes (i.e. emotional responses). This distinction between fear and danger control processes is also made in the extended parallel process model (Witte 1992), which proposes that attempts to reduce fear by engaging in defensive avoidance and message derogation (i.e. fear control processes) are initiated when the perceived threat is thought to be greater than one's efficacy to reduce the threat. In contrast, when perceived efficacy (i.e. response efficacy and self-efficacy) is greater than perceived threat (i.e. perceived severity and susceptibility), this leads to cognitive and behavioural responses in line with the recommended action to reduce the threat (i.e. danger control processes).

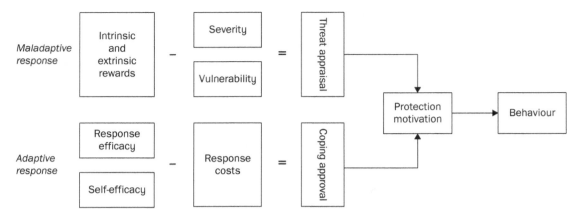

Figure 3.1 A schematic representation of the cognitive mediating processes of protection motivation theory

2 Description of the model

Protection motivation theory outlines the cognitive responses resulting from fear appeals (see Figure 3.1). Rogers (1983) proposed that various environmental (e.g. fear appeals) and intrapersonal (e.g. personality) sources of information can initiate two independent appraisal processes: threat appraisal and coping appraisal.

Threat appraisal focuses on the source of the threat and factors that increase or decrease the probability of maladaptive responses (e.g. avoidance, denial, wishful thinking). Individuals' perceptions of the *severity* of, and their *vulnerability* to, the threat are seen to inhibit maladaptive responses. For example, smokers may consider the seriousness of lung cancer and their chances of developing the disease. Fear is an additional, intervening variable, between perceptions of severity and vulnerability and the level of appraised threat. Thus, greater levels of fear will be aroused if an individual perceives him or herself to be vulnerable to a serious health threat, and this will increase their motivation to engage in protective behaviour. While perceptions of severity and vulnerability serve to inhibit maladaptive responses, there may be a number of *intrinsic* (e.g. pleasure) and *extrinsic* (e.g. social approval) *rewards* that increase the likelihood of maladaptive responses. For example, smokers may believe that smoking helps to regulate weight or that it facilitates social interaction.

Coping appraisal focuses on the coping responses available to the individual to deal with the threat and factors that increase or decrease the probability of an adaptive response, such as following behavioural advice. Both the belief that the recommended behaviour will be effective in reducing the threat (i.e. *response efficacy*) and the belief that one is capable of performing the recommended behaviour (i.e. *self-efficacy*) increase the probability of an adaptive response. For example, smokers may consider the extent to which quitting smoking may reduce their chances of developing lung cancer and whether they are capable of doing so. While perceptions of response efficacy and self-efficacy serve to increase the probability of an adaptive response, there may be a number of *response costs* or barriers (e.g. availability of resources) that inhibit performance of the adaptive behaviour. For example, smokers may believe that quitting smoking may lead to increased craving.

Protection motivation (i.e. intention to perform a recommended behaviour) results from the two appraisal processes, and is a positive function of perceptions of severity, vulnerability, response efficacy, and self-efficacy, and a negative function of perceptions of the rewards associated with maladaptive responses and the response costs of the adaptive behaviour. For protection motivation to be elicited, perceptions of severity and vulnerability should outweigh the rewards associated with maladaptive responses. In addition, perceptions of response efficacy and self-efficacy should outweigh the response costs of the adaptive behaviour. However, most applications of PMT simply consider the additive effects of these variables on protection motivation. Protection motivation, which is typically equated with behavioural intention, is seen to direct and sustain protective behaviour. Protection motivation therefore operates as a mediating variable between the threat and coping appraisal processes and protective behaviour.

In the original version of PMT, perceived severity, vulnerability, and response efficacy were hypothesized to combine in a multiplicative fashion to elicit protection motivation, as it was assumed that protection motivation would not be elicited if the value of any of these three components was zero. Despite the intuitive appeal of such a combinational rule, empirical support has been lacking and, in the revised version, Rogers (1983) proposed a simpler additive model. Most applications of PMT only consider the main effects of perceptions of severity, vulnerability, response efficacy, self-efficacy, and response costs, while the rewards associated with maladaptive responses are rarely considered, as 'the conceptual distinction between the reward value of a risk behaviour and cost of a preventative measure may not be clear' (Abraham *et al.* 1994: 271). For example, the reward of 'increased sexual pleasure' associated with unprotected sex could be rephrased as a response cost associated with condom use (i.e. 'reduced sexual pleasure'). The following review of research on PMT therefore examines the predictive utility of the five main components of the model: perceptions of severity, vulnerability, response efficacy, self-efficacy, and response costs.

3 Summary of research

Tests of PMT have typically taken two forms. First, PMT components are manipulated in persuasive communications and their effects on protection motivation and behaviour evaluated. Second, PMT is used as a model to predict health behaviour. Several narrative reviews of PMT (Rogers and Prentice-Dunn 1997; Conner and Norman 1998; Norman *et al.* 2005; Plotnikoff and Trinh 2010; Bui *et al.* 2013) as well as two meta-analyses (Floyd *et al.* 2000; Milne *et al.* 2000) have been conducted.

3.1 Meta-analyses

Floyd *et al.* (2000) conducted a meta-analysis of 65 studies measuring at least one PMT component and including intention and/or behaviour. Sixteen studies measured one PMT component only, 49 contained multiple PMT components, 27 measured intention only, 22 measured behaviour only, and 16 measured both intention and behaviour. Floyd *et al.* (2000) reported d_+ (sample weighted standardized mean differences) as an estimate of the effect size for each component, where d values of 0.20, 0.50, and 0.80 represent small, medium, and large effect sizes, respectively (Cohen 1992). Significant effects were found for all PMT components (see Table 3.1). The

Table 3.1 Summary of meta-analyses of protection motivation theory

| | Floyd et al. (2000) | Milne et al. (2000) | | |
	Intention and behaviour (d_+)	Intention (r_+)	Concurrent behaviour (r_+)	Future behaviour (r_+)
Severity	0.39***	0.10***	0.10***	0.07
Vulnerability	0.41***	0.16***	0.13***	0.12**
Response efficacy	0.54***	0.29***	0.17***	0.09
Self-efficacy	0.88***	0.33***	0.36***	0.22***
Response costs	−0.52***	−0.34***	−0.32***	−0.25***
Protection motivation	—	—	0.82***	0.40***

Note: Reported coefficients are d_+ = sample weighted standardized mean differences, and r_+ = sample weighted average correlations. **$p < 0.01$, ***$p < 0.001$.

effect sizes for the threat appraisal variables were in the small-to-medium range. In contrast, the effect sizes for the coping appraisal variables were in the medium-to-large range. Self-efficacy had the largest effect size. More detailed analyses were conducted to examine PMT across different behaviours. For example, the threat appraisal variables were found to have similar effect sizes for cessation (i.e. stopping smoking) and initiation behaviours (i.e. beginning breast self-examination). In contrast, the coping appraisal variables were found to have larger effect sizes for cessation behaviours than for initiation behaviours. Floyd *et al.* (2000) also compared the prediction of intention versus behaviour. Both the threat and coping appraisal variables had larger effect sizes when predicting intention than behaviour. Overall, the results suggest that coping appraisal variables, and especially self-efficacy, provide the strongest predictions of protection motivation (i.e. intention) and behaviour.

This pattern of results was, to a large extent, replicated in a more detailed meta-analysis conducted by Milne *et al.* (2000), who employed stricter inclusion criteria so that only empirical applications of PMT to health-related intentions, and concurrent behaviour or future behaviour were included (12 studies containing 13 independent samples). Most studies were concerned with the prediction of intention, while a minority focused on the prediction of behaviour. Milne *et al.* (2000) reported r_+ (sample weighted average correlations) as an estimate of the effect size for each component of PMT in relation to intention, concurrent behaviour, and future behaviour (see Table 3.1), where *r* values of 0.10, 0.30, and 0.50 represent small, medium, and large effect sizes, respectively (Cohen 1992).

Considering the prediction of intention, significant effects were found for all PMT components. Small effect sizes were found for the threat appraisal variables, whereas medium-to-large effect sizes were found for the coping appraisal variables. Response costs had the largest effect size, followed by self-efficacy. Milne *et al.* (2000) also reported *fail-safe N* (FSN) values that indicate the number of null findings that would be required to make a calculated effect non-significant. Interestingly, with the exception of self-efficacy, all the FSN values fell well short of Rosenthal's (1991) tolerance level (of $5k + 10$), suggesting the calculated effects are not robust and that they could be easily reduced to non-significance by unretrieved or future null results.

Results were similar for the prediction of concurrent behaviour. Again, all effects were significant, with small effect sizes for the threat appraisal variables and small-to-medium effect sizes for the coping appraisal variables. Self-efficacy had the largest effect size and was the only variable close to Rosenthal's (1991) tolerance level. In addition, the effect size for the correlation between protection motivation and concurrent behaviour was large and robust. Finally, a small number of studies examined the relationship between PMT and future behaviour. Only perceived vulnerability, self-efficacy, response costs, and protection motivation had significant effects, although these were somewhat attenuated compared with the effect sizes calculated for the prediction of intention and concurrent behaviour. Only the correlation between protection motivation and future behaviour approached robustness; however, the fact that the FSN values fell short of Rosenthal's (1991) tolerance level is most likely a consequence of the modest number of prospective PMT studies.

Overall, the results of these meta-analyses indicate that the coping appraisal variables provide stronger predictions of protection motivation and behaviour than do threat appraisal variables. The threat appraisal variables typically had small effect sizes, whereas the coping appraisal variables typically had medium effect sizes. In addition, protection motivation is typically a strong predictor of concurrent and, to a lesser extent, future behaviour. However, many of the relationships, while significant, were not robust, indicating the need for further replication. In addition, it is notable that the PMT variables are stronger predictors of intention than of future behaviour and that protection motivation is typically the strongest correlate of future behaviour. Such a pattern of results is consistent with the idea that protection motivation mediates the effects of threat and coping appraisals on behaviour.

These meta-analyses were based on the results of studies employing a wide range of methodologies. In particular, they included both experimental studies, in which the PMT components were manipulated and their effects evaluated, and correlational studies, in which PMT was used as a social cognition model to predict health behaviour. As a result, it is difficult to tease apart the predictive power of PMT as a social cognition model of health behaviour versus its utility as a framework for developing and evaluating interventions. The following narrative review of PMT studies therefore focuses solely on its use as a social cognition model to predict health behaviour (see Table 3.2 for example studies). Studies that have manipulated components of PMT are considered in Section 7.

3.2 Exercise

Protection motivation theory has been most frequently applied to the prediction of exercise intentions and behaviour. Considering studies using non-medical samples (e.g. community samples, students, older adults) (Plotnikoff and Higginbotham 2002; Norman *et al.* 2005; Leas and McCabe 2007; Yardley *et al.* 2007; Plotnikoff *et al.* 2009a; Tavares *et al.* 2009), regression and path analyses indicate that PMT explains between 25% and 53% of the variance in exercise intentions, with self-efficacy and, to a lesser extent, response efficacy emerging as the most consistent predictors. Protection motivation theory has been found to explain between 20% and 40% of the variance in exercise behaviour, with intention and self-efficacy emerging as the strongest predictors. These findings are mirrored in applications of PMT to the prediction of exercise intentions and behaviour in medical samples (e.g. cardiac, diabetes) (Plotnikoff and Higginbotham 1998; Blanchard *et al.* 2009; Plotnikoff *et al.* 2009b, 2010; Tulloch *et al.* 2009), although some

Table 3.2 Examples of studies applying protection motivation theory to predict health behaviour

Behaviour	References
Exercise	Plotnikoff and Higginbotham (1998, 2002), Norman *et al.* (2005), Leas and McCabe (2007), Yardley *et al.* (2007), Blanchard *et al.* (2009), Plotnikoff *et al.* (2009a, 2009b, 2010), Tavares *et al.* (2009), Tulloch *et al.* (2009)
Diet	Plotnikoff and Higginbotham (1995, 1998), Cox *et al.* (2004), Leas and McCabe (2007), Henson *et al.* (2010), Calder *et al.* (2011)
Smoking	Greening (1997), Ho (1998), Wright *et al.* (2006), Leas and McCabe (2007), Smerecnik *et al.* (2011), MacDonell *et al.* (2013), Thrul *et al.* (2013), Yan *et al.* (2014)
Alcohol	Ben-Ahron *et al.* (1995), Murgraff *et al.* (1999)
Safe sex	Aspinwall *et al.* (1991), Van der Velde and Van der Pligt (1991), Bakker *et al.* (1993), Abraham *et al.* (1994), Eppright *et al.* (1994), Bengel *et al.* (1996), Sheeran and Orbell (1996), Ho (2000), Greening *et al.* (2001), Li *et al.* (2004), Umeh (2004), Boer and Mashamba (2005, 2007), Yu *et al.* (2008), Lwin *et al.* (2010), Regan and Morisky (2013)
Cancer prevention	Seydel *et al.* (1990), Boer and Seydel (1996), Hodgkins and Orbell (1998), Orbell and Sheeran (1998), Grunfeld (2004), Azzarello *et al.* (2006), Naito *et al.* (2009), Inukai and Ninomiya (2010), Gu *et al.* (2012, 2013), Ch'ng and Glendon (2014), Hassani *et al.* (2014)
Medical adherence	Flynn *et al.* (1995), Taylor and May (1996), Bennett *et al.* (1998), Palardy *et al.* (1998), Rudman *et al.* (1999), Norman *et al.* (2003), Grindley *et al.* (2008), Levy *et al.* (2008), Beirens *et al.* (2010), Bassett and Prapavessis (2011)

effects are weaker. Protection motivation theory has been found to explain 23–53% of the variance in exercise intentions and 9–32% of the variance in exercise behaviour in patient samples. Self-efficacy and response efficacy are the most consistent predictors of exercise intentions, whereas intention and self-efficacy are the strongest predictors of exercise behaviour.

Tulloch *et al.* (2009), for example, applied PMT to the prediction of exercise intentions and behaviour at two, six, and 12 months following hospitalization for coronary heart disease. Using structural equation modelling, PMT was found to have good predictive utility for short-term, but not long-term, behaviour. Specifically, after controlling for age, gender, cardiac rehabilitation participation, and previous exercise levels, baseline PMT measures explained 23% of the variance in intentions at two months, with perceived severity, response efficacy, and self-efficacy emerging as significant predictors. Furthermore, intentions at two months and baseline self-efficacy were predictive of exercise behaviour at six months, with the PMT variables explaining 20% of the variance in behaviour. However, PMT failed to provide a good fit to the data when explaining behaviour at 12 months.

Despite some encouraging findings, applications of PMT to the prediction of exercise have suffered from three important methodological limitations. First, although many studies have included follow-up assessment of behaviour at six months (e.g. Blanchard *et al.* 2009; Taveres *et al.* 2009; Plotnikoff *et al.* 2010) and 12 months (e.g. Tulloch *et al.* 2009; Plotnikoff *et al.* 2010), others (Plotnikoff and Higginbotham 1998, 2002; Leas and McCabe 2007; Yardley *et al.* 2007) have employed cross-sectional designs. Second, some studies (Plotnikoff and Higginbotham 1998, 2002; Plotnikoff *et al.*, 2009a) have assessed exercise behaviour using a stage-based measure that may be confounded with intention (Sutton 2005). Third, few studies (Norman *et al.*

2005; Leas and McCabe 2007) have assessed response costs. Norman *et al.* (2005) reported that response costs had large correlations with both exercise intention and behaviour, although it was not significant in the multivariate analyses.

3.3 Dietary behaviour

Studies applying PMT to explain dietary intentions and behaviour in relation to eating a low-fat diet (Plotnikoff and Higginbotham 1995, 1998; Leas and McCabe 2007) have explained 46–55% of the variance in intentions and 27–39% of the variance in behaviour. For example, Plotnikoff and Higginbotham (1995) recruited samples in Australia from communities with high incidences of cardiovascular disease. Path analysis revealed that self-efficacy and response efficacy were predictive of intention to follow a low-fat diet. In turn, intention and self-efficacy were predictive of behaviour. In a subsequent study with a sample of cardiac patients, Plotnikoff and Higginbotham (1998) reported that self-efficacy was the sole predictor of intention, while intention, perceived vulnerability, and fear were predictive of dietary behaviour. Leas and McCabe (2007) recruited respondents without and with a mental illness (e.g. schizophrenia, depression) and examined associations between PMT and the consumption of low-fat foods. Self-efficacy was predictive of intention in both groups, along with response efficacy in those without a mental illness and perceived severity in those with a mental illness. Intention, in turn, was predictive of behaviour in both groups, with self-efficacy also predictive of behaviour in those without a mental illness.

The above studies suffered from three limitations. First, all three studies employed cross-sectional designs, meaning that only concurrent associations with dietary behaviour were examined. Second, Plotnikoff and Higginbotham (1995, 1998) employed a stage-based measure of behaviour. Third, only Leas and McCabe (2007) included a measure of response costs, although it was not a significant predictor in the regression analyses (bivariate correlations with intention and behaviour were not reported).

A number of studies have used PMT to examine intentions to consume foods and dietary supplements as a means of reducing future health risks (Cox *et al.* 2004; Henson *et al.* 2010; Calder *et al.* 2011). For example, Cox *et al.* (2004) examined intentions to consume four different foods or supplements to offset memory loss in middle-aged adults. Protection motivation theory explained 59–63% of the variance in intentions with perceived severity, response efficacy, and self-efficacy predictive of all four foods/supplements, whereas perceived vulnerability was only predictive of two. Similarly, Henson *et al.* (2010) found that PMT explained 76% of the variance in intentions to purchase foods and dietary supplements containing phytosterols in order to reduce the risk of coronary vascular disease, with coping appraisals, but not threat appraisals, predictive of purchasing intentions.

3.4 Smoking

A number of studies have applied PMT to the prediction of smoking intentions and behaviour in adolescent samples (Greening 1997; MacDonell *et al.* 2013; Thrul *et al.* 2013; Yan *et al.* 2014). For example, Yan *et al.* (2014) recruited a sample of more than 500 adolescents from secondary schools in China. The study used a previously developed scale to assess all of the PMT constructs, including measures of the intrinsic and extrinsic rewards of smoking (MacDonell *et al.* 2013). Protection motivation theory explained 19% of the variance in intentions to smoke, with perceived severity and intrinsic rewards emerging as significant predictors, and 31% of the variance in smoking behaviour over the previous 30 days, with intrinsic and extrinsic rewards and self-efficacy emerging as significant predictors. In a similar study, Thrul *et al.* (2013) assessed all of the PMT constructs (although the rewards measure was unreliable and not used in analyses) in a sample of 494 adolescents recruited from secondary schools in Germany and followed up at 10 weeks. Only self-efficacy was a significant predictor of baseline intention, which was the only significant predictor of intention at follow-up, which in turn was the only significant predictor of smoking behaviour at follow-up. Protection motivation theory explained 44%, 9%, and 14% of the variance in baseline intention, follow-up intention, and follow-up behaviour, respectively. Finally, Greening (1997) reported that PMT was predictive of concurrent smoking behaviour in a sample of adolescents in the USA. Smokers were more likely to downplay the health risks associated with smoking (i.e. perceived severity) and the response efficacy of not smoking, although they were also more likely to acknowledge greater personal vulnerability to smoking-related diseases.

Some studies have applied PMT to the prediction of smoking cessation intentions, explaining between 23% and 40% of the variance (Ho 1998; Leas and McCabe 2007). Ho (1998) found that only self-efficacy was a significant predictor of intentions to quit in young (aged ≤ 22 years) and older (aged ≥ 34 years) smokers, whereas Leas and McCabe (2007) found that both response efficacy and self-efficacy were significant predictors of intentions to quit in a sample of smokers with a mental illness.

Protection motivation theory has also been used to explore smokers' interest in, and the potential impact of, genetic testing (Wright *et al.* 2006; Smerecnik *et al.* 2011). Smerecnik *et al.* (2011) examined smokers' interest in genetic testing for nicotine susceptibility and their initial information-seeking behaviour. Protection motivation theory explained 74% of the variance in intentions and 33% of the variance in initial information-seeking behaviour. Both threat (perceived severity, perceived vulnerability) and coping appraisals (response efficacy, self-efficacy) were predictive of genetic testing intentions, which, in turn, were predictive of initial information-seeking behaviour. Wright *et al.* (2006) conducted an analogue study to examine the potential impact of genetic testing on smoking cessation intentions. Smokers were presented with one of three vignettes: a positive or negative result for a genetic test for susceptibility to heart disease, or standard smoking risk information. Participants then completed PMT measures. The results indicated that those who read the gene-positive vignette had stronger smoking cessation intentions, as did those with higher levels of self-efficacy.

Overall, PMT has been found to provide a useful theoretical framework for predicting smoking intentions and behaviour. Compared with other health behaviours, both threat appraisal (including rewards of the maladaptive behaviour) and coping appraisal variables have been found to be predictive, although self-efficacy is the strongest predictor. A notable strength of applications of the PMT in this area is the inclusion of measures of intrinsic and extrinsic rewards of smoking, which have been found to correlate with intentions (Yan *et al.* 2014) and behaviour (Greening 1997; Yan *et al.* 2014). However, there is a clear need for prospective studies to assess the ability of PMT to predict smoking cessation over extended follow-up periods (i.e. at least six months).

3.5 Alcohol

Few studies have applied PMT to the prediction of alcohol-related behaviour. Murgraff *et al.* (1999) used PMT to explain students' binge drinking behaviour. The PMT variables and past behaviour explained 31% of the variance in intention, with perceived severity, rewards of binge drinking, self-efficacy, and past behaviour emerging as significant predictors (although the significant result for perceived severity may have been due to a suppressor effect). Past behaviour was the only significant predictor of high-risk drinking behaviour at two-week follow-up, although the inclusion of past behaviour in the regression analysis may have masked the influence of the PMT variables. In an earlier cross-sectional study, Ben-Ahron *et al.* (1995) examined the ability of PMT to discriminate between students classified as binge and non-binge drinkers. All PMT constructs, except response efficacy (of drinking within safe daily limits), were found to discriminate between binge and non-binge drinkers, although a negative relationship was found for perceived severity. These two studies are noteworthy because they contained measures of the intrinsic and extrinsic rewards associated with binge drinking in addition to measures of other PMT constructs (including response costs). However, more research is needed on the use of PMT to predict alcohol-related behaviour despite these initial encouraging findings.

3.6 Safe sex

Protection motivation theory has been frequently applied to the prediction of sexual risk intentions and behaviour, although there are few prospective applications of the model. Aspinwall *et al.* (1991) examined the predictive utility of PMT in relation to a number of AIDS-risk reducing behaviours in gay men in the USA. After controlling for demographics, baseline behaviour, HIV status, and partner status, self-efficacy and perceived vulnerability were found to be predictive of reductions in the number of sexual partners at six-month follow-up. Self-efficacy was also predictive of reductions in the number of anonymous sexual partners, and response costs (i.e. barriers to change) were predictive of unprotected anal receptive intercourse over the same time period. Greening *et al.* (2001) examined the predictive utility of PMT over a one-year period in a sample of sexually active rural African-American female adolescents. Protection motivation theory was predictive of condom use at one-year follow-up, although only self-efficacy emerged as a significant predictor after controlling for baseline condom use. Contrary to predictions, low levels of self-efficacy were predictive of condom use. However, there was a lack of correspondence between the measure of self-efficacy (for preventing a pregnancy and using contraceptives) and the dependent variable (i.e. condom use); the study did not report the simple bivariate correlation between self-efficacy and condom use; the small sample size ($N = 61$) is likely to have resulted in the regression analysis being under-powered; and the negative relationship between self-efficacy and condom use found in the regression analysis may have been the result of a suppressor effect, given the strong effect observed for past behaviour.

Protection motivation theory has also been applied to sexual risk behaviour in studies using cross-sectional designs. Bengel *et al.* (1996) reported that response efficacy and self-efficacy were significant predictors of safer sex behaviour, and perceived vulnerability and self-efficacy were predictive of more frequent condom use. Similarly, Eppright *et al.* (1994) found that perceived vulnerability was positively related to the performance of both adaptive (i.e. being abstinent, avoiding sharing bodily fluids, using condoms) and maladaptive (i.e. reducing partners, being careful about selecting infection-free partners) behaviours in a student sample. The coping appraisal variables they considered (i.e. response efficacy, self-efficacy) were non-significant predictors, although it should be noted that there was a lack of correspondence between these measures and the dependent variables. More recently, Li *et al.* (2004) reported that all PMT constructs were predictive of level of sexual risk behaviour in a sample of rural-to-urban migrants in China, whereas Regan and Morisky (2013) reported that only perceived severity and response efficacy were predictive of consistent condom use in a sample of male clients of female sex workers in the Philippines.

Other PMT studies have focused solely on the prediction of intentions to use condoms (Van der Velde and Van der Pligt 1991; Bakker *et al.* 1993; Abraham *et al.* 1994; Sheeran and Orbell 1996; Ho 2000; Umeh 2004; Boer and Mashamba 2005, 2007; Yu *et al.* 2008; Lwin *et al.* 2010). For example, Van der Velde and Van der Pligt (1991) examined the condom use intentions of a sample heterosexual men and women and homosexual men with multiple partners. In the heterosexual sample, perceived vulnerability, response efficacy, and self-efficacy were all found to have direct positive effects on condom use intentions. In addition, perceived severity had an indirect effect on condom use intentions via fear. Similar results were found among the homosexual sample, with perceived severity, response efficacy, and self-efficacy having positive direct effects on safe sex intentions, although a negative relationship was found between perceived vulnerability and safe sex intentions. Boer and Mashamba (2005) applied PMT to explain the condom use intentions of black adolescents in South Africa. After controlling for age and gender, response efficacy was the only significant PMT predictor. Similar results have been reported in a subsequent study with black university students in South Africa (Boer and Mashamba 2007), which found that only response efficacy was predictive of condom use intentions in males, but that response efficacy and self-efficacy were predictive of condom use intentions in females.

Taken together, the above results suggest that PMT is a useful framework for understanding sexual risk intentions and behaviour. A notable strength of studies in this area is the number of applications of PMT in non-Western countries, including South Africa (Boer and Mashamba 2005, 2007), the Philippines (Regan and Morisky 2013), Singapore (Lwin *et al.* 2010), and China (Li *et al.* 2004). However, there are few prospective tests of PMT and a preponderance of studies have focused solely on safer sex (e.g. condom use) intentions. Nonetheless, the pattern of findings is consistent with self-efficacy and response efficacy typically found to be the most important predictors, with response costs and perceived severity also emerging as significant predictors in some studies. A conflicting pattern of results has been found for the vulnerability component, such that in some studies perceived vulnerability has a positive relationship with sexual risk intentions and behaviour, whereas in other studies the relationship is negative. Similar conclusions have been reached by Farin (1994) in a meta-analysis of PMT and HIV-protective behaviour. Self-efficacy and response efficacy emerged as the strongest predictors of HIV-protective behaviour, although they explained only 2.2% and 1.8% of the variance in such behaviour, respectively. Perceived severity was a weaker predictor, and a conflicting pattern of results was found for perceived vulnerability.

3.7 Cancer prevention

Protection motivation theory has been applied to the prediction of a range of cancer screening intentions and behaviour in women (Seydel *et al.* 1990; Boer and Seydel 1996; Hodgkins and Orbell 1998; Orbell and Sheeran 1998; Naito *et al.* 2009; Inukai and Ninomiya 2010; Gu *et al.* 2012, 2013; Hassani *et al.* 2014). Considering the uptake of cervical cancer screening, Orbell and Sheeran (1998) reported that perceived vulnerability, response efficacy (obtaining peace of mind), response costs (perceived potential negative emotional reactions to the test procedure), and self-efficacy were predictive of screening intentions in a sample of never-screened women in the UK. Intention was, in turn, predictive of actual uptake of screening at one-year follow-up, together with perceived vulnerability and response efficacy (belief that any abnormalities would be curable). In a cross-sectional study in the Netherlands, Seydel et al. (1990) found that perceived vulnerability, perceived severity, and self-efficacy were predictive of recent uptake of cervical cancer screening, and that response efficacy and self-efficacy were predictive of intentions to attend cervical cancer screening in the future. Gu et al. (2012, 2013) examined the screening intentions and behaviour of Chinese women using a cross-sectional design. None of the PMT measures were significantly associated with previous screening behaviour (Gu et al. 2012), although response efficacy was significantly associated with screening intentions (Gu et al. 2013).

Mixed findings have been reported for PMT in relation to uptake of breast cancer screening by mammography. Inukai and Ninomiya (2010) reported that self-efficacy and response costs were related to past uptake of mammography in Japanese women, whereas Naito et al. (2009) reported that PMT variables were unrelated to mammography screening intentions in Australian women after controlling for past behaviour. Using a prospective design in the Netherlands, Boer and Seydel (1996) reported that response efficacy and self-efficacy were predictive of screening intentions; however, PMT variables were unable to predict attendance at screening at two-year follow-up. Considering breast self-examination (BSE), Seydel et al. (1990) found that that response efficacy and self-efficacy were predictive of current BSE performance, and that perceived severity, response efficacy, and self-efficacy were predictive of future intentions to perform BSE. Using a prospective design, Hodgkins and Orbell (1998) examined BSE in a sample of young women (age 17–40 years) over a one-month period. In a path analysis, only self-efficacy was related to intention, which, in turn, was the only significant predictor of BSE performance at follow-up.

Several studies have also applied PMT to sun-protective intentions and behaviour (i.e. sunscreen use, avoiding midday sun) to reduce the risk of skin cancers (Grunfeld 2004; Azzarello et al. 2006; Ch'ng and Glendon 2014). Grunfeld (2004) found that PMT variables explained 21% of the variance in the sun-protective intentions of UK students, although perceived vulnerability was the sole predictor. Similarly, Azzarello et al. (2006) found that perceived vulnerability and self-efficacy correlated with concurrent sun-protective behaviour of people with a family history of melanoma. Finally, Ch'ng and Glendon (2014) reported that only response costs were correlated with sunscreen use in a sample of Australian beach-goers (although self-efficacy was not assessed).

Overall, the above results suggest that PMT is a useful framework for predicting cancer prevention behaviour. Self-efficacy and response efficacy consistently emerge as key predictors, especially of intention and concurrent behaviour, although threat appraisals (i.e. perceived severity and perceived vulnerability) and response costs have also been found to be important in some studies. Key strengths of PMT work in this area are the number of prospective studies and applications in non-Western countries.

3.8 Medical adherence

Protection motivation theory has been applied to predict adherence in a range of medical conditions, including asthma (Bennett et al. 1998), diabetes (Palardy et al. 1998), and following renal transplant (Rudman et al. 1999). In addition, several studies have focused on adherence to physiotherapy following injury (Taylor and May 1996; Grindley *et al.* 2008; Levy *et al.* 2008; Bassett and Prapavessis 2011). In a prospective study, Taylor and May (1996) applied PMT to the prediction of adherence to a physiotherapist's treatment recommendations (e.g. application of compression, hot/cold therapy, stretching and strengthening exercises) in a sports injury clinic. Patients completed a PMT questionnaire at the end of their initial appointment and treatment adherence was assessed at the second appointment (3–10 days later). Bivariate analyses revealed that the four main components of PMT (perceived vulnerability, perceived severity, response efficacy, self-efficacy) were each related to adherence, although in a regression analysis only perceived severity and self-efficacy emerged as significant predictors. Unfortunately, Taylor and May did not assess intention. Levy *et al.* (2008) also found that the four main components of PMT were correlated with adherence behaviour in patients with tendonitis injuries. Intention and self-efficacy were predictive of clinic-based adherence and attendance at clinic sessions (along with response efficacy). However, the PMT variables were unable to predict home-based adherence to physical therapy.

Protection motivation theory has also been used as a framework to predict actions taken by one individual (e.g. a parent) to protect another person's health (e.g. their child). For example, Norman *et al.* (2003) used a prospective design to examine parents' adherence to eye patching recommendations for children with amblyopia. Perceived vulnerability, response efficacy, and self-efficacy were predictive of adherence intentions at baseline, whereas perceived vulnerability and response costs were predictive of adherence behaviour at two-month follow-up. Interestingly, intention was unrelated to adherence behaviour at follow-up. Using an electronic measure of adherence to eye patching, Loudon *et al.* (2009) found that perceived vulnerability, self-efficacy, response costs, and intention were predictive of adherence. Flynn *et al.* (1995) examined parental adherence to physical therapy recommendations for children with muscular dystrophy. Self-efficacy and response efficacy were found to be predictive of adherence intentions, whereas self-efficacy was the sole predictor of adherence. Finally, Beirens *et al.* (2010) reported that (low) perceived vulnerability, self-efficacy, and response costs were predictive of the safe storage of medications in a sample of over 1700 parents of infants. The unexpected finding for perceived vulnerability is most likely due to the use of an unconditional measure of perceived vulnerability and the cross-sectional design (i.e. perceptions of vulnerability may reflect current behaviour).

Overall, the above studies suggest that PMT can be usefully employed to predict adherence to medical regimens. Both threat appraisal and coping appraisal variables have been found to be predictive of adherence intentions and behaviour. Despite some encouraging results, work in this area has suffered from two major shortcomings. First, self-report – rather than objective – measures of adherence behaviour are typically employed. Second, most studies have employed cross-sectional designs.

4 Developments

Five main areas for the future development of PMT as a social cognition model of health behaviour are outlined below. First, problems associated with interpreting correlations with perceived vulnerability are highlighted. Second, the role of fear in the model is considered. Third, the ability of PMT variables to predict maladaptive coping responses and the extent to which such responses may impede protection motivation is examined. Fourth, the extent to which protection motivation (i.e. intention) mediates the effects of other PMT variables on future behaviour is assessed. Finally, the sufficiency of the model is examined through a consideration of the impact of past behaviour on future behaviour.

4.1 Perceived vulnerability

Meta-analyses have found perceived vulnerability to be a relatively weak predictor of intention, concurrent behaviour, and future behaviour (Floyd *et al.* 2000; Milne *et al.* 2000). Moreover, the narrative review presented above reveals a mixed pattern of results. According to PMT, perceived vulnerability should be positively related to health-protective intentions and behaviour, as found in some studies (e.g. Grunfeld 2004; Li *et al.* 2004; Azzarello *et al.* 2006). However, a number of studies have reported significant negative correlations between perceived vulnerability and intentions to exercise (Plotnikoff and Higginbotham 2002), drink within safe limits (Ben-Ahron *et al.* 1995), use condoms (Van der Velde and Van der Pligt 1991), limit the number of sexual partners (Abraham *et al.* 1994), and participate in cancer screening (Seydel *et al.* 1990). Negative correlations have also been reported with concurrent behaviour in relation to binge drinking (Ben-Ahron *et al.* 1995), eating a low-fat diet (Plotnikoff and Higginbotham 1998), and participating in cervical cancer screening (Seydel *et al.* 1990). In contrast, when significant, perceived vulnerability is typically found to have a positive relationship with future protective behaviour (e.g. Aspinwall *et al.* 1991; Orbell and Sheeran 1998; Norman *et al.* 2003).

Negative relationships between perceived vulnerability and health-protective intentions/concurrent measures of behaviour are usually explained by reference to 'defensive avoidance' styles of coping (e.g. Seydel *et al.* 1990). Thus, individuals who feel particularly vulnerable to a health threat may experience high levels of anxiety and thereby engage in various maladaptive coping responses to deal with such anxiety (e.g. denial, avoidance). However, few studies have examined the relationships between PMT constructs and maladaptive coping strategies and, as a result, little evidence exists to support this interpretation.

Weinstein and Nicolich (1993) suggested that the results of many cross-sectional studies might have been misinterpreted. They argued that, to the extent that people use their current behaviour to make vulnerability judgements, a negative correlation is to be expected. For example, individuals who engage in regular exercise may infer that they are unlikely to develop cardiovascular disease in the future. However, Milne and colleagues' (2000) meta-analysis provides evidence against such a position, as a significant, but weak, positive correlation was found between perceived vulnerability and concurrent behaviour. In line with PMT, those currently engaging in a health-protective behaviour may be doing so because they believe themselves to be at risk. Unfortunately, it is difficult to tease apart these two rival positions, as some individuals may base their risk judgements on their current behaviour, whereas others may or may not engage in behaviour on the basis of their risk perceptions. Clearly, if these two opposing processes are operating in different sub-samples, then any correlation between perceived vulnerability and concurrent protective behaviour, positive or negative, is likely to be attenuated.

Weinstein and Nicolich (1993) proposed similar arguments regarding the relationship between perceived vulnerability and intention. According to PMT, individuals who feel vulnerable to a health threat should be more likely to intend to engage in a protective behaviour (i.e. a positive correlation). However, it can also be argued that individuals who intend to engage in a health-protective behaviour may feel less vulnerable to a health threat (i.e. a negative correlation). Again, it is difficult to disentangle whether perceptions of vulnerability drive health-protective intentions or whether these intentions are used to infer perceptions of vulnerability. The significant positive correlation between perceived vulnerability and intention found by Milne *et al.* (2000) in their meta-analysis would suggest that perceptions of vulnerability determine health-protective intentions, in line with PMT. Given the relatively small correlation, it is also possible that perceptions of vulnerability only determine health-protective intentions in some situations and/or among some individuals.

When considering the prediction of future behaviour, Weinstein and Nicolich (1993) only argued for the possibility of a positive relationship between perceived vulnerability and protective behaviour, as has been found in relation to reductions in the number of sexual partners (Aspinwall *et al.* 1991), the uptake of cervical cancer screening (Orbell and Sheeran 1998), and treatment adherence (Norman *et al.* 2003). In addition, Milne *et al.* (2000) reported a small, but significant, positive correlation between perceived vulnerability and future behaviour in their meta-analysis. These results are encouraging and suggest that perceptions of vulnerability may determine future protective behaviour. However, both Aspinwall *et al.* (1991) and Norman *et al.* (2003) reported that the significant effect of perceived vulnerability on future behaviour disappeared when past behaviour was included in the regression equation, suggesting that the 'apparent link between perceived risk and longitudinal changes in behavior is actually explained by the covariability of a sense of risk and behavior at [time] 1' (Joseph *et al.* 1987: 242).

Finally, Van der Velde *et al.* (1996) have advocated the use of conditional measures of perceived vulnerability when testing relationships with health-protective intentions and behaviour. In PMT studies, perceived vulnerability is typically measured by asking respondents to estimate the chances that an event will occur in the future (e.g. 'How likely is it that you will become infected with the AIDS virus in the next two years?'). Such questions are unconditional, as respondents can take into account an unspecified range of factors when responding. In contrast, conditional measures of perceived vulnerability ask respondents to estimate the chances that an event will occur in the future if preventive action is, or is not, taken (e.g. 'How likely is it that you will become infected with the AIDS virus in the next two years, if you don't use condoms?'). Van der Velde *et al.* (1996) argued that such conditional measures more closely resemble the perceived vulnerability construct as developed in PMT, as respondents estimate their vulnerability if no preventive action is taken. Conditional measures may also help to disentangle the nature of relationships with health-protective intentions and behaviour in cross-sectional studies. For example, Van der Velde *et al.* (1996) reported that a conditional measure of perceived vulnerability (for not using condoms) had a significant positive correlation with condom use intentions among STD clinic attendees (with both private partners and sex workers) in line with PMT predictions. In contrast, an unconditional measure had a significant negative correlation with condom use intentions with sex worker partners and a non-significant, positive, correlation with private partners.

4.2 Fear

Tanner *et al.* (1991) have questioned the extent to which PMT recognizes the importance of emotional responses to fear appeals. In particular, they argue that Rogers (1975) views fear as an insignificant by-product of the threat appraisal process that has no impact on ongoing appraisal and coping processes. However, Tanner *et al.* (1991) argue that fear arousal may increase motivation for health-protective behaviours. For example, Plotnikoff and Higginbotham (1995) found that a measure of fear arousal (i.e. '...how frightened you feel when you think about the possibility of having a heart attack') had a significant, though weak, effect on intention to follow a low-fat diet among an 'at-risk' community sample. Similarly, Van der Velde and Van der Pligt (1991) found that fear had a direct effect on condom use intentions among a sample of multiple-partner heterosexuals. In contrast, other studies have found non-significant relationships between fear and intentions to use condoms (Abraham *et al.* 1994; Ho 2000; Boer and Mashamba 2005, 2007), perform breast self-examination (Hodgkins and Orbell 1998), and attend cervical cancer screening (Gu *et al.* 2013). In their meta-analysis, Milne *et al.* (2000) reported significant average correlations between fear and intention ($r_+ = 0.20$) and concurrent behaviour ($r_+ = 0.26$), and a non-significant average correlation between fear and future behaviour ($r_+ = -0.04$). The effect sizes were small-to-medium, and associated *fail-safe N* values fell well short of recommended tolerance levels, indicating the effects are not robust.

Tanner *et al.* (1991) also argued that an emotional response, such as fear, may act as a source of feedback to heighten the processing of threat and coping information. The extended parallel process model (EPPM) includes a feedback loop between fear and message processing appraisals (Witte 1992) in line with this proposition. Lazarus and Folkman (1984: 227) state that, 'when information is appraised for our well-being, it becomes..."hot information"' and may increase attention to, and comprehension of, information related to the threat. Tanner *et al.* (1991) found that students exposed to a high threat essay that contained coping response information acquired more knowledge than those exposed to a low threat essay that contained coping response information. Tanner *et al.* (1991) therefore argue that the appraisal processes outlined in PMT should be viewed as sequential or ordered, such that coping appraisal processes are only activated when threat appraisal results in fear. A similar proposition is included in the EPPM (Witte 1992).

4.3 Maladaptive coping responses

In addition to assessing the ability of PMT to predict health-protective intentions and behaviour (i.e. adaptive coping responses), it is also possible to apply the model to the prediction of maladaptive coping responses. Thus, when individuals perceive a threat to their well-being in the absence of an effective coping response, they may engage in activities that reduce the fear associated with the threat without dealing with the threat itself. Such strategies may be termed 'maladaptive coping responses' (Rippetoe and Rogers 1987), and include strategies such as denial and avoidance. High levels of perceived vulnerability and severity and low levels of response efficacy and self-efficacy may therefore be expected to be associated with the adoption of maladaptive coping responses.

Ben-Ahron *et al.* (1995) considered a number of maladaptive coping responses in relation to binge drinking, including avoidance (e.g. not thinking about the adverse consequences of binge drinking), wishful thinking (e.g. hoping that medical breakthroughs will nullify the need for behaviour change), fatalism (e.g. believing that the adverse consequences are due to fate rather than personal action), and religious faith (e.g. trusting that God will provide protection). Using path analysis, a number of significant relationships with PMT variables were identified. Avoidance was predicted by perceived severity and self-efficacy (negative relationships), while the use of religious faith as a coping strategy was predicted by response efficacy and self-efficacy (negative relationships). Abraham *et al.* (1994) examined maladaptive coping responses in response to the threat of HIV/AIDS among a sample of adolescents and found negative relationships between response efficacy and wishful thinking, and between self-efficacy and both wishful thinking and denial. In addition, response costs associated with condom use predicted denial, fatalism, and irrational fear. Similarly, Hodgkins and Orbell (1998) found that the response costs associated with breast self-examination predicted use of avoidance as a coping strategy.

The above studies indicate that PMT can be usefully employed to predict maladaptive, as well as adaptive, coping responses. Future research may therefore seek to confirm these initial findings. In addition, Tanner *et al.* (1991) have argued that engaging in maladaptive coping responses may impede protection motivation and the adoption of actions to deal with the threat. Ben-Ahron *et al.* (1995) found that avoidance and religious faith were significant (negative) predictors of intentions to drink within safe limits. Similarly, measures of maladaptive coping (Ho 2000), denial (Abraham *et al.* 1994), and defensive avoidance (Van der Velde and Van der Pligt 1991) have been found to be significant (negative) predictors of condom use intentions. Finally, Hodgkins and Orbell (1998) reported that avoidance had a negative correlation with breast self-examination at one-month follow-up, although this effect became non-significant after controlling for PMT variables.

4.4 Mediating role of protection motivation

According to PMT, threat (i.e. perceived severity, perceived vulnerability, intrinsic and extrinsic rewards) and coping appraisals (i.e. response efficacy, self-efficacy, response costs) determine protection motivation (i.e. intention), which, in turn, determines future behaviour. Protection motivation theory is therefore a meditational model in that intention is the proximal predictor of future behaviour, mediating the effects of other PMT variables. The results of the meta-analyses conducted by Floyd *et al.* (2000) and Milne *et al.* (2000) indicate that the PMT variables have stronger relationships with intention than future behaviour, and that protection motivation is the strongest predictor of future behaviour. This pattern of results is consistent with the idea that protection motivation mediates the effects of threat and coping appraisals on behaviour. Some studies have reported that intention fully mediates the effects of PMT variables on future behaviour in relation to exercise (Norman *et al.* 2005) and breast self-examination (Hodgkins and Orbell 1998). However, other studies have found that both self-efficacy and intention are significant predictors of future exercise behaviour (Plotnikoff *et al.* 2009a, 2009b, 2010; Tavares *et al.* 2009; Tulloch *et al.* 2009), and clinic-based adherence to physiotherapy for tendonitis injuries (Levy *et al.* 2008). Such results suggest that PMT could be modified to include a direct link between self-efficacy and behaviour, as is also outlined in other models of health behaviour, such as social cognitive theory (Bandura 1986; Luszczynska and Schwarzer, Chapter 7 this volume).

4.5 Sufficiency of PMT

Relatively few PMT studies have examined the impact of past behaviour on health-protective intentions and behaviour. This is despite the fact that work on other social cognition models, such as the theory of planned behaviour (Ajzen 1988), has indicated that past behaviour is a strong predictor of future behaviour (Conner and Armitage 1998). Ouellette and Wood (1998) argue that strong past behaviour–future behaviour relations can be explained in two ways. First, past behaviour may affect future behaviour indirectly through its influence on intention (i.e. a conscious response). Past behaviour should shape individuals' beliefs about the behaviour, which, in turn, influence their intentions and subsequent behaviour. Thus, the effects of past behaviour should be mediated by PMT variables in line with Rogers' (1983) view of prior experience (i.e. past behaviour) as an intrapersonal source of information that may initiate the cognitive appraisal processes outlined in PMT. A direct effect of past behaviour on future behaviour therefore indicates that a model is not sufficient (Ajzen 1991), because if a model is sufficient (i.e. it contains all the important determinants of behaviour), the addition of past behaviour should not explain additional variance. Assuming that the determinants of a behaviour remain stable, the past behaviour–future behaviour correlation can be taken as an indication of the ceiling of a model's predictive validity. Second, past behaviour may affect future behaviour directly through the automatic repetition of established routines (i.e. an habitual response). As Triandis (1977) argues, repeated performance of a behaviour may result in the behaviour becoming under the influence of automatic processes that typify habitual processes (Eagly and Chaiken 1993). According to this account, when past behaviour is found to have a direct effect on future behaviour, this reflects the involvement of habitual processes.

Applications of PMT that include a measure of past behaviour typically find a strong, unmediated relationship with future behaviour. For example, several prospective PMT studies have found past behaviour to be the sole predictor of future exercise behaviour (Norman *et al.* 2005), binge drinking (Murgraff *et al.* 1999), and breast self-examination (Hodgkins and Orbell 1998). Other studies have found that past behaviour predicts future behaviour along with other PMT variables. For example, Plotnikoff *et al.* (2009b) found that self-efficacy and past behaviour predicted future exercise behaviour. Similarly, Aspinwall *et al.* (1991) reported that after controlling for demographics, HIV status, and partner status, both self-efficacy and past behaviour were predictive of reductions in the number of sexual partners at six-month follow-up. These results suggest that PMT is not a sufficient model of health behaviour and would benefit from the inclusion of additional variables. Given that PMT explains typically more of the variance in intention (i.e. protection motivation) than in future behaviour, it could be usefully extended by incorporating post-intentional (i.e. volitional) variables such as action and coping planning (see Schwarzer and Luszczynska, Chapter 8 this volume).

5 Operationalization of the model

In this section, the various steps to develop PMT measures are outlined. These broadly mirror the recommendations made by DeVellis (1991) for the development of reliable and valid scales. Most of the PMT studies reviewed in this chapter reported few details on the development of PMT measures, although there are a number of exceptions that are highlighted below.

The first stage in the development of a PMT questionnaire is to determine the content of items. This can be achieved in one of two ways. The first approach is to conduct a literature review of previous PMT studies on the health behaviour of interest to identify whether any previous, published or unpublished instruments exist. The second approach is to develop items specifically for the planned study. This involves generating an item pool to cover the PMT constructs, ideally achieved by conducting semi-structured interviews with a sample drawn from

Table 3.3   Example interview questions from Searle *et al.* (2000)

Severity
In your opinion, what are the potential consequences of your child's visual impairment?

Vulnerability
What are your thoughts about how your child's visual impairment will change over time?

Rewards of maladaptive response
Are there any benefits/advantages of not wearing a patch?

Response efficacy
What are the benefits/advantages of wearing a patch?

Self-efficacy
As a parent, to what extent do you feel that you can carry out the treatment requirements?

Response costs
What are the things/factors that hinder or prevent your child from wearing the patch?

---

the target population (e.g. 20–30 members) to determine the salient beliefs about the target health threat and health behaviour.

Few PMT studies have taken the latter approach. For example, in their study on treatment adherence, Norman *et al.* (2003) conducted pilot PMT-based semi-structured interviews (open-ended questions followed by prompts) with 20 parents of children who had been prescribed an eye patch for the treatment of amblyopia (see Table 3.3 for examples taken from Searle *et al.* 2000). Plotnikoff and Higginbotham (1995, 1998, 2002) conducted focus groups to supplement information obtained from interviews concerning exercise and dietary behaviour in response to the threat of cardiovascular disease. Hassani *et al.* (2014) conducted focus groups with women about cervical cancer screening in conjunction with a literature review and interviews with experts to generate a PMT item pool. Rather than conduct interviews, an alternative approach is to conduct an elicitation study. Hodgkins and Orbell (1998) administered a short questionnaire to a sample of 40 women to ascertain salient cognitions about breast cancer and performing breast self-examination. For example, for perceived severity, women were asked, 'In what way would you consider contracting breast cancer would affect your life?' The most frequently mentioned (i.e. modal) beliefs for each PMT construct were included in the resultant questionnaire and used in the main study. Orbell and Sheeran (1998) used a similar approach in their study of cervical cancer screening.

Having generated an item pool, items are reviewed to ensure adequate coverage of each PMT construct, as well as face and content validity, which can be achieved by obtaining expert ratings. For example, Hassani *et al.* (2014) asked expert judges to rate the necessity and relevance (i.e. congruence) of each item to the target construct. Content validity index (Polit and Beck 2006) and content validity ratio (Lawshe 1975) scores were then calculated to assess agreement among raters.

The next stage of questionnaire development is to administer the items to a pilot sample. This allows an opportunity to check respondents' comprehension of the items and to detect any potential difficulties that are likely to occur when respondents complete the questionnaire in the main study. In addition, a number of data checks can be conducted. For example, individual items can be assessed for range and skewness. Items can then be combined to form scales to measure each PMT construct. Psychometric properties including internal consistency (Cronbach's alpha; Cronbach 1951), test–retest reliability, and construct validity (i.e. how the scales relate to each other and additional variables) can also be examined. Finally, factor analyses – exploratory (to identify latent constructs) or confirmatory (to assess the degree of fit with PMT constructs) – can be conducted to assess the factorial validity of the scales (Comrey 1988).

Few PMT studies have included a pilot study when developing PMT measures. Some studies have reported pre-testing questionnaires with a small number of participants to check the wording and understanding of items (e.g. Grunfeld 2004; Li *et al.* 2004; Beirens *et al.* 2010; Henson *et al.* 2010; Gu *et al.* 2012). Plotnikoff and Higginbotham (2002, see also 1995, 1998 for similar procedures) conducted a pilot test of their questionnaire with 95 people from the target population, with an additional 46 respondents interviewed to establish adequate comprehension of the questionnaire instructions and response formats. Taylor and May (1996) piloted a PMT questionnaire with 267 patients from a wide range of sports injury clinics, and then factor analysed the responses to ensure that the items mapped onto the four main PMT constructs. Reliable scales were subsequently constructed. Similarly, Murgraff *et al.* (1999) developed a PMT questionnaire on binge drinking by administering a pilot questionnaire to 169 students. First, the means and standard deviations of individual items were calculated to ensure adequate spread. Second, scales to measure each of the PMT constructs were constructed and the item–total correlations were examined in order to delete items that reduced the scale's internal reliability. Third, the retained items were subjected to an exploratory factor analysis (i.e. principal components analysis), which confirmed the structure of PMT.

An alternative approach not involving a pilot study is to factor analyse questionnaire items employed in the main study using either the full (e.g. Norman *et al.* 2003) or restricted range of PMT constructs. For example, Plotnikoff and Higginbotham (1995) factor analysed the perceived vulnerability, response efficacy, self-efficacy, and protection motivation items, whereas elsewhere the same authors (Plotnikoff and Higginbotham 1998, 2002) factor analysed only the response efficacy, self-efficacy, and protection motivation items. Sheeran and Orbell (1996) only factor analysed items assessing the response cost items (of using condoms) and rewards (of not using condoms), but found that they were uni-dimensional. Other studies have reported factor analyses of items measuring specific constructs. MacDonell *et al.* (2013) separately factor analysed the threat (i.e. perceived severity, perceived vulnerability, intrinsic rewards, extrinsic rewards) and coping (i.e. response efficacy, self-efficacy, response costs) appraisal items. Abraham *et al.* (1994) conducted separate factor analyses on items measuring perceptions of vulnerability and response costs in relation to the AIDS virus. The vulnerability items were found to load onto two factors (at a personal and group level). The response cost items also loaded onto two factors reflecting pleasure loss and reputation concerns. Finally, Orbell and Sheeran (1998) factor analysed items assessing various expectancies associated with cervical cancer screening and identified three factors reflecting response efficacy, response costs, and the possibility of finding abnormal cells and/or another health problem.

When PMT items are subjected to a factor analysis, they tend to load onto factors in line with the structure of PMT (e.g. Taylor and May 1996; Murgraff *et al.* 1999; Norman *et al.* 2003). However, most factor analyses are exploratory. Given the problems associated with exploratory factor analysis and the fact that researchers are able to specify, *a priori*, which items should load onto which factors, there is a strong case for the use of confirmatory factor analysis, as has been reported in several studies (e.g. Ho *et al.* 2000; MacDonell *et al.* 2013; Hassani *et al.* 2014). Future studies should routinely report factor analyses of PMT items to demonstrate that they load onto factors in line with the structure of PMT, rather than simply report the internal reliability (i.e. alpha coefficients) of scales used to measure PMT variables.

A range of items has been used to measure PMT constructs in applications of the model. Considering perceived severity, many studies have used single items (e.g. Orbell and Sheeran 1998; Plotnikoff and Higginbotham 1998; Tulloch *et al.* 2009; Regan and Morisky 2013). Multi-item scales often have poor internal reliability (e.g. Abraham *et al.* 1994; Boer and Seydel 1996; Taylor and May 1996; Grunfeld 2004), although other studies have reported reliable multi-item scales (e.g. Sheeran and Orbell 1996; Boer and Hashamba 2007; Yu *et al.* 2008; Thrul *et al.* 2013; Hassani *et al.* 2014). Perceived severity items typically focus on the physical severity of the health threat (e.g. 'How serious a health problem is a heart attack?'; Plotnikoff and Higginbotham 2002). However, other aspects of the seriousness of the health threat have been considered, including the potential impact on psychological well-being (e.g. 'Even if I was infected by HIV, I would still lead a happy life'; Sheeran and Orbell 1996), finances (e.g. 'Having heart disease would seriously affect my financial situation'; Henson *et al.* 2010), and involvement in normal activities (e.g. 'Skin cancer would disrupt my daily life'; Ch'ng and Glendon 2014).

Some studies have assessed perceived vulnerability using single items (e.g. Leas and McCabe 2007; Tulloch *et al.* 2009; Regan and Morisky 2013), but in the main studies report using multi-item scales with good levels of internal reliability. The perceived vulnerability items tend to focus on the individual's chances of experiencing the health threat in the future (e.g. 'My chances of developing breast cancer in the future are... very low/very high'; Hodgkins and Orbell 1998). Some studies ask respondents to consider their vulnerability on the basis of their current and past behaviour (e.g. 'Considering my present and past behaviour, my chances of getting health problems from binge drinking are very high'; Murgraff *et al.* 1999). Such a wording is consistent with Weinstein and Nicolich's (1993) argument that people may use their current behaviour to inform vulnerability judgements. An alternative approach is to ask respondents to provide vulnerability ratings if a behaviour is not performed (e.g. 'If I do not use condoms, I will run a high risk of getting HIV/AIDS'; Boer and Mashamba 2005, 2007). As Van der Velde *et al.* (1996) have argued, such a conditional measure of perceived vulnerability may provide a more accurate assessment of perceived vulnerability as outlined in PMT. Finally, some perceived vulnerability items measure fear or worry (e.g. 'How worried are you about the possibility of catching AIDS?'; Eppright *et al.* 1994).

Intrinsic and extrinsic rewards have not been assessed in many studies. Abraham *et al.* (1994) argue that any reward associated with not performing the recommended behaviour (e.g. 'Sex would be *more* exciting *without* a condom') can be rephrased as a response cost of performing the recommended behaviour (i.e. 'Sex would be *less* exciting *with* a condom'). In support of such a position, Sheeran and Orbell (1996) found only one factor underlying items measuring various response costs of using condoms and rewards of not using condoms. Nonetheless, some studies have reported using reliable measures of intrinsic and extrinsic rewards (e.g. Murgraff *et al.* 1999; Grunfeld 2004). Other studies have assessed intrinsic and extrinsic rewards separately with reliable scales (e.g. Li *et al.* 2004; MacDonnel *et al.* 2013). Items assessing intrinsic rewards tend to focus on the personal advantages of the maladaptive behaviour (e.g. 'Smoking helps people concentrate'; MacDonnel *et al.* 2013), whereas items assessing extrinsic rewards tend to focus on social aspects of the maladaptive behaviour (e.g. 'Smoking is good for social networking'; MacDonnel *et al.* 2013)

Most studies have used reliable multi-item measures to assess response efficacy, although some studies have employed single-item measures (e.g. Eppright *et al.* 1994; Greening 1997; Murgraff *et al.* 1999). Such items typically focus on the effectiveness of the behaviour to reduce the threat (e.g. 'Regular exercise will reduce my chances of having a heart attack'; Plotnikoff and Higginbotham 2002). However, other positive outcomes of performing the behaviour have been measured (e.g. 'The test will give me peace of mind'; Orbell and Sheeran 1998; Gu *et al.* 2013). Often, general perceived effectiveness is rated (e.g. 'Using a condom is effective in preventing a man passing the AIDS virus to a woman'; Abraham *et al.* 1994), rather than in relation to the individual performing the behaviour (e.g. 'The rehabilitation programme designed for me will ensure my complete recovery from this injury'; Taylor and May 1996).

Self-efficacy is typically assessed with multi-item scales with good levels of internal reliability. The self-efficacy items focus on individuals' overall levels of confidence (e.g. 'I am capable of starting and continuing drinking at safe levels'; Murgraff *et al.* 1999), or on their perceptions of the ease or difficulty of performing the behaviour (e.g. 'I would find it easy to suggest using a condom to a new partner'; Abraham *et al.* 1994). Some studies ask respondents to rate their confidence that they can perform a behaviour when faced with specific obstacles (e.g. 'I will have the pap test even if it is painful'; Hassani *et al.* 2014). Alternatively, respondents may indicate the extent to which specific obstacles may prevent performance of the behaviour (e.g. Boer and Seydel 1996; Orbell and Sheeran 1998).

Response costs have been measured in fewer PMT studies, although they tend to be assessed with reliable multi-item scales (e.g. Smerecnik *et al.* 2011; Thrul *et al.* 2013). Some studies have reported scales with low reliability (e.g. Li *et al.* 2004; Yu *et al.* 2008), which might reflect a disparate range of potential response costs. Items typically focus on various negative aspects of performing the behaviour, including psychological (e.g. 'The test will make me feel anxious'; Orbell and Sheeran 1998), physical (e.g. 'Applying sunscreen can be messy'; Ch'ng and Glendon 2014), and financial (e.g. 'If I undergo a genetic test it will be harder to get a mortgage or life insurance'; Smerecnik *et al.* 2011) response costs.

Finally, protection motivation is typically equated with intention to perform a behaviour. Studies have employed a mixture of single-item and reliable multi-item measures that ask respondents to indicate whether they intend/plan/are likely/are willing to engage in a behaviour (e.g. 'Do you plan to follow a low-fat diet for at least the next six months?'; Plotnikoff and Higginbotham 1998). Questions may refer to the future (e.g. 'In the future I will use dental floss regularly'; Sheeran and Orbell 1996) or not specify a timeframe (e.g. 'I intend to drink within safe limits as a regular habit'; Murgraff *et al.* 1999). Few studies include a specific timeframe (e.g. 'I intend to carry out BSE in the next month'; Hodgkins and Orbell 1998).

Although many studies have employed multi-item scales, with adequate internal reliability, to assess PMT constructs, a number of measurement issues can be highlighted. First, few studies have conducted an elicitation study to identify the salient beliefs about the threat and behaviour under consideration in the target population. Second, factor analyses are rarely reported. Future studies should therefore address these two shortcomings to ensure the construction of reliable multi-item measures. This, in turn, is likely to increase the statistical power of subsequent analyses (Lipsey 1990). Third, the measurement of perceived vulnerability would be improved by the use of conditional vulnerability measures that ask respondents to indicate their vulnerability if a recommended behaviour is not followed (cf. Van der Velde *et al.* 1996). Fourth, many items that have been used to measure coping appraisal and protection motivation have failed to specify an appropriate timeframe. As a result, measures may have a low level of correspondence, thus attenuating the size of subsequent correlations (Fishbein and Ajzen 1975). Finally, PMT has considerable overlap with other social cognition models of health behaviour reviewed in this book. For example, measures of perceived severity and vulnerability are also included in the health belief model, while intention is a key variable in the theory of planned behaviour, and self-efficacy is the cornerstone of social cognitive theory. Recommendations for the measurement of these variables are therefore also outlined in other chapters (Abraham and Sheeran, Chapter 2 this volume; Conner and Sparks, Chapter 5 this volume; Luszczynska and Schwarzer, Chapter 7 this volume).

6 Intervention studies

Milne *et al.* (2000) distinguish between two types of PMT intervention studies can be distinguished: (1) experimental manipulations of specific PMT variables, and (2) health behaviour interventions that are broadly based on PMT. In this section we consider different ways that PMT variables have been targeted and previous reviews of PMT interventions, before considering the results of PMT-based experimental and health behaviour intervention studies in more detail.

6.1 Designing PMT interventions

Experimental tests directly manipulate specific variables. In these studies, participants typically read a persuasive communication manipulating specific PMT variables. Most of these studies seek to manipulate specific variables through the presentation of information designed to produce high versus low levels of the targeted construct – for example, one condition designed to increase perceptions of vulnerability and the other condition designed to decrease perceived vulnerability. Fruin *et al.* (1992) is a good example of this approach. Participants were presented with material about exercise in which response efficacy, response costs, and self-efficacy were independently manipulated resulting in a $2 \times 2 \times 2$ between-subjects factorial design with two levels (high vs. low) for each factor. After reading the information, participants completed a PMT questionnaire. Other studies seek to manipulate specific PMT variables in order to encourage health-protective behaviour (i.e. present vs. absent). For example, Wurtele and Maddux (1987) presented essays to sedentary female undergraduates recommending beginning a regular exercise programme. Perceptions of vulnerability, severity, response efficacy, and self-efficacy were independently manipulated, such that the specific manipulation was either present or absent. After reading the essays, participants completed a PMT questionnaire.

Specific PMT constructs have been manipulated in a variety of ways in experimental studies. Considering threat appraisal variables, Stainback and Rogers (1983) manipulated the perceived severity of excessive drinking by arguing that it may cause either severe injury (i.e. high severity) or minor irritation (i.e. low severity) to internal organs. In a study designed to increase dietary intake of calcium among female students, Wurtele (1988) manipulated perceptions of vulnerability to osteoporosis. Many studies have combined perceived severity and vulnerability so that the potential threat of an illness/disease is manipulated. Rippetoe and Rogers (1987) manipulated the perceived threat of breast cancer by presenting women with either a high- or low-threat essay.

The high-threat essay graphically described breast cancer and highlighted college-age women's vulnerability to breast cancer, whereas the low-threat essay described breast cancer as less severe and rare in college-aged women.

Considering coping appraisal variables, response efficacy has been manipulated in essays that argue that there is an effective method to prevent or treat a disease or that there is no such method. For example, Fruin *et al.* (1992) presented high school students with essays on cardiovascular disease and exercise. The high response efficacy essay emphasized the effectiveness of regular exercise in reducing their risk of developing cardiovascular disease. In contrast, the low response efficacy essay stated that 'Many people do not believe that regular exercise is effective in preventing cardiovascular disease' (p. 60). Rippetoe and Rogers (1987) manipulated self-efficacy by providing information, in the high self-efficacy essay, that emphasized a woman's ability to perform breast self-examination and to incorporate it into her health routine. In contrast, the low self-efficacy essay highlighted the difficulty of performing a good breast self-examination and accurately detecting a lump. Finally, Fruin *et al.* (1992) manipulated the response costs of regular exercise. In the high response costs essay the possible negative side-effects were highlighted, whereas the low response costs essay stated that any negative side-effects are 'quite minor and easily overcome' (p. 60).

In health behaviour intervention studies, the intervention group receives information about a health threat and recommended action, whereas the control group receives information on an unrelated topic or receives no information. The intervention typically provides general factual information on the health threat and an appropriate coping response, based on PMT. For example, in an intervention to encourage participation in mammography screening (Boer and Seydel 1996), women in the intervention group were sent a PMT-based leaflet that described the relative high vulnerability of older women to breast cancer and the high response efficacy of mammography screening. In addition, by explaining that mammography is a straightforward procedure with little discomfort, feelings of self-efficacy towards participating in the screening programme were encouraged.

6.2 Meta-analysis

Milne *et al.* (2000) reviewed experimental tests of PMT through a meta-analysis of cognition changes following manipulations of specific PMT variables. Their meta-analysis consisted of eight studies that included specific manipulations of constructs and considered the effects of the manipulations on corresponding cognitions (effect sizes were expressed in terms of r_+). Manipulations of the threat appraisal variables led to significant changes in corresponding perceptions of severity ($r_+ = 0.66$) and vulnerability ($r_+ = 0.63$). These effect sizes are large according to Cohen's (1992) guidelines. The effect sizes for manipulations of response efficacy ($r_+ = 0.42$) and self-efficacy ($r_+ = 0.32$) though smaller, were significant and in the medium-to-large range. Only manipulations of response costs ($r_+ = 0.09$) were unable to produce a significant effect, although it should be noted that only one study was included in the meta-analysis (Fruin *et al.* 1992). Furthermore, for all the significant effect sizes with the exception of self-efficacy, the *fail-safe N* values were well above recommended tolerance levels, indicating the effects to be robust. It is noteworthy that the experimental manipulations tend to be more successful at changing threat than coping appraisal cognitions.

There were too few health behaviour intervention studies to be able to conduct a meaningful meta-analysis. Milne *et al.* (2000) therefore conducted a vote count of the percentage of times

Table 3.4 Examples of intervention studies based on protection motivation theory

Behaviour	Experimental studies	Health behaviour interventions
Exercise	Stanley and Maddux (1986), Wurtele and Maddux (1987), Fruin et al. (1992), Courneya and Hellsten (2001)	Milne et al. (2002), Prestwich et al. (2008), Zhang and Cooke (2012)
Diet	Wurtele (1988)	Boeka et al. (2010), Zhang and Cooke (2012)
Smoking	Maddux and Rogers (1983)	
Alcohol	Stainback and Rogers (1983)	
Safe sex	Tanner et al. (1989), Kyes (1995), Yzer et al. (2001), Smerecnik and Ruiter (2010)	Stanton et al. (1996, 1998, 2004, 2005, 2006), Kaljee et al. (2005), Chen et al. (2009, 2010), Gong et al. (2009), Li et al. (2008), Lin et al. (2010), Pham et al. (2012)
Cancer prevention	Rippetoe and Rogers (1987), McMath and Prentice-Dunn (2005), Prentice-Dunn et al. (2009)	Steffen (1990), Boer and Seydel (1996), McClendon and Prentice-Dunn (2001), Milne and Sheeran (2002), Fry and Prentice-Dunn (2006)
Medical adherence		Bassett and Prapavessis (2011)

the interventions produced significant changes in PMT cognitions. The health behaviour interventions were unable to produce significant changes in perceptions of severity and vulnerability (0% significance ratios), although there was some evidence of an impact of such interventions on response efficacy (50% significance ratio) and self-efficacy (100% significance ratio). These findings can be contrasted with a similar vote count conducted for experimental manipulations of specific PMT variables that revealed 100% significance ratios for manipulations of the four main PMT constructs. However, it is clear that there are too few studies at this stage to make any reliable conclusions on the effectiveness of PMT-based health behaviour interventions to change threat and coping appraisal cognitions.

The analyses conducted by Milne et al. (2000) only considered the impact of interventions on changes in threat and coping appraisals. Of more importance is the impact of such interventions on protection motivation (i.e. intention) and behaviour. This is reviewed narratively below (see Table 3.4).

6.3 Experimental studies

A number of experimental studies have focused on exercise. For example, Courneya and Hellsten (2001) presented students with essays that manipulated each of the four main PMT constructs. Only the perceived severity manipulation was found to have a significant effect on exercise intentions. However, most other studies have reported significant effects for self-efficacy manipulations on intentions (Stanley and Maddux 1986; Wurtele and Maddux 1987; Fruin et al. 1992), and significant effects have also been reported for perceived vulnerability (Wurtele and Maddux 1987) and response efficacy (Stanley and Maddux 1986) manipulations.

Considering experimental studies that have focused on safe sex intentions, Yzer et al. (2001) presented female undergraduate students with newspaper articles that manipulated perceptions of vulnerability to AIDS and self-efficacy to engage in safe sex practice. Only the self-efficacy manipulation was found to have a significant effect on safe sex intentions. Tanner *et al.* (1989) also found a self-efficacy manipulation to have a significant effect on condom use intentions. In contrast, manipulating other PMT constructs has been found to have little effect on safe sex intentions (e.g. Kyes 1995). Smerecnik and Ruiter (2010) manipulated threat and coping appraisals for condom use. Only the coping message had a significant effect on condom use intentions, although this was qualified by an interaction with the threat message such that the high coping essay was most effective when used in conjunction with the high threat message.

Some studies have manipulated PMT constructs in relation to cancer prevention behaviours. For example, Ripptoe and Rogers (1987) manipulated threat of breast cancer as well as response efficacy and self-efficacy for performing breast self-examination (BSE). All three manipulations were found to impact on BSE intentions. McMath and Prentice-Dunn (2005) manipulated threat and coping appraisals in relation to sun-protection. The high-threat essay had a significant effect on intentions, although the effect of the coping essay was only marginally significant. In a subsequent study (Prentice-Dunn *et al.* 2009), both conditions were found to have significant effects on intentions, but not on requests for skin cancer-related items (e.g. sunscreen, brochures).

Few experimental studies have focused on other health behaviours. Maddux and Rogers (1983) manipulated the main PMT constructs and found that response efficacy and self-efficacy had significant effects on intentions to quit smoking. In research into osteoporosis, Wurtele (1988) found that the perceived vulnerability manipulation had significant effects on women's calcium consumption intentions and behaviour. The response efficacy manipulation was only found to have a significant effect on calcium consumption intentions. Beck and Lund (1981) investigated periodontal disease. Only the severity manipulation, and not the vulnerability manipulation, impacted on intentions to use disclosing tablets and, at four-week follow-up, dental flossing behaviour. Finally, Stainback and Rogers (1983) presented alcohol-related high- versus low-threat information to high school students, which they found to influence intentions to remain abstinent and to not drink and drive.

6.4 Health behaviour intervention studies

There have been several PMT-based health behaviour interventions. Milne *et al.* (2002) reported that a PMT-based health behaviour intervention had a significant effect on exercise intentions but not behaviour in university students. Zhang and Cooke (2012) found a significant effect on exercise intentions and behaviour over a four-week period, although the effect on behaviour was heightened when combined with a volitional intervention (i.e. action and coping planning). Similar effects were also found on dietary intentions and behaviour. Prestwich *et al.* (2008) also found that a PMT-based intervention had a significant effect on intentions to reduce saturated fat intake as well as on dietary behaviour at one-month follow-up. The effect on behaviour was also augmented by an implementation intention (i.e. planning) intervention.

Protection motivation theory has been used as the theoretical basis for a successful adolescent HIV-prevention intervention programme: 'Focus on Kids' is a community-based intervention delivered in groups over eight weekly sessions (Galbraith *et al.* 1996; Stanton *et al.* 1996). Developed in the 1990s in the USA, it has been evaluated through several randomized controlled trials (RCTs) (Stanton *et al.* 1996, 2004, 2005, 2006) and has been included by the Centers for

Disease Control and Prevention in its 'Diffusion of Effective Behavioural Interventions' portfolio (Lyles *et al.* 2007). In the original RCT among low-income African-American adolescents in Baltimore, Maryland, Stanton *et al.* (1996) reported that the intervention produced significant effects on condom use intentions and behaviour at six-month, but not 12-month, follow-up. When tested in West Virginia (Stanton *et al.* 2006), significant intervention effects were found on response efficacy, self-efficacy, and response costs, but not on behaviour, at six-month follow-up.

Adaptations of the programme have been developed and tested in several other countries, including the Bahamas (Chen *et al.* 2009, 2010; Gong *et al.* 2009), Namibia (Stanton *et al.* 1998), Vietnam (Kaljee *et al.* 2005; Pham *et al.* 2012), and China (Li *et al.* 2008; Lin *et al.* 2009, 2010). For example, Chen *et al.* (2010) reported that the intervention increased condom use intentions and behaviour at 36-month follow-up in the Bahamas. Lin *et al.* (2010) adapted the programme for female rural-to-urban workers in China, reporting that the intervention had significant effects on perceived vulnerability, response efficacy, self-efficacy, and condom use intentions and behaviour at four-month follow-up.

Considering cancer prevention behaviour, Steffen (1990) evaluated a leaflet on testicular self-examination (TSE) among undergraduates. The intervention was found to increase intentions to perform TSE, compared with the control group. Milne and Sheeran (2002) reported similar results, finding that a PMT-based leaflet had a significant effect on TSE intentions but not behaviour. Fry and Prentice-Dunn (2006) also found that a PMT-based intervention increased intentions to perform BSE immediately after the session, but not on intentions or behaviour at three-month follow-up. Boer and Seydel (1996) found that a mammography screening intervention among an older community sample increased intentions; however, it was not possible to assess the impact on behaviour as attendance was extremely high in both groups. McClendon and Prentice-Dunn (2001) found that a PMT intervention had a significant effect on sun-protective intentions than was maintained at one-month follow-up. A significant intervention effect was also found on skin tone (as judged by raters blind to condition at follow-up).

Bassett and Prapavessis (2011) reported that a video designed to increase adherence to physiotherapy after injury had a significant effect on perceptions of vulnerability, severity, and response efficacy. However, the video had no effect on intention or behaviour. Finally, Boeka *et al.* (2010) found that an intervention to increase adherence to eating guidelines after bariatric surgery had no significant impact on cognitions or intentions.

6.5 Summary and discussion

Experimental tests of PMT have shown that manipulating specific constructs typically produces changes in corresponding cognitions (Milne *et al.* 2000). Interestingly, larger effect sizes are typically found for manipulations of perceived severity and vulnerability than for manipulations of response efficacy and self-efficacy, thereby indicating that attempts to change threat appraisals have been more successful than those to change coping appraisals. However, when the effects of manipulating specific variables on intentions are considered, manipulations of self-efficacy are typically more effective than manipulations of other constructs. In terms of motivating people to engage in health behaviour, these results suggest that interventions should attempt to change perceptions of self-efficacy, even though such perceptions are difficult to change. Experimental tests of PMT typically only assess the immediate impact of PMT manipulations on cognitions and intentions and, as a result, are likely to overestimate their impact.

Analyses of the longer-term impact of such manipulations on PMT cognitions or behaviour are rarely conducted (for exceptions, see Beck and Lund 1981; Wurtele 1988).

Studies evaluating PMT-based interventions have reported some encouraging findings with significant effects often found on intentions and, to a lesser extent, on behaviour. A notable strength of these studies is the assessment of PMT variables at follow-up. Encouragingly, the effects of interventions on cognitions, intentions, and behaviour have been observed over extended follow-up periods, suggesting that changes in cognitions and behaviour following interventions may be relatively stable over time. Furthermore, many interventions have been evaluated in non-Western countries.

Few studies have tested whether the effects of PMT interventions are mediated by PMT variables. Some studies have reported correlations between manipulated variables and intention (e.g. Stanley and Maddux 1986; Courneya and Hellsten 2001), but not full mediation analyses (cf. Baron and Kenny 1986). A notable exception is Rippetoe and Rogers' (1987) experimental study that assessed the impact of manipulating threat, response efficacy, and self-efficacy on breast self-examination (BSE) intentions. The manipulations had significant effects on corresponding cognitions and BSE intentions. Path analysis provided support for a mediation model, as no direct effects were found for the PMT manipulations on BSE intentions; instead, the effects were mediated by corresponding PMT variables. Similarly, Chen *et al.* (2010) reported that a HIV-prevention programme for adolescents increased response efficacy, self-efficacy, condom use intentions, and behaviour at 36 months. Path analyses indicated that response efficacy and self-efficacy mediated the effect of the intervention on intention and that self-efficacy mediated the effect of the intervention on condom use. Such findings suggest that PMT interventions influence health-protective intentions through changing PMT variables, thereby providing good support for the model.

In addition to assessing the impact of PMT interventions on health-protective intentions and behaviour, it is also possible to assess their impact on maladaptive coping responses. Thus, individuals may engage in various strategies in order to reduce the fear associated with the threat without dealing with the threat itself. Few studies have examined the impact of PMT interventions on maladaptive coping (e.g. Rippetoe and Rogers 1987; Yzer *et al.* 2001; Fruin *et al.* 1992; McMath and Prentice-Dunn 2005; Fry and Prentice-Dunn 2006). For example, Rippetoe and Rogers (1987) examined the impact of threat, response efficacy, and self-efficacy manipulations on BSE. The threat manipulation increased the likelihood of both adaptive and maladaptive coping, consistent with the idea that threat appraisal is a necessary, but not sufficient, condition for protection motivation. In contrast, the coping appraisal manipulations were found to have significant effects on specific coping responses. For example, women who read the high self-efficacy essay were more likely to engage in adaptive responses, whereas those who read the low self-efficacy essay were more likely to feel hopeless. Similarly, Fry and Prentice-Dunn (2006) reported that an intervention to promote BSE increased rational problem-solving and BSE intentions (i.e. adaptive responses), but also reduced maladaptive responses such as avoidance and fatalistic religiosity.

Milne *et al.* (2002) noted that there is good evidence that experimental manipulations of specific PMT variables are able to change corresponding cognitions and intentions. However, applying such manipulations to real-world health behaviour interventions may be difficult, as it is not generally ethical to manipulate specific variables in a high versus low level in such settings because to do so would involve providing some individuals with false information. One solution to this problem is to either provide or not provide information on the specific PMT variables (i.e. present vs. absent), as has been done in some experimental studies (e.g. Yzer *et al.* 2001). Alternatively, it may be more appropriate to test the impact of a single intervention (relative to a control group) in which all PMT components are addressed together. However, the disadvantage of such an approach is that it is not possible to assess the relative impact of different components of the intervention and, as a result, it is not possible to identify the 'active ingredients'. Moreover, such an approach may provide only limited information for the future theoretical development of PMT.

7 Future directions

Protection motivation theory includes many of the key social cognitive determinants of health behaviour reviewed in this book. It shares a number of similarities with the health belief model (Rosenstock 1974; Abraham and Sheeran, Chapter 2 this volume) that also includes perceived vulnerability and severity. Furthermore, the perceived benefits of, and barriers to, performing a health-protective action are analogous to the response efficacy and response costs constructs of PMT. However, PMT also includes self-efficacy and protection motivation (i.e. intention). These variables are among the most powerful predictors of health behaviour and are included in the theory of planned behaviour (Ajzen 1988; Conner and Sparks, Chapter 5 this volume) and social cognitive theory (Bandura 1986; Luszczynska and Schwarzer, Chapter 7 this volume). In addition, PMT posits that protection motivation acts as a mediating variable between the threat and coping appraisal variables and health behaviour, again in line with the theory of planned behaviour. Given that PMT includes a range of threat and coping appraisal variables that have been found to be important in other models, it is not surprising that PMT has been found to be a useful model for predicting intentions and behaviour. Nonetheless, there are a number of issues that need to be addressed in future research.

There is a need for more prospective tests. This would assist the theoretical development of PMT in three important ways. First, the use of prospective designs provides an opportunity to examine the proposed mediating role of protection motivation (i.e. intention) in more detail. According to PMT, the threat and coping appraisal variables should be mediated by intention. Meta-analyses (Floyd *et al.* 2000; Milne *et al.* 2000) indicate that the threat and coping appraisal variables provide only weak predictions of future behaviour, whereas intention is a consistent, and moderately strong, predictor of future behaviour. This pattern of results is consistent with a mediation hypothesis; however, relatively few formal mediation tests have been reported in the literature. While some studies have found that intention fully mediates the effects of PMT variables on future behaviour (e.g. Hodgkins and Orbell 1998; Norman *et al.* 2005), other studies have indicated that self-efficacy often emerges as a significant predictor of future behaviour along with intention (e.g. Levy *et al.* 2008; Plotnikoff *et al.* 2009a, 2010; Tavares *et al.* 2009; Tulloch *et al.* 2009). As a result, there is a case to be made for modifying PMT to include a direct link between self-efficacy and behaviour, as included in social cognitive theory (Bandura 1986; Luszczynska and Schwarzer, Chapter 7 this volume) and analogous to the direct link between perceived behavioural control and future behaviour in the theory of planned behaviour (Ajzen 1988; Conner and Sparks, Chapter 5 this volume). Second, the use of prospective designs would provide a more appropriate test of the relationship between perceived vulnerability and health behaviour. As Weinstein and Nicolich (1993) argue, in cross-sectional studies it is unclear whether a positive or negative correlation should be expected between perceived vulnerability and health behaviour. Prospective designs, coupled with the use of conditional measures of perceived vulnerability (Van der Velde *et al.* 1996), are required to disentangle the nature of this relationship. Third, the use of prospective designs would allow the sufficiency of the model to be assessed in more detail, by examining whether PMT fully mediates the impact of past behaviour on future behaviour.

One of the strengths of PMT is that it has been subjected to numerous experimental tests. In their meta-analysis of cognition changes following experimental manipulations of specific variables, Milne *et al.* (2000) found large effect sizes for the threat appraisal variables and medium-to-large effect sizes for the coping appraisal variables. Furthermore, their meta-analysis indicated that self-efficacy manipulations have the weakest impact on corresponding cognitions, whereas the narrative review of experimental studies presented earlier suggests that self-efficacy manipulations have the most consistent impact on intentions. Future work should therefore consider additional ways of manipulating self-efficacy (cf. Bandura 1991), especially given that self-efficacy is the strongest PMT predictor of intentions. Protection motivation theory has also been used as the theoretical framework for health behaviour interventions in which constructs are targeted in a single intervention and compared with a control condition. Such interventions have been found to have significant effects on intentions and behaviour.

Despite some encouraging results from both experimental and intervention studies, future research needs to address two key issues. First, most experimental tests only measure cognitions and intentions immediately post-manipulation (for exceptions, see Boer and Seydel 1996; Milne *et al.* 2002) and fail to consider impacts on subsequent behaviour (for exceptions, see Beck and Lund 1981; Wurtele and Maddux 1987; Wurtele 1988; Milne *et al.* 2002). Future experimental studies therefore need to assess the longer-term impact of manipulating PMT variables. Encouragingly, PMT-based interventions have assessed cognitions, intentions, and behaviour over extended follow-up periods, finding that effects are often sustained over time. Second, few studies have tested whether effects on intention and behaviour are mediated by PMT variables. This is true for both experiments and interventions, although there are some exceptions (e.g. Rippetoe and Rogers 1987; Chen *et al.* 2010). Thus, future research should routinely conduct mediation analyses, which will help to identify the 'active ingredients' needed to change health behaviour.

In conclusion, PMT has received strong support from correlational studies that have used PMT as a social cognition model to predict health behaviour and, to a lesser extent, from experimental and health behaviour intervention studies that have sought to change health-related cognitions, intentions, and behaviour. Moreover, given its sound theoretical foundation and its overlap with other social cognition models, PMT is likely to continue to be an important model of health behaviour. In addition, as outlined above, there are various issues that require attention in future studies and these are likely to stimulate further research on PMT.

References

Abraham, C.S., Sheeran, P., Abrams, D. and Spears, R. (1994) Exploring teenagers' adaptive and maladaptive thinking in relation to the threat of HIV infection, *Psychology and Health*, 9, 253–72.

Ajzen, I. (1988) *Attitudes, Personality and Behavior*. Buckingham: Open University Press.

Ajzen, I. (1991) The theory of planned behavior, *Organizational Behavior and Human Decision Processes*, 50, 179–211.

Aspinwall, L.G., Kemeny, M.E., Taylor, S.E., Schneider, S.G. and Dudley, J.P. (1991) Psychosocial predictors of gay men's AIDS risk-reduction behavior, *Health Psychology*, 10, 432–44.

Azzarello, L.M., Dessureault, S. and Jacobsen, P.B. (2006) Sun-protective behavior among individuals with a family history of melanoma, *Cancer Epidemiology, Biomarkers and Prevention*, 15, 142–5.

Bakker, A., Buunk, B. and Siero, F. (1993) Condom use among heterosexuals: a comparison of the theory of planned behavior, the health belief model and protection motivation theory, *Gedrag en Gezondheid*, 21, 238–54.

Bandura, A. (1986) *Social Foundations of Thought and Action: A Cognitive Social Theory.* Englewood Cliffs, NJ: Prentice-Hall.

Bandura, A. (1991) Self-efficacy mechanism in physiological activation and health-promoting behavior, in J. Madden (ed.) *Neurobiology of Learning, Emotion and Affect* (pp. 229–70). New York: Raven Press.

Baron, R.M. and Kenny, D.A. (1986) The moderator–mediator variable distinction in social psychological research: conceptual, strategic, and statistical considerations, *Journal of Personality and Social Psychology*, 51, 1173–82.

Bassett, S.F. and Prapavessis, H. (2011) A test of an adherence-enhancing adjunct to physiotherapy steeped in the protection motivation theory, *Physiotherapy Theory and Practice*, 27, 360–72.

Beck, K.H. and Lund, A.K. (1981) The effects of health threat seriousness and personal efficacy upon intentions and behavior, *Journal of Applied Social Psychology*, 11, 401–15.

Beirens, T.M., van Beeck, E.F., Brug, J., den Hertog, P. and Raat, H. (2010) Why do parents with toddlers store poisonous products safely? *International Journal of Pediatrics*, 2010, article 702827.

Ben-Ahron, V., White, D. and Phillips, K. (1995) Encouraging drinking at safe limits on single occasions: the potential contribution of protection motivation theory, *Alcohol and Alcoholism*, 30, 633–9.

Bengel, J., Belz-Merk, M. and Farin, E. (1996) The role of risk perception and efficacy cognitions in the prediction of HIV-related preventive behavior and condom use, *Psychology and Health*, 11, 505–25.

Bennett, P., Rowe, A. and Katz, D. (1998) Reported adherence with preventive asthma medication: a test of protection motivation theory, *Psychology, Health and Medicine*, 3, 347–54.

Blanchard, C.M., Reid, R.D., Morrin, L.I., McDonnell, L., McGannon, K., Rhodes, R.E. *et al.* (2009) Does protection motivation theory explain exercise intentions and behavior during home-based cardiac rehabilitation? *Journal of Cardiopulmonary Rehabilitation and Prevention*, 29, 188–92.

Boeka, A.G., Prentice-Dunn, S. and Lokken, K.L. (2010) Psychosocial predictors of intentions to comply with bariatric surgery guidelines, *Psychology, Health and Medicine*, 15, 188–97.

Boer, H. and Mashamba, M.T. (2005) Psychosocial correlates of HIV protection motivation among black adolescents in Venda, South Africa, *AIDS Education and Prevention*, 17, 590–602.

Boer, H. and Mashamba, M.T. (2007) Gender power imbalance and differential psychosocial correlates of intended condom use among male and female adolescents from Venda, South Africa, *British Journal of Health Psychology*, 12, 51–63.

Boer, H. and Seydel, E.R. (1996) Protection motivation theory, in M. Conner and P. Norman (eds.) *Predicting Health Behaviour* (pp. 95–120). Buckingham: Open University Press.

Bui, L., Mullan, B. and McCaffery, K. (2013) Protection motivation theory and physical activity in the general population: a systematic literature review, *Psychology, Health and Medicine*, 18, 522–42.

Calder, S.C., Davidson, G.R. and Ho, R. (2011) Intentions to consume omega-3 fatty acids: a comparison of protection motivation theory and ordered protection motivation theory, *Journal of Dietary Supplements*, 8, 115–34.

Ch'ng, J.W. and Glendon, A.I. (2014) Predicting sun protection behaviors using protection motivation variables, *Journal of Behavioral Medicine*, 37, 245–56.

Chen, X., Lunn, S., Deveaux, L., Li, X., Brathwaite, N., Cottrell, L. *et al.* (2009) A cluster randomized controlled trial of an adolescent HIV prevention program among Bahamian youth: effect at 12 months post-intervention, *AIDS and Behavior*, 13, 499–508.

Chen, X., Stanton, B., Gomez, P., Lunn, S., Deveaux, L., Brathwaite, N. *et al.* (2010) Effects on condom use of an HIV prevention programme 36 months postintervention: a cluster randomized controlled trial among Bahamian youth, *International Journal of STD and AIDS*, 21, 622–30.

Cohen, J. (1992) A power primer, *Psychological Bulletin*, 112, 155–9.

Comrey, A.L. (1988) Factor-analytic methods of scale development in personality and clinical psychology, *Journal of Consulting and Clinical Psychology*, 56, 754–61.

Conner, M. and Armitage, C.J. (1998) Extending the theory of planned behavior: a review and avenues for further research, *Journal of Applied Social Psychology*, 28, 1429–64.

Conner, M. and Norman, P. (1998) Health behavior, in D.W. Johnston and M. Johnston (eds.) *Comprehensive Clinical Psychology, Vol. 8: Health Psychology* (pp. 1–37). Oxford: Pergamon Press.

Courneya, K.S. and Hellsten, L.-A. (2001) Cancer prevention as a source of exercise motivation: an experimental test using protection motivation theory, *Psychology, Health and Medicine*, 6, 59–64.

Cox, D., Koster, A. and Russell, C. (2004) Predicting intentions to consume functional foods and supplements to offset memory loss using an adaptation of protection motivation theory, *Appetite*, 43, 55–64.

Cronbach, L.J. (1951) Coefficient alpha and the internal structure of tests, *Psychometrika*, 16, 297–334.

DeVellis, R.F. (1991) *Scale Development: Theory and Applications*. Newbury Park, CA: Sage.

Eagly, A.H. and Chaiken, S. (1993) *The Psychology of Attitudes*. Fort Worth, TX: Harcourt Brace Jovanovich.

Eppright, D.R., Tanner, J.F., Jr. and Hunt, J.B. (1994) Knowledge and the ordered protection motivation model: tools for preventing AIDS, *Journal of Business Research*, 30, 13–24.

Farin, E. (1994) Eine Metaanalyse Empirischer Studien zum Prädiktiven Wert Kognitiver Variablen der HIV-Bezogenen Risikowahrnehmung und-Verabeitung für das HIV-Risikoverhalten. Dissertation, Universität Freiburg.

Fishbein, M. and Ajzen, I. (1975) *Belief, Attitude, Intention, and Behavior*. New York: Wiley.

Floyd, D.L., Prentice-Dunn, S. and Rogers, R.W. (2000) A meta-analysis of research on protection motivation theory, *Journal of Applied Social Psychology*, 30, 407–29.

Flynn, M.F., Lyman, R.D. and Prentice-Dunn, S. (1995) Protection motivation theory and adherence to medical treatment regimens for muscular dystrophy, *Journal of Social and Clinical Psychology*, 14, 61–75.

Fruin, D.J., Pratt, C. and Owen, N. (1992) Protection motivation theory and adolescents' perceptions of exercise, *Journal of Applied Social Psychology*, 22, 55–69.

Fry, R.B. and Prentice-Dunn, S. (2006) Effects of a psychosocial intervention on breast self-examination attitudes and behaviors, *Health Education Research*, 21, 287–95.

Galbraith, J., Ricardo, I., Stanton, B., Black, M., Feigelman, S. and Kaljee, L. (1996) Challenges and rewards of involving community in research: an overview of the 'Focus on Kids' HIV Risk Reduction Program, *Health Education and Behavior*, 23, 383–94.

Gong, J., Stanton, B., Lunn, S., Deveaux, L., Li, X., Marshall, S. *et al.* (2009) Effects through 24 months of an HIV/AIDS prevention intervention program based on protection motivation theory among preadolescents in the Bahamas, *Pediatrics*, 123, e917–28.

Greening, L. (1997) Adolescents' cognitive appraisals of cigarette smoking: an application of the protection motivation theory, *Journal of Applied Social Psychology*, 27, 1972–85.

Greening, L., Stoppelbein, L. and Jackson, M. (2001) Health education programs to prevent teen pregnancy, *Journal of Adolescent Health*, 28, 257–8.

Grindley, E.J., Zizzi, S.J. and Nasypany, A.M. (2008) Use of protection motivation theory, affect, and barriers to understand and predict adherence to outpatient rehabilitation, *Physical Therapy*, 88, 1529–40.

Grunfeld, E.A. (2004) What influences university students' intentions to practice safe sun exposure behaviors? *Journal of Adolescent Health*, 35, 486–92.

Gu, C., Chan, C.W., He, G.-P., Choi, K. and Yang, S.-B. (2013) Chinese women's motivation to receive future screening: the role of social-demographic factors, knowledge and risk perception of cervical cancer, *European Journal of Oncology Nursing*, 17, 154–61.

Gu, C., Chan, C.W., Twinn, S. and Choi, K.C. (2012) The influence of knowledge and perception of the risk of cervical cancer on screening behavior in mainland Chinese women, *Psycho-Oncology*, 21, 1299–1308.

Hassani, L., Dehdari, T., Hajizadeh, E., Shojaeizadeh, D., Abedini, M. and Nedjat, S. (2014) Development of an instrument based on the protection motivation theory to measure factors influencing women's intention to first pap test practice, *Asian Pacific Journal of Cancer Prevention*, 15, 1227–32.

Henson, S., Cranfield, J. and Herath, D. (2010) Understanding consumer receptivity towards foods and non-prescription pills containing phytosterols as a means to offset the risk of cardiovascular disease: an application of protection motivation theory, *International Journal of Consumer Studies*, 34, 28–37.

Ho, R. (1998) The intention to give up smoking: disease versus social dimensions, *Journal of Social Psychology*, 138, 368–80.

Ho, R. (2000) Predicting intention for protective health behaviour: a test of the protection versus the ordered protection motivation model, *Australian Journal of Psychology*, 52, 110–18.

Hodgkins, S. and Orbell, S. (1998) Can protection motivation theory predict behaviour? A longitudinal test exploring the role of previous behaviour, *Psychology and Health*, 13, 237–50.

Hovland, C., Janis, I.L. and Kelley, H. (1953) *Communication and Persuasion*. New Haven, CT: Yale University Press.

Inukai, S. and Ninomiya, K. (2010) Cognitive factors relating to mammographic breast cancer screening, *Japanese Journal of Public Health*, 57, 796–806 [in Japanese].

Janis, I.L. (1967) Effects of fear arousal on attitude change: recent developments in theory and experimental research, *Advances in Experimental Social Psychology*, 3, 166–224.

Joseph, J.G., Montgomery, S.B., Emmons, C.A., Kirscht, J.P., Kessler, R.C., Ostrow, D.G. *et al.* (1987) Perceived risk of AIDS: assessing the behavioral and psychosocial consequences in a cohort of gay men, *Journal of Applied Social Psychology*, 17, 231–50.

Kaljee, L.M., Genberg, B., Riel, R., Cole, M., Tho, L.H., Thoa, L.T.K. *et al.* (2005) Effectiveness of a theory-based risk reduction HIV prevention program for rural Vietnamese adolescents, *AIDS Education and Prevention*, 17, 185–99.

Kyes, K.B. (1995) Using fear to encourage safer sex: an application of protection motivation theory, *Journal of Psychology and Human Sexuality*, 7, 21–37.

Lawshe, C.H. (1975) A quantitative approach to content validity, *Personnel Psychology*, 28, 563–75.

Lazarus, R.S. and Folkman, S. (1984) *Stress, Appraisal, and Coping*. New York: Springer.

Leas, L. and McCabe, M. (2007) Health behaviors among individuals with schizophrenia and depression, *Journal of Health Psychology*, 12, 563–79.

Leventhal, H. (1970) Findings and theory in the study of fear communications, *Advances in Experimental Social Psychology*, 5, 119–86.

Levy, A., Polman, R. and Clough, P. (2008) Adherence to sport injury rehabilitation programs: an integrated psycho-social approach, *Scandinavian Journal of Medicine and Science in Sports*, 18, 798–809.

Li, X., Stanton, B., Fang, X., Lin, D., Mao, R., Wang, J. *et al.* (2004) HIV/STD risk behaviors and perceptions among rural-to-urban migrants in China, *AIDS Education and Prevention*, 16, 538–56.

Li, X., Stanton, B., Wang, B., Mao, R., Zhang, H., Qu, M. *et al.* (2008) Cultural adaptation of the Focus on Kids program for college students in China, *AIDS Education and Prevention*, 20, 1–14.

Lin, D., Li, X., Stanton, B., Fang, X., Lin, X., Xu, X. *et al.* (2010) Theory-based HIV-related sexual risk reduction prevention for Chinese female rural-to-urban migrants, *AIDS Education and Prevention*, 22, 344–55.

Lipsey, M.W. (1990) *Design Sensitivity: Statistical Power for Experimental Research*. Beverly Hills, CA: Sage.

Loudon, S., Passchier, J., Chaker, L., de Vos, S., Fronius, M., Harrad, R. *et al.* (2009) Psychological causes of non-compliance with electronically monitored occlusion therapy for amblyopia, *British Journal of Ophthalmology*, 93, 1499–1503.

Lwin, M.O., Stanaland, A.J. and Chan, D. (2010) Using protection motivation theory to predict condom usage and assess HIV health communication efficacy in Singapore, *Health Communication*, 25, 69–79.

Lyles, C.M., Kay, L.S., Crepaz, N., Herbst, J.H., Passin, W.F., Kim, A.S. *et al.* (2007) Best-evidence interventions: findings from a systematic review of HIV behavioral interventions for US populations at high risk, 2000–2004, *American Journal of Public Health*, 97, 133–43.

MacDonell, K., Chen, X., Yan, Y., Li, F., Gong, J., Sun, H. *et al.* (2013) A protection motivation theory-based scale for tobacco research among Chinese youth, *Journal of Addiction Research and Therapy*, 4, article 154.

Maddux, J.E. and Rogers, R.W. (1983) Protection motivation and self-efficacy: a revised theory of fear appeals and attitude change, *Journal of Experimental Social Psychology*, 19, 469–79.

McClendon, B.T. and Prentice-Dunn, S. (2001) Reducing skin cancer risk: an intervention based on protection motivation theory, *Journal of Health Psychology*, 6, 321–8.

McMath, B.F. and Prentice-Dunn, S. (2005) Protection motivation theory and skin cancer risk: the role of individual differences in responses to persuasive appeals, *Journal of Applied Social Psychology*, 35, 621–43.

Milne, S. and Sheeran, P. (2002) Combining motivational and volitional interventions to prevent testicular cancer, presentation to the *13th General Meeting of the European Association of Experimental Social Psychology*, San Sebastian, Spain, June.

Milne, S., Orbell, S. and Sheeran, P. (2002) Combining motivational and volitional interventions to promote exercise participation: protection motivation theory and implementation intentions, *British Journal of Health Psychology*, 7, 163–84.

Milne, S., Sheeran, P. and Orbell, S. (2000) Prediction and intervention in health-related behavior: a meta-analytic review of protection motivation theory, *Journal of Applied Social Psychology*, 30, 106–43.

Murgraff, V., White, D. and Phillips, K. (1999) An application of protection motivation theory to riskier single-occasion drinking, *Psychology and Health*, 14, 339–50.

Naito, M., O'Callaghan, F.V. and Morrissey, S. (2009) Understanding women's mammography intentions: a theory-based investigation, *Women and Health*, 49, 101–18.

Norman, P., Boer, H. and Seydel, E.R. (2005) Protection motivation theory, in M. Conner and P. Norman (eds.) *Predicting Health Behaviour* (pp. 81–126). Buckingham: Open University Press.

Norman, P., Searle, A., Harrad, R. and Vedhara, K. (2003) Predicting adherence to eye patching in children with amblyopia: an application of protection motivation theory, *British Journal of Health Psychology*, 8, 67–82.

Orbell, S. and Sheeran, P. (1998) 'Inclined abstainers': a problem for predicting health-related behaviour, *British Journal of Social Psychology*, 37, 151–65.

Ouellette, J.A. and Wood, W. (1998) Habit and intention in everyday life: the multiple processes by which past behavior predicts future behavior, *Psychological Bulletin*, 124, 54–74.

Palardy, N., Greening, L., Ott, J., Holderby, A. and Atchison, J. (1998) Adolescents' health attitudes and adherence to treatment for insulin-dependent diabetes mellitus, *Journal of Developmental and Behavioral Pediatrics*, 19, 31–7.

Pham, V., Nguyen, H., Tho, L.H., Minh, T.T., Lerdboon, P., Riel, R. *et al.* (2012) Evaluation of three adolescent sexual health programs in Ha Noi and Khanh Hoa Province, Vietnam, *AIDS Research and Treatment*, 2012 [DOI: 10.1155/2012/986978].

Plotnikoff, R.C. and Higginbotham, N. (1995) Predicting low-fat diet intentions and behaviors for the prevention of coronary heart disease: an application of protection motivation theory among an Australian population, *Psychology and Health*, 10, 397–408.

Plotnikoff, R.C. and Higginbotham, N. (1998) Protection motivation theory and the prediction of exercise and low-fat diet behaviours among Australian cardiac patients, *Psychology and Health*, 13, 411–29.

Plotnikoff, R.C. and Higginbotham, N. (2002) Protection motivation theory and exercise behaviour change for the prevention of heart disease in a high-risk, Australian representative community sample of adults, *Psychology, Health and Medicine*, 7, 87–98.

Plotnikoff, R.C. and Trinh, L. (2010) Protection motivation theory: is this a worthwhile theory for physical activity promotion? *Exercise and Sport Sciences Reviews*, 38, 91–9.

Plotnikoff, R.C., Lippke, S., Trinh, L., Courneya, K.S., Birkett, N. and Sigal, R.J. (2010) Protection motivation theory and the prediction of physical activity among adults with type 1 or type 2 diabetes in a large population sample, *British Journal of Health Psychology*, 15, 643–61.

Plotnikoff, R.C., Rhodes, R.E. and Trinh, L. (2009a) Protection motivation theory and physical activity: a longitudinal test among a representative population sample of Canadian adults, *Journal of Health Psychology*, 14, 1119–34.

Plotnikoff, R.C., Trinh, L., Courneya, K.S., Karunamuni, N. and Sigal, R.J. (2009b) Predictors of aerobic physical activity and resistance training among Canadian adults with type 2 diabetes: an application of the protection motivation theory, *Psychology of Sport and Exercise*, 10, 320–8.

Polit, D.F. and Beck, C.T. (2004) *Nursing Research: Principles and Practice* (46th edn.). Philadelphia, PA: Wolters Kluwer Health.

Prentice-Dunn, S., McMath, B.F. and Cramer, R.J. (2009) Protection motivation theory and stages of change in sun protective behavior, *Journal of Health Psychology*, 14, 297–305.

Prestwich, A., Ayres, K. and Lawton, R. (2008) Crossing two types of implementation intentions with a protection motivation intervention for the reduction of saturated fat intake: a randomized trial, *Social Science and Medicine*, 67, 1550–8.

Regan, R. and Morisky, D.E. (2013) Perceptions about HIV and condoms and consistent condom use among male clients of commercial sex workers in the Philippines, *Health Education and Behavior*, 40, 216–22.

Rippetoe, P.A. and Rogers, R.W. (1987) Effects of components of protection-motivation theory on adaptive and maladaptive coping with a health threat, *Journal of Personality and Social Psychology*, 52, 596–604.

Rogers, R.W. (1975) A protection motivation theory of fear appeals and attitude change, *Journal of Psychology*, 91, 93–114.

Rogers, R.W. (1983) Cognitive and physiological processes in fear appeals and attitude change: a revised theory of protection motivation, in J.T. Cacioppo and R.E. Petty (eds.) *Social Psychophysiology: A Source Book* (pp. 153–76). New York: Guilford Press.

Rogers, R.W. and Deckner, C.W. (1975) Effects of fear appeals and physiological arousal upon emotion, attitudes, and cigarette smoking, *Journal of Personality and Social Psychology*, 32, 222–30.

Rogers, R.W. and Prentice-Dunn, S. (1997) Protection motivation theory, in D.S. Gochman (ed.) *Handbook of Behavior Research: Personal and Social Determinants* (pp. 113–32). New York: Plenum Press.

Rosenstock, I.M. (1974) Historical origins of the health belief model, *Health Education Monographs*, 2, 1–8.

Rosenthal, R. (1991) *Meta-Analytic Procedures for Social Research* (2nd edn.). Newbury Park, CA: Sage.

Rudman, L.A., Hope Gonzales, M. and Borgida, E. (1999) Mishandling the gift of life: noncompliance in renal transplant patients, *Journal of Applied Social Psychology*, 29, 834–51.

Searle, A., Vedhara, K., Norman, P., Frost, A. and Harrad, R. (2000) Compliance with eye patching in children and its psychosocial effects: a qualitative application of protection motivation theory, *Psychology, Health and Medicine*, 5, 43–54.

Seydel, E., Taal, E. and Wiegman, O. (1990) Risk-appraisal, outcome and self-efficacy expectancies: cognitive factors in preventive behaviour related to cancer, *Psychology and Health*, 4, 99–109.

Sheeran, P. and Orbell, S. (1996) How confidently can we infer health beliefs from questionnaire responses? *Psychology and Health*, 11, 273–90.

Smerecnik, C., Quaak, M., van Schayck, C.P., van Schooten, F.-J. and de Vries, H. (2011) Are smokers interested in genetic testing for smoking addiction? A socio-cognitive approach, *Psychology and Health*, 26, 1099–112.

Smerecnik, C.M. and Ruiter, R.A. (2010) Fear appeals in HIV prevention: the role of anticipated regret, *Psychology, Health and Medicine*, 15, 550–9.

Stainback, R.D. and Rogers, R.W. (1983) Identifying effective components of alcohol abuse prevention programs: effects of fear appeals, message style, and source expertise, *Substance Use and Misuse*, 18, 393–405.

Stanley, M.A. and Maddux, J.E. (1986) Cognitive processes in health enhancement: investigation of a combined protection motivation and self-efficacy model, *Basic and Applied Social Psychology*, 7, 101–13.

Stanton, B., Cole, M., Galbraith, J., Li, X., Pendleton, S., Cottrel, L. *et al.* (2004) Randomized trial of a parent intervention: parents can make a difference in long-term adolescent risk behaviors, perceptions, and knowledge, *Archives of Pediatrics and Adolescent Medicine*, 158, 947–55.

Stanton, B., Guo, J., Cottrell, L., Galbraith, J., Li, X., Gibson, C. *et al.* (2005) The complex business of adapting effective interventions to new populations: an urban to rural transfer, *Journal of Adolescent Health*, 37, 17–26.

Stanton, B.F., Harris, C., Cottrell, L., Li, X., Gibson, C., Guo, J., Pack, R., Galbraith, J., Pendleton, S., and Wu, Y. (2006) Trial of an urban adolescent sexual risk-reduction intervention for rural youth: a promising but imperfect fit, *Journal of Adolescent Health*, 38, 55. e25-55.

Stanton, B.F., Li, X., Kahihuata, J., Fitzgerald, A.M., Neumbo, S., Kanduuombe, G. *et al.* (1998) Increased protected sex and abstinence among Namibian youth following a HIV risk-reduction intervention: a randomized, longitudinal study, *AIDS*, 12, 2473–80.

Stanton, B.F., Li, X., Ricardo, I., Galbraith, J., Feigelman, S. and Kaljee, L. (1996) A randomized, controlled effectiveness trial of an AIDS prevention program for low-income African-American youths, *Archives of Pediatrics and Adolescent Medicine*, 150, 363–72.

Steffen, V.J. (1990) Men's motivation to perform the testicle self-exam: effects of prior knowledge and an educational brochure, *Journal of Applied Social Psychology*, 20, 681–702.

Sutton, S. (1982) Fear-arousing communications: a critical examination of theory and research, in J.R. Eiser (ed.) *Social Psychology and Behavioural Medicine* (pp. 303–37). London: Wiley.

Sutton, S. (2005) Stage theories of health behaviour, in M. Conner and P. Norman (eds.) *Predicting Health Behaviour* (pp. 223–75). Buckingham: Open University Press.

Tanner, J.F., Jr., Day, E. and Crask, M.R. (1989) Protection motivation theory: an extension of fear appeals theory in communication, *Journal of Business Research*, 19, 267–76.

Tanner, J.F., Jr., Hunt, J.B. and Eppright, D.R. (1991) The protection motivation model: a normative model of fear appeals, *Journal of Marketing*, 55, 36–45.

Tavares, L.S., Plotnikoff, R.C. and Loucaides, C. (2009) Social-cognitive theories for predicting physical activity behaviours of employed women with and without young children, *Psychology, Health and Medicine*, 14, 129–42.

Taylor, A.H. and May, S. (1996) Threat and coping appraisal as determinants of compliance with sports injury rehabilitation: an application of protection motivation theory, *Journal of Sports Sciences*, 14, 471–82.

Thrul, J., Stemmler, M., Bühler, A. and Kuntsche, E. (2013) Adolescents' protection motivation and smoking behaviour, *Health Education Research*, 28, 683–91.

Triandis, H.C. (1977) *Interpersonal Behavior*. Monterey, CA: Brooks-Cole.

Tulloch, H., Reida, R., D'Angeloa, M.S., Plotnikoff, R.C., Morrina, L., Beatona, L. *et al.* (2009) Predicting short- and long-term exercise intentions and behaviour in patients with coronary artery disease: a test of protection motivation theory, *Psychology and Health*, 24, 255–69.

Umeh, K. (2004) Cognitive appraisals, maladaptive coping, and past behaviour in protection motivation, *Psychology and Health*, 19, 719–35.

Van der Velde, F.W. and Van der Pligt, J. (1991) AIDS-related health behavior: coping, protection motivation, and previous behavior, *Journal of Behavioral Medicine*, 14, 429–51.

Van der Velde, F.W., Hooykaas, C. and van der Pligt, J. (1996) Conditional versus unconditional risk estimates in models of AIDS-related risk behaviour, *Psychology and Health*, 12, 87–100.

Weinstein, N.D. and Nicolich, M. (1993) Correct and incorrect interpretations of correlations between risk perceptions and risk behaviors, *Health Psychology*, 12, 235–45.

Witte, K. (1992) Putting the fear back into fear appeals: the extended parallel process model, *Communications Monographs*, 59, 329–49.

Wright, A.J., French, D.P., Weinman, J. and Marteau, T.M. (2006) Can genetic risk information enhance motivation for smoking cessation? An analogue study, *Health Psychology*, 25, 740–52.

Wurtele, S.K. (1988) Increasing women's calcium intake: the role of health beliefs, intentions, and health value, *Journal of Applied Social Psychology*, 18, 627–39.

Wurtele, S.K. and Maddux, J.E. (1987) Relative contributions of protection motivation theory components in predicting exercise intentions and behavior, *Health Psychology*, 6, 453–66.

Yan, Y., Jacques-Tiura, A.J., Chen, X., Xie, N., Chen, J., Yang, N. *et al.* (2014) Application of the protection motivation theory in predicting cigarette smoking among adolescents in China, *Addictive Behaviors*, 39, 181–8.

Yardley, L., Donovan-Hall, M., Francis, K. and Todd, C. (2007) Attitudes and beliefs that predict older people's intention to undertake strength and balance training, *Journals of Gerontology Series B: Psychological Sciences and Social Sciences*, 62B, 119–25.

Yu, S., Marshall, S., Cottrell, L., Li, X., Liu, H., Deveaux, L. *et al.* (2008) Longitudinal predictability of sexual perceptions on subsequent behavioural intentions among Bahamian preadolescents, *Sexual Health*, 5, 31–9.

Yzer, M.C., Siero, F.W. and Buunk, B.P. (2001) Bringing up condom use and using condoms with new sexual partners: intentional or habitual? *Psychology and Health*, 16, 409–21.

Zhang, Y. and Cooke, R. (2012) Using a combined motivational and volitional intervention to promote exercise and healthy dietary behaviour among undergraduates, *Diabetes Research and Clinical Practice*, 95, 215–23.

Chapter **4**

Self-determination theory

Martin S. Hagger and Nikos L.D. Chatzisarantis

1 General background

Self-determination theory has received considerable attention in the literature on predicting and changing health behaviour (Hagger and Chatzisarantis 2007a; Ng *et al.* 2012; Teixeira *et al.* 2012b). Self-determination theory is really a meta-theory comprising four sub-theories: cognitive evaluation theory, causality orientations theory, basic psychological needs theory, and organismic integration theory. Each theory contributes a set of key testable hypotheses as part of the overarching meta-theory, which aims to provide a comprehensive explanation of human motivation. The theory has its origins in humanistic and organismic theories of motivation, intention and free will (Lewin 1951), personal causation and effectance (DeCharms 1968), competence (White 1959), and control (Weiner *et al.* 1972). Despite its humanistic roots, the theory has been developed based on evidence from quantitative, experimental, and social cognitive methodological traditions. For example, initial evidence for the theory was based on a series of experiments on the key constructs of intrinsic motivation, perceived causality of behaviour, persistence, and contingencies that facilitate or undermine intrinsic motivation. This evidence provided for the first incarnation of the theory, known as cognitive evaluation theory (Deci and Ryan 1985b). Since then, the theory has undergone substantial development and application to achieve its status as a leading meta-theory of human motivation (Deci and Ryan 2000, 2002; Ryan and Deci 2008), with considerable application in many domains where self-directed motivation and self-regulation are pertinent (Ryan *et al.* 2008), including health-related behaviours (Deci and Ryan 2012).

The purpose of the theory is to explain human motivation and behaviour on the basis of individual differences in motivational orientations, contextual influences on motivation, and interpersonal perceptions. Central to self-determination theory is the distinction between self-determined or *autonomous* forms of motivation relative to non-self-determined or *controlling* forms of motivation. The *cognitive evaluation sub-theory* outlines the environmental or contextual contingencies that either support or thwart self-determined motivation. The *organismic integration sub-theory* explains the processes by which people 'take in' or internalize behaviours that may have been initially performed for controlling or non-self-determined reasons and integrate them into their sense of self so that they are performed for more autonomous or self-determined reasons. The *basic psychological needs sub-theory* provides a framework for explaining the origins of self-determined forms of motivation on the basis of innate psychological needs. Finally, the *causality orientations sub-theory* explains how individual differences in the perceived origins of behaviour affect motivation and associated behavioural outcomes. The purpose of this chapter is to provide an overview of the application of self-determination theory to health behaviour including its major hypotheses and predictions, applications, and contributions to health behaviour interventions, as well as outlining future avenues for research.

2 Description of the model

2.1 Theory origins and cognitive evaluation theory

Self-determination theory (SDT) arose from experimental inquiry into how rewards affect motivation in educational contexts. Studies on the effects of rewards and intrinsic motivation on behaviour led to the development of cognitive evaluation theory – an early 'version' and sub-theory of SDT (Deci 1971, 1972). The theory hypothesizes that an individual performing a behaviour for external contingencies like money or fame will persist provided the reward is omnipresent. The withdrawal of the reward is likely to result in desistance. This is known as the 'undermining effect' and occurs because the administration of the reward significantly lowers levels of intrinsic motivation. According to the theory, the mechanism responsible for this is that participants experience a shift in their perceptions of the cause or control of their behaviour (Deci and Ryan 1985b). The person no longer performs the behaviour for intrinsic reasons and the perceived cause or 'origin' of the behaviour shifts from 'within' the person (e.g. as if emanating from the self) to 'outside' the person (i.e. caused by external events). The individual does not, therefore, engage in the behaviour for its own sake and the inherent satisfaction and interest derived from the behaviour itself, but instead engages in it to obtain the reward or externally referenced contingency. A related effect is the 'over-justification' hypothesis, which is conceptually similar to the undermining effect in that the reward or external contingency provides an additional and usually superfluous reason for engaging in the behaviour and, therefore, 'over-justifies' the rationale for engaging in it, but results in the same shift from an internal to external reason for engaging in the behaviour (Lepper *et al.* 1973; Tang and Hall 1995). Perceptions of the cause or origin of a behaviour by individuals became known as the 'perceived locus of causality'.

External contingencies such as rewards, according to SDT, do not always have to lead to decrements in intrinsic motivation. The undermining effect of rewards can be offset by the informational function of the reward. Presenting rewards in such a way that they are merely informative of competence rather than contingent on the behaviour has been found to moderate the undermining effect (Ryan 1982; Ryan *et al.* 1983). Ryan's critical experiments involved providing participants with rewards for engaging in interesting tasks, just as Deci did in his original free-choice paradigm experiments. However, Ryan also included a condition in which participants received competence-related feedback in conjunction with the reward. The competence-related feedback highlighted that the reward was for 'doing well' on the task and that participants were performing according to their own targets. Participants in the feedback condition did not exhibit the undermining effect relative to participants provided with the reward alone. This provided the basis for an extension of cognitive evaluation theory to incorporate the role of social agents in the environment in the promotion or undermining of intrinsic motivation. The extension had important ramifications for the development of the theory and, in particular, its potential as a means to modify and change behaviour.

While the undermining effect and informational function of the reward in cognitive evaluation theory has been found to be a robust effect in social psychology (Tang and Hall 1995; Deci *et al.* 1999a, 1999b; Lepper *et al.* 1999), there are few direct applications of the theory in applied settings such as health behaviour. A probable reason for this is that health behaviours are unlikely to be performed solely for extrinsic rewards or external contingencies. Rather, other forms of contingencies and effects of extrinsic or controlling forms of motivation may be implicated in the control of behaviour in health-related contexts. Cognitive evaluation theory, therefore, provides a starting point for understanding the environmental effects on behaviours, including health behaviour, but the subsequently developed and expanded form of the theory that incorporates additional sub-theories provides the basis of more comprehensive explanations of motivated behaviour and multiple influences (Deci and Ryan 2000). These additional sub-theories provide explanations for the process by which activities are internalized and become autonomously motivated in organismic integration theory, the origins of different forms of motivation in basic needs theory, and the role of individual differences in autonomous and controlled motivational orientation on behaviour in causality orientations theory.

2.2 Organismic integration theory

Organismic integration theory extends the essential distinction between intrinsic and extrinsic forms of motivation outlined in cognitive evaluation theory, and seeks to provide an explanation for the processes by which people assimilate behaviours that are externally regulated and incorporate them into their repertoire of behaviours that are self-determined. Central to organismic integration theory is the perceived locus of causality, which represents a graduated multi-faceted conceptualization of motivational styles or *regulations*, rather than the bivariate distinction outlined in cognitive evaluation theory. These motivational styles are purported to delineate a continuum characterized by two relatively autonomous forms of motivation – *intrinsic motivation* and *identified regulation*, and two relatively controlling forms of motivation – *external regulation* and *introjected regulation* (Ryan and Connell 1989). The distinction between autonomous and controlling forms of motivation, and the more nuanced forms of motivation on the perceived locus of causality continuum, is illustrated in Figure 4.1, points 1 and 2, respectively.

The defining features of the different regulation types are outlined in Figure 4.1, point 3. Specifically, *intrinsic motivation* is the prototypical form of autonomous motivation and reflects engaging in behaviour for the intrinsic satisfaction of the behaviour itself and for no external contingency. *Identified regulation* is also an autonomous form of motivation but is, strictly speaking, extrinsic in nature because behaviour is motivated by the pursuit of personally valued outcomes rather than for the behaviour itself. Pursuing behaviours for external contingencies such as gaining extrinsic rewards or avoiding punishment characterizes *external regulation*. *Introjected regulation* refers to an extrinsic form of motivation in which behavioural control

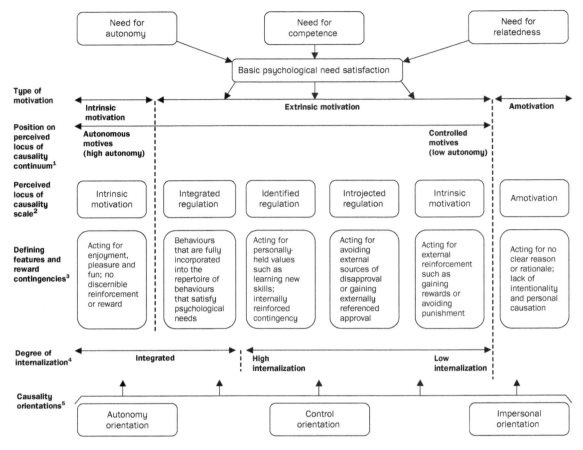

Figure 4.1 Diagrammatic representation of self-determination theory illustrating the components from three of the sub-theories: basic psychological needs theory, organismic integration theory, and causality orientations theory

arises from contingencies administered by the self, such as the pursuit of contingent self-worth or the avoidance of negative affective states such as guilt or shame. Intrinsic motivation and identified regulation lie adjacent to each other at the autonomous extreme of the perceived locus of causality continuum, whiles external regulation and introjected regulation are located alongside each other at the controlling extreme of the continuum (see Figure 4.1, point 2; Ryan and Connell 1989). Importantly, research has supported the discriminant and construct validity of the taxonomy of motivational regulations offered by the perceived locus of causality. For example, intercorrelations among the constructs are proposed to be ordered in a simplex-like pattern (Ryan and Connell 1989). In this pattern, the strongest correlations are exhibited by constructs immediately adjacent to each other on the continuum, with correlations declining in size among constructs in proportion to their relative distance from the construct at the far extremes of the continuum. This means that the correlations of intrinsic motivation with identified regulation and external regulation will be the strongest, while those of intrinsic motivation with introjected and external regulation will be progressively weaker, with the same principle applying to the pattern of correlations of external regulation with identified and external regulation.

The perceived locus of causality continuum has been further differentiated in recent incarnations of organismic integration theory to include the constructs of *integrated regulation* and *amotivation* (see Figure 4.1, points 2 and 3). Researchers have proposed that the process of internalization necessitates the introduction of integrated regulation, which reflects engaging in behaviour because it is completely consistent with one's true sense of self (see Figure 4.1, point 4; Wilson *et al.* 2006a; Duncan *et al.* 2010). This type of regulation reflects behaviours that may have previously been performed for controlled reasons, but have been fully internalized by the individual. Research has demonstrated that integrated regulation achieves discriminant validity with intrinsic motivation and identified regulation, although correlations are substantial (McLachlan *et al.* 2011). Amotivation is a further addition to the continuum. Amotivation is a form of motivation that reflects engaging in tasks for no discernible reason and, effectively, reflects non-intentionality when it comes to acting (Markland and Tobin 2004). This form of motivation has been characterized as a controlling form of motivation, but, probably more correctly, it lies outside the continuum as it has the unique distinguishing feature of having no reason for behaving. Not surprisingly, amotivation is not expected to predict engagement and persistence with tasks and is likely to be unrelated to other forms of regulation on the continuum (Levesque *et al.* 2007).

2.3 Basic needs theory

Basic needs theory is a key sub-theory of the self-determination approach. Deci and Ryan (2000) proposed that the origins of self-determined motivation stem from individuals' innate propensity to satisfy three basic psychological needs: *autonomy*, *competence*, and *relatedness*. These needs are perceived to be *fundamental* to all humans and people approach behaviours in an autonomously motivated fashion because they perceive them to be effective in satisfying psychological needs. The satisfaction of basic psychological needs as a 'driver' of the type of motivational regulations in SDT is illustrated in Figure 4.1. Need satisfaction is depicted at the top of the schematic to illustrate its overarching influence on motivation in multiple contexts. The existence of these basic psychological needs has been justified empirically and research has illustrated that these needs are pervasive across different cultures (Sheldon *et al.* 2001). Basic needs theory is linked with organismic integration theory because it charts the origins of autonomous or self-determined motivational regulations. The perceived locus of causality from organismic integration theory reflects the degree to which behaviours have become internalized or 'taken in', the most complete form of which is integrated regulation (Figure 4.1, point 4). Behaviours that have the propensity to fulfil personally relevant, autonomous goals that individuals value (e.g. exercising to improve fitness or eating healthily to gain more energy for other daily activities), and are perceived as efficacious in satisfying psychological needs, are more likely to be enacted and maintained. Increased participation in such behaviours leads to the behaviour being internalized and finally integrated into the person's repertoire of behaviours that can satisfy these needs. As a result, people may not perform the behaviour for the activity itself as in the 'classic' definition of intrinsic motivation. Rather, they perform it to achieve an intrinsic 'outcome' that is highly valued and perceived to be part of the person's 'true self'.

It is also important to note that the three basic needs are complementary – that is, optimal functioning and truly integrated behaviour can only result if all three psychological needs are supported. For example, competence alone – that is, mastering a technique or skilled action – is not sufficient for a behaviour to be perceived to be need satisfying. Competence coupled with a perception that the behaviour is performed out of a true sense of self – without external contingency, perceived or real, and out of choice and volition (i.e. autonomously regulated) – and that behavioural engagement is supported by others (i.e. relatedness) is necessary for an action to be fully integrated and to support psychological needs. Research has suggested that the basic needs tend to be strongly correlated (Ntoumanis 2005; Standage *et al.* 2005) and can be subsumed by a single global factor (Hagger *et al.* 2006a). Furthermore, interventions that provide synergistic support for the needs of autonomy, competence, and relatedness tend to result in greater behavioural engagement than support for each individual need alone (Deci *et al.* 1994). Overall, the satisfaction of basic psychological needs has been shown to be related to autonomous forms of motivation from the perceived locus of causality consistent with SDT (Hagger *et al.* 2006a; Edmunds *et al.* 2007b; Standage *et al.* 2007), and interventions supporting autonomous motivation have been found to increase psychological need satisfaction as well as motivational regulations (Edmunds *et al.* 2007b).

2.4 Causality orientations theory

A final sub-theory of SDT is causality orientations theory (Deci and Ryan 1985a). Unlike the other sub-theories that focus on the effects of the environment on motivation or the types and quality of motivation experienced towards tasks and behaviours in specific contexts, causality orientations theory adopts an individual difference approach to forms of motivation. The theory proposes that individuals vary in the extent to which they interpret situations and cues in the environment as autonomous or controlled. A distinction is made between *autonomy orientation*, in which individuals have a generalized tendency to interpret ambiguous events as choiceful, interesting, self-determined, and emanating from the self, and *control orientation*, in which individuals tend to interpret events as imposed, pressured, determined by external events, and emanating from outside the self. A third causality orientation has also been identified, labelled *impersonal orientation*, in which individuals tend to view tasks and actions as non-intentional and that their actions are ineffectual in bringing about outcomes. These constructs are considered generalized, stable, and enduring (i.e. trait-like) and likely affect the interpretation of cues and actions in multiple domains (Deci and Ryan 1985a). As with other traits like personality that have the same characteristics, the effects of causality orientations are expected to be relatively weak but consistent across domains (Ferguson 2013; Ferguson *et al.* 2013). The generalized influence of causality orientations on motivational regulations is illustrated in Figure 4.1, point 5. Like need satisfaction, causality orientations are depicted as a global, distal influence on the motivational regulations across multiple contexts. Individuals with an autonomous motivational orientation are likely to align their motivational regulations so that they are consistent with their orientation and, therefore, experience activities and behaviours as more autonomous or intrinsically motivating (Koestner and Zuckerman 1994; Wong 2000; Hagger *et al.* 2014a, 2015). Furthermore, they are also likely to view behaviours as satisfying their basic psychological needs. Importantly, recent evidence suggests that an autonomous motivational orientation is an interpersonal bias that leads individuals to interpret even controlling events such as rewards as more autonomous (Hagger and Chatzisarantis 2011). An autonomy orientation, therefore, offers protection from the deleterious effects of extrinsic or controlling contingencies on intrinsic motivation and serves as a potentially adaptive bias in the interpretation of events.

3 Summary of research

The SDT approach has provided a comprehensive system to explain health-related behaviour in three key areas. First, it has identified motivational constructs that form the antecedents and predictors of health behaviour. The factors include the environmental (e.g. rewards, informational feedback, instruction style) and interpersonal (e.g. basic psychological need satisfaction) factors that affect motivational style or regulation in health behavioural contexts, actual health behaviour, and key psychological outcomes (e.g. intentions to engage in behaviour in the future, psychological well-being). Second, it provides an explanation for the mechanisms by which the antecedent constructs influence health behaviour and other key outcomes; these include mediation and moderation effects. Finally, it provides guidelines on the constructs that interventionists in the field of health promotion can target in order to develop effective strategies that can be incorporated into behavioural modification interventions.

Most studies in health-related contexts have adopted correlational designs and examined the effects of the perceived locus of causality from organismic integration theory on behavioural and psychological outcomes. Research has shown that autonomous forms of regulation are positively related to adaptive behavioural and psychological outcomes in health contexts. For example, research has associated autonomous forms of motivation with increased engagement in, and persistence with, a number of health-related behaviours, including physical activity (Chatzisarantis *et al.* 1997, 2002, 2003; Pelletier *et al.* 2004; Vansteenkiste *et al.* 2004; Fortier and Kowal 2007), healthy eating (Hagger *et al.* 2006b; Mata *et al.* 2009; Jacobs *et al.* 2011), alcohol consumption and drinking alcohol moderately (Neighbors *et al.* 2003; Chawla *et al.* 2009; Hagger *et al.* 2012), and smoking cessation (Williams *et al.* 2002a). As an illustration of the kinds of studies that have been conducted to provide evidence for the predictive validity of SDT in health behaviour contexts, Pelletier *et al.* (2004) demonstrated that autonomous forms of motivation were strongly related to healthy eating with a strong effect size, while controlled forms were related to dysfunctional eating patterns and actually had a weak negative effect on healthy eating. One criticism of this research was that it predicted concurrent behaviour, which, in effect, represents a measure of past rather than future behavioural engagement, which brings into question the direction of the effect (Liska 1984). This has been addressed in other correlational tests of SDT using a prospective design in which motivational constructs from the theory have predicted behaviour measured at a subsequent point in time. For example, Chatzisarantis *et al.* (2002) demonstrated that school pupils' autonomous motivation towards physical activity was significantly related to their participation in physical activity five weeks later mediated by attitudes, intentions, and effort. These studies, and many others, have demonstrated the predictive validity of measures from SDT in accounting for variance in behaviour, and other variables related to behaviour engagement such as intentions. In addition, autonomous motivation has also been associated with adaptive psychological outcomes such as psychological well-being, vitality, and positive emotions (Bartholomew *et al.* 2011; Waaler *et al.* 2012). This is in line with the notion in SDT that autonomous behavioural engagement is consistent with an individual's true 'sense of self' and optimal psychological functioning (Ryan and Deci 2000), as opposed to actions that are not self-endorsed and reflect pressured or coerced reasons for engaging in behaviour, which likely leads to reactance and avoidance if reinforcing contingencies are not omnipresent (Bartholomew *et al.* 2009, 2011).

In addition, autonomous motivation has been shown to be related to key psychological health-related outcomes such as intentions to engage in health behaviour (Hagger *et al.* 2003; Phillips *et al.* 2003; Wilson and Rodgers 2004; Standage *et al.* 2005; Hagger and Chatzisarantis 2007b) and psychological well-being (Pelletier *et al.* 2004; Edmunds *et al.* 2007a; Wilson and Rodgers 2007; Moustaka *et al.* 2012; Standage *et al.* 2012). Furthermore, environmental antecedents such as autonomy support (Edmunds *et al.* 2007b) and people's perceptions that the motivational context is supportive of their autonomous motivation (Hagger *et al.* 2003, 2005; Koka and Hein 2003; Standage *et al.* 2005; Hein and Koka 2007) have also been linked with autonomous motivational regulations, that is, the direct antecedents of intentions and behaviour (see Section 6).

These findings have been supported by recent meta-analyses and systematic reviews of the effects of motivational regulations from the perceived locus of causality on behaviour and outcomes in health settings (Chatzisarantis *et al.* 2003; Ng *et al.* 2012; Teixeira *et al.* 2012a). Chatzisarantis *et al.* (2003) were the first to meta-analyse relations between the motivational orientations from SDT and a health behaviour, namely, sport, exercise, and physical activity contexts. The researchers collected 21 studies from a database literature search and conducted a cumulative synthesis of relations among the intrinsic motivation, identified regulation, introjected regulation, external regulation, and amotivation constructs from the perceived locus of causality and between these constructs and perceived competence towards, and intentions to engage in, sport, exercise, and physical activity behaviours, broadly defined. The authors conducted a path analysis using the meta-analytically derived correlations among these variables and tested a process model in which the effect of perceived competence on sport, exercise, and physical activity intentions was mediated by the perceived locus of causality constructs. Results indicated that the intrinsic motivation construct had the strongest effects on intentions and also mediated the effect of perceived competence on intentions, consistent with hypotheses but, interestingly, there were very weak effects of identified regulation, another autonomous form of regulation, on intentions. This was the first meta-analysis of SDT in health behaviour, and provided support for the role of one form of autonomous motivation, intrinsic motivation, on behaviour. A limitation of this analysis was the exclusive focus on a single category of health behaviour and a relatively small number of studies.

A subsequent systematic review conducted by Teixeira *et al.* (2012a) encompassed a larger sample of studies ($k = 66$, with 72 independent samples) and examined relations between constructs from an extended perceived locus of causality that included integrated motivation based on organismic integration theory and physical activity behaviour, measured using self-report and other objective measures such as accelerometry and pedometry. In addition, the analysis also encompassed relations between exercise regulations and satisfaction of psychological needs of autonomy, competence, and relatedness from basic needs theory, and the autonomy, control, and impersonal causality orientations from causality orientations theory. The review also analysed relations between physical activity and other important variables derived from SDT, including intrinsic, fitness, and body-related motives derived from the Exercise Motivations Inventory (Markland and Hardy 1993). The research also examined the frequency of statistically significant associations between the SDT constructs and physical activity behaviour and other outcomes. Teixeira *et al.* reported consistent relations between autonomous forms of motivation with physical activity behaviour. They also reported that identified regulation was more effective in predicting initial and short-term participation in physical activity, while intrinsic motivation was the stronger predictor of long-term exercise adherence. In addition, competence need satisfaction and intrinsic motives were most effective in predicting physical activity behaviour in multiple samples and settings. Despite the comprehensive literature search, larger sample, and wider array of SDT variables derived from the sub-theories, the analysis had the serious limitation of relying exclusively on null-hypothesis significance testing (Cumming 2014) and did not account for artefacts of error using meta-analytic techniques when sufficient data were available (Hunter and Schmidt 1994; Hagger 2006).

The most comprehensive cumulative analysis of self-determination theory in health contexts to date was conducted by Ng *et al.* (2012). These researchers adopted meta-analytic methods identical to those used by Chatzisarantis *et al.* (2003) and applied them to SDT research from multiple health behaviours (including physical activity, weight loss, smoking abstinence, glycaemic control, medication adherence, eating a healthy diet, and dental hygiene) and used the meta-analytically derived correlations to test specific relations among the variables. They also analysed relations among SDT variables and key health-related outcomes other than behaviour, including negative affect (e.g. depression, anxiety), positive affect (e.g. vitality), and quality of life. They also conducted a comprehensive literature search and identified 184 independent data sets from 166 studies that included published and unpublished data. An additional advance of this analysis was that the authors also examined the effects of interventions based on SDT on health behaviour and also tested process models of relations among SDT variables.

The results of Ng *et al.* (2012) provided further support for the relationship between autonomous motivation and health-related behaviour and behavioural outcomes. In particular, autonomous forms of motivation, such as regulation styles from organismic integration theory and satisfaction of psychological needs from basic psychological needs theory, were statistically significantly and positively related to adaptive health outcomes including 'positive' mental health (meta-analytic correlation (r) range: $r_+ = 0.22$ to 0.62) and physical health, including health behaviours such as physical activity, weight loss, and eating a healthy diet (correlation range: $r_+ = 0.07$ to 0.67). Most important were the intrinsic and identified forms of motivational regulation, which were statistically significantly related to health-related behaviours including physical activity (intrinsic motivation, $r_+ = 0.32$; identified regulation, $r_+ = 0.36$), weight loss (intrinsic motivation, $r_+ = 0.24$; identified regulation, $r_+ = 0.30$), and eating a healthy diet (intrinsic motivation, $r_+ = 0.41$; identified regulation, $r_+ = 0.43$). Ng and colleagues' results provide the most comprehensive support to date for autonomous forms of motivation across multiple mental and physical health-related outcomes, including health-related behaviour, and patterns of relations across studies for autonomous forms of motivation are consistent with hypotheses from SDT. The analysis is also the first to provide these relations for variables related to autonomous motivation from the sub-theories of SDT, including the motivational regulations from organismic integration theory and basic psychological need satisfaction from basic needs theory.

In addition to examining links between SDT constructs and health outcomes, including health behaviour, meta-analytic reviews of SDT have also supported the simplex-like pattern of relations among the regulation styles from organismic integration theory as well as links between constructs from the different sub-theories derived from SDT. Such relations are important in providing empirical support for the proposed links between different components from within the sub-theories (e.g. the 'continuum' or regulation styles from organismic theory), as well as links between constructs between sub-theories (e.g. links between basic psychological need satisfaction and behavioural regulation styles). Overall, studies have generally corroborated hypotheses proposed in the key sub-theories of SDT in research applied to health-behaviour contexts. Chatzisarantis and co-workers' (2003) meta-analysis is the only analysis to date to test a model representing the continuum arrangement of relations among the regulation styles from organismic integration theory. Specifically, they tested a model in which each regulation style predicted the next construct in line from the continuum ranging from external regulation to intrinsic motivation using meta-analytically derived correlations. Results were not entirely consistent with Ryan and Connell's (1989) proposed 'simplex-like' order of relations among the regulation styles, because although strong relations were present between constructs at the extremes (i.e. between external regulation and introjected regulation and between identified regulation and intrinsic motivation), much stronger relations were found between identified and introjected forms of regulation (the regulations in the middle between more autonomous and controlled forms of regulation). However, the indirect effects from the extreme constructs (e.g. external regulation) on other extreme constructs (e.g. intrinsic motivation) were smaller than the indirect effect of more proximal constructs (e.g. introjected regulation on intrinsic motivation). The authors concluded that their data provided some support for the simplex-like relationships, but the pattern was not unequivocal.

Similarly, Ng *et al.* (2012) found theoretically plausible and statistically significant relations among constructs from the different sub-theories of SDT. Specifically, they found statistically significant and positive relations among autonomy-supportive health care 'climate' and basic psychological need satisfaction variables (correlation range: $r_+ = 0.31$ to 0.48), and between autonomy-supportive climate and behavioural regulations from autonomous forms of regulation from organismic integration theory (correlation range: $r_+ = 0.22$ to 0.59). They also found negative relations between basic psychological need satisfaction and controlled forms of regulation (correlation range: $r_+ = -0.05$ to -0.35). These results are consistent with hypotheses from SDT and indicate that relations among measures tapping the constructs from the various sub-theories exhibit theoretically consistent patterns of relations across studies.

4 Developments

Recent research in the health behavioural domain has provided some important innovations to the theories adopting the self-determination approach. Such research is extremely useful, as it not only advances understanding of the motivational antecedents of health behaviour, but also tests the processes and mechanisms proposed in the theory and, therefore, serves to support its predictive and nomological validity. The next sections of this chapter will focus on three areas that have been the subject of recent research in the application of self-determination theory to health contexts: testing process models of the theory, adopting implicit as well as explicit measures of self-determined motivation, and developing integrated approaches using the theory of planned behaviour to provide complementary explanations of self-determined motivation in health contexts.

4.1 Process models of self-determined motivation in health behaviour

The domain of health behaviour has proven an effective 'testing ground' for assessing the predictive validity and mechanisms and processes proposed in SDT. Recent research has attempted go beyond mere tests of relations between the perceived locus of causality from organismic integration theory and health behaviour to test models that integrate the premises of the sub-theories that comprise SDT in a single process model. Process models provide a framework to explain how the different sub-theories complement each other, particularly relations among the core concepts of the sub-theories, including perceived autonomous support and motivational regulations from organismic integration theory and psychological need satisfaction from basic needs theory.

One of the most prominent models is the self-determination process model developed in health care contexts proposed by Williams *et al.* (2002a, 2002b, 2006b) and an elaborated model proposed by Ryan *et al.* (2008). Both models propose that agentic support for autonomous motivation predicts autonomous motivation, which, in turn, predicts key physical and mental health outcomes, particularly engagement in health behaviour and psychological well-being. The effect of autonomy support on the outcomes is proposed to be mediated by autonomous forms of motivation, which corroborates a core hypothesis of SDT that support for autonomous motivation from social agents likely results in positive behavioural and psychological outcomes because it engenders autonomous motivation. The proposed mediational model is depicted in Figure 4.2. Ryan and co-workers' (2008) elaborated process model specifies the exact same pattern of effects, but also includes the satisfaction of needs as a mediator of the effect of autonomy support on autonomous motivation. The model therefore identifies need satisfaction as the mechanism by which autonomy support predicts autonomous forms of motivational regulations (see Figure 4.3). The proposed mechanism indicates that autonomy support leads to autonomous motivation towards engaging in a target behaviour because it provides information that the behaviour is likely to satisfy needs for autonomy, competence, and relatedness. The model therefore provides a nomological framework that integrates two sub-theories of SDT, namely, basic needs theory and organismic integration theory.

Various tests of the models have been conducted in health behaviour contexts and have largely supported the nomological validity of the model. A recent meta-analysis used sample-corrected correlations among components from the theory of planned behaviour to estimate path models testing the proposed pattern of effects in the integrated model (Ng *et al.* 2012). The analysis provideds a robust test of effects in each model because it is based on a relatively large sample ($N = 13,356$ for Williams and co-workers' [2002a, 2006b] model and $N = 8,893$ for Ryan and co-workers' [2008] elaborated model), examines the relative contribution of effects when accounting for the other factors in the model, uses estimates that are ostensibly free of (corrected for) measurement error, and

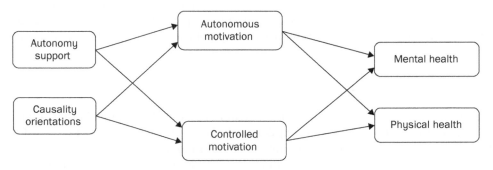

Figure 4.2 Williams and co-workers' (2002a, 2006b) process model based on self-determination theory

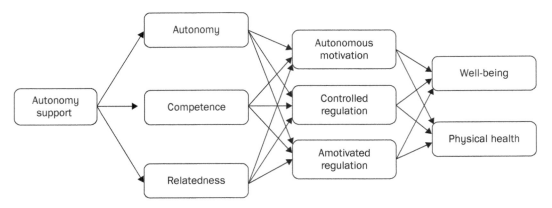

Figure 4.3 Ryan and co-workers' (2008) elaborated process model based on self-determination theory

includes tests of the key mediation processes in the model. Results support the proposed pattern of effects of both models. Specifically, there were direct effects of autonomy support on satisfaction of all three basic psychological needs and indirect effects of autonomy support on autonomous motivation, but not controlled forms of motivation, each mediated by the psychological needs in the elaborated model. This was corroborated in Williams and co-workers' (2002a, 2006b) process model, which confirmed the links between autonomy support and behavioural regulations. In both models, autonomous behavioural regulations were associated with key outcomes including physical health and psychological well-being.

Importantly, while the conceptualization of Ryan and co-workers' (2008) elaborated process model specified multiple indices of physical health including objective measures of behavioural coping with illness (e.g. glycaemic control for diabetics and weight loss in obese and overweight individuals) and engagement in health behaviours (e.g. taking medication, physical activity participation, healthy eating, smoking cessation, and dental hygiene behaviours), studies included in the analysis were confined to healthy eating and physical activity. This points to the need for future research to examine the effects of motivational regulations on a broader range of health-related behaviours. This will not only assist researchers in inferring the generalizability of the proposed effects in the model across multiple health behavioural contexts, which has implications for interventions, but also corroborate a key defining characteristic of social cognitive and motivational models that the processes underpinning the theories represent generalized, universal processes based on information processing metaphors for the effects of cognition on behaviour.

4.2 Importance of implicit processes

There has been a progressive shift in social psychology away from models that focus exclusively on deliberative, intentional, and explicit influences on behaviour in favour of models that also account for the non-conscious, impulsive, and implicit influences on human behaviour (Bargh and Chartrand 1999; Greenwald *et al.* 2002; Kehr 2004; Strack and Deutsch 2004; Nosek *et al.* 2007). Such approaches have given rise to *dual systems* models of motivation that recognize that behaviour is a function of deliberative, volitional, and planned inferences as well as those that are automatic, non-conscious, and unplanned (Strack and Deutsch 2004). Research adopting measures of implicit constructs, such as implicit attitudes towards health behaviours and outcomes, alongside more traditional self-report measures of social cognitive variables has illustrated that behaviour is influenced by both explicit and implicit processes and these effects are relatively independent (Perugini 2005; Spence and Townsend 2007).

Given the increasing attention being paid to implicit processes, researchers have endeavoured to examine the role of implicit processes in self-determined motivation and behaviour. It may be that implicit processes mirror underlying individual differences that predispose individuals to adopt specific motivational styles and responses across multiple behavioural domains. In the context of SDT, implicit motives may reflect the autonomy and control causality orientations specified in the causality orientations sub-theory. Implicit motives may, therefore, account for recent evidence from process models of motivation based on SDT that have found stable, generalized constructs such as basic need satisfaction predict health behaviour directly, independent of contextual motivational orientations and intentions (Hagger *et al.* 2006a; Barkoukis *et al.* 2010). Assuming the indirect effects of the individual difference variables on health behaviour mediated by the explicit motivational and intentional variables reflect more deliberative, intentional pathways to action, the direct effects likely reflect implicit processes and affect behaviour via a process that is beyond the awareness of the individual.

Recent research has included implicit motivational constructs in the prediction of behaviour adopting a SDT approach. Levesque and Pelletier (2003) adopted priming techniques used in previous studies examining implicit processes to activate either autonomous or non-autonomous (termed *heteronomous*) motivational orientations. Using this method they found that priming autonomous and heteronomous motivation influenced participants' perceptions of intrinsic motivation, choice, and competence as well as persistence with subsequent problem-solving tasks consistent with explicit, consciously regulated motivational orientations. Similarly, Burton *et al.* (2006) used a lexical decision task to measure implicit autonomous motivation and found that this measure predicted psychological well-being and academic performance independent of explicit measures of autonomous motivation. Together these studies suggest that the motivational influences from SDT can influence behaviour and other outcomes implicitly and these effects are independent of explicit motivational orientations.

Keatley *et al.* (2012, 201) have recently extended this research to health behavioural contexts by adopting measures of implicit motivational orientations from SDT and included them in the process models of motivation alongside explicit measures of autonomous motivation. In one study, two implicit measures of self-determined motivational orientations based on the implicit association test (IAT) and the Go/NoGo Task (GNAT) were developed. The extent to which the implicit motives tapped by the new measures accounted for variance in health behaviours was tested in a predictive study (Keatley *et al.* 2012). The IAT requires individuals to classify stimuli representing the target category ('autonomous motivation' vs. 'controlled motivation') into an attribute that is related to the self ('me') or others ('others'). The dependent variable is the difference in response time in matching the category stimuli with either the 'self' or 'others', with participants faster in matching 'autonomous' stimuli with the 'self' high in autonomous orientation. The GNAT measure is similar but dichotomizes autonomous and controlled motivation into two constructs rather than viewing them as a continuum, resulting in separate measures of implicit autonomous and controlled motivation. In two studies, implicit measures of motivation from

SDT were included alongside traditional self-report measures of explicit motivational styles as predictors of intentions to perform the health behaviour in the future and self-reported behavioural engagement four weeks later for 20 different health behaviours.

Results indicated that the explicit measures of autonomous and controlling motivational regulations were consistently related to intentions and behaviour in multiple health contexts (Keatley *et al.* 2012). Furthermore, the effects for the explicit measures were mediated by intentions consistent with dual systems theories. There was comparatively weaker support for the direct effects of implicit measures of motivation on behaviour across the set of health behaviours. For example, there were independent effects of implicit autonomous motivation from the GNAT on tooth brushing and sitting with correct posture, effects of implicit autonomous motivation from the IAT on physical activity, and effects of implicit controlled motivation from the GNAT on alcohol consumption and caffeine reduction. Results do not unequivocally support a dual systems approach for all behaviours but do suggest that implicit measures may have unique effects above and beyond explicit measures in some health behaviours. Additionally, results are consistent with our contention derived from individual difference research that such trait-like constructs have comparatively weaker effects on behaviour than domain-specific motivational styles. Future research needs to identify the most effective means to tap implicit forms of autonomous motivation. In addition, although there is some evidence for the predictive validity of implicit motivation from SDT on behaviour, results are preliminary and further corroboration and identification of potential moderators is necessary before confirming the value and implications of these predictions for intervention.

4.3 Theoretical integration

One recent approach to the prediction of health behaviour has been the integration of SDT with the theory of planned behaviour. An integrated model may have utility in addressing the limitations and boundary conditions inherent in each theory: one theory may assist in explaining a process that is unspecified or under-specified in the other. One of the limitations of SDT is that it does not specify precisely how autonomous motivation leads to future behavioural engagement. In other words, it does not specify the psychological mediators of the effect of motivational orientations, such as the behavioural regulations from organismic integration theory, on behaviour. Similarly, the theory of planned behaviour (see Conner and Sparks, Chapter 5 this volume) explains considerable variance in intentions and health behaviour, but is relatively silent on the antecedents of the belief-based constructs that give rise to intentions, namely, attitudes, subjective norms, and perceived behavioural control (Hagger and Chatzisarantis 2007c).

Consideration of the integration of SDT and the theory of planned behaviour is based on Deci and Ryan's (1985b) and Ajzen's (1985) original conceptualization of the respective theories and was pioneered by Chatzisarantis and colleagues (Chatzisarantis *et al.* 1997; Chatzisarantis and Biddle 1998; Hagger *et al.* 2002). Ajzen proposed that the belief-based antecedents of intention, namely, attitudes, subjective norms, and perceived behavioural control, tended to be developed over time and through previous experience, but did not formally specify the process. Deci and Ryan (1985b: 228) state that: 'Cognitive theories [such as the theory of planned behaviour] begin their analysis with...a motive, which is a cognitive representation of some future desired state. What is missing, of course, is the consideration of the conditions of the organism that makes these future states desired.' Therefore, motivational orientations that reflect the extent to which behaviours might permit the satisfaction of psychological needs may drive the formation of beliefs that underpin future action. Analogously, Deci and Ryan also propose that self-determined forms of motivation predict subsequent behaviour by bringing their systems of beliefs and cognition into line with their motivational orientations. Taken together, motives from SDT and the satisfaction of basic psychological needs may serve as antecedents of the belief-based proximal predictors of intention and those beliefs, along with intentions, may act as mediators explaining the process by which motivational orientations lead to behavioural engagement.

The rationale underpinning the integrated mediational model in which the effects of motives from SDT predict behaviour mediated by the belief-based constructs from the theory of planned behaviour is derived from the processes of psychological need satisfaction and internalization. If an individual experiences an activity as autonomously motivated and has internalized it into his or her repertoire of behaviours likely to satisfy psychological needs, he or she is likely to actively pursue opportunities to engage in the activity to further experience the satisfaction of needs derived from the activity. Forming beliefs aligned with the motives is, therefore, adaptive because doing so will likely lead to intentions to pursue the need-satisfying activity in future. Furthermore, beliefs regarding the extent to which engaging in the activity will lead to important personally relevant outcomes (attitudes) and beliefs regarding capacity to engage in the activity (perceived behavioural control) are sets of beliefs that have been shown to be aligned with autonomous motivation (Sheeran *et al.* 1999; McLachlan and Hagger 2010, 2011). This is because autonomous motivation reflects engaging in activities out of a true sense of self, consistent with personal beliefs about outcomes, and engaging in activities to feel an effective agent in the environment, consistent with beliefs about control. Subjective norms are less likely to be aligned with autonomous motivation because the belief is conceptualized as social pressure to engage in the activity, and is therefore more consistent with controlling forms of motivation.

The proposed integrated model is illustrated in Figure 4.4. On the far left of the figure, perceived autonomy support, representing the extent to which individuals perceive social agents in their environment provide support for autonomy in a particular context (e.g. a school pupil's perception that their physical education teacher supports their autonomy), is depicted as predicting self-determined forms of motivation. This represents a test of the hypothesis that autonomous motivation is derived, in part, from the extent to which the individual's environment supports their autonomy. Self-determined motivation is presented as a predictor of the social cognitive antecedents of intention, namely, attitudes, subjective norms, and perceived behavioural control, derived from the theory of planned behaviour. This is consistent with the hypothesis that individuals motivated to engage in a health behaviour for autonomous reasons will report sets of beliefs that are aligned with their motives. Consistent with the theory of planned behaviour, the antecedents of intentions predict health behaviour mediated by intention, with the exception of perceived behavioural control, which also has a direct effect on behaviour. The model presents the 'motivational sequence' such that autonomous motivation, the belief-based antecedents from the theory of planned behaviour, and intentions serve to mediate the indirect effect from perceived autonomy support to behaviour.

Considerable research has supported the role of autonomous motivational orientations – that is, motivation to engage in behaviours that fulfil psychological need-satisfying outcomes – as an influence on intentions and behaviour for a number of health behaviours (e.g. Chatzisarantis *et al.* 2002; Phillips *et al.* 2003; Standage *et al.* 2003; Hagger and Armitage 2004; Wilson and Rodgers 2004; Hagger *et al.* 2006a, 2012; Edmunds *et al.* 2008). A meta-analysis of the health behaviour research

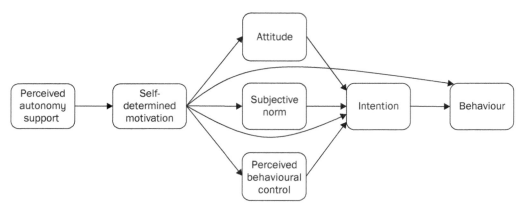

Figure 4.4 Integrated model of self-determination theory and the theory of planned behaviour based on Hagger and Chatzisarantis (2009)

examining effects of autonomous forms of motivation from SDT on intentions, behavioural engagement, and the belief-based antecedents of intentions from the theory of planned behaviour, found a remarkable degree of consistency in the effects across studies (Hagger and Chatzisarantis 2009). Specifically, a path analytic model using the meta-analytically derived correlations provided support for the mediational model depicted in Figure 4.4. There were statistically significant, positive, and medium-sized effects of perceived autonomy support on self-determined motivation (standardized path coefficient, $\beta = 0.31$), of self-determined motivation on attitudes ($\beta = 0.45$) and perceived behavioural control ($\beta = 0.38$), of attitude ($\beta = 0.37$) and perceived behavioural control ($\beta = 0.26$) on intention, and of intention on behaviour ($\beta = 0.27$). The effects of self-determined motivation on subjective norms ($\beta = 0.14$), and subjective norms on intentions ($\beta = 0.06$), were also statistically significant but substantially smaller in size. There was also a statistically significant, albeit small, direct effect of self-determined motivation on intention ($\beta = 0.10$). Most importantly, there was a statistically significant medium-sized indirect effect of self-determined motivation on intentions ($\beta = 0.27$) and a small statistically significant effect of self-determined motivation on behaviour ($\beta = 0.10$) mediated by the motivational sequence, including intentions and its belief-based antecedents (Hagger and Chatzisarantis 2007b). Overall, results provided robust support across studies for the proposed motivational sequence outlined in the integrated model across studies when correcting for sources of bias and controlling for past behaviour.

The utility of the integrated model lies in its potential to provide multiple means for intervention to change health behaviour. The model identifies two potential 'routes' that interventionists can adopt to target behaviour change. The first is through promoting autonomous motivation and the other is through persuasive communication and information provision to change the belief-based antecedents of intention. Chatzisarantis and Hagger (2009) demonstrated the effectiveness of an intervention based on the integrated model in increasing exercise behaviour in young people. The intervention included techniques or strategies that targeted the constructs involved in the different 'routes' to behaviour: an autonomy-supportive intervention involving perceived autonomy support and autonomous motivation from SDT as the mediator of the effect of the intervention of physical activity, and a belief-based intervention involving attitudes and perceived behavioural control from the theory of planned behaviour as mediators of the effect of the intervention on physical activity. The specific techniques involved in these interventions will be reviewed in Section 6 of this chapter. Results indicated that the effects of the autonomy-supportive intervention on physical activity were mediated by perceived autonomy support and autonomous motivation. Similarly, there were independent effects of the theory of planned behaviour (belief-based) intervention on physical activity mediated by attitudes. These findings supported the integrated model and indicated that intervention techniques could be isolated that changed health behaviour by acting on the different, theory-specific, mediating variables.

5 Operationalization of the model

Self-determination theory has typically been operationalized in health behaviour contexts as mediational models that integrate key components from the different sub-theories. Prototypical forms of the mediational models include the models outlined by Williams *et al.* (2002a, 2006b) and Ryan *et al.* (2008) that have been tested in Ng and co-workers' (2012) meta-analysis (see Section 4). Consistent with other models of social cognition, the process models based on SDT are usually tested using cross-sectional or longitudinal correlational studies that adopt self-report measures of model constructs. Operationalization of the constructs used in the process models should begin with the identification of the key model components. The following components should be considered 'core' to the operationalization of the models: forms of behavioural regulations and perceived autonomy support from organismic integration theory, and basic psychological need satisfaction from basic needs theory. As is the case in most tests of social cognitive and motivational models, measures of behavioural engagement or salient health-related outcomes related to behaviour are also important for a meaningful test (cf. Baumeister *et al.* 2007). Finally, tests of the model adopting this design should be analysed using path analysis or structural equation modelling in order to simultaneously test the proposed network or pattern of effects proposed in the model. Such tests provide the most effective means to evaluate the nomological validity of the proposed model (Bagozzi 1981; McLachlan *et al.* 2011).

Standardized measures of all of the core constructs in the process model are available for use in health-behaviour contexts and accessible and readily adaptable for researchers to apply and test the models in health-behaviour contexts, whether or not the measures have been used with the particular behaviour previously. We provide a taxonomy of the measures in Table 4.1, including the construct to which each measure pertains, the sub-theory of SDT from which the construct is derived, a description of the construct scale and sample item, and a typical inventory developed to measure the construct in a health context. All of these scales have been found to be relatively flexible for minor modifications to the specified behavioural context without losing meaning or face validity or violating the psychometric integrity of the scales. Consistent with psychometric scales tapping social cognitive constructs, all of the measures used to tap constructs of the process models use 4- to 7-point response scales. We detail each construct in turn in the following sections.

5.1 Perceived autonomy support

Perceived autonomy support is central to organismic integration theory as it assesses the extent to which individuals believe salient social agents in their environment engender or

Table 4.1 Measures used to tap constructs from self-determination theory, the sub-theory to which they pertain, sample items, and example inventories

Construct	Sub-theory	Description	Sample item	Example inventory
Perceived autonomy support	OIT	The extent to which respondents report that the social agents in the environment (e.g. teacher, parent, medical practitioner, physician) support their autonomous motivation	'I feel that [social agent] understands me'	Health Care Climate Questionnaire (Williams *et al.* 1999)
Intrinsic motivation	OIT	Acting out of external contingency or reinforcement and for the inherent enjoyment and satisfaction derived from the activity itself	'I participate in [health behaviour] because I enjoy it'	Behavioural Regulation in Exercise Questionnaire (Mullan *et al.* 1997)
Integrated regulation	OIT	Acting because the behaviour is consistent with one's true sense of self	'I participate in [health behaviour] because it is an important part of who I am'	Modified Behavioural Regulation in Exercise Questionnaire (McLachlan *et al.* 2011)
Identified regulation	OIT	Acting out of personally valued outcomes	'I participate in [health behaviour] because it is important to me'	Behavioural Regulation in Exercise Questionnaire (Mullan *et al.* 1997)
Introjected regulation	OIT	Acting to gain (e.g. contingent self-esteem) or avoid (e.g. shame or guilt) an externally referenced outcome	'I participate in [health behaviour] because I will feel guilty if I don't'	Behavioural Regulation in Exercise Questionnaire (Mullan *et al.* 1997)
External regulation	OIT	Acting out of external contingency or reinforcement	'I participate in [health behaviour] because I will be punished if I don't'	Behavioural Regulation in Exercise Questionnaire (Mullan *et al.* 1997)
Amotivation	OIT	Acting for no apparent reason or intention	'I don't really see why I participate in [health behaviour]'	Modified Behavioural Regulation in Exercise Questionnaire (Markland and Tobin 2004).
Autonomy need satisfaction	BPNT	Perception that acting is consistent with one's genuine sense of self and the self is the origin of one's actions	'I feel free to do [health behaviour]'	Psychological Need Satisfaction in Exercise Scale (Wilson *et al.* 2006b)
Competence need satisfaction	BPNT	Perception of feeling effective in producing behavioural outcomes	'I feel very capable in doing [health behaviour]'	Psychological Need Satisfaction in Exercise Scale (Wilson *et al.* 2006b)

Table 4.1 *Continued*

Construct	Sub-theory	Description	Sample item	Example inventory
Relatedness need satisfaction	BPNT	Perception that salient social agents provide support for one's actions consistent with self-determined reasons for acting	'I feel close and connected with people who do [health behaviour]'.	Psychological Need Satisfaction in Exercise Scale (Wilson *et al.* 2006b)

Note: OIT = organismic integration theory; BPNT = basic psychological needs theory.

create a 'climate' that supports their motivation. Measures of perceived autonomy support have typically adopted the Health Care Climate Questionnaire (Williams *et al.* 1999), or variants of it (Hagger *et al.* 2007), a measure that requires respondents to report the extent to which social agents display specific behaviours likely to foster autonomous motivation in health care contexts. Items reflect the defining features typically thought to engender autonomous motivation, such as support for choice, encouraging the setting of personally relevant goals, adopting a questioning approach, and providing positive feedback (see Table 4.1 for examples). The measures have typically been used in correlational tests of process models such as those proposed by Williams *et al.* (2002a, 2006b), Ryan *et al.* (2008), and Hagger and Chatzisarantis (2009).

5.2 Behavioural regulations

Measures of the behavioural regulations from organismic integration theory have typically used adapted forms of Ryan and Connell's (1989) questionnaire, originally developed in an educational context, which taps the key constructs from the motivational continuum (e.g. Mullan *et al.* 1997). The core constructs include measures of intrinsic motivation and identified, introjected, and external regulations (see Table 4.1 for examples). These measures include Mullan and colleagues' (1997) Behavioural Regulations in Exercise Questionnaire and the Treatment Self-Regulation Questionnaire (Ryan *et al.* 1995). These inventories are all based on the original measures of constructs from the perceived locus of causality continuum first developed by Ryan and Connell (1989). Various authors have subsequently augmented the measures to include additional constructs important to the theory. The first is *integrated regulation*, which is a more nuanced form of identified regulation (e.g. McLachlan *et al.* 2011). Integrated regulation is defined as the extent to which behaviours have not only been internalized but integrated into the sets of behaviours that satisfy psychological needs and are consistent with the individual's true sense of self. A second added construct is *amotivation* (e.g. Markland and Tobin 2004), which reflects engaging in tasks for no discernible reason. Both of these feature in modified versions of the scale (see Table 4.1 for examples). The behaviour regulations feature heavily in research examining relations between autonomous and controlled forms of motivation in process models of SDT, particularly tests of organismic integration theory. They are typically used to measure the extent to which health behaviours are incorporated into sets of behaviours that service psychological needs and are, therefore, likely to be persisted with. They are also used to determine the extent to which health behaviours are not internalized or integrated as satisfying psychological needs and are, therefore, perceived as being controlled by external contingencies and less likely to be persisted with in the absence of the controlling contingency.

5.3 Basic psychological need satisfaction

Basic psychological need satisfaction has been typically measured in health behavioural contexts using modified versions of the scales developed by Sheldon and colleagues (e.g. Sheldon *et al.* 2001; Sheldon and Bettencourt 2002) to tap the extent to which respondents perceive their psychological needs for autonomy, competence, and relatedness are satisfied (see Table 4.1 for examples). The scales are generally tailored towards the particular behaviour, and there are variants that have been tested extensively in physical activity (Hagger *et al.* 2006a, 2006b; Chatzisarantis *et al.* 2012) and healthy eating (Hagger *et al.* 2006a) behaviours. Although more generalized versions of the need satisfaction scales exist, these are perhaps less desirable in tests of the process model in health contexts and more generalized scales typically produce substantially smaller effects. Although confirmatory factor analyses of measures of the three basic psychological needs constructs support the discriminant validity of the constructs, they are typically strongly correlated and can be subsumed by a single higher-order factor, consistent with the notion that satisfaction of the needs is complementary (Hagger *et al.* 2006a).

5.4 Study designs

Study designs testing the process model are typically cross-sectional and such tests have utility in that they provide some corroboration for the proposed model effects. However, the correlational nature of such tests limits their value in determining the causes of health behaviour and an increasing body of research is adopting longitudinal (Hagger *et al.* 2006b), cross-lagged panel (Guay *et al.* 2003), and experimental designs (Burton *et al.* 2006) to better infer causality among constructs, a typical problem encountered in tests of social cognition models (see Conner and Norman, Chapter 1 this volume). Researchers are therefore advised to be mindful of the relative contribution a correlational study can make in terms of understanding the processes of the model and design their study accordingly. We strongly recommend the adoption of panel or experimental designs. Both forms of data are more demanding to collect than cross-sectional correlational research given the need to take measurements at multiple time points or administer manipulations of the typical variables. However, the pay-off is substantial given that cross-lagged panel and experimental designs permit better inference of the causal arrangement of variables and are often rated of higher quality than cross-sectional data (Hagger *et al.* 2003; Nouwen *et al.* 2011; Fortier *et al.* 2012).

A major problem faced by researchers when testing the proposed effects in process models based on SDT in health behaviour is the relatively large number of constructs, which adds complexity to path and structural equation models based on the theory. This presents problems when testing models in comparatively small samples, as the statistical power is substantially reduced raising the possibility of type 2 errors, namely, an inability to find true effects and reject the null hypothesis. An obvious solution would be to ensure that the study is adequately powered in terms of sample size. However, obtaining an adequately powered study with a sufficiently large sample size presents a challenge when it comes to collecting data from hard-to-reach clinical samples where numbers of participants may be limited. In addition, other problems arise with the inclusion of measures of constructs that have considerable conceptual and empirical overlap, such as the identified regulation, integrated regulation, and intrinsic motivation constructs and external regulation, introjected regulation, and amotivation constructs on the perceived locus of causality. The issue of complexity notwithstanding, the relatively high correlations among measures of these constructs may introduce problems of multicollinearity in models based on regression such as path analysis and structural equation modelling. Such problems cause inaccurate and unstable estimates of effects in the model and make it difficult to ascertain their true pattern of interrelationship.

A relatively elegant solution to the problem of multiple constructs has been to reduce their number by aggregating them into single, global constructs. This is based on the proposed simplex-like pattern of relations among constructs on the continuum, with constructs situated farther away from intrinsic motivation, the prototypical form of autonomous regulation, reflecting progressively lower levels of intrinsic motivation. A typical approach has been to use weighted composites that represent the global construct of interest. This includes the self-determination index or relative autonomy index, which is a single construct representing the degree of autonomous motivation or self-determination an individual experiences for the target behaviour. It is computed by assigning weights to scores on each construct according to their position on the continuum and then aggregating the weighted scores on each form of regulation into a single score. As the index is supposed to reflect degree of autonomy, autonomous forms of motivation are assigned positive weights and controlled forms of regulation are assigned negative weights. For example, intrinsic motivation, integrated regulation, and identified regulation are typically assigned weights of +3, +2, and +1, respectively and amotivation, extrinsic regulation, and introjected regulation weights of –3, –2, and –1, respectively (Pelletier and Sarrazin 2007). This approach has been used in many studies adopting SDT in health contexts in order to increase the parsimony and minimize analytic difficulties when testing the model (Guay *et al.* 2003; Ntoumanis 2005; Hagger *et al.* 2006a, 2006b; Chan and Hagger 2012b; Standage *et al.* 2012). However, problems have been identified with the proposal that the measures from scales based on the perceived locus of causality represent a continuum and follow a simplex-like pattern. Chemolli and Gagné (2014) demonstrated that the proposed pattern was violated in many cases; for example, introjected and identified regulation frequently correlated together significantly and with stronger effect size than with their respective adjacent constructs intrinsic and external regulations, respectively. Chemolli and Gagné proposed that if weighted composites are to be used, they should reflect separate autonomous and controlled forms of regulation, such that the weighted constructs of the autonomous and controlled forms of regulation from the 'continuum' are grouped together to form two separate autonomous and controlled constructs. This approach has also been used effectively in numerous studies and allows for testing the independent effects of autonomous and controlled forms of regulation (e.g. Pelletier *et al.* 2004; Chan and Hagger 2012a; Chan *et al.* 2014). The use of separate autonomous and controlling constructs is more in keeping with the original conceptualization of the locus of causality and with the proposed structure of Williams and co-workers' (2002a, 2006b) and Ryan and co-workers' (2008) process models (see Figures 4.1 and 4.2).

6 Intervention studies

Intervention and experimental studies testing relations among variables in the process models based on SDT (Williams *et al.* 2002b, 2006a; Ryan *et al.* 2008) through the manipulation of one or more model variables and observing their effects on others are very rare in health behaviour contexts, but the value of such data should be rated highly. Most studies that have manipulated variables from the process models are best characterized as interventions. This is because they have typically been conducted in applied settings and used manipulations that are programmes of autonomy support rather than isolating single strategies or techniques matched to specific mediating variables. They have also been conducted in applied health care settings where control over extraneous factors is less stringent than is typically expected in experimental contexts. There is therefore a need for experimental research in health contexts, which can perhaps best be characterized as 'field experiments' that allow for formal manipulations of the process model variables (Mullan *et al.* 2014). Factorial designs would be considered gold standard in this regard in that they typically isolate one or more manipulations that aim to affect change in a single mediator and its effects on behaviour, similar to the design adopted by Sniehotta (2009) for the theory of planned behaviour. For example, a replication of Deci and co-workers' (1994) classic 'autonomy-support' experiment in which components of autonomy support, namely, provision of choice, providing rationale, and acknowledging conflict, were manipulated alone or in synergy is needed in a health behaviour context. Such tests will elevate the level of support for the causal nature of the effects in the model, including the proposed mediators.

There are good examples of field experiments of self-determination theory focusing on careful manipulation of autonomy support as a means to promote autonomous motivation and the effects of the manipulation on behaviour. To qualify as a field experiment, the research requires careful control of the key variable in a health-related context, with very strong control over extraneous factors such as the potential for additional information to change or contaminate the data and variations in the way in which the intervention was administered. Chatzisarantis *et al.* (2012), for example, examined the effects of an autonomy-support message in promoting gym attendance in young people. Participants ($N = 152$) were randomly allocated to three conditions: an autonomy-support condition, a comparison condition receiving only one component of autonomy support, and a control condition. For the autonomy-support condition, researchers administered clearly defined text-based messages to participants that provided a rationale for attending the gym, acknowledged the difficulties involved, and provided choice over whether or not to engage in the intervention. These components are the three hallmarks of autonomy support as they foster self-determined perceptions and highlight the autonomous function of the behaviour. In the comparison condition, participants were provided with a message that provided a rationale (only one of the components of autonomy support) without the acknowledgement of conflict or choice components. Participants allocated to the control or 'forced-choice' condition were provided with instructions to comply with gym attendance with no support. The messages were presented in a controlled manner in a laboratory environment via written communication in experimental cubicles in the laboratory. This demonstrates extreme control over the manipulations, hence the study is classified as a field experiment. Behaviour was measured objectively using gym attendance. Results indicated that participants allocated to both the autonomy-support and rationale-only conditions were more likely to attend the gym compared with those allocated to the forced-choice control condition. These results are important, as they demonstrate the effectiveness of an intervention including components from SDT, relative to non-self-determined controlling components, in promoting health-related behaviour. It also adopts a factorial design to test isolated components that comprise autonomy-supportive interventions, in this case the condition adopting three autonomy-support components (autonomy-support condition) and the condition adopting a single component (rationale only).

Interventions to promote increased engagement in health behaviour based on SDT have focused on the core construct of autonomy support. The role that social agents play in promoting self-directed behavioural engagement by increasing autonomous motivation is central to SDT. Autonomy support encapsulates a set of key behaviours that social agents would be expected to display that make the psychological need-satisfying aspects of the behaviour salient to the individual and, thereby, foster autonomous motivation. Research has identified numerous behaviours aligned with one or more of the basic psychological needs from the theory and they form the basis of autonomy-support interventions. This work has also been accompanied by training programmes aimed at instructing social agents such as teachers and health practitioners precisely how to implement the autonomy-supportive behaviours in practice. There is also evidence that interventions using print communication to deliver the autonomy-supportive intervention are effective (e.g. Chatzisarantis and Hagger 2009; Jacobs et al. 2011; Chatzisarantis et al. 2012). The cornerstone of autonomy-supportive interventions are behaviours that engender a motivational 'climate' in which individuals feel their needs are being supported but are also not undermined by controlling contingencies such as deadlines, negative feedback, and rewards.

Cheon et al. (2012) have recently developed a comprehensive autonomy-support training programme encompassing an array of autonomy-supportive behaviours with the goal of nurturing 'inner' motivational resources by supporting psychological needs, providing explanations and rationales for acting and highlighting the personal utility of the action or behaviour, and acknowledging potential conflict or negative affects accompanying some courses of action. Behaviours typically expected to be displayed by a social agent adopting an autonomy-supportive style to promote a health behaviour include providing a choice over activities and courses of action wherever possible, offering encouragement, providing a meaningful rationale for acting and prompting the development of personal rationales for engaging in the behaviour, adopting a questioning rather than didactic approach, providing informational feedback, being responsive to questions, and acknowledging the perspective of the person. It is also important that the social agent avoids (i) controlling language, (ii) a focus on externally referenced feedback and contingencies for behaviour (e.g. rewards), and (iii) a didactic approach. These autonomy-supportive programmes have typically been delivered verbally by the social agent such as a health care professional. The principles of autonomy support, however, can also be delivered using print communication through the language used in delivering the health messages (e.g. using supportive and avoiding controlling language) and content (e.g. providing rationale, acknowledging conflict) (e.g. Chatzisarantis et al. 2012). Autonomy-supportive interventions would be expected to adopt a number of these stylistic or content components.

Autonomy-supportive interventions based on SDT have shown utility in promoting engagement in health behaviours. Autonomy-supportive interventions delivered by health care professionals have resulted in significantly greater behavioural engagement in numerous health contexts, including smoking cessation (Williams et al. 2002a, 2006a, 2006b; Niemiec et al. 2009), engaging in self-care behaviours in diabetics (Williams et al. 1998, 2004), participating in physical activity (Silva et al. 2010), and fruit and vegetable consumption (Resnicow et al. 2008). The interventions have generally adopted appropriate randomized controlled designs and interventions that target multiple components from SDT to change behaviour, and have not included the strict controls adopted in 'field experiments' such as that reported by Chatzisarantis *et al.* (2012). However, their design features include validated outcome measures variables that are clearly linked to the target health behaviour.

Williams and colleagues' research adopting autonomy-supportive interventions in clinical settings to promote more effective health behaviour serves as a prime example of intervention studies based on self-determination theory. In one study, Williams *et al.* (2006a) randomly allocated nicotine-dependent patients to two conditions, an autonomy-supportive condition and a control condition. Participants allocated to the autonomy-supportive condition received an 'intensive' intervention including print messages from a quit-smoking campaign and autonomy-supportive counselling from a trained counsellor on smoking cessation. Participants allocated to the control 'community care' condition received the print quit-smoking messages only and were encouraged to seek help by visiting their physician. The counsellors in the autonomy-supportive condition received training on autonomy support and were instructed on how to adopt an autonomy-supportive interpersonal style to encourage patients to make their own choices and to support competence for quitting smoking by establishing a clear cessation plan. The primary dependent variable was rates of cessation among participants at both one- and six-month follow-up. Cessation was measured using a biochemically validated self-report point-prevalence measure asking participants to report whether or not they had smoked in the previous seven days. The measure was validated against measures of serum cotinine. Secondary dependent variables were behavioural regulations measured by the Health Care Climate Questionnaire, and these were also hypothesized mediators of the effects of the intervention on the primary dependent measure of smoking abstinence.

Results indicated statistically significant effects of the autonomy-support intervention on smoking abstinence measured at six-month follow-up. Participants allocated to the intervention condition exhibited statistically significantly higher rates of abstinence (11.8%) relative to those allocated to the community-care condition (4.1%). The authors also tested a process model using structural equation modelling in which baseline and follow-up measures of autonomous motivation and perceived competence were set as predictors of smoking cessation at six-month follow-up and compared the effects across the intervention and control group. Results revealed that the autonomous motivation and competence perceptions significantly predicted the abstinence outcomes in both community samples, with perceived competence having a stronger effect in the intervention group than the community care group.

The intervention is an effective one with strong design features that means the data are of high quality. These design features include: (1) the adoption of a randomized controlled design with a clear and valid comparison or control group; (2) an intention-to-treat analysis; (3) the use of an objectively validated measure reflecting a clinically significant outcome related to the target behaviour of smoking cessation; and (4) the test of a SDT process model in which the effects of theory-based psychological variables predicted smoking cessation and its effects compared across intervention conditions. These features are good examples of the components that should be included in evaluations of health behaviour interventions adopting components from SDT. Limitations of the study included differences in the amount and level of support across the intervention and control groups, with the intervention group receiving more 'intensive' intervention relative to the control group, making it difficult to ascertain whether the intervention components themselves (i.e. autonomy-supportive style adopted by the counsellor) or the intensiveness of the intervention were responsible for the intervention effects.

In terms of overall evidence for the effectiveness of autonomy support on health-related outcomes, Ng *et al.* (2012) examined the effects of autonomy-supportive conditions, based on SDT, on health behavioural outcomes in their meta-analysis. Results revealed small-to-medium effect sizes for the effect of autonomy support on health behaviour. Specifically, Ng *et al.* identified that autonomy-supportive conditions were statistically significantly related to mental health outcomes (correlation range: $r_+ = 0.22$ to 0.37) and physical health including health-related behaviours (correlation range: $r_+ = 0.08$ to 0.39). The strongest effect was between autonomy support for dental hygiene ($r_+ = 0.39$), eating a healthy diet ($r_+ = 0.29$), physical activity behaviour ($r_+ = 0.23$), and weight loss ($r_+ = 0.28$), with much weaker effects for medication adherence ($r_+ = 0.08$), smoking abstinence ($r_+ = 0.12$), and glycaemic control ($r_+ = 0.08$). However, it must be stressed that few of these were experimental or intervention studies and no moderation analysis of the autonomy support–autonomous motivation relationship by study type (intervention/experimental vs. correlational) was reported. Nevertheless, it would appear that interventions based on SDT have utility in promoting health behaviour consistent with theoretical predictions. It must be emphasized that, relative to other models, the number of interventions based on SDT in health care contexts is small, and further assessment of the effectiveness of SDT interventions is needed.

It is also important to note that the components of SDT interventions have not been fully isolated and itemized in taxonomies of behaviour change techniques that have been employed to isolate the active components of behaviour change interventions (Michie *et al.* 2013). This is an important omission and one that will not only have implications for SDT and interventions based on it, but also for the taxonomies themselves. This is because key components of SDT-based interventions are communicated through interpersonal style rather than content (Hagger and Hardcastle 2014). Taxonomies of techniques tend to be content-based, and very little has been written about the style in which the techniques should be delivered. While some autonomy-supportive techniques are content-oriented, such as those providing a meaningful rationale and feedback or offering choice, techniques such as using autonomy-supportive language and avoiding controlling language focus on interpersonal style. Such 'stylistic' techniques may require a modification or revision of taxonomies to recognize that techniques relating to interpersonal style such as those from SDT can be applied to content-related behaviour change techniques. For example, incentives such as rewards or feedback can be presented in an autonomy-supportive or controlling manner (Hagger *et al.* 2014b). According to SDT, this will determine whether the reward maintains or undermines intrinsic motivation, which will have implications for behavioural persistence. Further work is needed to classify the behaviour change techniques, both content and interpersonal style components, and examine their effects on behaviour.

7 Future directions

There are numerous gaps in the literature on SDT applied to health behaviour contexts and these issues are priority areas for future research. Key areas for future research include the need for factorial designs to isolate the specific components of autonomy-support programmes that impact on health behaviour, providing further replications of autonomy-support interventions in multiple domains of health behaviour, and testing more elaborate process models that incorporate constructs from the sub-theories that comprise SDT and implicit processes. We will elaborate on these future research directions in this section.

7.1 Factorial experimental designs

Factorial experimental designs are necessary to elucidate the precise mechanisms by which the multiple components that comprise autonomy support affect health behaviour. As we outlined earlier, much of the research that has adopted SDT to change health behaviour has adopted an intervention approach, which usually means including a raft of autonomy-supportive techniques and behaviours delivered by social agents. A good example of this is the autonomy-support training programme proposed by Cheon *et al.* (2012) that comprises multiple techniques and behaviours. While the effects of these interventions on health behaviour have been shown to be significant and substantive and mediated by the relevant variable from the theory (i.e. perceived autonomy support), the studies testing these effects do not provide a fully satisfactory process evaluation of the effectiveness of the intervention. The fact that autonomy support comprises multiple techniques and behaviours means that such interventions cannot isolate the individual technique(s) and or behaviour(s) that lead to behaviour change. Of course, there is the possibility that all of the techniques and behaviours may have unique effects on health behaviour, but until the independent effect of each has been tested, it is not possible to provide unequivocal confirmation. Furthermore, it may be that different techniques act synergistically in changing behaviour, but these cannot be distinguished in designs that include all the techniques in a single manipulation. The differentiation of intervention components into single, unique techniques and behaviours is consistent with taxonomies of behaviour change that have aimed to break down interventions into the fundamental components that cannot be further separated and works towards process evaluation of the effectiveness of interventions (Michie and Johnston 2012; Hagger and Hardcastle 2014). The use of factorial designs in which individual techniques are manipulated independently and, potentially, interactively alongside each other is the solution. There is already some precedent for this in laboratory studies of autonomy support. For example, Deci *et al.* (1994) demonstrated the independent effects of providing choice, providing rationale, and acknowledging conflict, and the synergistic effects of these techniques on novel behaviours in a laboratory setting. A similar approach was taken by Sniehotta (2009) in adopting a factorial design to test the independent effects of techniques to change components from the theory of planned behaviour on health behaviour. A future experiment could, for example, include separate manipulations of provision of choice and provision of positive feedback (two components of autonomy supportive interventions) on health behaviours in a 2×2 design, which would permit a test of each component alone and together with the absence of both as a control condition. Theory predicts that both would have independent effects, but the relative strength of the effect or potential interaction would be of interest and may provide an indication as to whether either one or both of these components is best targeted in an intervention.

7.2 Need for replication

Replications of autonomy-support interventions are also needed in multiple health behaviours. Ng *et al.* (2012) indicated that interventions adopting autonomy-support techniques have been successful with small-to-medium effect sizes, but the effects have been confined to two behaviours, healthy eating and physical activity participation, with relatively small numbers of studies ($k < 10$). Further research is needed to replicate these findings in the same domains in order to provide more robust findings, but also to extend the test to a wider range of behavioural domains. Such research will not only provide a stronger basis to ascertain the true size of the effect, but will also contribute to the theoretical development by testing the relative generality of effects. A key premise of SDT and other social cognition models is that its effects extend to the population and reflect generalized, universal processes consistent with information-processing metaphors for cognition and behaviour (Chatzisarantis *et al.* 2012). To the extent that the effects of autonomy support are relatively homogenous and invariant across behaviours, we will gain confirmatory evidence for this generality hypothesis.

7.3 Implicit processes

A final suggested future direction for research is to further examine the role of implicit motivational orientations from SDT on health behaviour. While there is evidence for some relatively modest effects of implicit measures of motivation on health behaviour, the effects were relatively weak, restricted to a small number of behaviours, and did not have the pervasive effects of explicitly measured forms of motivation (Keatley *et al.* 2012, 2013). However, this does not mean the current tests should provide sufficient evidence to abandon inquiry into implicit processes in health behaviour models based on SDT. Research is needed to better validate the measures of implicit autonomous motivation, which are in their infancy. Furthermore, establishing the types of behaviours likely to be subject to more implicit processes is a fruitful endeavour. There is also the need to evaluate the effects of autonomous motivation on health behaviour in light of key individual-difference variables from SDT, namely, causality orientations (Deci and Ryan 1985a). If implicit self-determined constructs are congruent with individual differences in autonomy and controlled orientations and their effects on health behaviour, the implicit motives could be conceptualized as mediators of the effects of those variables on behaviour. The mediating role of implicit motives would provide an explanation why causality orientations lead to biases in behavioural engagement, as they reflect underlying implicit motives that affect behaviour beyond the awareness of the individual. The value of establishing the extent to which behaviours are predicted by implicit motives, and individual differences in causality orientations, lies in enabling interventionists to appropriately target intervention efforts that match the underlying biases of the individuals and establish the extent to which individuals require additional support to overcome the bias.

7.4 Summary

Despite its relative complexity, SDT has been shown to be effective in explaining variance in a number of health behaviours and has shown efficacy as a basis for interventions. The construct of autonomy support has been shown to be particularly efficacious in this regard with auton- omy-supportive training programmes based on the theory developed to provide interventionists with the necessary skills and techniques to implement theory-based interventions in multiple health behaviour contexts. Future research on the long-term efficacy of the theory in predict- ing behaviour, perhaps using panel designs, in a wider range of health behaviours is warranted, given Ng and co-workers' (2012) finding that the majority of tests of the theory have been confined to a relatively narrow set of behaviours. Developing factorial designs that can isolate the active ingredients of autonomy-support interventions and elucidating the role of implicit constructs in the context of the theory are also avenues that would merit further investigation. Self-determination theory is receiving increased attention from researchers and practitioners in health contexts because of its unique focus on self-directed behaviour change, through the key person-centred construct of autonomous motivation. This means that the future of the theory as a way of predicting and changing health behaviour is bright.

References

Ajzen, I. (1985) From intentions to actions: a theory of planned behavior, in J. Kuhl and J. Beckmann (eds.) *Action-Control: From Cognition to Behavior*. Heidelberg: Springer.

Bagozzi, R.P. (1981) An examination of the validity of two models of attitude, *Multivariate Behavioral Research*, 16, 323–59.

Bargh, J.A. and Chartrand, T.L. (1999) The unbearable automaticity of being, *American Psychologist*, 54, 462–79.

Barkoukis, V., Hagger, M.S., Lambropoulos, G. and Torbatzoudis, H. (2010) Extending the trans-contextual model in physical education and leisure-time contexts: examining the role of basic psychological need satisfaction, *British Journal of Educational Psychology*, 80, 647–70.

Bartholomew, K.J., Ntoumanis, N. and Thøgersen-Ntoumani, C. (2009) A review of controlling motivational strategies from a self-determination theory perspective: implications for sports coaches, *International Review of Sport and Exercise Psychology*, 2, 215–33.

Bartholomew, K.J., Ntoumanis, N., Ryan, R.M., Bosch, J.A. and Thøgersen-Ntoumani, C. (2011) Self-determination theory and diminished functioning: the role of interpersonal control and psychological need thwarting, *Personality and Social Psychology Bulletin*, 37, 1459–73.

Baumeister, R.F., Vohs, K.D. and Funder, D.C. (2007) Psychology as the science of self-reports and finger movements: whatever happened to actual behavior? *Perspectives on Psychological Science*, 2, 396–403.

Burton, K.D., Lydon, J.E., D'Alessandro, D.U. and Koestner, R. (2006) The differential effects of intrinsic and identified motivation on well-being and performance: prospective, experimental, and implicit approaches to self-determination theory, *Journal of Personality and Social Psychology*, 91, 750–62.

Chan, D.K.C. and Hagger, M.S. (2012a) Self-determined forms of motivation predict sport injury prevention and rehabilitation intentions, *Journal of Science and Medicine in Sport*, 15, 398–406.

Chan, D.K.C. and Hagger, M.S. (2012b) Trans-contextual development of motivation in sport injury prevention among elite athletes, *Journal of Sport and Exercise Psychology*, 34, 661–82.

Chan, D.K.C., Fung, Y.-K., Xing, S. and Hagger, M.S. (2014) Myopia prevention, near work, and visual acuity of college students: integrating the theory of planned behavior and self-determination theory, *Journal of Behavioral Medicine*, 37, 369–80.

Chatzisarantis, N.L.D. and Biddle, S.J.H. (1998) Functional significance of psychological variables that are included in the theory of planned behaviour: a self-determination theory approach to the study of attitudes, subjective norms, perceptions of control and intentions, *European Journal of Social Psychology*, 28, 303–22.

Chatzisarantis, N.L.D. and Hagger, M.S. (2009) Effects of an intervention based on self-determination theory on self-reported leisure-time physical activity participation, *Psychology and Health*, 24, 29–48.

Chatzisarantis, N.L.D., Biddle, S.J.H. and Meek, G.A. (1997) A self-determination theory approach to the study of intentions and the intention–behaviour relationship in children's physical activity, *British Journal of Health Psychology*, 2, 343–60.

Chatzisarantis, N.L.D., Hagger, M.S., Biddle, S.J.H. and Karageorghis, C. (2002) The cognitive processes by which perceived locus of causality predicts participation in physical activity, *Journal of Health Psychology*, 7, 685–99.

Chatzisarantis, N.L.D., Hagger, M.S., Biddle, S.J.H., Smith, B. and Wang, J.C.K. (2003) A meta-analysis of perceived locus of causality in exercise, sport, and physical education contexts, *Journal of Sport and Exercise Psychology*, 25, 284–306.

Chatzisarantis, N.L.D., Hagger, M.S., Kamarova, S. and Kee, A.Y.H. (2012) When effects of the universal psychological need for autonomy on health behaviour extend to a large proportion of individuals: a field experiment, *British Journal of Health Psychology*, 17, 785–97.

Chawla, N., Neighbors, C., Logan, D., Lewis, M.A. and Fossos, N. (2009) The perceived approval of friends and parents as mediators of the relationship between self-determination and drinking, *Journal of Studies on Alcohol and Drugs*, 70, 92–100.

Chemolli, E. and Gagné, M. (2014) Evidence against the continuum structure underlying motivation measures derived from self-determination theory, *Psychological Assessment*, 26, 575–85.

Cheon, S.H., Reeve, J. and Moon, I. (2012) Experimentally based, longitudinally designed, teacher-focused intervention to help physical education teachers be more autonomy supportive toward their students, *Journal of Sport and Exercise Psychology*, 34, 365–96.

Cumming, G. (2014) The new statistics: why and how, *Psychological Science*, 25, 7–29.

DeCharms, R. (1968) *Personal Causation: The Internal Affective Determinants of Behavior*. New York: Academic Press.

Deci, E.L. (1971) Effects of externally mediated rewards on intrinsic motivation, *Journal of Personality and Social Psychology*, 18, 105–15.

Deci, E.L. (1972) Intrinsic motivation, extrinsic motivation, and inequity, *Journal of Personality and Social Psychology*, 22, 113–20.

Deci, E.L. and Ryan, R.M. (1985a) The general causality orientations scale: self-determination in personality, *Journal of Research in Personality*, 19, 109–34.

Deci, E.L. and Ryan, R.M. (1985b) *Intrinsic Motivation and Self-determination in Human Behavior*. New York: Plenum Press.

Deci, E.L. and Ryan, R.M. (2000) The 'what' and 'why' of goal pursuits: human needs and the self-determination of behavior, *Psychological Inquiry*, 11, 227–68.

Deci, E.L. and Ryan, R.M. (2002) An overview of self-determination theory: an organismic-dialectical perspective, in E.L. Deci and R.M. Ryan (eds.) *Handbook of Self-determination Research*. New York: University of Rochester Press.

Deci, E.L. and Ryan, R. (2012) Self-determination theory in health care and its relations to motivational interviewing: a few comments, *International Journal of Behavioral Nutrition and Physical Activity*, 9: 24.

Deci, E.L., Eghrari, H., Patrick, B.C. and Leone, D.R. (1994) Facilitating internalization: the self-determination theory perspective, *Journal of Personality*, 62, 119–42.

Deci, E.L., Koestner, R. and Ryan, R.M. (1999a) A meta-analytic review of experiments examining the effects of extrinsic rewards on intrinsic motivation, *Psychological Bulletin*, 125, 627–68.

Deci, E.L., Koestner, R. and Ryan, R.M. (1999b) The undermining effect is a reality after all: extrinsic rewards, task interest, and self-determination. Reply to Eisenberger, Pierce, and Cameron (1999) and Lepper, Henderlong, and Gingras (1999), *Psychological Bulletin*, 125, 692–700.

Duncan, L.R., Hall, C.R., Wilson, P.M. and Jenny, O. (2010) Exercise motivation: a cross-sectional analysis examining its relationships with frequency, intensity, and duration of exercise, *International Journal of Behavioral Nutrition and Physical Activity*, 7: 7.

Edmunds, J.K., Ntoumanis, N. and Duda, J.L. (2007a) Adherence and well-being in overweight and obese patients referred to an exercise prescription scheme: a self-determination theory perspective, *Psychology of Sport and Exercise*, 8, 722–40.

Edmunds, J.K., Ntoumanis, N. and Duda, J.L. (2007b) Perceived autonomy support and psychological need satisfaction in exercise, in M.S. Hagger and N.L.D. Chatzisarantis (eds.) *Intrinsic Motivation and Self-determination in Exercise and Sport*. Champaign, IL: Human Kinetics.

Edmunds, J.K., Ntoumanis, N. and Duda, J.L. (2008) Testing a self-determination theory based teaching style in the exercise domain, *European Journal of Social Psychology*, 38, 375–88.

Ferguson, E. (2013) Personality is of central concern to understand health: towards a theoretical model for health psychology, *Health Psychology Review*, 7, S32–70.

Ferguson, E., Ward, J.W., Skatova, A., Cassaday, H.J., Bibby, P.A. and Lawrence, C. (2013) Health specific traits beyond the Five Factor Model, cognitive processes and trait expression: replies to Watson (2012), Matthews (2012) and Haslam, Jetten, Reynolds, and Reicher (2012), *Health Psychology Review*, 7, S85–103.

Fortier, M. and Kowal, J. (2007) The flow state and physical activity behaviour change as motivational outcomes: a self-determination theory perspective, in M.S. Hagger and N.L.D. Chatzisarantis (eds.) *Intrinsic Motivation and Self-determination Theory in Exercise and Sport*. Champaign, IL: Human Kinetics.

Fortier, M.S., Sweet, S.N., Tulloch, H., Blanchard, C.M., Sigal, R.J., Kenny, G.P. *et al.* (2012) Self-determination and exercise stages of change: results from the Diabetes Aerobic and Resistance Exercise Trial, *Journal of Health Psychology*, 17, 87–99.

Greenwald, A.G., Banaji, M.R., Rudman, L.A., Farnham, S.D., Nosek, B.A. and Mellott, D.S. (2002) A unified theory of implicit attitudes, stereotypes, self-esteem, and self-concept, *Psychological Review*, 109, 3–25.

Guay, F., Mageau, G.A. and Vallerand, R.J. (2003) On the hierarchical structure of self-determined motivation: a test of top-down, bottom-up, reciprocal, and horizontal effects, *Personality and Social Psychology Bulletin*, 29, 992–1004.

Hagger, M.S. (2006) Meta-analysis in sport and exercise research: review, recent developments, and recommendations, *European Journal of Sport Science*, 6, 103–15.

Hagger, M.S. and Armitage, C. (2004) The influence of perceived loci of control and causality in the theory of planned behavior in a leisure-time exercise context, *Journal of Applied Biobehavioral Research*, 9, 45–64.

Hagger, M.S. and Chatzisarantis, N.L.D. (2007a) Advances in self-determination theory research in sport and exercise, *Psychology of Sport and Exercise*, 8, 597–9.

Hagger, M.S. and Chatzisarantis, N.L.D. (2007b) Self-determination theory and the theory of planned behavior: an integrative approach toward a more complete model of motivation, in L.V. Brown (ed.) *Psychology of Motivation*. Hauppauge, NY: Nova Science.

Hagger, M.S. and Chatzisarantis, N.L.D. (2007c) The trans-contextual model of motivation, in M.S. Hagger and N.L.D. Chatzisarantis (eds.) *Intrinsic Motivation and Self-determination in Exercise and Sport*. Champaign, IL: Human Kinetics.

Hagger, M.S. and Chatzisarantis, N.L.D. (2009) Integrating the theory of planned behaviour and self-determination theory in health behaviour: a meta-analysis, *British Journal of Health Psychology*, 14, 275–302.

Hagger, M.S. and Chatzisarantis, N.L.D. (2011) Causality orientations moderate the undermining effect of rewards on intrinsic motivation, *Journal of Experimental Social Psychology*, 47, 485–9.

Hagger, M.S. and Hardcastle, S.J. (2014) Interpersonal style should be included in taxonomies of behaviour change techniques, *Frontiers in Psychology*, 5, 254.

Hagger, M.S., Chatzisarantis, N.L.D. and Biddle, S.J.H. (2002) The influence of autonomous and controlling motives on physical activity intentions within the theory of planned behaviour, *British Journal of Health Psychology*, 7, 283–97.

Hagger, M.S., Chatzisarantis, N.L.D., Barkoukis, V., Wang, C.K.J. and Baranowski, J. (2005) Perceived autonomy support in physical education and leisure-time physical activity: a cross-cultural evaluation of the trans-contextual model, *Journal of Educational Psychology*, 97, 376–90.

Hagger, M.S., Chatzisarantis, N.L.D. and Harris, J. (2006a) From psychological need satisfaction to intentional behavior: testing a motivational sequence in two behavioral contexts, *Personality and Social Psychology Bulletin*, 32, 131–8.

Hagger, M.S., Chatzisarantis, N.L.D. and Harris, J. (2006b) The process by which relative autonomous motivation affects intentional behavior: comparing effects across dieting and exercise behaviors, *Motivation and Emotion*, 30, 306–20.

Hagger, M.S., Chatzisarantis, N.L.D., Culverhouse, T. and Biddle, S.J.H. (2003) The processes by which perceived autonomy support in physical education promotes leisure-time physical activity intentions and behavior: a trans-contextual model, *Journal of Educational Psychology*, 95, 784–95.

Hagger, M.S., Chatzisarantis, N.L.D., Hein, V., Pihu, M., Soos, I. and Karsai, I. (2007) The Perceived Autonomy Support Scale for Exercise Settings (PASSES): development, validity, and cross-cultural invariance in young people, *Psychology of Sport and Exercise*, 8, 632–53.

Hagger, M.S., Hardcastle, S.J., Chater, A., Mallett, C., Pal, S. and Chatzisarantis, N.L. (2014a) Autonomous and controlled motivational regulations for multiple health-related behaviors: between- and within-participants analyses, *Health Psychology and Behavioral Medicine*, 2, 565–601.

Hagger, M.S., Keatley, D.A., Chan, D.K.C., Chatzisarantis, N.L., Dimmock, J.A., Jackson, B. *et al.* (2014b) The goose is (half) cooked: a consideration of the mechanisms and interpersonal context is needed to elucidate the effects of personal financial incentives on health behaviour, *International Journal of Behavioral Medicine*, 21, 197–201.

Hagger, M.S., Koch, S. and Chatzisarantis, N.L.D. (2015) The effect of causality orientations and positive competence-enhancing feedback on intrinsic motivation: aA test of additive and interactive effects, *Personality and Individual Differences*, 72, 107–11.

Hagger, M.S., Lonsdale, A.J., Hein, V., Koka, A., Lintunen, T., Pasi, H. *et al.* (2012) Predicting alcohol consumption and binge drinking in company employees: an application of planned behaviour and self-determination theories, *British Journal of Health Psychology*, 17, 379–407.

Hein, V. and Koka, A. (2007) Perceived feedback and motivation in physical education and physical activity, in M.S. Hagger and N.L.D. Chatzisarantis (eds.) *Intrinsic Motivation and Self-determination in Exercise and Sport*. Champaign, IL: Human Kinetics.

Hunter, J.E. and Schmidt, F. (1994) *Methods of Meta-analysis: Correcting Error and Bias in Research Findings* (2nd edn.). Newbury Park, CA: Sage.

Jacobs, N., Hagger, M.S., Streukens, S., De Bourdeaudhuij, I. and Claes, N. (2011) Testing an integrated model of the theory of planned behaviour and self-determination theory for different energy-balance related behaviours and intervention intensities, *British Journal of Health Psychology*, 16, 113–34.

Keatley, D.A., Clarke, D.D. and Hagger, M.S. (2012) Investigating the predictive validity of implicit and explicit measures of motivation on condom use, physical activity, and healthy eating, *Psychology and Health*, 27, 550–69.

Keatley, D.A., Clarke, D.D. and Hagger, M.S. (2013) The predictive validity of implicit measures of self-determined motivation across health-related behaviours, *British Journal of Health Psychology*, 18, 2–17.

Kehr, H.M. (2004) Implicit/explicit motive discrepancies and volitional depletion among managers, *Personality and Social Psychology Bulletin*, 30, 315–27.

Koestner, R. and Zuckerman, M. (1994) Causality orientations, failure, and achievement, *Journal of Personality*, 62, 321–46.

Koka, A. and Hein, V. (2003) Perceptions of teacher's feedback and learning environment as components of motivation in physical education, *Psychology of Sport and Exercise*, 4, 333–46.

Lepper, M.R., Greene, D. and Nisbett, R.E. (1973) Undermining children's intrinsic interest with extrinsic rewards: a test of the 'overjustification' hypothesis, *Journal of Personality and Social Psychology*, 28, 129–37.

Lepper, M.R., Henderlong, J. and Gingras, I. (1999) Understanding the effects of extrinsic rewards on intrinsic motivation – uses and abuses of meta-analysis: comment on Deci, Koestner, and Ryan (1999), *Psychological Bulletin*, 125, 669–76.

Levesque, C.S. and Pelletier, L.G. (2003) On the investigation of primed and chronic autonomous and heteronomous motivational orientations, *Personality and Social Psychology Bulletin*, 29, 1570–84.

Levesque, C.S., Williams, G.C., Elliot, D., Pickering, M.A., Bodenhamer, B. and Finley, P.J. (2007) Validating the theoretical structure of the Treatment Self-Regulation Questionnaire (TSRQ) across three different health behaviors, *Health Education Research*, 22, 691–702.

Lewin, K. (1951) Intention, will, and need, in D. Rapaport (ed.) *Organisation and Pathology of Thought*. New York: Columbia University Press.

Liska, A.E. (1984) A critical examination of the causal structure of the Fishbein/Ajzen attitude–behavior model, *Social Psychology Quarterly*, 47, 61–74.

Markland, D. and Hardy, L. (1993) The Exercise Motivations Inventory: preliminary development and validity of a measure of individuals' reasons for participation in regular physical exercise, *Personality and Individual Differences*, 15, 289–96.

Markland, D. and Tobin, V. (2004) A modification to the Behavioural Regulation in Exercise Questionnaire to include an assessment of amotivation, *Journal of Sport and Exercise Psychology*, 26, 191–6.

Mata, J., Silva, M.N., Vieira, P.N., Carraca, E.V., Andrade, A.M., Coutinho, S.R. *et al.* (2009) Motivational 'spill-over' during weight control: increased self-determination and exercise intrinsic motivation predict eating self-regulation, *Health Psychology*, 28, 709–16.

McLachlan, S. and Hagger, M.S. (2010) Associations between motivational orientations and chronically-accessible outcomes in leisure-time physical activity: are appearance-related outcomes controlling in nature? *Research Quarterly for Exercise and Sport*, 81, 102–7.

McLachlan, S. and Hagger, M.S. (2011) Do people differentiate between intrinsic and extrinsic goals in physical activity behavior? *Journal of Sport and Exercise Psychology*, 33, 273–88.

McLachlan, S., Spray, C. and Hagger, M.S. (2011) The development of a scale measuring integrated regulation in exercise, *British Journal of Health Psychology*, 16, 722–43.

Michie, S. and Johnston, M. (2012) Theories and techniques of behaviour change: developing a cumulative science of behaviour change, *Health Psychology Review*, 6, 1–6.

Michie, S., Richardson, M., Johnston, M., Abraham, C., Francis, J., Hardeman, W. *et al.* (2013) The behavior change technique taxonomy (v1) of 93 hierarchically clustered techniques: building an international consensus for the reporting of behavior change interventions, *Annals of Behavioral Medicine*, 46, 81–95.

Moustaka, F.C., Vlachopoulos, S.P., Kabitsis, C. and Theodorakis, Y. (2012) Effects of an autonomy-supportive exercise instructing style on exercise motivation, psychological well-being, and exercise attendance in middle-age women, *Journal of Physical Activity and Health*, 9, 138–50.

Mullan, B.A., Todd, J., Chatzisarantis, N.L.D. and Hagger, M.S. (2014) Experimental methods in health psychology in Australia: implications for applied research, *Australian Psychologist*, 49, 104–9.

Mullan, E., Markland, D.A. and Ingledew, D.K. (1997) A graded conceptualisation of self-determination in the regulation of exercise behaviour: development of a measure using confirmatory factor analysis, *Personality and Individual Differences*, 23, 745–52.

Neighbors, C., Walker, D.D. and Larimer, M.E. (2003) Expectancies and evaluations of alcohol effects among college students: self-determination as a moderator, *Journal of Studies in Alcohol*, 64, 292–300.

Ng, J.Y.Y., Ntoumanis, N., Thögersen-Ntoumani, C., Deci, E.L., Ryan, R.M., Duda, J.L. *et al.* (2012) Self-determination theory applied to health contexts, *Perspectives on Psychological Science*, 7, 325–40.

Niemiec, C.P., Ryan, R.M., Deci, E.L. and Williams, G.C. (2009) Aspiring to physical health: the role of aspirations for physical health in facilitating long-term tobacco abstinence, *Patient Education and Counseling*, 74, 250–7.

Nosek, B.A., Greenwald, A.G. and Banaji, M.R. (2007) The Implicit Association Test at age 7: a methodological and conceptual review, in J.A. Bargh (ed.) *Automatic Processes in Social Thinking and Behavior*. New York: Psychology Press.

Nouwen, A., Ford, T., Balan, A.T., Twisk, J., Ruggiero, L. and White, D. (2011) Longitudinal motivational predictors of dietary self-care and diabetes control in adults with newly diagnosed type 2 diabetes mellitus, *Health Psychology*, 30, 771–9.

Ntoumanis, N. (2005) A prospective study of participation in optional school physical education based on self-determination theory, *Journal of Educational Psychology*, 97, 444–53.

Pelletier, L.G. and Sarrazin, P. (2007) Measurement issues in self-determination theory and sport, in M.S. Hagger and N.L.D. Chatzisarantis (eds.) *Intrinsic Motivation and Self-determination in Exercise and Sport*. Champaign, IL: Human Kinetics.

Pelletier, L.G., Dion, S.C., Slovinec-D'Angelo, M. and Reid, R. (2004) Why do you regulate what you eat? Relationships between forms of regulation, eating behaviors, sustained dietary behavior change, and psychological adjustment, *Motivation and Emotion*, 28, 245–77.

Perugini, M. (2005) Predictive models of implicit and explicit attitudes, *British Journal of Social Psychology*, 44, 29–45

Phillips, P., Abraham, C. and Bond, R. (2003) Personality, cognition, and university students' examination performance, *European Journal of Personality*, 17, 435–48.

Resnicow, K., Davis, R.E., Zhang, G., Konkel, J., Strecher, V.J., Shaikh, A.R. *et al.* (2008) Tailoring a fruit and vegetable intervention on novel motivational constructs: results of a randomized study, *Annals of Behavioral Medicine*, 35, 159–69.

Ryan, R.M. (1982) Control and information in the intrapersonal sphere: an extension of cognitive evaluation theory, *Journal of Personality and Social Psychology*, 43, 450–61.

Ryan, R.M. and Connell, J.P. (1989) Perceived locus of causality and internalization: examining reasons for acting in two domains, *Journal of Personality and Social Psychology*, 57, 749–61.

Ryan, R.M. and Deci, E.L. (2000) The darker and brighter sides of human existence: basic psychological needs as a unifying concept, *Psychological Inquiry*, 11, 319–38.

Ryan, R.M. and Deci, E.L. (2008) From ego depletion to vitality: theory and findings concerning the facilitation of energy available to the self, *Social and Personality Psychology Compass*, 2, 702–17.

Ryan, R.M., Mims, V. and Koestner, R. (1983) Relation of reward contingency and interpersonal context to extrinsic motivation: a review and test using cognitive evaluation theory, *Journal of Personality and Social Psychology*, 45, 736–50.

Ryan, R.M., Patrick, H., Deci, E.L. and Williams, G.C. (2008) Facilitating health behaviour change and its maintenance: interventions based on self-determination theory, *European Health Psychologist*, 10, 2–5.

Ryan, R.M., Plant, R.W. and O'Malley, S. (1995) Initial motivations for alcohol treatment: relations with patient characteristics, treatment involvement and dropout, *Addictive Behaviors*, 20, 279–97.

Sheeran, P., Norman, P. and Orbell, S. (1999) Evidence that intentions based on attitudes better predict behaviour than intentions based on subjective norms, *European Journal of Social Psychology*, 29, 403–6.

Sheldon, K.M. and Bettencourt, B.A. (2002) Psychological need-satisfaction and subjective well-being within social groups, *British Journal of Social Psychology*, 41, 25–38.

Sheldon, K.M., Elliot, A.J., Kim, Y. and Kasser, T. (2001) What is satisfying about satisfying events? Testing 10 candidate psychological needs, *Journal of Personality and Social Psychology*, 80, 325–39.

Silva, M.N., Vieira, P.N., Coutinho, S.R., Minderico, C.S., Matos, M.G., Sardinha, L.B. *et al.* (2010) Using self-determination theory to promote physical activity and weight control: a randomized controlled trial in women, *Journal of Behavioral Medicine*, 33, 110–22.

Sniehotta, F.F. (2009) An experimental test of the theory of planned behavior, *Applied Psychology: Health and Well-being*, 1, 257–70.

Spence, A. and Townsend, E. (2007) Predicting behaviour towards genetically modified (GM) food using implicit and explicit attitudes, *British Journal of Social Psychology*, 46, 437–57.

Standage, M., Duda, J.L. and Ntoumanis, N. (2003) A model of contextual motivation in physical education: using constructs from self-determination and achievement goal theories to predict physical activity intentions, *Journal of Educational Psychology*, 95, 97–110.

Standage, M., Duda, J.L. and Ntoumanis, N. (2005) A test of self-determination theory in school physical education, *British Journal of Educational Psychology*, 75, 411–33.

Standage, M., Gillison, F.B. and Treasure, D.C. (2007) Self-determination and motivation in physical education, in M.S. Hagger and N.L.D. Chatzisarantis (eds.) *Intrinsic Motivation and Self-Determination in Exercise and Sport.* Champaign, IL: Human Kinetics.

Standage, M., Gillison, F.B., Ntoumanis, N. and Treasure, G.C. (2012) Predicting students' physical activity and health-related well-being: a prospective cross-domain investigation of motivation across school physical education and exercise settings, *Journal of Sport and Exercise Psychology*, 34, 37–60.

Strack, F. and Deutsch, R. (2004) Reflective and impulsive determinants of social behavior, *Personality and Social Psychology Review*, 8, 220–47.

Tang, S.H. and Hall, V.C. (1995) The overjustification effect: a meta-analysis, *Applied Cognitive Psychology*, 9, 365–404.

Teixeira, P.J., Carraca, E., Markland, D.A., Silva, M.N. and Markland, D.A. (2012a) Exercise, physical activity, and self-determination theory: a systematic review, *International Journal of Behavioral Nutrition and Physical Activity*, 9: 78.

Teixeira, P.J., Palmeira, A. and Vansteenkiste, M. (2012b) The role of self-determination theory and motivational interviewing in behavioral nutrition, physical activity, and health: an introduction to the IJBNPA special series, *International Journal of Behavioral Nutrition and Physical Activity*, 9: 17.

Vansteenkiste, M., Simons, J., Soenens, B. and Lens, W. (2004) How to become a persevering exerciser? Providing a clear, future intrinsic goal in an autonomy-supportive way, *Journal of Sport and Exercise Psychology*, 26, 232–49.

Waaler, R., Halvari, H., Skjesol, K. and Bagoien, T.E. (2012) Autonomy support and intrinsic goal progress expectancy and its links to longitudinal study effort and subjective wellbeing: the differential mediating effect of intrinsic and identified regulations and the moderator effects of effort and intrinsic goals, *Scandinavian Journal of Educational Research*, 57, 325–41.

Weiner, B., Heckhausen, H., Meyer, W.U. and Cook, R.E. (1972) Causal ascriptions and achievement motivation: a conceptual analysis and reanalysis of locus of control, *Journal of Personality and Social Psychology*, 21, 239–48.

White, R.W. (1959) Motivation reconsidered: the concept of competence, *Psychological Review*, 66, 297–333.

Williams, G.C., Cox, E.M., Kouides, R. and Deci, E.L. (1999) Presenting the facts about smoking to adolescents: the effects of an autonomy supportive style, *Archives of Pediatrics and Adolescent Medicine*, 153, 959–64.

Williams, G.C., Freedman, Z.R. and Deci, E.L. (1998) Supporting autonomy to motivate glucose control in patients with diabetes, *Diabetes Care*, 21, 1644–51.

Williams, G.C., Gagné, M., Ryan, R.M. and Deci, E.L. (2002a) Facilitating autonomous motivation for smoking cessation, *Health Psychology*, 21, 40–50.

Williams, G.C., McGregor, H.A., Sharp, D., Kouides, R.W., Lévesque, C.S., Ryan, R.M. *et al.* (2006a) A self-determination multiple risk intervention trial to improve smokers' health, *Journal of General Internal Medicine*, 21, 1288–94.

Williams, G.C., McGregor, H.A., Sharp, D., Lévesque, C.S., Kouides, R.W., Ryan, R.M. *et al.* (2006b) Testing a self-determination theory intervention for motivating tobacco cessation: supporting autonomy and competence in a clinical trial, *Health Psychology*, 25, 91–101.

Williams, G.C., McGregor, H.A., Zeldman, A., Freedman, Z.R. and Deci, E.L. (2004) Testing a self-determination theory process model for promoting glycemic control through diabetes self-management, *Health Psychology*, 23, 58–66.

Williams, G.C., Minicucci, D.S., Kouides, R.W., Lévesque, C.S., Chirkov, V.I., Ryan, R.M. *et al.* (2002b) Self-determination, smoking, diet and health, *Health Education Research*, 17, 512–21.

Wilson, P.M. and Rodgers, W.M. (2004) The relationship between perceived autonomy support, exercise regulations and behavioral intentions in women, *Psychology of Sport and Exercise*, 5, 229–42.

Wilson, P.M. and Rodgers, W.M. (2007) Self-determination theory, exercise and well-being, in M.S. Hagger and N.L.D. Chatzisarantis (eds.) *Intrinsic Motivation and Self-determination in Exercise and Sport*. Champiagn, IL: Human Kinetics.

Wilson, P.M., Rodgers, W.M., Loitz, C.C. and Scime, G. (2006a) 'It's who I am…really!' The importance of integrated regulation in exercise contexts, *Journal of Applied Biobehavioral Research*, 11, 79–104.

Wilson, P.M., Rogers, W.T., Rodgers, W.M. and Wild, T.C. (2006b) The psychological need satisfaction in exercise scale, *Journal of Sport and Exercise Psychology*, 28, 231–51.

Wong, M.M. (2000) The relations among causality orientations, academic experience, academic performance, and academic commitment, *Personality and Social Psychology Bulletin*, 36, 315–26.

Chapter 5

The theory of planned behaviour and the reasoned action approach

Mark Conner and Paul Sparks

1 General background

The theory of planned behaviour (TPB; Ajzen 1988, 1991) is an extension of the earlier theory of reasoned action (TRA; Fishbein and Ajzen 1975; Ajzen and Fishbein 1980), which continues to attract attention in psychology (Fishbein and Ajzen 2010). Both models emphasize, but are not restricted to, a deliberative processing of available information in the formation of intentions. The origins of the TRA are in Fishbein's work on the psychological processes by which attitudes cause behaviour (Fishbein 1967), and in an analysis of the failure to predict behaviour from individuals' attitudes. The former work (Fishbein 1967) used an expectancy-value framework (Peak 1955) to explain relationships between beliefs and attitudes, and interposed a mediating variable, behavioural intention, between attitudes and behaviour; the latter work (Fishbein and Ajzen 1975) generated a powerful explanation of the conditions under which strong attitude–behaviour relationships might be expected.

Based on an analysis of previous studies of the relationship between attitudes and behaviour, Fishbein and Ajzen (1975; Ajzen and Fishbein 1977) developed the principle of compatibility (Ajzen 1988).[1] This principle holds that each attitude and behaviour has the four elements of action, target, context, and time (sometimes referred to as TACT by reversing the order of first two elements), and states that correspondence between attitudes (or other cognitions) and behaviour will be greatest when both are measured at the same degree of specificity with respect to each element (for discussions, see Ajzen and Fishbein 2005; Fishbein and Ajzen 2010). Hence, any behaviour consists of (a) an action (or behaviour), (b) performed on or towards a target or object, (c) in a particular context, (d) at a specified time or occasion. For example, a person concerned about oral hygiene (a) brushes (b) her teeth (c) in the bathroom (d) every morning after breakfast. In the study of health behaviours, it is usually the repeated and often regular performance of a single behaviour (e.g. teeth brushing) or general category of behaviours (e.g. healthy eating) across contexts and times that we wish to predict (Ajzen 1988). Attitudes and behaviour will be most strongly related when both are assessed at the same level of specificity with regard to these four elements. Thus, general attitudes should predict general categories of behaviours and specific attitudes should predict specific behaviours. Considerations of compatibility are particularly important in developing appropriate measures for all components of the TRA/TPB (see Section 5).

2 Description of the model

The TRA suggests that the proximal determinant of volitional behaviour is one's behavioural intention to engage in that behaviour. Behavioural intention represents a person's motivation in the sense of her or his conscious plan, decision or self-instruction to exert effort to perform the target behaviour. Attitudes towards a specific behaviour impact on performance of that behaviour via intention. Thus in the TRA the issue of how the unobservable attitude is transformed into observable action is clarified by interposing another psychological event: the formation of an intention between the attitude and the behaviour. However, the theory is less clear about the factors translating attitudes into intentions. One possibility is that the anticipated opportunity to perform the behaviour promotes the formation of an intention. The TRA includes a second determinant of intention: subjective norm. This component reflects one form of social influence (i.e. what others would want one to do) on performance of the target behaviour. The TRA restricts itself to the prediction of volitional behaviours. Behaviours that require skills, resources or opportunities that are not freely available are not within the domain of the TRA and so are likely to be poorly predicted by it (Fishbein 1993).

The TPB was developed to broaden the applicability of the TRA beyond purely volitional behaviours by incorporating explicit considerations of perceptions of control over performance of the behaviour as an additional predictor (Ajzen 1988, 1991). Consideration of perceptions of control, or perceived behavioural control (PBC), is important because PBC extends the applicability of the theory beyond easily performed, volitional behaviours to those complex goals and behaviours that are dependent on performance of a complex series of other behaviours, but of considerable importance in terms of health outcomes (e.g. healthy eating). It is the lack of actual control that attenuates the power of intention to predict behaviour (Ajzen and Fishbein 2005). However, given the myriad of problems defining and measuring actual control (Ajzen and Fishbein 2005; Fishbein and Ajzen 2010), PBC has tended to be employed as a direct predictor of behaviour and an indirect predictor of behaviour via intention. To the extent that PBC accurately reflects actual control, it should provide good predictions of behaviour. Inclusion of PBC in the TPB provides information about potential constraints on action as perceived by the actor, and explains why intentions do not always predict behaviour.

The TPB depicts behaviour as a linear regression function of behavioural intention and perceived behavioural control:

$$B = w_1BI + w_2PBC \tag{1}$$

where B is behaviour, BI is behavioural intention, PBC is perceived behavioural control, and w_1 and w_2 are regression weights. Contrary to some commentators' misconceptions, the value of these regression weights needs to be empirically determined and will likely vary as a function of both the behaviour and population examined.

The link between intention and behaviour reflects the fact that people tend to engage in behaviours they intend to perform. However, the link between PBC and behaviour is more complex. Perceived behavioural control is held to exert both direct and interactive (with behavioural intentions) effects on behaviour. This is based on the rationale that however strongly held, the implementation of an intention into action is at least partially influenced by personal and environmental barriers. Thus, the 'addition of perceived behavioral control should become increasingly useful as volitional control over behavior decreases' (Ajzen 1991: 185). Therefore, in situations where prediction of behaviour from intention is likely to be hindered by the level of actual (i.e. volitional) control, PBC should (a) facilitate the implementation of behavioural intentions into action, and (b) predict behaviour directly (Armitage and Conner 2001). Ajzen (1988) is explicit in stating that it is actual control which is important here, in that people will tend to perform (and exert additional effort to perform) desirable behaviours they have control over, and not perform desirable behaviours they have little or no control over. Perceived behavioural control will predict behaviour directly to the extent that the measure matches actual control (Ajzen 1988). In their review, Armitage and Conner (2001) showed the interaction between intentions and PBC to be significant in approximately half of reported tests, while Sheeran *et al.* (2003) showed that where PBC was accurate it provided stronger predictions of behaviour and moderated the intention–behaviour relationship (higher PBC was associated with stronger intention—behaviour relationships).

2.1 Determinants of intention

In the TRA, attitudes are one predictor of behavioural intention. Attitudes are the overall evaluations of the behaviour by the individual. Fishbein and Ajzen (1975: 6) define an attitude as 'a learned disposition to respond in a consistently favorable or unfavorable manner with respect to a given object'. Applying the principle of compatibility, the relevant attitudes are those towards performance of the behaviour, assessed at a similar level of specificity to that used in the assessment of behaviour. The TRA also specifies subjective norms as the other determinant of intentions. Subjective norms consist of a person's beliefs about whether significant others (i.e. referents) think he or she should engage in the behaviour. Significant others are individuals or groups whose opinions about a person's behaviour in this domain are important to him or her. Subjective norms are assumed to assess the 'social pressures' (from salient referents) that individuals feel to perform or not perform a particular behaviour. The TPB incorporates a third predictor of intentions, PBC, which is the individual's perception of the extent of control over performance of the behaviour. Perceived behavioural control is seen as a continuum with easily executed behaviours (e.g. walking up stairs) at one end and behavioural goals demanding resources, opportunities, and specialized skills (e.g. running 120 miles a week) at the other end. Hence, behavioural intention is a linear regression function of attitudes, subjective norms, and perceived behavioural control:

$$\text{BI} = w_3\text{A} + w_4\text{SN} + w_5\text{PBC} \tag{2}$$

where BI is behavioural intention, A is attitude towards the behaviour, SN is subjective norm, PBC is perceived behavioural control, and w_3, w_4, and w_5 are empirical weights indicating the relative importance of the determinants of intention. The equation indicates that intentions are a function of one's evaluation of personally engaging in the behaviour, one's perception that significant others think one should or should not perform the behaviour, and perceptions of one's control over performance of the behaviour. Without the PBC component, equation (2) represents the TRA. The PBC–intention link represents the fact that, in general, individuals are more disposed (i.e. intend) to engage in positively valued behaviours that are believed to be achievable (cf. Bandura 2000).

The weights in equation (2) are assumed to vary. Ajzen (1991: 188) states that the 'relative importance of attitude, subjective norm, and perceived behavioral control in the prediction of intention is expected to vary across behaviors and situations'. Research also indicates that there may be individual differences in the weights placed on the different components, with some individuals tending to base their intentions on attitudes and others on norms across behaviours (Trafimow and Findlay 1996). Indirect evidence for this has been found in studies that have shown that measures of attitude strength (e.g. Sparks *et al.* 1992) and individual differences in sociability (e.g. Trafimow and Findlay 1996) increase the relative predictive power of attitudes and subjective norms, respectively. In addition, in situations where, for example, attitudes are strong, or where normative influences are powerful, PBC may be less predictive of intentions.

2.2 Determinants of attitudes

Just as intentions are held to have determinants, so the attitude, subjective norm, and PBC components are also held to have their own determinants. The determinants are sometimes referred to as indirect measures. However, it is worth noting that both the direct and indirect measures of each of the components are considered to be measures of one and the same construct (Ajzen and Fishbein 1980). Attitude is a function of salient behavioural beliefs, each of which represents the perceived likelihood that performance of the behaviour will lead to a particular outcome or is associated with a particular attribute. Following expectancy-value conceptualizations (Peak 1955), expectancy-value products are composed of the multiplicative combination of beliefs about the likelihood of each behavioural outcome and the evaluation of that outcome. These expectancy-value products are then summed over the various salient outcomes:

$$A = \sum_{i=1}^{i=p} b_i \cdot e_i \qquad (3)$$

where b_i is the behavioural belief that performing the behaviour leads to some consequence i (thus b_i is the subjective probability that the behaviour has the consequence i), e_i is the evaluation of consequence i, and p is the number of salient consequences over which these values are summed. It is not claimed that an individual performs such calculations each time he or she is faced with a decision about performing a behaviour, but rather that the results of such considerations are maintained in memory and retrieved and used when necessary (Ajzen and Fishbein 1980: 245). However, it is also possible for the individual to retrieve the relevant individual beliefs and evaluations when necessary. Fishbein (1993) claims equation (3) is not a model of a process but is a computational representation aimed to capture the output of a process that occurs automatically as a function of learning (see Ajzen and Fishbein 2000). This part of the model, the relationship between attitudes and beliefs, is based on Fishbein's (1967a, 1967b) *summative model of attitudes*. It is assumed that a person may possess a large number of beliefs about a particular behaviour, but that at any one time only a limited number are likely to be salient. It is

Table 5.1 A meta-analysis of meta-analyses of relationships in the TRA/TPB for health behaviours

Relationship	k	N	r_+
BI–B	423	112 100	0.42
PBC–B	353	97 613	0.28
A–B	340	88 410	0.30
SN–B	325	84 545	0.18
PB-B	149	41 975	0.44
A–BI	467	138 781	0.45
SN–BI	472	142 671	0.35
PBC–BI	426	132 872	0.44
PB-BI	142	45 222	0.46
SN–A	315	89 763	0.30
PBC–A	293	87 724	0.37
PB–A	142	41 948	0.33
PBC–SN	281	85 179	0.24
PB-SN	139	41 611	0.21
PB-PBC	134	41 450	0.30
BB–A	90	27 027	0.49
NB–SN	88	23 785	0.47
CB–PBC	54	17 605	0.23

Note: Included meta-analyses had *k*, *N*, and r_+ values available: Hausenblas *et al.* (1997); Sheeran and Taylor (1999); Albarracin *et al.* (2001); Armitage and Conner (2001); Hagger *et al.* (2002); Cooke and French (2008); Rodgers *et al.* (2008); McEachan *et al.* (2011); Cooke *et al.* (in press).
k = number of studies, *N* = total sample size; r_+ = frequency weighted correlation; BI = behavioural intention; B = behaviour; PBC = perceived behavioural control; A = attitude; SN = subjective norm; PB = past behaviour; BB = behavioural beliefs; NB = normative beliefs; CB = control beliefs.

the salient beliefs that are assumed to determine a person's attitude. This link between attitudes and behavioural beliefs is generally strong (Table 5.1).

2.3 Determinants of subjective norm

Subjective norm is a function of normative beliefs, which represent perceptions of specific significant others' preferences about whether one should or should not engage in a behaviour. This is quantified in the model as the subjective likelihood that specific salient groups or individuals (referents) think the person should or should not perform the behaviour, multiplied by the person's motivation to comply with that referent's expectation. Motivation to comply is the extent to which the person wishes to comply with the specific wishes of the referent on this issue. These products are then summed across salient referents:

$$\text{SN} = \sum_{j=1}^{j=q} \text{nb}_j \cdot \text{mc}_j$$

(4)

where SN is the subjective norm, nb_j is the normative belief (i.e. a subjective probability) that some referent j thinks one should perform the behaviour, mc_j is the motivation to comply with referent j, and q is the number of salient referents. It should be noted that the distinction between behavioural beliefs and normative beliefs is somewhat arbitrary (i.e. both are outcome expectancies; Miniard and Cohen 1981) and there is often considerable correlation between the two (O'Keefe 1990). However, it has been argued that there is some merit in maintaining a distinction between the determinants of behaviour that are attributes of the person and those which are attributes of the social environment (see Eagly and Chaiken 1993: 171; Trafimow and Fishbein 1995). The expectancy-value nature of equation (4) has been noted by a number of authors (e.g. Eagly and Chaiken 1993) and is supported by strong correlations between normative beliefs and subjective norms (Table 5.1).

2.4 Determinants of perceived behavioural control

Judgements of PBC are influenced by beliefs concerning whether one has access to the necessary resources and opportunities to perform the behaviour successfully, weighted by the perceived power of each factor (Ajzen 1988, 1991). The perceptions of factors likely to facilitate or inhibit the performance of the behaviour are referred to as control beliefs. These factors include both internal (information, personal deficiencies, skills, abilities, emotions) and external (opportunities, dependence on others, physical constraints) control factors. People who perceive they have access to the necessary resources and perceive that there are opportunities (or lack of obstacles) to perform the behaviour are likely to perceive a high degree of behavioural control (Ajzen 1991). Ajzen (1991) has suggested that each control factor is weighted by its perceived power to facilitate or inhibit performance of the behaviour. The model quantifies these control beliefs by multiplying the frequency or likelihood of occurrence of the factor by the subjective perception of the power of the factor to facilitate or inhibit the performance of the behaviour:

$$\text{PBC} = \sum_{k=1}^{k=r} c_k \cdot p_k \tag{5}$$

where PBC is perceived behavioural control, c_k is the perceived frequency or likelihood of occurrence of factor k, p_k is the perceived facilitating or inhibiting power of factor k, and r is the number of control factors. The similarity of equation (5) to an expectancy-value computation is again worth noting. Correlations between control beliefs and PBC is generally supportive of the multiplicative composite (Table 5.1).

2.5 Commentary and the reasoned action approach

The causal model the TPB represents is illustrated in Figure 5.1. The model is held to be a complete theory of behaviour in that any other influences on behaviour (i.e. external influences such as demographic variables, personality traits or environmental influences) have their impact on behaviour via influencing components of the TPB. However, it is perhaps more correctly regarded as a theory of the *proximal* determinants of behaviour. Although not illustrated in Figure 5.1 the theory does allow for feedback loops from behaviour (Fishbein and Ajzen 2010: 218). The assumption is that unanticipated consequences, reactions from others, difficulties or

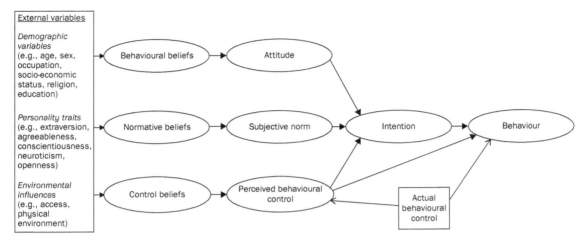

Figure 5.1 The theory of planned behaviour

facilitating factors experienced when performing a behaviour can change behavioural, normative or control beliefs and thus affect future intentions and actions.

The TPB as represented in Figure 5.1 is one part of a broader reasoned action approach (RAA; Fishbein and Ajzen 2010). As Fishbein (2008: 834) states, 'what the reasoned action approach attempts to do is to identify a relatively small set of variables that can account for a substantial proportion of the variance in any given behavior'. As Head and Noar (2014) usefully point out, there have been four chronological phases of research within the RAA. The initial phase was work on the TRA by Fishbein and Ajzen. The second phase was work on the TPB by Ajzen that added perceived behavioural control to the TRA. The third phase was Fishbein's work on extending the TRA to include self-efficacy as a predictor of intention and a number of other predictors of behaviour (e.g. skills, environmental constraints) (see discussion of the major theorists' model in Conner and Norman, Chapter 1 this volume). The fourth and final phase is represented by Fishbein and Ajzen's more recent collaboration that attempted to reconcile the differences between their two approaches (Fishbein and Ajzen 2010). One contribution of this latest phase of the RAA and renewed collaboration between Fishbein and Ajzen (Ajzen and Fishbein 2005; Fishbein and Ajzen 2010) has been a further consideration of different components of attitude, subjective norms, and perceived behavioural control (see Figure 5.2 and Section 4 of this chapter).

3 Summary of research

The TRA/TPB has been applied to the prediction of a wide variety of different behaviours, including a broad range of health-related behaviours, with varying degrees of success. There are a number of narrative reviews (e.g. Liska 1984; Eagly and Chaiken 1993; Sparks 1994; Manstead and Parker 1995; Jonas and Doll 1996; Fishbein and Ajzen 2010) as well as quantitative reviews of the TRA (e.g. Sheppard *et al.* 1988) and TPB (e.g. McEachan *et al.* 2011). Here, we summarize meta-analytic reviews of the TPB, discuss key issues raised, and summarize applications to health behaviours.

3.1 Meta-analytic reviews of the TPB

A series of meta-analyses have now been reported for the TPB, including general reviews (e.g. Ajzen 1991; Armitage and Conner 2001; Trafimow *et al.* 2002), those focusing on health behaviours (Godin and Kok 1996; McEachan *et al.* 2011), and those focusing on specific health behaviours (e.g. exercise: Blue 1995; Hausenblas *et al.* 1997; Hagger *et al.* 2002; condom use: Sheeran and Taylor 1999; Albarracin *et al.* 2001; alcohol consumption: Cooke *et al.* in press).

In a review of early studies using the TPB, Ajzen (1991) reported the multiple correlation between intentions (BI) and attitude (A), subjective norm (SN), and perceived behavioural control (PBC) to be 0.71 (across 16 studies). Similarly, Van den Putte (1991) computed a value of $R = 0.64$ across 37 studies, but noted a marked variation between behaviours. Trafimow *et al.* (2002), in a review of studies distinguishing between two aspects of PBC (difficulty and control), reported $R = 0.66$. Finally, in one of the most comprehensive reviews, Armitage and Conner (2001) reported $R = 0.63$ across 154 studies. Other reviews have focused on health behaviours. For example, in a review of 76 applications of the TPB to health behaviours, Godin and Kok (1996) reported $R = 0.64$, while noting considerable variation between studies. McEachan *et al.* (2011) reviewed up to 237 prospective tests of the TPB and reported $R = 0.67$. Overall, attitude, subjective norm, and PBC account for between 40% and 50% of the variance in intentions across studies. When considering sample weighted mean correlations (r_+), attitude and PBC generally emerged as stronger predictors than subjective norm (e.g. Armitage and Conner 2001: A–BI, $r_+ = 0.49$; SN–BI, $r_+ = 0.34$; PBC–BI, $r_+ = 0.43$), although all equate to medium-to-large effect sizes (Cohen 1992).

In relation to the prediction of behaviour (B), Ajzen (1991) reported a mean $R = 0.51$ between behavioural intention, PBC, and behaviour, while Van den Putte (1991) computed a value of 0.46. Similar values are reported by the reviews of Trafimow *et al.* (2002; $R = 0.60$), Armitage and Conner (2001; $R = 0.52$), Godin and Kok (1996; $R = 0.58$), and McEachan *et al.* (2011; $R = 0.44$). Thus overall, behavioural intention and PBC account for between 19% and 36% of the variance in behaviour. Godin and Kok (1996) noted considerable variation in this figure across behaviours, from 16% for clinical screening behaviours to 41% for addictive behaviours. In the majority of reviews, intention accounts for more variance in behaviour than PBC (e.g. Armitage and Conner 2001: BI–B, $r_+ = 0.47$; PBC–B, $r_+ = 0.37$), although the Armitage and Conner (2001) review also indicated that on average PBC predicts a significant *additional* 2% variance in behaviour after controlling for intentions.

In order to summarize the overall size of relationships among variables in the TRA/TPB, we conducted a meta-analysis of meta-analyses that considered relationships in the TRA/TPB (cf. Sutton 1998) and focused on health behaviours. We only used meta-analyses that focused on the TRA or TPB and included the sample-weighted mean correlation (r_+) between TRA/TPB components together with total number of participants included in the analyses (N) and the number of hypotheses tested (k). Given the overlap in included studies between meta-analyses, we should be cautious in interpreting the findings. The findings summarized in Table 5.1 give some indication of the overall size of relationships among variables in the TRA/TPB. Based on Cohen's (1992) power primer, the majority of relationships are in the medium ($r_+ \sim 0.3$) to large ($r_+ \sim 0.5$) range. It is worth noting that the correlations between the direct and indirect measures (e.g. attitudes and behavioural beliefs) varied between 0.23 and 0.49. The lower value for the relationship between control beliefs and PBC might suggest the need for further work to better understand the basis on which PBC forms.

Regression analysis of the meta-analytic data presented in Table 5.1 indicated that attitude, subjective norm, and PBC explained 32.3% of the variance in intentions with each being a significant predictor. Adding past behaviour explained an additional 6.7% of the variance in intentions, although all the other predictors remained significant. Intention and PBC explained 18.8% of the variance in behaviour with both variables being significant. The addition of attitudes and subjective norms explained an additional 1.1% of the variance in behaviour, while the addition of past behaviour explained a further 6.5% of the variance in behaviour. At this final step, intention, PBC, attitude, and past behaviour were significant predictors of behaviour, although subjective norm was not.

The TPB generally explains less variance in behaviour than intentions. Indeed, the lack of a perfect correlation between intentions and behaviour (or the intention–behaviour 'gap') has been the focus of considerable research attention (e.g. Sheeran 2002). Fishbein and Ajzen (2010: 53–63) provide a useful discussion of the many problems that may contribute to this 'gap' in the context of the TRA/TPB. Important factors include changes in intentions between their assessment and the opportunity to act (one of the identified limitations of the TRA/TPB), unanticipated obstacles to action, and differences in the beliefs that are accessible between when TPB components are measured and when the behaviour is performed. In contrast, the fact that the TPB does not fully account for the variance in intentions is partly attributable to measurement error in the assessment of the predictors of intentions (Ajzen 2014).

3.2 Key issues raised in reviews of the TPB

Applications of the TRA and TPB have tended to rely on self-reports, despite evidence suggesting the vulnerability of such data to self-presentational biases (e.g. Gaes *et al.* 1978). Armitage and Conner (2001) reported that the TPB accounted for large, highly significant proportions of the variance in prospective measures of both objective ($R^2 = 0.20$, $k = 19$) and self-reported ($R^2 = 0.31$, $k = 44$) behaviour. McEachan *et al.* (2011) reported values of $R^2 = 0.12$ and $R^2 = 0.26$, respectively, for objective and self-reported health behaviours in prospective designs. Researchers should be cognizant of the problems of self-report data, and wherever possible take accurate and objective measures of behaviour.

Figure 5.1 recognizes the importance of background or distal factors such as socio-demographic variables within the TPB but assumes they are mediated by TPB variables that are more proximal determinants of behaviour. A number of studies have explored the idea that socio-demographic variables might influence health behaviour alongside TPB variables via direct, mediated or moderated pathways. For example, Conner *et al.* (2013b) showed that socio-economic status moderated the intention–behaviour relationship across three health behaviours. In each case, increasing socio-economic status was associated with stronger intention–behaviour relationships. The majority of studies have demonstrated that background/distal factors influence intentions and behaviour only indirectly through TPB beliefs (i.e. their effects are fully mediated; for reviews, see Ajzen and Fishbein 2005; Fishbein and Ajzen 2010).

One common criticism of the TRA/TPB has been that it assumes that all behaviour is rational and fails to take account of other non-cognitive, non-conscious or irrational determinants of human behaviour (e.g. van der Pligt and de Vries 1998; Churchill *et al.* 2008; Sniehotta *et al.* 2014; Gibbons *et al.*, Chapter 6 this volume). Ajzen (2014) makes the point that the TPB does not propose that people are rational or behave in a rational manner. The TPB makes no assumptions about the objectivity or veridicality of behavioural, normative or control beliefs. Various non-cognitive, non-conscious or irrational factors may influence the formation of these beliefs. The TPB only assumes that people's attitudes, subjective norms, and perceptions of control follow reasonably and consistently from these beliefs, and in this way influence intentions and behaviour. Relatedly, Ajzen and Fishbein (2005) note that typical applications of the TRA/TPB devote little attention to the role of affect/emotion, which may be relevant to a range of health behaviours. Such emotions would be considered background variables in the TRA/TPB and might be expected to influence intentions and behaviour via their impact on beliefs. However, this criticism highlights potential problems with the way in which typical TRA/TPB studies are conducted. In particular, differences may exist between the contemplation of a behaviour (e.g. when filling in a TPB questionnaire) and its actual performance in a real-life context. It may be that the beliefs activated when completing the questionnaire are different from the ones accessible at the point of performing the behaviour (Fishbein and Ajzen 2010), leading to the attitudes, norms, PBC, and intentions being poor representations of those which exist in the behavioural situation and thus poor predictors of action. It may be particularly difficult for individuals to correctly anticipate the strong emotions that drive their behaviour in real life (Ajzen and Fishbein 2005). This would lead to problems with incorporating emotional factors within typical TRA/TPB applications. Nevertheless, it should be noted that there is usually considerable consistency between intentions and behaviours where one might expect considerable differences in emotional state between the context in which the questionnaire is completed and the one in which the behaviour is performed (e.g. condom use: Albarracin *et al.* [2001] report intention–behaviour $r_+ = 0.45$ across 96 data sets, although mainly based on self-reported behaviour).

3.3 Review of applications of the TPB to health behaviours

The relatively large number of TPB studies on health behaviours allows consideration of its application to different types of behaviour. To structure our presentation, we use a common distinction among types of health behaviours (e.g. Roysamb *et al.* 1997) that has been used in some recent reviews of the TPB (Conner *et al.* 2014). This distinguishes between protection (e.g. physical activity), risk (e.g. smoking), and detection (e.g. screening) health behaviours. In each case, we summarize the overall findings as presented in relevant meta-analyses and provide example studies.

3.3.1 Protection behaviours

The TPB has been applied to a diverse range of health protection behaviours, including supplement use (Conner *et al.* 2001), sun protection (White *et al.* 2008), and blood donation (Godin *et al.* 2007). Owing to the large number of studies, there have been reviews of the application of the TPB to categories of protection behaviours such as physical activity/exercise (Hausenblas *et al.* 1997; Hagger *et al.* 2002; Downs and Hausenblas 2005), dietary behaviours (McEachan *et al.* 2011), and safe sex (Sheeran and Taylor 1999; Albarracin *et al.* 2001). McEachan *et al.* (2011) provide the most comprehensive review across a broad range of protection behaviours and included 148 prospective studies. Across studies, a frequency-weighted average of 37% of the variance in behavioural intention was explained by attitude, subjective norm, and PBC, with attitude the strongest predictor ($r_+ = 0.51$), followed by PBC ($r_+ = 0.46$) and subjective norm ($r_+ = 0.34$). Across the same studies, a frequency-weighted average of 19% of the variance in behaviour was explained by behavioural intention and PBC, with behavioural intention the stronger predictor ($r_+ = 0.42$) and PBC the weaker predictor ($r_+ = 0.30$).

Within protection behaviours, participation in physical activity/exercise has been a particularly prominent focus. Studies of the TPB in this area have looked at exercise (Rhodes and Courneya 2005), physical activity (Hagger *et al.* 2001), and walking (Galea and Bray 2006) in a variety of samples. Reviews of applications of the TPB to physical activity include Godin and Kok (1996) and Hausenblas *et al.* (1997). However, the two most comprehensive reviews to date have been performed by Hagger *et al.* (2002) in a review of 72 independent studies and McEachan *et al.* (2011) in a review of 103 independent studies. Across these two reviews, attitude, subjective norm, and PBC explained 45–46% of the variance in intentions, with attitude ($r_+ = 0.48$–0.51) and PBC ($r_+ = 0.44$-0.47) stronger predictors than subjective norm ($r_+ = 0.25$–0.32). Behavioural intention and PBC accounted for an average of 24–27% of the variance in behaviour across studies, with intention ($r_+ = 0.42$–0.45) having slightly more predictive power than PBC ($r_+ = 0.31$–0.34).

The TPB has also been applied to a range of dietary behaviours, including low fat consumption (Armitage and Conner 1999), fruit and vegetable consumption (Blanchard *et al.* 2009), and healthy eating (Conner *et al.* 2002). McEachan *et al.* (2011) identified 30 prospective TPB studies examining dietary behaviours. Across studies, a frequency-weighted average of 50% of the variance in behavioural intention was explained by attitude, subjective norm, and PBC, with attitude the strongest predictor ($r_+ = 0.52$), followed by PBC ($r_+ = 0.44$) and subjective norm ($r_+ = 0.35$). A frequency-weighted average of 21% of the variance in behaviour was explained by behavioural intention and PBC, with intention the stronger predictor ($r_+ = 0.38$) and PBC the weaker predictor ($r_+ = 0.30$).

The TPB has also been applied to a number of sexual behaviours, including using condoms (Morrison *et al.* 1998) and various safe sex behaviours (De Wit *et al.* 2000). In addition, a range of different population groups have been examined, including general populations, heterosexual and homosexual samples, and sex workers. There have been several reviews of the application of the TPB to sexual behaviours (Godin and Kok 1996) or condom use (Sheeran and Taylor 1999). Albarracin *et al.* (2001) report the most inclusive review of the application of the TRA and TPB to condom use, which included a maximum of 96 datasets. Across studies, attitude, subjective norm, and PBC explained 50% of the variance in intentions, with attitude ($r_+ = 0.58$) and PBC ($r_+ = 0.45$) stronger predictors than subjective norm ($r_+ = 0.39$). Behavioural intention and PBC accounted for an average 30% of the variance in behaviour, with the intention–behaviour relationship ($r_+ = 0.45$) considerably stronger than the PBC–behaviour relationship ($r_+ = 0.25$). Indeed, in this review, across studies, PBC failed to increase significantly the amount of variance explained in condom use over and above that explained by intentions. McEachan *et al.* (2011) identified 15 prospective studies. Across these studies, a frequency-weighted average of 51% of the variance in intentions was explained by attitude, subjective norm, and PBC, with attitude the strongest predictor ($r_+ = 0.51$), followed by subjective norm ($r_+ = 0.45$) and PBC ($r_+ = 0.44$). A frequency-weighted average of 14% of the variance in behaviour was explained by behavioural intention and PBC, with intention the stronger predictor ($r_+ = 0.34$) and PBC the weaker predictor ($r_+ = 0.21$).

3.3.2 Risk behaviours

Fewer TPB studies have been applied to risk behaviours. However, the existing studies have focused on a diverse range of risk behaviours, including overall alcohol use (Conner *et al.* 1999), binge drinking (Norman *et al.* 2007), illicit drug use (McMillan and Conner 2003), smoking initiation

(Conner *et al.* 2006) and quitting (Moan and Rise 2005), and various risk-related driving violations such as exceeding the posted speed limit in cars (Elliott and Armitage 2009). Cooke *et al.* (in press) provided a meta-analysis of up to 40 TPB studies on alcohol. Attitude was the strongest predictor ($r_+ = 0.62$), followed by subjective norm ($r_+ = 0.47$) and PBC ($r_+ = 0.31$). Behavioural intention was a strong predictor of behaviour ($r_+ = 0.54$), although PBC was not ($r_+ = -0.05$). McEachan *et al.* (2011) provide the most comprehensive review of risk behaviours and included 42 prospective studies. Across these studies, a frequency-weighted average of 33% of the variance in intentions was explained by attitude, subjective norm, and PBC, with attitude the strongest predictor ($r_+ = 0.46$), followed by PBC ($r_+ = 0.43$) and subjective norm ($r_+ = 0.38$). A frequency-weighted average of 14% of the variance in behaviour was explained by behavioural intention and PBC, with intention the stronger predictor ($r_+ = 0.37$) and PBC the weaker predictor ($r_+ = 0.23$).

McEachan *et al.* (2011) also distinguish between simple risk behaviours (e.g. unhealthy snacking; Verplanken 2006) and abstinence behaviours (e.g. quitting smoking; Van den Putte *et al.* 2009). Twenty-nine prospective studies of risk behaviours were identified. Across these studies, a frequency-weighted average of 40% of the variance in intentions was explained by attitude, subjective norm, and PBC, with attitude the strongest predictor ($r_+ = 0.46$), followed by PBC ($r_+ = 0.43$) and subjective norm ($r_+ = 0.40$). A frequency-weighted average of 15% of the variance in behaviour was explained by behavioural intention and PBC, with intention the stronger predictor ($r_+ = 0.37$) and PBC the weaker predictor ($r_+ = 0.22$). There were also 13 prospective studies of abstinence behaviours. Across these studies, a frequency-weighted average of 37% of the variance in intentions was explained by attitude, subjective norm, and PBC, with attitude the strongest predictor ($r_+ = 0.47$), followed by PBC ($r_+ = 0.43$) and subjective norm ($r_+ = 0.33$). A frequency-weighted average of 15% of the variance in behaviour was explained by behavioural intention and PBC, with intention the stronger predictor ($r_+ = 0.35$) and PBC the weaker predictor ($r_+ = 0.26$).

3.3.3 Detection behaviours

The TPB has been used in a number of studies to investigate detection behaviours, including self-examination (Lechner *et al.* 2004), cervical screening attendance (Sandberg and Conner 2009), and breast cancer screening (Rutter 2000). McEachan *et al.* (2011) reviewed 17 prospective applications of the TPB to detection behaviours. Across studies, a frequency-weighted average of 40% of the variance in behavioural intention was explained by attitude, subjective norm, and PBC, with attitude the strongest predictor ($r_+ = 0.45$), followed by PBC ($r_+ = 0.45$) and subjective norm ($r_+ = 0.33$). A frequency-weighted average of 15% of the variance in behaviour was explained by behavioural intention and PBC, with intention the stronger predictor ($r_+ = 0.37$) and PBC the weaker predictor ($r_+ = 0.20$). Cooke and French (2008) reviewed 33 applications of the TPB to screening attendance (although the overall variance explained in intentions and behaviour was not reported). Attitude was the strongest predictor ($r_+ = 0.51$) of intentions, followed by PBC ($r_+ = 0.46$) and subjective norm ($r_+ = 0.41$). Behavioural intention was the strongest predictor ($r_+ = 0.37$) and PBC the weaker predictor ($r_+ = 0.19$) of behaviour.

3.3.4 Conclusions from studies applying the TPB to health behaviours

The TPB has been applied to a wide range of health behaviours. In some cases, the number of studies is considerable; for example, Hagger *et al.* (2002) identified over 70 applications of the TPB to physical activity. In the vast majority of cases, these have been successful applications in that the TPB has been able to explain considerable proportions of variation in intentions and behaviours. In relation to behaviour, this is despite the fact that there is commonly a considerable time gap between the measurement of TPB variables and subsequent behaviour. However, it is also the case that there is significant variation in the findings between studies. Some of this variation appears to be attributable to differences between behaviours (see Godin and Kok 1996; McEachan *et al.* 2011). In addition, relationships with behavior are generally stronger when using self-report as opposed to objective measures of behavior, and when the time interval between measurement of cognitions and behavior is shorter (McEachan *et al.* 2011).

4 Developments

In this section, we comment on two related areas of development concerning the role of additional predictors in the TPB: new predictors incorporated through reconceptualizations of each of the major constructs (Ajzen 2002a; Hagger and Chatzisarantis 2005), and new predictors that constitute useful additions to the model (Conner and Armitage 1998).

4.1 Multiple component view of the TPB – the reasoned action approach

4.1.1 Components of intentions

The construct of intention is central to the TRA/TPB. Intentions capture the motivational factors that influence a behaviour: how hard people are willing to try, how much effort they are willing to exert to perform the behaviour (Ajzen 1991: 181) or the self-instructions individuals give themselves to act (Triandis 1977). There has been some variation in how the intention construct has been operationalized in TRA/TPB studies. Warshaw and Davis (1985) made the distinction between measures of behavioural intentions (e.g. 'I intend to perform behaviour X') and self-predictions (e.g. 'How likely is it that you will perform behaviour X?'). Sheppard and colleagues' (1988) meta-analysis indicated the latter to be more predictive of behaviour. Beyond this, Bagozzi (1992) has suggested that attitudes may first be translated into desires (e.g. 'I want to perform behaviour X'), which then develop into intentions to act, which direct action (see Perugini and Bagozzi 2003). In their meta-analysis, Armitage and Conner (2001) specifically considered the role of intentions, desires, and self-predictions in the context of the TPB. Intentions and self-predictions were stronger predictors of behaviour than desires when PBC was included as a predictor. The meta-analytic data indicated that the most variance in behaviour was explained by employing measures of intentions and PBC. When added to the clearer causal argument that can be made for intentions in determining behaviour, this provides strong support for employing a measure of intentions rather than one of self-predictions or desires. However, given the commonly very high level of correlation between measures of desire, intention, and expectation, it is perhaps not surprising that the majority of studies reviewed by Armitage and Conner (2001) employed mixed measures of intention (combining measures of intention, self-prediction, and/or desire). The extent to which a second-order factor (i.e. motivation) might usefully account for the more differentiated components of intentions, expectations, and desires has yet to be examined in the literature.

4.1.2 Components of attitudes

As noted earlier, reviews of the TRA/TPB often demonstrate attitudes to be the best predictor of intentions. In the TRA/TPB, attitudes towards behaviours are measured by semantic differential scales (Osgood *et al.* 1957). However, research on attitudes towards objects has used such measures to distinguish between affective and cognitive measures of attitudes, with the suggestion that the former are more closely related to behaviour (e.g. Breckler and Wiggins 1989; Eagly *et al.* 1994). It is now recognized that similar components of an attitude towards a behaviour can be distinguished in the TRA/TPB. In particular, it has been noted that an attitude may contain instrumental or cognitive (e.g. desirable–undesirable, valuable–worthless) as well as experiential or affective (e.g. pleasant–unpleasant, interesting–boring) aspects (see Ajzen and Driver 1992; Crites *et al.* 1994). However, research with the TPB has been criticized for focusing on the instrumental/cognitive aspects of attitudes to the detriment of affective/experiential aspects. This is problematic because research has indicated that intentions may be more closely related to affective than cognitive measures of attitudes. For example, Ajzen and Driver (1992) reported affective measures of attitudes (e.g. pleasant–unpleasant) to be more closely related to intentions than were instrumental (e.g. useful–useless) measures in four of five behaviours studied (see also Ajzen and Timko 1986; Ajzen and Driver 1992; Chan and Fishbein 1993; Manstead and Parker 1995). Similarly, Lawton *et al.* (2009) showed affective attitudes to be significantly stronger predictors of intentions and behaviour across a number of health behaviours.

Ajzen and Fishbein (2005) have recently indicated that appropriate attitude measures for use in the TPB should contain items representing both the instrumental/cognitive and affective/experiential components of attitudes (see also Fishbein 1993). The two components do tend to be correlated with one another but can be discriminated based on their underlying belief systems (Trafimow and Sheeran 1998), their different functions (Breckler and Wiggins 1989), experimental manipulations (Conner *et al.* 2011), and empirical differences (Eagly and Chaiken 1993). Ajzen (2002a) has suggested that in order to maintain the parsimony of the TPB, it is useful to distinguish between a higher-order construct of attitude and these differentiated components of attitude at a lower order (Ajzen 2002a). One approach would then be to use this higher-order attitude measure as a predictor of intentions and behaviour alongside other components of the TPB. Such a higher-order construct has the advantages of parsimony (i.e. not increasing the number of predictors) and explaining the shared variance between two lower-order components of attitudes. The higher-order construct is not measured directly from observed data but is indicated by the first-order constructs (i.e. instrumental/cognitive and experiential/affective attitudes), which are so named because they are derived from the observed data (Bollen 1989). However, a problem of such an approach is the need for further theorizing about the relationship between the higher- and lower-order components – that is, which causes which (Ajzen 2002a; Rhodes and Courneya 2003a; Hagger and Chatzisarantis 2005). An alternative approach has been to consider the lower-order components as independent predictors of intentions and behaviour. This approach is less parsimonious but does allow us to examine which is the more important predictor. The growing number of studies taking this approach has prompted meta-analyses of such TPB studies.

As part of a study examining the overlap between affective attitude and anticipated regret, Conner *et al.* (2014) report a meta-analysis of 16 prospective studies on health behaviours involving 6121 participants. They report a frequency-weighted correlation between cognitive/instrumental attitudes and affective/experiential attitudes of 0.51, and note that affective/experiential attitudes were stronger correlates of behaviour than instrumental/cognitive attitudes ($r_+ = 0.27$ vs. $r_+ = 0.18$) but showed similar correlations with intentions ($r_+ = 0.40$ vs. $r_+ = 0.41$). McEachan *et al.* (submitted) report a meta-analysis of 45 prospective studies on health behaviours involving 12,125 participants. The frequency-weighted correlation between cognitive/instrumental attitudes and affective/experiential attitudes was 0.46. In this review, affective/experiential attitudes were stronger predictors than instrumental/cognitive attitudes of both intentions ($r_+ = 0.57$ vs. $r_+ = 0.42$) and behaviour ($r_+ = 0.31$ vs. $r_+ = 0.24$).

In the TRA/TPB, attitudes are held to be determined by underlying salient behavioural beliefs (Fishbein 1967). It is assumed that a person may possess a large number of beliefs about a particular behaviour, but that at any one time only some of these are likely to be salient. It is the salient beliefs that are assumed to determine a person's attitude. However, Towriss (1984) noted that while the theory would suggest the use of individually salient beliefs, respondents are normally presented with modal salient beliefs based on pilot work, following the procedures outlined by Ajzen and Fishbein (1980). This procedure has a number of disadvantages. First, procedures (e.g. asking for advantages and disadvantages of the behaviour) for sampling 'behavioural beliefs' about specific behaviours may sample an excessively cognitive subset (i.e. instrumental beliefs) of the influences that actually play on people's attitudes (Wilson et al. 1989), and fail to elicit beliefs that are more difficult to articulate (e.g. affective/experiential or moral influences; Sparks 1994), yet are potentially important influences on attitude formation. A second problem is that the TPB is primarily concerned with individuals' beliefs. The supply of beliefs by researchers may not adequately capture the beliefs salient to the individual no matter how extensive the pilot work. Studies have explored the use of individually generated beliefs within the TRA (e.g. Rutter and Bunce 1989). For example, in a study of individually generated and modal beliefs about condom use, Agnew (1998) reported that individually generated beliefs were marginally significantly more strongly related to overall attitudes ($r = 0.46$ vs. 0.38, $p_{diff} < 0.10$). This does not compare favourably with the moderately strong correlation between modal behavioral beliefs and attitudes more commonly reported (Table 5.1). Thus, while the use of individually generated beliefs is more consistent with the TRA/TPB, it does not appear to reduce measurement error sufficiently to increase levels of prediction of attitudes and so compensate for the additional effort required in data collection.

Another problem related to the use of modal beliefs concerns the relative importance of beliefs. Although some studies have suggested that just the outcome expectancy needs to be measured (Gagne and Godin 2000; Rhodes et al. 2009), the summative model of attitudes used in the TPB suggests that each outcome expectancy is weighted by a corresponding outcome evaluation (see Section 2.2). Alternatively, some authors have suggested that the prediction of attitudes might be improved by adding a measure of importance or relevance of the attribute to the attitude towards the behaviour, although the evidence is mixed (e.g. Agnew 1998). Nevertheless, information about belief importance could usefully inform the design of interventions to change behaviour in segments of the population stratified by key beliefs (Van der Pligt and de Vries 1998; for a discussion, see Van der Pligt et al. 2000). A further approach to dealing with differences in the relative importance of beliefs is to group beliefs on theoretical grounds (Bandura 2000; Rhodes and Conner 2010) and examine their predictive power. For example, beliefs about more proximal outcomes have been found to be more important determinants of intentions and behaviour than those concerned with more distal outcomes (Goldberg et al. 2002); similarly, beliefs about affective/experiential outcomes have been found to be more predictive of intentions and behaviour than those concerned with instrumental/cognitive outcomes (Lawton et al. 2007).

4.1.3 Components of norms

A number of researchers have argued that more attention needs to be paid to the concept of normative influences within the TRA/TPB (e.g. Conner and Armitage 1998). For example, Armitage and Conner (2001) noted that subjective norms were the weakest predictor of intentions in the TPB. Similarly, Sheppard *et al.* (1988) and Van den Putte (1991) noted that subjective norms were weak predictors of intentions across the TRA studies they reviewed. Although this could merely reflect the lesser importance of normative factors as determinants of intentions in the behaviours studied, a number of alternative explanations for such weak effects are possible.

Armitage and Conner (2001) suggested that the weaker predictive power of subjective norms might, in part, be attributable to the use of single-item measures with lower reliability. Their meta-analysis indicated that where studies employed reliable multi-item measures, subjective norms were significantly stronger predictors of intentions, although still weaker than attitudes or PBC.

Another explanation of the weak predictive power of normative measures in the TRA/TPB is the conceptualization of norms used (Cialdini *et al.* 1991). Cialdini *et al.* (1991) call the normative beliefs used in the TRA/TPB injunctive social norms, as they concern the social approval of others, which motivates action through social reward/punishment, and distinguish them from descriptive social norms, which describe perceptions of what others do (see Deutsch and Gerard 1955). The relative predictive power of these normative components is an issue of some debate.

De Vries *et al.* (1995) reported that measures of injunctive and descriptive norms significantly predicted smoking. Rivis and Sheeran (2003a) have reported a meta-analysis of the role of descriptive norms in the TPB. Across 14 tests with a total $N = 5810$, they reported $r_+ = 0.46$ for the descriptive norm–intention correlation. In addition, across studies descriptive norms were found to explain a highly significant additional 5% of variance in intentions after taking account of attitudes, subjective norms, and PBC. Manning (2009) also reported a meta-analysis of TPB studies measuring both injunctive and descriptive norms and reported injunctive compared to be stronger correlates of intentions than descriptive norms ($r_+ = 0.51$, $k = 160$ vs. $r_+ = 0.40$, $k = 17$), although the pattern was reversed for predictions of behaviour ($r_+ = 0.28$, $k = 156$ vs. $r_+ = 0.34$, $k = 17$).

Fishbein (1993), Ajzen and Fishbein (2005), and Fishbein and Ajzen (2010) have all suggested that subjective norms and descriptive norms be both considered indicators of the same underlying concept, social influence. Similar to attitudes, one might conceive of social pressure as a higher-order factor with injunctive and descriptive norms as lower-order measures. However, it is unclear whether a formative model with injunctive and descriptive norms producing overall social pressure or a reflective model with social pressure producing injunctive and descriptive norms is more appropriate. The moderate correlation between the two [subjective norm–descriptive norm correlation: Rivis and Sheeran (2003a) report $r_+ = 0.38$; Manning (2009) report $r_+ = 0.59$] might be interpreted as supporting the former. A number of TPB studies have measured both injunctive and descriptive norms and used them as independent predictors of intentions and behaviour. McEachan *et al.* (submitted) report a meta-analysis of prospective studies of the TPB applied to health behaviours, and show the two to be only moderately related across 19 tests ($r_+ = 0.26$). Similar to Manning (2009), injunctive norms were found to be stronger correlates of intentions than descriptive norms ($r_+ = 0.39$, $k = 41$ vs. $r_+ = 0.35$, $k = 41$), although the pattern was reversed for predictions of behaviour ($r_+ = 0.22$, $k = 40$ vs. $r_+ = 0.26$, $k = 39$).

A further distinction in relation to the normative component of the TPB has been made by researchers adopting a social identity theory/self-categorization approach (e.g. Terry and Hogg 1996). For example, Terry and Hogg (1996) demonstrated that group norm measures were more predictive of intentions when they employed a measure of group identification (e.g. 'I identify with my friends with regard to smoking') rather than motivation to comply. In two studies, norms only influenced intentions for those who strongly identified with their 'in-group'.

Group norms have been operationalized as either what members of the group are perceived to do (e.g. 'Most of my friends smoke'; i.e. descriptive norms) or to think (e.g. 'Most of my friends think smoking is a good thing to do' [see Johnston and White 2003], sometimes referred to as group attitude). Studies using this approach sometimes report interactive effects between group norms and group identification rather than main effects (e.g. Terry *et al.* 1999). However, where the target group is strongly associated with the behaviour (e.g. my smoking friends), then main effects of group identification on intentions have been reported (e.g. Fekadu and Kraft 2001). Research is required to disentangle further the different social-normative influences on intentions. We believe that evidence strongly supports the use of measures that tap both injunctive and descriptive norms. Whether additional measures of either group attitude or group identification would increase the predictive power of a second-order normative construct requires further research. In particular, for referent groups not defined by the behaviour, an interactive model between group attitude (or descriptive norm) and group identification may be appropriate.

Research has also examined normative beliefs. It should be noted that the distinction between behavioural beliefs and normative beliefs is somewhat arbitrary (Miniard and Cohen 1981), and a strong correlation between the two has often been found (O'Keefe 1990). Miniard and Cohen (1981) point out that the impact of another person's behaviour can equally be assessed as a behavioural belief (e.g. 'Using a condom would please my partner') or a normative belief (e.g. 'My partner thinks I should use a condom'). However, as we noted earlier, it has been argued that there is merit in maintaining a distinction between the determinants of behaviour that are attributes of the person and those that are attributes of the social environment (see Eagly and Chaiken 1993: 171; Trafimow 1998). Trafimow and Fishbein (1995) present a number of experiments that support the distinction (for a review, see Trafimow 1998).

Other researchers have suggested that, rather than the way normative influence is tapped, it is measurement of compliance with this pressure that requires attention. In the TRA/TPB, this is tapped by measures of motivation to comply with the perceived pressure from each salient source of social influence. Typically, such items tap the extent to which the individual wants to do what this individual or group wishes them to in general (Fishbein and Ajzen 1975: 306). There has been debate about the most appropriate level of specificity to use in the wording of the motivation to comply item (e.g. O'Keefe 1990). For example, should motivation to comply specify a group of behaviours in general, or be specific to the behaviour in question (the principle of compatibility might suggest this last alternative)? Alternatively, as we noted earlier in relation to social identity theory, a measure of group identification (e.g. 'I identify with my friends with regard to smoking') rather than motivation to comply might be more appropriate. Such an approach would also suggest combining such identification with a different measure of group norm (i.e. descriptive norm or group attitude rather than injunctive norm). Furthermore, Gibbons and Gerrard (1997) draw upon ideas of behavioural prototypes (e.g. the typical smoker) and suggest that positive evaluation and perceived similarity to such prototypes may represent another way in which social influence and comparison processes operate. Rivis and Sheeran (2003b) provide support for this idea in relation to engaging in exercise behaviour. Prototype similarity but not prototype evaluation had an independent effect on both intentions and behaviour in the context of TPB variables, descriptive norms, and past behaviour. Alternatively, if both injunctive norm and descriptive norm measures are taken in relation to specific referents to tap *perceived norms,* then the added predictive value of weighting either or both by motivation to comply or a related measure in such models is unclear.

4.1.4 Components of PBC

The difference between the TRA and TPB lies in the control component (i.e. PBC) of the TPB. We noted earlier that meta-analytic evidence has generally supported the power of PBC to explain additional variance in intentions and behaviour after controlling for the components of the TRA. The overlap in definition of PBC with Bandura's (1977: 192) definition of self-efficacy, '…the conviction that one can successfully execute the behavior required to produce the outcomes', is striking. Ajzen (1991) argued that the PBC and self-efficacy constructs were synonymous and more recently 'quite similar' (Ajzen 2002a). Congruent with this view of a conceptual overlap between PBC and self-efficacy, several researchers (e.g. De Vries *et al.* 1995) have advocated the use of measures of self-efficacy in place of PBC within the TPB. However, this has proved problematic because of differences in the way the two constructs have been operationalized. This latter issue reflects a broader controversy surrounding the nature and measurement of PBC, which has a number of threads. A first thread concerns disparities in the definitions and operationalizations used with respect to PBC and the possibility that it represents a multidimensional construct (for reviews, see Ajzen 2002a; Trafimow *et al.* 2002; Rodgers *et al.* 2008). A second thread has questioned the discriminant validity of some operationalizations of PBC as distinct from other components of the TPB.

Early definitions of the PBC construct were intended to encompass perceptions of factors that were both internal (e.g. knowledge, skills, willpower) and external (e.g. time availability, cooperation of others) to the individual. For example, Ajzen and Madden (1986: 457) defined PBC as: '…the person's belief as to how easy or difficult performance of the behavior is likely to be'. However, the items used to tap PBC included both perceptions of difficulty and perceptions of control over the behaviour (see Sparks *et al.* 1997). In the majority of early applications of the TPB, researchhers tended to employ 'mixed' measures of PBC that included both components. However, opinion appears to have coalesced around the idea of PBC being a multidimensional construct consisting of two separate but related components (Ajzen 2002a; Trafimow *et al.* 2002; Rodgers *et al.* 2008). In particular, Ajzen (2002a) argues that PBC can be considered as a second-order construct that consists of two components, which he labels perceived self-efficacy and perceived controllability. Trafimow *et al.* (2002) label these terms perceived difficulty and perceived control, and provide experimental and meta-analytic support for distinguishing the two. Rodgers *et al.* (2008) distinguish between self-efficacy, perceived difficulty, and perceived control and provide evidence supporting the greater predictive power of self-efficacy measures. There seems to be little evidence that these different components show any simple mapping onto control factors that are internal versus external to the individual (Ajzen 2002a).

The *self-efficacy* or perceived confidence component of PBC '…deals with the ease or difficulty of performing a behavior, with people's confidence that they can perform it if they want to do so' (Ajzen 2002c). Ajzen (2002a) has suggested that this component of PBC can be tapped by two types of items: first, the perceived difficulty of the behaviour, e.g. 'For me to quit smoking would be…' (very difficult–very easy); second, the perceived confidence the individual has that he or she can perform the behaviour, e.g. 'I am confident that I could quit smoking' (definitely false–definitely true). It is clear that perceived confidence items most closely resemble the 'can-do cognitions' involved in assessing self-efficacy (Bandura 2000; Luszczynska and Schwarzer, Chapter 7 this volume). Ajzen (2002c) suggests that the *perceived control* component of PBC 'involves people's beliefs that they have control over the behavior, that performance or non-performance of the behavior is up to them'. Again, two types of items can be distinguished: first, perceived control over performance of the behaviour, e.g. 'How much control do you believe you have over quitting smoking?' (no control–complete control); second, perceptions of where control resides, e.g. 'It is mostly up to me whether or not I quit smoking' (strongly disagree–strongly agree).

Kraft *et al.* (2005) note that in the majority of TPB studies, PBC has been assessed by a mixture of these four different types of items. This might explain why low internal reliabilities have been reported for such measures of PBC (see Notani 1998). Ajzen (2002a) has suggested that formative research could allow the selection of a set of items that adequately tap PBC and show good internal reliability. This might avoid the complexity of employing a second-order PBC factor based on separate measures of perceived self-efficacy and perceived controllability.

A second thread to research with the PBC construct has focused on discriminant validity. Fishbein and colleagues (Chan and Fishbein 1993; Fishbein 1997; Leach *et al.* 2001) suggest two problems with employing perceived difficulty items to tap PBC: first, there is no necessary association between an individual's perceptions of how difficult a behaviour is held to be and how much they perceive control over performing it; second, easy–difficult items overlap conceptually and empirically with semantic-differential items designed to tap affective attitudes. The argument is that an individual is likely to hold a positive affective attitude towards an easy-to-perform behaviour and a negative affective attitude towards a difficult-to-perform behaviour. Leach *et al.* (2001) showed that perceived difficulty items appeared to tap both attitudes and self-efficacy in relation to condom use. Kraft *et al.* (2005) also provided evidence for an empirical overlap between perceived difficulty items and affective attitude for physical activity and recycling behaviours.

This review of existing research suggests at least three possibilities in relation to measuring PBC within the TPB. First, Ajzen (2002a) has suggested that the use of formative research within a behavioural domain can result in the appropriate selection of items with a unidimensional structure. Such items might reflect perceived difficulty, perceived confidence, and/or perceived control, as appropriate. Second, measures can explicitly tap the two components of PBC identified by Ajzen (2002a): perceived self-efficacy and perceived controllability. Ajzen and Fishbein (2005) argue that items concerned with the ease or difficulty of performing a behaviour, or confidence in one's ability to perform it, tend to load on the former, whereas items that address control over the behaviour, or the extent to which its performance is up to the actor, load on the second factor. Research could then either explore the relative predictive power of these two components (see Trafimow *et al.* 2002) or, as Ajzen (2002a) suggested, explore the power of a second-order factor of PBC based on these two components (e.g. see Hagger and Chatzisarantis 2005). Third, measures of PBC could be selected that explicitly avoid perceived difficulty items because of concerns about overlap with affective attitudes. Such measures might be selected to be unidimensional (i.e. PBC) or bidimensional (i.e. perceived self-efficacy and perceived controllability). Armitage and Conner (1999) provided evidence to support a distinction between self-efficacy and 'perceived control over behaviour', utilizing measures that do not rely on perceived ease or difficulty.

Research is needed to explore further these different possibilities and their implications. Evidence from previous meta-analyses is mixed. For example, while Armitage and Conner (2001) report evidence that measures of self-efficacy are better than measures of controllability at predicting intentions $(r_+ = 0.44$ vs. $0.23)$ and behaviour $(r_+ = 0.35$ vs. $0.18)$, self-efficacy was no better than unidimensional measures of PBC for predicting intentions $(r_+ = 0.44$ vs. $0.44)$ or behaviour $(r_+ = 0.35$ vs. $0.40)$. Similarly, Trafimow *et al.* (2002) showed perceived difficulty to be more strongly correlated than perceived control with both intentions $(r_+ = 0.53$ vs. $0.27)$ and behaviour

($r_+ = 0.48$ vs. 0.27). In their meta-analysis of prospective studies of the TPB applied to health behaviours, McEachan *et al.* (submitted) reported that perceived self-efficacy was more strongly correlated than perceived control with both intentions ($r_+ = 0.60$, $k = 35$ vs. $r_+ = 0.29$, $k = 30$) and behaviour ($r_+ = 0.39$, $k = 35$ vs. $r_+ = 0.20$, $k = 30$). Thus it is clear that measures tapping perceived self-efficacy tend to be more predictive than measures tapping perceived controllability. In contrast, Rhodes and Courneya (2003b) have argued for a focus on controllability because it shows better discriminant validity with intention than does self-efficacy. In contrast, Ajzen (2002a) suggests that a reliable unidimensional measure of PBC or a second-order measure of PBC based on perceived self-efficacy and perceived controllability would provide the strongest prediction of intentions and behaviour.

Another issue in relation to the PBC component of the TPB is the assessment of underlying control beliefs. There has been some variation in how such beliefs have been tapped (Manstead and Parker 1995). Ajzen (1991: 196) suggests that control beliefs 'assess the presence or absence of requisite resources and opportunities'. These beliefs are assumed to be based upon various forms of previous experience with the behaviour. These factors might be elicited in a pilot study by the question, 'What factors might prevent or help you perform behavior X?' However, there has been some variation in how modal control beliefs have been operationalized. Ajzen and Madden (1986) assessed PBC based upon the sum of frequency of occurrence of various facilitators and inhibitors. Others (e.g. Godin and Gionet 1991) have employed a formulation closer to that used to assess self-efficacy to gauge the extent to which a particular barrier will make performance of the behaviour more difficult, e.g. 'How likely is being drunk to inhibit your use of a condom?' (likely–unlikely). Ajzen (1991) suggests a formulation closer to that employed to assess the other beliefs in the TPB. Control beliefs are tapped by items assessing the frequency with which a facilitator or inhibitor of the behaviour occurs, e.g. 'I can climb in an area that has good weather' (likely–unlikely) weighted by its perceived power to facilitate or inhibit performance of the behaviour, e.g. 'Good weather makes mountain climbing...' (easier–more difficult), with both items scored as bipolar items. This format has been employed by several authors (e.g. Ajzen and Driver 1992; Parker *et al.* 1995). Future research might usefully assess the relationship of underlying beliefs to overall perceptions of control and whether different sets of control beliefs underlie the different dimensions of PBC. For example, Armitage and Conner (1999) provided evidence to suggest that control beliefs were antecedents of self-efficacy, but correlated only weakly with perceived control. Finally, as we have noted in relation to behavioural and normative beliefs, research that tests the predictive value of each component against the multiplicative combination is required.

4.1.5 Multi-component TPB

Integrating the above distinctions into the TPB produces a multi-component TPB, extended TPB (McEachan *et al.* submitted) or reasoned action approach (see Figure 5.2) that appears to be endorsed by Ajzen and Fishbein (Ajzen and Fishbein 2005; Conner and Sparks 2005; Fishbein and Ajzen 2010; Head and Noar 2014). Each of attitude, perceived norm, and perceived behavioural control are represented as breaking down into two sub-components. Although Fishbein and Ajzen (2010) have argued for retaining overall measures of attitude, perceived norm, and PBC based on the sub-components, a growing number of researchers separately measure each of the sub-components. Meta-analyses of TPB studies examining affective versus cognitive attitudes (Conner *et al.* 2014), injunctive versus descriptive norms (Manning 2009), and perceived control versus self-efficacy (Rodgers *et al.* 2008) have been published. More recently McEachan *et al.*

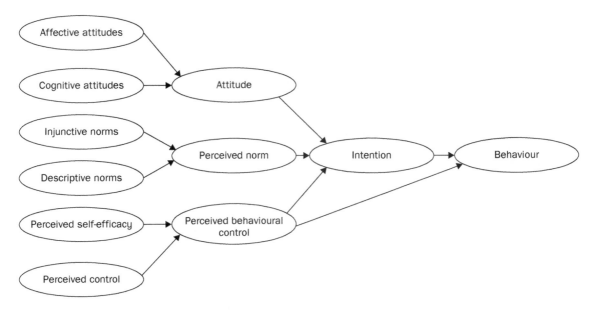

Figure 5.2 Multi-component theory of planned behaviour

(submitted) reported a meta-analysis of tests of the full extended TPB (Table 5.2). Regression analysis of this meta-analytic data indicated that the six variables explain 51.0% of the variance in intentions, with all except perceived control being significant predictors. Intention plus the six variables explained 25.1% of the variance in behaviour with intention, perceived self-efficacy, affective attitudes, and descriptive norms being significant. There were several striking features of this meta-analysis: first, the strong predictive power of perceived self-efficacy compared with perceived control measures in predicting both behaviour and intentions (despite their relatively strong intercorrelation); second, the stronger correlations for affective/experiential attitudes than instrumental/cognitive attitudes with both intentions and behaviour (Table 5.2); third, the fact that descriptive norm was a significant predictor of both intentions and behaviour, whereas injunctive norm was mainly a predictor of intentions (despite their relatively strong intercorrelation). Together these findings might suggest that measures of perceived control add relatively little to predictions of intentions or behaviour, and that a direct path (bypassing intentions) from affective attitudes and descriptive norm to behaviour might be usefully added to the model.

4.2 Additional predictors

The sufficiency of the TRA/TPB has received considerable attention (Eagly and Chaiken 1993: 168–93; see Conner and Armitage 1998), and a number of potential additional predictors have been proposed. Ajzen (1991: 199) suggested the openness of the TPB to such developments: 'The theory of planned behavior is, in principle, open to the inclusion of additional predictors if it can be shown that they capture a significant proportion of variance in intention or behavior after the theory's current variables have been taken into account.' In this section, we consider four additional constructs: anticipated affective reactions, moral norms, self-identity, and past

Table 5.2 A meta-analysis of the multi-component theory of planned behaviour (from McEachan *et al.* submitted)

Relationship	k	N	r_+
Intention–Behaviour	82	21 008	0.48
Perceived self-efficacy–Behaviour	35	6 844	0.39
Perceived control–Behaviour	30	6 201	0.20
Affective attitude–Behaviour	46	12 490	0.30
Cognitive attitude–Behaviour	46	12 490	0.19
Injunctive norm–Behaviour	40	12 696	0.22
Descriptive norm–Behaviour	39	11 934	0.26
Perceived self-efficacy–Intention	35	7 131	0.60
Perceived control–Intention	30	6 348	0.29
Affective attitude–Intention	47	12 756	0.55
Cognitive attitude–Intention	47	12 756	0.39
Injunctive norm–Intention	43	20 880	0.39
Descriptive norm–Intention	43	20 861	0.35

behaviour. In each case, theoretical (Fishbein 1993) and empirical (Ajzen 1991) justifications for their inclusion in the TPB are considered. Although a range of other constructs (e.g. personality dimensions; Conner and Abraham 2001) have been addressed sporadically in the literature, there is insufficient published research to evaluate their contribution. As the TRA/TPB 'has the great virtue of parsimony' (Charng *et al.* 1988: 303), we argue that the evidence needs to be strong to justify serious consideration of any additional variables.

4.2.1 Anticipated affective reactions

As noted earlier, the traditional method for eliciting behavioural beliefs may fail to elicit affective outcomes associated with performance of the behaviour (see Manstead and Parker 1995; Van der Pligt and de Vries 1998). Such anticipated affective reactions to the performance or non-performance of a behaviour may be important determinants of attitudes and intentions (Triandis 1977; Van der Pligt and de Vries 1998), especially where the consequences of the behaviour are unpleasant or negatively affectively laden. Emotional outcomes are commonly factored into decision-making. One type of anticipated affective reaction that has received particular attention is anticipated regret. Anticipated regret is a negative, cognitive-based emotion that is experienced when we realize or imagine that the present situation could have been better had we acted differently. This concept of anticipated regret has been considered in a number of TPB studies (for a review, see Sandberg and Conner 2008).

Factor analytic studies (Richard *et al.* 1996; Sheeran and Orbell 1999; Conner *et al.* 2013a) have demonstrated that regret is distinct from the other components of the TPB (attitude, subjective norm, and PBC). Studies have shown anticipated regret to add to the prediction of intentions over and above the components of the TPB for a range of behaviours, including eating junk foods, using soft drugs, and alcohol use (Richard *et al.* 1996). In a meta-analysis of TPB studies using regret, Sandberg and Conner (2008) found the correlation between anticipated regret and intentions to be $r_+ = 0.47$ ($N = 11\ 098$ participants, $k = 24$ studies). More importantly, regret explained an additional 7.0% of the variance in intentions after attitude, subjective norm, and PBC were taken into account ($p < 0.0001$) (see also Rivis *et al.* 2009). More recently, Conner *et al.* (2014) reported a meta-analysis of anticipated regret and affective/experiential attitude studies. Across 16 studies involving 6121 participants, affective attitudes and anticipated regret were only moderately related ($r_+ = 0.35$) and had similar correlations with intentions ($r_+ = 0.27$ and $r_+ = 0.23$, respectively) and behaviour ($r_+ = 0.40$ and $r_+ = 0.47$, respectively). Ajzen and Sheikh (2013; see also Fishbein and Ajzen 2010) argue that studies measuring regret tend to examine regret about not doing the behaviour when the TPB variables are measured in relation to performing the behaviour (or vice versa). When all are measured in relation to the same behaviour (doing or not doing), regret was shown to have little impact on intentions. While this criticism does appear to apply to many tests of adding anticipated regret to the TPB, some positive results have been obtained when regret is measured in relation to the same behaviour as the TPB variables (Sandberg 2005). Ajzen and Sheikh's argument also raises interesting issues about the added value of measuring TPB and other variables in relation to both doing the behaviour and not doing the behaviour (see Richetin *et al.* 2011).

4.2.2 Moral norms

Cialdini *et al.* (1991) distinguished between injunctive, descriptive, and moral norms. We have commented on how the first two might usefully be considered components of a social norm construct. The latter are the individual's perception of the moral correctness or incorrectness of performing a behavior and take account of '…personal feelings of…responsibility to perform, or refuse to perform, a certain behavior' (Ajzen 1991: 199). Moral norms might be expected to have an important influence on the performance of those behaviours with a moral or ethical dimension (e.g. Beck and Ajzen 1991). Ajzen (1991) suggested that moral norms work in parallel with attitudes, subjective norms, and PBC, and directly influence intentions. For example, Beck and Ajzen (1991) included a measure of moral norm in their analysis of dishonest actions, and found that it significantly increased the amount of variance accounted for in each intention (by 3–6%). Conner and Armitage (1998) reported the correlation between moral norms and intentions to be $r_+ = 0.50$ across 11 TPB studies. Moral norm added, on average, a significant 4% to the prediction of intention. Rivis *et al.* (2009) reported a meta-analysis of 47 TPB studies with 16 420 participants in which they also measured moral norms. The frequency-weighted correlation between moral norms and intentions was found to be $r_+ = 0.47$, with moral norms explaining an additional 3% of variance in intentions after controlling for TPB variables. Any effects of moral norms on behaviour were found to be fully mediated by intentions. These findings imply that moral norms could be a useful addition to the TPB, at least for those behaviours where moral considerations are likely to be important (see Godin *et al.* 2005). Manstead (2000) provides a more detailed review of research with the moral norm construct.

4.2.3 Self-identity

Baumeister and Muraven (1996: 406) describe identity as 'a set of meaningful definitions that are ascribed or attached to the self, including social roles, reputation, a structure of values and priorities, and a conception of one's potentiality'. It may reflect, for example, the extent to which an actor sees him or herself fulfilling the criteria for any societal role, e.g. 'someone who is concerned with green issues' (Sparks and Shepherd 1992: 392). Several authors have addressed the extent to which self-identity might be a useful addition to the TRA/TPB (e.g. Sparks and Shepherd 1992). Conner and Armitage (1998) reported that across six TPB studies, self-identity had a correlation of $r_+ = 0.27$ with intentions and only explained an additional 1% of variance in intentions after accounting for other TPB variables. Rise *et al.* (2010) report a meta-analysis of 40 TPB studies with a combined total of 11 607 participants that included a measure of self-identity and showed self-identity and intentions to have a correlation of $r_+ = 0.47$. Regressions indicated that self-identity explained an additional 6% of variance in intentions after controlling for TPB variables, although effects on behaviour appeared to be mediated by intentions. Rise *et al.* interpreted their findings as providing support for the role of self-identity as a useful addition to the TPB. However, Ajzen and Fishbein (2005) suggest self-identity might be better considered as an alternative measure of intentions. The overlap between self-identity and frequency of past behaviour is also noteworthy. Despite these mixed views on the value of adding self-identity to the TPB, given the findings of authors such as Sparks and Shepherd (1992), it is reasonable to assume that there are certain behaviours where self-identity will provide additional predictions of intentions. Further research is needed to identify the characteristics of behaviours or the conditions (e.g. for predicting maintenance of a behaviour) under which self-identity becomes a useful addition to the TPB. A strong theoretical rationale for self-identity effects has also not been forthcoming (but see Terry and Hogg 1996; Sparks 2013; Case *et al.* in press) and developments in this regard would seem to be especially important given the concerns that have been raised about measurement issues in relation to this construct (Fishbein and Ajzen 2010).

4.2.4 Past behaviour

The influence of past behaviour on future behaviour is an issue that has attracted considerable attention (for reviews, see Eagly and Chaiken 1993: 178–82; Fishbein and Ajzen 2010: 285–90). It is argued that many behaviours are better predicted by one's previous behaviour rather than cognitions such as described in the TRA/TPB (Sutton 1994). This argument is based on the results of a number of studies showing past behaviour to be the best predictor of future behaviour (e.g. Mullen *et al.* 1987). Conner and Armitage (1998) provide an empirical review of the impact of past behaviour within the TPB. They reported relatively large past behaviour–future behaviour, past behaviour–intention, past behaviour–attitude, and past behaviour–PBC correlations. Ajzen (1991) regards the role of past behaviour as a test of sufficiency of the TPB and that its effects should be mediated by PBC: repetition of behaviour should lead to enhanced perceptions of control. On this basis, one might predict that past behaviour should be most strongly correlated with PBC, although this was not supported in the review of Conner and Armitage (1998). What is of particular interest is the contribution of past behaviour to the predictions of intentions and behaviour once the TPB variables are taken into account. Ajzen (1991) reports that across three studies, the amount of variance added to the prediction of behavior by past behaviour (mean 2.1%) was so small as to reflect common method variance due to use of similar response formats for the two measures. Conner *et al.* (1999) manipulated the degree of similarity in response formats for the two measures of behaviour but found this to explain only a modest amount of variance. Conner and Armitage (1998) found that after taking account of attitude, subjective norm, and PBC, past behaviour, on average, explained a further 7.2% of the variance in intentions (across 12 studies). Similarly, past behaviour explained a mean 13.0% of variance in behaviour after taking account of intentions and PBC (across seven studies) (see also Ouellette and Wood

1998). In their meta-analysis, McEachan *et al.* (2011) included 86 studies on health behaviours that reported past behaviour–behaviour relationships. After taking account of TPB variables, past behaviour, on average, explained a further 5.3% of the variance in intentions and 10.9% of the variance in behaviour. Despite these strong effects of past behaviour within the TPB, we should be cautious in giving past behaviour the same status as other predictors in the TPB. It is clear that past behaviour cannot be used to explain future performance of an action (i.e. individuals do not perform a behaviour *because* they have performed it in the past). However, various automatic processes could explain why past behaviour has such a strong impact on future behaviour. For example, the Reflective Impulsive Model of Strack and Deutsch (2004) suggests a number of such processes that might become important as the behaviour becomes more habitual with frequent performance. Measures of habit strength have been shown to be strong predictors of behaviour (see Norman and Conner, Chapter 12 this volume).

Ajzen (2002b) provides a stimulating review of the effects of past behaviour on later behaviour. He notes that the residual impact of past behaviour on later behaviour after taking account of intentions noted in a number of studies is influenced by several factors. In particular, weaker effects are observed when measures of intention and behaviour are matched on the principle of compatibility. Also, strong, well-formed intentions appear to be associated with an attenuation of the effect of past behaviour. In addition, where expectations are realistic and specific plans for implementation of intentions have been developed, little impact of past behaviour on later behaviour is observed after controlling for intentions (Ajzen 2002b). Finally, experience of the behaviour may itself lead to a change in intentions and reversion to a previous pattern of behaviour (Ajzen and Fishbein 2005). Stable intentions and planning have also been suggested as attenuating the effect of past behaviour and increasing the strength of intentions. For example, Conner *et al.* (2002) showed that as intentions became more stable, their power to predict behaviour six years later increased, while the power of past behaviour decreased

5 Operationalization of the model

In this section, we describe the formulation of measures of each of the model components. Extensive details of applying the TRA can be found in Ajzen and Fishbein (1980), while Ajzen (1991) provides examples of applications of the TPB. Fishbein and Ajzen (2010) provide examples and a guide to measuring components of the multi-component TPB. For those wishing to construct a TPB questionnaire, we recommend that the current section is read in conjunction with the Fishbein and Ajzen (2010) text, so that similarities and differences within question formulation can be identified and considered. It is also worth referring to Ajzen's website (http://people.umass.edu/~aizen/) for his up-to-date views on measurement issues.

While the examples provided in Fishbein and Ajzen (2010) provide a clear demonstration of how to construct a questionnaire assessing 'exercising for at least 20 minutes, three times per week, for the next three months', the examples provided here relate to a series of different behaviours around the broader theme, or behavioural category, of exercising. Thus, Fishbein and Ajzen (2010) provide a comprehensive example of measures for a particular behaviour so that the reader can see how to construct a questionnaire (concerning that specific behaviour) that complies with the *principle of compatibility* requirement. The present text, on the other hand, provides some examples of measures from published research so that the reader can see (a) examples of measures applied to somewhat different behaviours within the same common theme, and (b) the variation between research studies in the level of specificity and in adherence to the target, action, context, time (TACT) principle.

5.1 Behaviour

> Selecting and assessing a behavioral criterion is often the most difficult part of any behavioral study.
>
> (Fishbein 1997: 81)

In considering the development of appropriate measures of each of the components of the TPB, it is important to begin by developing a clear conceptualization of the behaviour or behavioural categories we wish to predict. The principle of compatibility indicates that measures of behaviours and components of the TPB need to be formulated at the same level of specificity with regard to action, target, context, and time. Hence, we need to make an unambiguous decision about the level at which we wish to predict behaviour with regard to these four elements. Specification of the action, target, context, and timeframe for the behaviour will greatly assist the specification of the TPB measures. For example, we may wish to predict running (action) a marathon (target) in Berlin (context) in September next year (timeframe), or walking (action) for an hour (target) in the countryside (context) later today (timeframe).[2] In the latter example, the TPB measures would be taken on one day and the measure of behaviour would need to be taken at a later stage (e.g. the next day). Obviously, aggregation of behaviours across timeframes, contexts, targets, and actions is possible. The minimum specification would require an action to be stated. Such clear specification allows easy application of the principle of compatibility with respect to the TPB measures. Assessment of such a behaviour might involve simple self-reports of whether the behaviour was performed in the specified context over the appropriate time period (in this example, the behaviour is assessed on the following day):

I walked for an hour in the countryside yesterday.   Yes □   No □

Ideally, of course, one would take more objective behaviour measures. Sparks *et al.* (2004), for example, made use of computer records of attendance at a health club; but more often than not, it is either difficult or impossible to obtain appropriate objective behaviour measures (even in this case, the measure was not one of actual exercise behaviour!). The reliability of self-report measures may be expected to vary as a function of the behaviour and context in question, with some (perhaps more 'sensitive' in one way or other) behaviours raising the suspicion that self-reports may be less than accurate (Ajzen and Fishbein 2005).

5.2 Behavioural intention

Behavioural intention measures tend to use a number of standard wordings that incorporate the same level of specificity with respect to action, target, context, and timeframe, as used in the behaviour measure. For example:

I intend to exercise at X health club at least four times each week during the next two weeks.

Definitely do ☐ ☐ ☐ ☐ ☐ ☐ ☐ *Definitely do not*

How likely is it that you will exercise at X health club at least four times each week during the next two weeks?

Very unlikely ☐ ☐ ☐ ☐ ☐ ☐ ☐ *Very likely*

I will try to exercise at X health club at least four times each week during the next two weeks.

Definitely will not ☐ ☐ ☐ ☐ ☐ ☐ ☐ *Definitely will*

Do you intend to exercise at X health club at least four times each week during the next two weeks?

Definitely do ☐ ☐ ☐ ☐ ☐ ☐ ☐ *Definitely do not*
(Adapted from Sparks *et al.* 2004)

From a psychometric point of view, multiple-item measures are more appropriate than single-item measures because of increased reliability.

5.3 Attitudes

Attitudes are a person's evaluation of the target behaviour and are typically measured by using items such as:

My taking regular physical activity over the next 6 months would be:

Harmful	☐ ☐ ☐ ☐ ☐ ☐ ☐	Beneficial
Foolish	☐ ☐ ☐ ☐ ☐ ☐ ☐	Wise
Unpleasant	☐ ☐ ☐ ☐ ☐ ☐ ☐	Pleasant
Unenjoyable	☐ ☐ ☐ ☐ ☐ ☐ ☐	Enjoyable
Bad	☐ ☐ ☐ ☐ ☐ ☐ ☐	Good

(Adapted from Norman *et al.* 2000)

Here participants evaluate the behaviour described at the appropriate level of specificity on a series of semantic differentials (taken from the evaluative dimension of Osgood *et al.* 1957). Typically, 4–6 such differentials are used and these tend to show high internal reliability (alpha > 0.9). While at one stage it was suggested that researchers need only ensure that such items were evaluative and formed a single factor, several dimensions have been identified in a number of studies (Ajzen and Driver 1992). More recently, Ajzen (2002c) has suggested that steps be taken to ensure that both cognitive/instrumental (e.g. harmful–beneficial; foolish–wise;

unimportant–important) and affective/experiential (e.g. unpleasant–pleasant; unenjoyable–enjoyable; unsatisfying–satisfying) items should be included within attitude measures.

Attitudes can also be assessed by simply asking respondents more direct questions about their attitudes (see Ajzen and Fishbein 1980: 55). For example:

My attitude towards my exercising at X health club is…

Extremely unfavourable ☐ ☐ ☐ ☐ ☐ ☐ ☐ *Extremely favourable*
Extremely negative ☐ ☐ ☐ ☐ ☐ ☐ ☐ *Extremely positive*

(Adapted from Sparks *et al.* 2004)

Zanna and Rempel (1988) recommend this latter, 'more purely evaluative' method for measuring attitudes, since it allows research participants to express their general evaluation of the behaviour without the researcher prejudging what the basis (e.g. cognitive or affective) of that attitude might be.

5.4 Subjective norm/perceived norm

In early descriptions of the subjective norm construct, it was both described as a 'person's… perception that most people who are important to him think he should or should not perform the behavior in question' (Ajzen and Fishbein 1980: 57), and a 'person's perception of the social pressures put on him to perform or not perform the behavior in question' (p. 6). There is a difference in these two definitions (consider the example of voting for a particular political party in a secret ballot!) but the construct has traditionally been operationalized as the person's subjective judgement concerning whether significant others would want him or her to perform the behaviour or not, using items such as:

Most people who are important to me think I:

Should ☐ ☐ ☐ ☐ ☐ ☐ ☐ *Should not*

take regular physical activity over the next 6 months. (Adapted from Norman *et al.* 2000)

There are a number of well-known problems with the use of single items (see Armitage and Conner 2001) and additional items have been suggested to make a multi-item scale, although there is little reliability data on such measures.

People who are important to me would:

Approve ☐ ☐ ☐ ☐ ☐ ☐ ☐ *Disapprove*

of my taking regular physical activity over the next 6 months.

People who are important to me want me to take regular physical activity over the next 6 months.

Likely ☐ ☐ ☐ ☐ ☐ ☐ ☐ *Unlikely*

(Adapted from Norman *et al.* 2000)

More recently, Fishbein and Ajzen (2010) have suggested that the notion of perceived norm (reflecting injunctive normative influences, as indicated above) needs to be complemented by an acknowledgement of descriptive normative influences (such as the items given below, which reflect what significant others are perceived to do with respect to the behaviour in question):

People who are important to me exercise regularly.

Strongly disagree   □ □ □ □ □ □ □   *Strongly agree*

How many of the people important to you exercise regularly?

None   □ □ □ □ □ □ □   *All*

5.5 Perceived behavioural control

Perceived behavioural control represents the overall control an individual perceives him or herself to have over performance of the behaviour. Typical items used to measure PBC would be the following:

How much control do you have over whether or not you exercise for at least 20 minutes, three times per week for the next fortnight?

No control   □ □ □ □ □ □ □   *Complete control*

I feel in complete control of whether or not I exercise for at least 20 minutes, three times per week for the next fortnight.

Completely false   □ □ □ □ □ □ □   *Completely true*

For me to exercise for at least 20 minutes, three times per week for the next fortnight would be...

Very easy   □ □ □ □ □ □ □   Very difficult

I am confident that I could exercise for at least 20 minutes, three times per week for the next fortnight.

Strongly disagree   □ □ □ □ □ □ □   *Strongly agree*
(Adapted from Norman *et al.* 2000)

The internal reliability of PBC items has frequently been found to be low (e.g. Sparks 1994; Ajzen 2002a), such that separate assessment of controllability (e.g. the first two items above) and self-efficacy (e.g. the latter two items above) is now recommended (Ajzen 2002a). The problem of the adequate measurement of PBC has received a good deal of attention in recent years (e.g. Ajzen 2002a). For example, if we consider the sorts of items that are currently used to assess the construct, part of the problem with inter-item reliability may be due to differences in the way lay people conceptualize the notion of 'control' and the notion of 'difficulty' (Chan and Fishbein 1993; Sparks *et al.* 1997). People may consider the performance of a behaviour to be 'under their control' yet at the same time consider it to be difficult to carry out. Mixing unipolar and bipolar scales among PBC items may also contribute to this problem.

5.6 Behavioural beliefs

In the TRA/TPB, the relevant behavioural beliefs are those salient to the individual. However, most applications of these models employ modal salient beliefs derived from pilot studies with a representative sample of individuals drawn from the population of interest (for an exception, see Rutter and Bunce 1989). The pilot studies typically consist of semi-structured interviews or questionnaire studies in which participants are asked to list the characteristics, qualities, and attributes of the object or behaviour (Ajzen and Fishbein 1980: 64–71). For example, participants are asked 'What do you see as the advantages and disadvantages of [behaviour]?' The most frequently mentioned (modal) beliefs are then used in the final questionnaire, with commonly between six and 12 beliefs being employed.

Examples of belief strength and outcome evaluation items are given below. Belief strength assesses the subjective probability that a particular outcome will be a consequence of performing the behaviour. Such items commonly use response formats such as 'unlikely–likely', 'improbable–probable' or 'false–true', which are scored in a bipolar fashion (e.g. –3 to +3, on a 7-point scale) or unipolar fashion (e.g. 1 to 7, on a 7-point scale) (for a discussion, see Ajzen 2002c). Outcome evaluations assess the overall evaluation of that outcome and are generally treated as bipolar (–3 'negative evaluation' to +3 'positive evaluation') and responded to on 'bad–good' response formats (Ajzen and Fishbein 1980). Belief strength and outcome evaluation are then multiplicatively combined and summed (equation 3) to give an indirect measure of attitude. The problem with such calculations with interval level data has been noted (e.g. French and Hankins 2003), although no completely satisfactory solution has been found. Ajzen (2002c) has recommended the use of optimal rescaling techniques in order to avoid this problem, but this practice is currently not common in published research and has attracted criticism (French and Hankins 2003).

Belief strength

My taking regular physical activity would make me feel healthier.

Unlikely ☐ ☐ ☐ ☐ ☐ ☐ ☐ *Likely*

My taking regular physical activity would make me lose weight.

Unlikely ☐ ☐ ☐ ☐ ☐ ☐ ☐ *Likely*

Outcome evaluation

Feeling healthier would be…	*Bad* ☐ ☐ ☐ ☐ ☐ ☐ ☐	*Good*
Losing weight would be…	*Bad* ☐ ☐ ☐ ☐ ☐ ☐ ☐	*Good*

(Adapted from Norman *et al.* 2000)

5.7 Normative beliefs

As with behavioural beliefs, most studies employ modal rather than individually salient referent groups as the basis of normative items and derive these from pilot studies with a representative sample of individuals from the population of interest (for an exception, see Steadman *et al.* 2002). Ajzen and Fishbein (1980: 74–5) suggest that we ask about the groups or individuals who would approve or disapprove of you performing the behaviour or who come to mind when thinking about the target behaviour. For example, participants might be asked, 'Are there any groups or individuals who come to mind when thinking about behaviour X?' The most frequently mentioned (modal) referents are then incorporated in the final questionnaire. Typically, two to six referent groups are included. Below we give examples of normative belief and motivation to comply items. Normative beliefs (i.e. 'injunctive normative beliefs') are the person's perceptions of whether specific referents would want him or her to perform the behaviour under consideration. These items are typically responded to on a 'should not–should' or 'unlikely–likely' response format and scored in a bipolar fashion (i.e. –3 'strong negative pressure to perform' to +3 'strong positive pressure to perform'). Motivation to comply is operationalized as the person's willingness to comply with the expectations of the specific referents. Such items are typically responded to on 'not at all–strongly' or 'unlikely–likely' response formats and treated as unipolar scales (i.e. +1 'low motivation to comply' to +7 'strong motivation to comply'). This scoring procedure is used because people are considered unlikely to be motivated to do the opposite of what they perceive significant others want them to do. The relevant normative beliefs and motivations to comply are then multiplicatively combined and summed (equation 4) to give an indirect measure of normative pressure.

Injunctive normative beliefs

My friends think I should take regular physical activity.

Unlikely □ □ □ □ □ □ □ *Likely*

Health experts think I should take regular physical activity.

Unlikely □ □ □ □ □ □ □ *Likely*

Motivation to comply

With regard to physical activity, I want to do what my friends think I should.

Strongly disagree □ □ □ □ □ □ □ *Strongly agree*

With regard to physical activity, I want to do what health experts think I should.

Strongly disagree □ □ □ □ □ □ □ *Strongly agree*
(Adapted from Norman *et al.* 2000)

As noted above, in addition to (injunctive) normative beliefs, Fishbein and Ajzen (2010) acknowledge that descriptive norms (which reflect what salient referents actually do) are also likely to be a powerful source of social influence (Ajzen and Fishbein 2005). Underpinning these descriptive norms, descriptive normative beliefs might be measured in the following way, for example:

Descriptive normative beliefs

How many of your friends take regular physical activity?

None ☐ ☐ ☐ ☐ ☐ ☐ *All of them*

How many health experts take regular physical activity?

None ☐ ☐ ☐ ☐ ☐ ☐ *All of them*

Fishbein and Ajzen (2010) suggest that these descriptive normative beliefs might be weighted by the degree of identification with each of the referents (such as, in the above examples, friends and health experts) in order to help predict descriptive norms. This idea is awaiting empirical exploration.

5.8 Control beliefs

For control beliefs, the few studies that have reported these items have also used modal control beliefs derived from pilot studies with samples representative of the target population, although presumably salient control factors are the most appropriate measures. Ajzen and Driver (1992) suggest that individuals are asked to list the factors and conditions that make it easy or difficult to perform the target behaviour, with the most frequently mentioned (modal) items being used in the final questionnaire. For example, participants might be asked, 'What factors might prevent you or help you take regular physical activity?' However, perhaps because of their infrequent use to date, there has been some variation in how control beliefs have been operationalized. Below we give examples of both control belief and power items. Control beliefs assess the presence or absence of facilitating or inhibiting factors and are commonly scored on 'never–frequently', 'false–true', 'unavailable–available' or 'unlikely–likely' response formats. Ajzen (1991) suggests that control is best treated as a bipolar scale (–3 'inhibits' to +3 'facilitates'), although a unipolar scoring appears more appropriate for certain response formats (e.g. +1 'never' to +7 'frequently'). Perceived power items assess the power of the item to facilitate or inhibit performance of the behaviour. Power items are also problematic: response formats include 'less likely–more likely', 'more difficult–easier', and 'not important–very important'. Ajzen (1991) reports mixed evidence concerning whether these should be scored as unipolar or bipolar, although the wording of the response format may suggest the most appropriate scoring to use. The relevant items are then multiplicatively combined and summed (equation 5) to give an indirect measure of perceived behavioural control. This offers an opportunity to identify those factors that underpin people's perceptions of control. However, precisely how these control beliefs combine to influence PBC requires more attention, since this research is currently at a preliminary stage.

Control beliefs

I have free time…	*Never* ☐ ☐ ☐ ☐ ☐ ☐	*Frequently*
I am near sports facilities…	*Never* ☐ ☐ ☐ ☐ ☐ ☐	*Frequently*

Power

Having free time makes taking regular physical activity...

Less likely ☐ ☐ ☐ ☐ ☐ ☐ *More likely*

Being near sports facilities makes taking regular physical activity...

Less likely ☐ ☐ ☐ ☐ ☐ ☐ *More likely*

(Adapted from Norman *et al.* 2000)

6 Intervention studies

The title of Ajzen and Fishbein's (1980) seminal work on the theory of reasoned action made reference to the theory's role in 'understanding' and 'predicting' behaviour, while Fishbein and Ajzen (2010) make reference to 'predicting' and 'changing' behaviour. Because of its popularity in applied research, it is not surprising that the issue of the theory's possible additional role in behavioural interventions has been raised. In fact, Eagly (1992: 705) has been quite explicit in stating that 'interest in attitude theory is widespread and quite intense because of the desire of many groups to change attitudes and behaviors'. Nevertheless, Ajzen (2014: 3) is quite clear: '...the TPB is in fact not a theory of behaviour change. Instead it is meant to help explain and predict people's intentions and behaviour. Nevertheless, the theory can serve as a useful framework for designing effective behaviour change interventions.'

Ajzen and Fishbein (1980) suggested a number of ways in which the TRA can be used to change behavioural intentions and behaviour (see also Ajzen 2011). A first step is an application of the TPB in the behaviour and population of interest to help identify whether we need to target increasing intentions (low to moderate mean intentions) or, if intentions are sufficiently strong (high intentions), target helping individuals enact their intentions. If the former, such a study can also help identify the need to focus on changing attitudes, subjective norms or perceptions of control as the means to increase intentions. In such situations, the TPB approach focuses on the targeting of underlying beliefs. Ajzen and Fishbein (1980) argue that changing these underlying beliefs should bring about long-lasting change in intentions and behaviour. Ajzen (2014) suggests that there are five key stages to developing an intervention to change beliefs: (1) eliciting easily accessible behavioural, normative, and control beliefs in a representative sample of the target population; (2) selecting specific existing accessible beliefs or perhaps novel beliefs to target in the intervention; (3) designing an intervention that changes the selected beliefs; (4) testing that the intervention produces large changes in the targeted belief and does not produce any negative effects on other beliefs; and (5) demonstrating that the intervention had significant effects on the aggregate of behavioural, normative, and/or control beliefs (i.e. the aggregate of accessible beliefs are significantly more favourable towards the behaviour compared with aggregate scores before the intervention). In general, the intervention can target changing either component of behavioural, normative or control beliefs (e.g. for behavioural beliefs, it could be outcome likelihood and/or outcome evaluation that is targeted) or try to introduce novel beliefs. Pilot work can be used to identify which strategy is likely to be most effective. Sutton (2002) provides a more detailed consideration of changing behaviour through targeting beliefs.

In contrast, where it is established that many people have positive intentions about the behaviour but fail to act on them, Ajzen (2014) suggests a different approach to changing behaviour. Here investigators are advised to: (1) try to ensure that the beliefs that are accessible in the context in which the behaviour is to be performed do not differ substantially from the accessible beliefs identified in the elicitation phase; (2) that participants have the means, skills, and other resources to perform the target behaviour; (3) that potential barriers to performance of the behaviour have been removed; and (4) that no unanticipated events or new information have led to revised intentions. The difficulty of achieving all four steps should not be underestimated.

The TPB has been used in intervention studies for a range of health behaviours, including smoking (Conner *et al.* 2006), road safety behaviours (Parker *et al.* 1996), exercise (Rhodes and Courneya 2003a), dietary change (Beale and Manstead 1991), and testicular self-examination (Brubaker and Fowler 1990). As an example of research that has used the TPB[3] as a basis for intervention designed to influence people's motives to engage in health-related behaviours, we consider the work of Brubaker and Fowler (1990) on testicular self-examination (TSE). Brubaker and Fowler (1990) were concerned about an increase in the incidence of testicular cancer in the USA and the lack of knowledge young men had about carrying out TSE in order to detect the disease. They consequently designed a study in which they attempted 'to evaluate the effect of a persuasive message based on the theory of reasoned action on the performance of TSE' (p. 1413). Male undergraduate students ($n = 114$) were randomly assigned to one of three conditions:

1. In the *theory-based message* group, participants heard a message based on the TRA/ TPB.
2. In the *informational message* group, participants heard a message containing more general information about, for example, the incidence of testicular cancer and how it can be treated.
3. In the *no-message* group, participants received no message at all.

The information that participants received was presented in the form of an audiotaped dialogue lasting for about 10 minutes between, ostensibly, a doctor and some students (these roles were taken, in fact, by actors). For the *theory-based message* group, the dialogue consisted of the actors 'challenging misconceptions' about TSE that had been identified in previous research in the form of beliefs that had differentiated between males who performed TSE and males who did not. Brubaker and Fowler (1990) give the following examples as beliefs that were addressed in this way: 'TSE is difficult to perform; TSE can lead to early detection of cancer; TSE does not take a lot of time to perform'.

A subsequent questionnaire, focused on performing TSE during the next month, assessed, for example, intentions, attitudes, subjective norm, self-efficacy, behavioural beliefs, normative beliefs, outcome evaluations, and motivation to comply. In follow-up telephone calls one week and four weeks later, participants were asked for a self-report of their TSE behaviour since the experimental procedure. The results clearly showed differences between participants who received messages and those who did not (e.g. the former reported more TSE, greater intentions, and more positive attitudes). However, there was no evidence of differences between the *theory-based message* group and the *informational message* group on the key dependent variables (i.e. intentions and behaviour). Despite the lack of clear findings, it is important to note that this study sought to modify the structure of people's beliefs about the behaviour in question.

This is in line with how Ajzen and Fishbein would propose the TRA and TPB should be used in interventions aimed at influencing people's behavioural motives. However, we would reiterate our earlier comment that the method by which this is effected is an issue beyond the remit of the TPB/TRA. Researchers may select ineffective methods, or may influence model components that they did not intend to influence, or may discover effective strategies which they had not expected to work. The range of methods open to them is very broad (Fishbein and Ajzen 2004; Ajzen 2011), and the effectiveness of different methods may be expected to be highly context-dependent. However, while some attitudes and behaviours may be amenable to change, others may be more entrenched and intransigent.

Hardeman *et al.* (2002) reviewed studies using the TPB to promote behaviour change. A total of 24 intervention studies were identified, although the TPB was used to develop the intervention in only half the studies. In the other half of the studies, the TPB was only used in relation to assessing the effects of the intervention. Where the results were reported, the interventions were effective in changing intentions in approximately half the studies and behaviour in approximately two-thirds, although the effect sizes tended to be small. However, two main problems with interpreting these findings are apparent. First, many studies did not conduct an initial TPB study to identify appropriate targets for intervention. Second, many studies did not test the effectiveness of interventions in changing targeted cognitions before examining impacts on intentions and behaviour. Hardeman *et al.* (2002: 149) indicate that many interventions they examined appeared to be poorly designed, that 'interventions were seldom explicitly developed to target specific components of the model', and that this area should focus more on whether any observed effects are mediated by changes in TPB components. Fishbein and Ajzen (2010) also emphasize the problems with the majority of studies Hardeman *et al.* (2002) reviewed, and note that only four studies conformed to the requirements of the TPB (Brubaker and Fowler 1990; Murphy and Brubaker 1990; Sanderson and Jemmott 1996; Jemmott *et al.* 1998). They note that consideration of these four studies only produces more encouraging results with strong effects on the targeted theoretical components and on behaviour. Ajzen (2014) also notes good support for the theory in other studies (see Rutter and Quine 2002) not included in Hardeman and co-workers' review. Tyson *et al.* (2014) report a meta-analysis of TPB intervention studies focusing on reducing heterosexual risk behaviours. Only studies with strong designs (randomized controlled trials or quasi-experimental studies) were included. Across 34 tests in relation to condom use, a small but significant effect size was reported ($d_+ = 0.126$). However, it was unclear the extent to which all studies conformed to the requirements of the TPB and whether this moderated the effect size observed. Despite some promising findings, the limited number of studies providing appropriate tests of using interventions targeting beliefs in a way consistent with the TPB is noteworthy.

What, then, should we make of the role of the TPB in behavioural change interventions? At one level, the use of the TPB as a means to identify appropriate target cognitions for interventions seems a useful contribution. At another level, the approach to changing these target cognitions through changing underlying beliefs has weaknesses. Although there are intervention studies designed to be consistent with the TPB that show effects on behaviour, the number of such studies is small. Given the widespread interest in health behaviour change, it is unclear why there have been so few interventions that appropriately test the approach advocated by the TPB. Increased understanding of the approach advocated by the TPB, such as that provided by Ajzen (2011), may help remove one barrier to such testing. Another barrier that is more difficult to address is the fact that the TPB does not provide specific advice about how to change beliefs. As Ajzen (2004: 2) puts it, 'The theory of planned behavior can provide general guideline [*sic*] …but it does not tell us what kind of intervention will be most effective'. This is a problem common to a number of social cognition models employed in the health area and has partly driven interest in testing effective behavior change techniques (BCTs). We would want to see a greater number of well-designed tests of the TPB approach before reaching a firm conclusion about the effectiveness of this approach for changing health behaviour.

Another way in which the TPB can be used for interventions is in relation to helping identify the appropriate targets for such interventions. In this way, it is similar to many other social cognition models. A standard application of the TPB to the target behaviour in the population of interest is the first step in this process. This helps identify the appropriate cognitions to target in an intervention. A growing body of research has examined the effects of various interventions in changing constructs identified in the TPB and impacts on subsequent intentions and action. For example, Webb and Sheeran (2006) reviewed studies that significantly changed intentions ($d_+ = 0.66$) and reported medium-sized effects on behaviour ($d_+ = 0.36$, $k = 47$). Importantly, this research identified those BCTs (see Michie and Wood, Chapter 11 this volume) that were most successful in changing intentions (e.g. incentives, environmental changes, planning implementation). More recently, Sheeran *et al.* (submitted) have examined the impacts of changing attitudes, norms, and self-efficacy on intentions and behaviour. They again focused on examining studies that had successfully changed these components. Changes in attitudes, norms, and self-efficacy were associated with medium-sized changes in intentions ($d_+ = 0.50$, $k = 47$; $d_+ = 0.41$, $k = 11$; $d_+ = 0.50$, $k = 39$, respectively) and small- to medium-sized changes in behaviour ($d_+ = 0.37$, $k = 55$; $d_+ = 0.20$, $k = 11$; $d_+ = 0.46$, $k = 76$, respectively). Using a combination of a TPB study to identify what determinants to target and then employing BCTs shown to be effective in changing the identified determinants may prove to be a powerful way to produce change in both intentions and behaviour.

7 Future directions

7.1 Mediation effects

The TPB contains a number of assumed mediated effects. For example, the impact of variables internal to the theory (e.g. attitude and subjective norm) on behaviour is assumed to be fully mediated by intentions, while the impact of various external variables (e.g. demographic variables, personality variables) on intentions and behaviour is assumed to be fully mediated by attitude, subjective norm, and PBC. In general, the majority of studies would appear to support such assumed mediation. However, in relation to internal variables, most TPB studies do not report direct effects of attitude or subjective norm on behaviour after controlling for intentions. As noted earlier, distinguishing among components of attitudes and norms may reveal more direct paths (e.g. direct effects of affective/experiential attitude and descriptive norms on behaviour). Future research might usefully explore the factors (e.g. types of behaviour, populations, and other moderating variables) influencing the significance of such direct effects for internal variables before we reach any definitive conclusions about the importance of adding such direct effects to the theory. Similarly, although a number of studies do report direct effects of external variables on intentions and behaviour (for example, Conner *et al.* [2009] examined personality variables), the majority of studies have not reported such effects. We should be cautious about adding external variables as direct predictors of intentions or behaviour without sufficient evidence about the generality of such effects across behaviours and populations or the key moderators of when such effects occur. A key strength of the TPB has been its parsimony in predicting so many different behaviours across different populations using only a limited number of variables.

7.2 Moderator variables

A significant body of work in recent years has examined the role of moderator variables within the TPB (i.e. variables that influence the magnitude of relationships between TPB constructs). The value of this work for applied researchers lies in identifying the conditions that maximize the relationships between TPB variables. From a theoretical perspective, such moderators help elucidate the range of conditions under which the theory works. A range of moderator variables has been examined in relation to the TPB. These can be broadly split into additional variables and properties of components of the TPB. The former include anticipated regret, moral norms, and past behaviour; the latter include accessibility, direct experience, involvement, certainty, ambivalence, affective-cognitive consistency, and temporal stability (for a review of 44 such studies, see Cooke and Sheeran 2004).

For example, anticipated regret has been posited as a moderator of intention–behaviour relationships on the basis that high levels of anticipated regret may bind people to their intentions and so strengthen their intentions because failing to act would be associated with aversive affect (Sheeran and Orbell 1999). Several studies have demonstrated this effect in relation to exercising (Sheeran and Abraham 2003; Sandberg and Conner 2011) and smoking initiation (Conner *et al.* 2006, Study 2). Moreover, Abraham and Sheeran (2003, Study 1) manipulated regret and demonstrated similar moderation effects.

The predominant basis on which intentions are formed has also been examined as a moderator of intention–behaviour relationships in a number of studies. For example, Sheeran *et al.* (1999) showed that intentions more aligned with attitudes than with subjective norms were significantly stronger predictors of behaviour. It was argued that this was because attitudinally aligned intentions were more intrinsically motivated (Ryan *et al.* 1996). Relatedly, Keer *et al.* (2014) showed intentions based on affective/experiential attitudes were stronger predictors of behaviour than those based on cognitive/instrumental attitudes. Godin *et al.* (2005) demonstrated across a number of studies that intentions that were most closely aligned with moral norms were significantly stronger predictors of behaviour. It was argued that such intentions were more consistent with an individual's core self-identity.

Several studies have also examined various external variables as moderators of TPB relationships. For example, Norman *et al.* (2000) found PBC to be a significantly stronger predictor of exercise behaviour for those who had exercised frequently in the past. This was interpreted as being attributable to PBC being more accurate for those who had more experience of exercise (i.e. had exercised more frequently in the past). Relatedly, studies have also examined whether habit strengths moderate the intention–behaviour relationship. Gardner (2014) reviewed 24 studies that had tested this hypothesis and found that 18 reported evidence that intention became a weaker predictor of behaviour as habit strength increased. Other studies have examined personality measures as moderators of relationships in the TPB. For example, Conner *et al.* (2009)

reported the personality dimension of conscientiousness to moderate the relationship between intentions and smoking behaviour such that intentions were stronger predictors of behaviour among those high in conscientiousness (for a review, see Rhodes and Dickau 2013).

In relation to properties of components of the TPB, the main focus has been on attitudes and intentions. In Cooke and Sheeran's (2004) meta-analytic review, accessibility, direct experience, certainty, ambivalence, and affective-cognitive consistency all significantly moderated the attitude–behaviour relationship, while ambivalence, certainty, and involvement all moderated the attitude–intention relationship. All these properties plus certainty also significantly moderated the intention–behaviour relationship. In each case, greater accessibility, greater involvement, more direct experience, more certainty, less ambivalence, and greater affective-cognitive consistency were associated with significantly stronger relationships.

Temporal stability appears to be a particularly important moderator of relationships with behaviour. In Cooke and Sheeran's (2004) review, it emerged as the strongest moderator. As Ajzen (1996: 389) has argued: '...to obtain accurate prediction of behavior, intentions...must remain reasonably stable over time until the behavior is performed'. Intentions measured prior to performance of a behaviour may change as a result of new information or unforeseen obstacles resulting in a reduced predictive power. The moderating role of temporal stability has been addressed in several recent studies of health behaviours. Conner *et al.* (2002) found a significant intention stability moderation effect in relation to healthy eating over a period of six years, such that intentions were stronger predictors of behaviour when intentions were stable. Similar results have been reported in relation to smoking initiation (Conner *et al.* 2006), attending health screening, eating a low-fat diet (Conner *et al.* 2000), and exercising (Sheeran and Abraham 2003). Sheeran and Abraham (2003) found intention stability both to moderate the intention–behaviour relationship for exercising and, more importantly, to mediate the impacts of various other moderators of the intention–behaviour relationship (e.g. anticipated regret, certainty). This suggests that a number of these other moderators may have their effect on intention–behaviour relationships through changing the temporal stability of intentions. Nevertheless, the stability of intentions is an emergent property of an individual's intention, and future research may well show it to be dependent on other more directly modifiable aspects of intention (e.g. prioritizing one particular intention/goal over other competing intentions/goals).

7.3 Conclusion

A rather critical stance towards the TPB has been taken here, since we believe that this is the best foundation on which to make progress (see discussions by Sarver 1983; Liska 1984; Eagly and Chaiken 1993; Ajzen 2014; Sniehotta *et al.* 2014; see also Norman and Conner, Chapter 12 this volume, for consideration of critiques of the social cognition approach). Its contribution may be seen as significant, but limited, for health behaviours: significant because at one level of analysis it increases our understanding of many health-related behaviours; limited because in the broad social environment there will be a number of influences on people's health and on their behaviour – any of these that do not impinge on people's perceptions of control will not be accessible to analysis via the TPB. Health behaviours need to be understood not only in terms of people's beliefs, values, perceived norms, and perceived control but also in terms of the individual's behavioural history and the broader social influences that may be operating. While we have to acknowledge the role of the broader social structure within which these influences develop, the

TPB provides a strong account of the proximal psychological influences on behaviour that may mediate these other influences and so constitute an appropriate focus for interventions.

Notes

1. This was originally called the principle of correspondence (Fishbein and Ajzen 1975; Ajzen and Fishbein 1977).
2. As Ajzen (2002c) notes, 'Defining the TACT elements is somewhat arbitrary' (p. 2).
3. Brubaker and Fowler's (1990) study is, in fact, a study of an extended TRA incorporating a measure of self-efficacy.

References

Abraham, C. and Sheeran, P. (2003) Evidence that anticipated regret strengthens intentions, enhances intention stability, and improves intention–behaviour consistency, *British Journal of Health Psychology*, 9, 269–78.

Agnew, C. (1998) Modal versus individually-derived behavioural and normative beliefs about condom use: comparing measurement alternatives of the cognitive underpinnings of the theories of reasoned action and planned behaviour, *Psychology and Health*, 13, 271–87.

Ajzen, I. (1988) *Attitudes, Personality and Behavior*. Buckingham: Open University Press.

Ajzen, I. (1991) The theory of planned behavior, *Organizational Behavior and Human Decision Processes*, 50, 179–211.

Ajzen, I. (1996) The directive influence of attitudes on behavior, in P. Gollwitzer and J.A. Bargh (eds.) *Psychology of Action* (pp. 385–403). New York: Guilford Press.

Ajzen, I. (2002a) Perceived behavioural control, self-efficacy, locus of control, and the theory of planned behaviour, *Journal of Applied Social Psychology*, 32, 1–20.

Ajzen, I. (2002b) Residual effects of past on later behavior: habituation and reasoned action perspectives, *Personality and Social Psychology Review*, 6, 107–22.

Ajzen, I. (2002c) Constructing a TpB questionnaire: conceptual and methodological considerations [www.people. umass.edu/aizen/pdf/tpb.measurement.pdf, accessed 12 July 2004].

Ajzen, I. (2004) Behavioral interventions based on the theory of planned behavior [http://www.people.umass.edu/ aizen/pdf/tpb.intervention.pdf, accessed 12 July 2004].

Ajzen, I. (2011) Behavioral interventions: design and evaluation guided by the theory of planned behavior, in M.M. Mark, S.I. Donaldson and B. Campbell (eds.) *Social Psychology for Program and Policy Evaluation* (pp. 74–100). New York: Guilford Press.

Ajzen, I. (2014) The theory of planned behaviour is alive and well, and not ready to retire: a commentary on Sniehotta, Presseau, and Araujo-Soares, *Health Psychology Review* [DOI: 10.1080/17437199.2014.883474].

Ajzen, I. and Driver, B.L. (1992) Application of the theory of planned behavior to leisure choice, *Journal of Leisure Research*, 24, 207–224.

Ajzen, I. and Fishbein, M. (1977) Attitude–behavior relations: a theoretical analysis and review of empirical research, *Psychological Bulletin*, 84, 888–918.

Ajzen, I. and Fishbein, M. (1980) *Understanding Attitudes and Predicting Social Behavior*. Englewood-Cliffs, NJ: Prentice-Hall.

Ajzen, I. and Fishbein, M. (2000) Attitudes and the attitude–behavior relation: reasoned and automatic processes, *European Review of Social Psychology*, 11, 1–33.

Ajzen, I. and Fishbein, M. (2005) The influence of attitudes on behavior, in D. Albarracin, B.T. Johnson and M.P. Zanna (eds.) *Handbook of Attitudes and Attitude Change: Basic Principles* (pp. 173–221). Mahwah, NJ: Erlbaum.

Ajzen, I. and Madden, T.J. (1986) Prediction of goal directed behavior: attitudes, intentions and perceived behavioral control, *Journal of Experimental Social Psychology*, 22, 453–74.

Ajzen, I. and Sheik, S. (2013) Action versus inaction: anticipated affect in the theory of planned behavior, *Journal of Applied Social Psychology*, 43, 155–62.

Ajzen, A. and Timko, C. (1986) Correspondence between health attitudes and behavior, *Journal of Basic and Applied Social Psychology*, 7, 259–76.

Albarracin, D., Johnson, B.T., Fishbein, M. and Muellerleile, P.A. (2001) Theories of reasoned action and planned behavior as models of condom use: a metaanalysis, *Psychological Bulletin*, 127, 142–61.

Armitage, C.J. and Conner, M. (1999) Distinguishing perceptions of control from self-efficacy: predicting consumption of a low fat diet using the theory of planned behavior, *Journal of Applied Social Psychology*, 29, 72–90.

Armitage, C.J. and Conner, M. (2001) Efficacy of the theory of planned behaviour: a meta-analytic review, *British Journal of Social Psychology*, 40, 471–99.

Bagozzi, R.P. (1992) The self-regulation of attitudes, intentions and behaviour, *Social Psychology Quarterly*, 55, 178–204.

Bandura, A. (1977) Self-efficacy: toward a unifying theory of behavioural change, *Psychological Review*, 84, 191–215.

Bandura, A. (2000) Health promotion from the perspective of health-related behaviour change, in P. Norman, C. Abraham and M. Conner (eds.) *Understanding and Changing Health Behaviour: From Health Beliefs to Self-regulation* (pp. 299–339). Amsterdam: Harwood Academic.

Baumeister, R.F. and Muraven, M. (1996) Identity as adaptation to social, cultural, and historical context, *Journal of Adolescence*, 19, 405–16.

Beale, D.A. and Manstead, A.S.R. (1991) Predicting mothers' intentions to limit frequency of infants' sugar intake: testing the theory of planned behavior, *Journal of Applied Social Psychology*, 21, 409–31.

Beck, L. and Ajzen, I. (1991) Predicting dishonest actions using the Theory of Planned Behavior, *Journal of Research in Personality*, 25, 285–301.

Blanchard, C.M., Fisher, J., Sparling, P.B., Shanks, T.H., Nehl, E., Rhodes, R.E. *et al.* (2009) Understanding adherence to 5 servings of fruits and vegetables per day: a theory of planned behavior perspective, *Journal of Nutrition Education and Behavior*, 41, 3–10.

Blue, C.L. (1995) The predictive capacity of the theory of reasoned action and the theory of planned behavior in exercise research: an integrated literature review, *Research in Nursing and Health*, 18, 105–21.

Bollen, K.A. (1989) *Structural Equations with Latent Variables*. New York: Wiley.

Breckler, S.J. and Wiggins, E.C. (1989) Affect versus evaluation in the structure of attitudes, *Journal of Experimental Social Psychology*, 25, 253–71.

Brubaker, R.G. and Fowler, C. (1990) Encouraging college males to perform testicular self-examination: evaluation of a persuasive message based on the revised theory of reasoned action, *Journal of Applied Social Psychology*, 17, 1411–22.

Case, P., Sparks, P. and Pavey, L.J. (in press) Identity appropriateness and the structure of the theory of planned behaviour, *British Journal of Social Psychology*.

Chan, D.K. and Fishbein, M. (1993) Determinants of college women's intentions to tell their partners to use condoms, *Journal of Applied Social Psychology*, 23, 1455–70.

Charng, H.-W., Piliavin, J.A. and Callero, P.L. (1988) Role identity and reasoned action in the prediction of repeated behavior, *Social Psychology Quarterly*, 51, 303–17.

Churchill, S., Jessop, D.C. and Sparks, P. (2008) Impulsive and/or planned behaviour: can impulsivity contribute to the predictive utility of the theory of planned behaviour? *British Journal of Social Psychology*, 47, 631–46.

Cialdini, R.B., Kallgren, C.A. and Reno, R.R. (1991) A focus theory of normative conduct: a theoretical refinement and re-evaluation of the role of norms in human behaviour, *Advances in Experimental Social Psychology*, 24, 201–34.

Cohen, J. (1992) A power primer, *Psychological Bulletin*, 112, 155–9.

Conner, M. and Abraham, C. (2001) Conscientiousness and the theory of planned behavior: towards a more complete model of the antecedents of intentions and behavior, *Personality and Social Psychology Bulletin*, 27, 1547–61.

Conner, M. and Armitage, C.J. (1998) Extending the theory of planned behavior: a review and avenues for further research, *Journal of Applied Social Psychology*, 28, 1430–64.

Conner, M. and Sparks, P. (2005) The theory of planned behaviour and health behaviours, in M. Conner and P. Norman (eds.) *Predicting Health Behaviour: Research and Practice with Social Cognition Models* (2nd edn., pp. 170–222). Maidenhead: Open University Press.

Conner, M., Godin, G., Sheeran, P. and Germain, M. (2013a) Some feelings are more important: cognitive attitudes, affective attitudes, anticipated affect and blood donation, *Health Psychology*, 32, 264–72.

Conner, M., Grogan, S., Fry, G., Gough, B. and Higgins, A.R. (2009) Direct, mediated and moderated impacts of personality variables on smoking initiation in adolescents, *Psychology and Health*, 24, 1085–1104.

Conner, M., Kirk, S.F.L., Cade, J.E. and Barrett, J.H. (2001) Why do women use dietary supplements? The use of the theory of planned behaviour to explore beliefs about their use, *Social Science and Medicine*, 52, 621–33.

Conner, M., McEachan, R., Jackson, C., McMillan, B., Woolridge, M., and Lawton, R. (2013b) Moderating effect of socioeconomic status on the relationship between health cognitions and behaviors, *Annals of Behavioral Medicine*, 46, 19–30.

Conner, M., McEachan, R., Taylor, N., O'Hara, J. and Lawton, R. (2014) Role of affective attitudes and anticipated affective reactions in predicting health behaviors, *Health Psychology* [DOI: 10.1037/hea0000143].

Conner, M., Norman, P. and Bell, R. (2002) The Theory of Planned Behavior and healthy eating, *Health Psychology*, 21, 194–201.

Conner, M., Rhodes, R., Morris, B., McEachan, R. and Lawton, R. (2011) Changing exercise through targeting affective or cognitive attitudes, *Psychology and Health*, 26, 133–49.

Conner, M., Sandberg, T., McMillan, B. and Higgins, A. (2006) Role of anticipated regret in adolescent smoking initiation, *British Journal of Health Psychology*, 11, 85–101.

Conner, M., Sheeran, P., Norman, P. and Armitage, C.J. (2000) Temporal stability as a moderator of relationships in the theory of planned behaviour, *British Journal of Social Psychology*, 39, 469–93.

Conner, M., Warren, R., Close, S. and Sparks, P. (1999) Alcohol consumption and the theory of planned behavior: an examination of the cognitive mediation of past behavior, *Journal of Applied Social Psychology*, 29, 1675–703.

Cooke, R. and French, D.P. (2008) How well do the theory of reasoned action and theory of planned behaviour predict intentions and attendance at screening programmes? A meta-analysis, *Psychology and Health*, 23, 745–65.

Cooke, R. and Sheeran, P. (2004) Moderation of cognition–intention and cognition–behaviour relations: a meta-analysis of properties of variables from the theory of planned behaviour, *British Journal of Social Psychology*, 43, 159–86.

Cooke, R., Dahdah, M. and Norman, P. (in press) How well does the theory of planned behaviour predict alcohol consumption? A systematic review and meta-analysis. *Health Psychology Review* [DOI: 10.1080/17437199.2014.947547].

Crites, S.L., Fabrigar, L.R. and Petty, R.E. (1994) Measuring the affective and cognitive properties of attitudes: conceptual and methodological issues, *Personality and Social Psychology Bulletin*, 20, 619–34.

Deutsch, M. and Gerard, H.B. (1955) A study of normative and informational social influences upon human judgment, *Journal of Abnormal and Social Psychology*, 51, 629–36.

De Vries, H., Backbier, E., Kok, G. and Dijkstra, M. (1995) The impact of social influences in the context of attitude, self-efficacy, intention and previous behaviour as predictors of smoking onset, *Journal of Applied Social Psychology*, 25, 237–57.

De Wit, J.B.F., Stroebe, W., De Vroome, E.M.M., Sandfort, T.G.M. and Van Griensven, G.J.P. (2000) Understanding aids preventive behaviour with casual and primary partners in homosexual men: the theory of planned behaviour and the information–motivation-behavioural-skills model, *Psychology and Health*, 15, 325–40.

Downs, D.S. and Hausenblas, H.A. (2005) The theories of reasoned action and planned behavior applied to exercise: a meta-analytic update, *Journal of Physical Activity and Health*, 2, 76–97.

Eagly, A.H. (1992) Uneven progress: social psychology and the study of attitudes, *Journal of Personality and Social Psychology*, 63, 693–710.

Eagly, A.H. and Chaiken, S. (1993) *The Psychology of Attitudes*. Fort Worth, TX: Harcourt Brace Jovanovich.

Eagly, A.H., Mladinic, A. and Otto, S. (1994) Cognitive and affective bases of attitudes towards social groups and social policies, *Journal of Experimental Social Psychology*, 30, 113–37.

Elliott, M.A. and Armitage, C.J. (2009) Promoting drivers' compliance with speed limits: testing an intervention based on the theory of planned behaviour, *British Journal of Psychology*, 100, 111–32.

Fekadu, Z. and Kraft, P. (2001) Expanding the theory of planned behaviour: the role of social norms and group identification, *Journal of Health Psychology*, 7, 33–43.

Fishbein, M. (1967a) Attitude and the prediction of behavior, in M. Fishbein (ed.) *Readings in Attitude Theory and Measurement* (pp. 477–92). New York: Wiley.

Fishbein, M. (1967b) A behavior theory approach to the relations between beliefs about an object and the attitude toward the object, in M. Fishbein (ed.) *Readings in Attitude Theory and Measurement* (pp. 389–400). New York: Wiley.

Fishbein, M. (1993) Introduction, in D.J. Terry, C. Gallois and M. McCamish (eds.) *The Theory of Reasoned Action: Its Application to AIDS-preventive Behaviour* (pp. xv–xxv). Oxford: Pergamon Press.

Fishbein, M. (1997) Predicting, understanding, and changing socially relevant behaviors: lessons learned, in C. McGarty and S.A. Haslam (eds.) *The Message of Social Psychology* (pp. 77–91). Oxford: Blackwell.

Fishbein, M. (2008) A reasoned action approach to health promotion, *Medical Decision Making*, 28, 834–44.

Fishbein, M. and Ajzen, I. (1975) *Belief, Attitude, Intention, and Behavior*. New York: Wiley.

Fishbein, M. and Ajzen, I. (2004) Theory-based behavior change interventions: comments on Hobbis and Sutton (2004), *Journal of Health Psychology*, 10, 27–31.

Fishbein, M. and Ajzen, I. (2010) *Predicting and Changing Behavior: The Reasoned Action Approach*. New York: Psychology Press.

French, D.P. and Hankins, M. (2003) The expectancy-value muddle in the theory of planned behaviour – and some proposed solutions, *British Journal of Health Psychology*, 8, 37–55.

Gaes, G.G., Kalle, R.J. and Tedeschi, J.I. (1978) Impression management in the forced compliance situation: two studies using the bogus pipeline, *Journal of Experimental Social Psychology*, 9, 491–501.

Gagne, C. and Godin, G. (2000) The theory of planned behavior: some measurement issues concerning belief-based variables, *Journal of Applied Social Psychology*, 30, 2173–93.

Galea, M.N. and Bray, S.R. (2006) Predicting walking intentions and exercise in individuals with intermittent claudication: an application of the theory of planned behaviour, *Rehabilitation Psychology*, 51, 299–305.

Gardner, B. (2014) A review and analysis of the use of 'habit' in understanding, predicting and influencing health-related behaviour, *Health Psychology Review*, 8, 1–19.

Gibbons, F.X. and Gerrard, M. (1997) Health images and their effects on health behavior, in B.P. Buunk and F.X. Gibbons (eds.) *Health, Coping, and Social Comparisons* (pp. 63–94). Hillsdale, NJ: Erlbaum.

Godin, G. and Gionet, N.J. (1991) Determinants of an intention to exercise of an electric power commission's employees, *Ergonomics*, 34, 1221–230.

Godin, G. and Kok, G. (1996) The theory of planned behavior: a review of its applications to health-related behaviors, *American Journal of Health Promotion*, 11, 87–98.

Godin, G., Conner, M. and Sheeran, P. (2005) Bridging the intention-behavior 'gap': the role of moral norm, *British Journal of Social Psychology*, 44, 497–512.

Godin, G., Conner, M., Sheeran, P., Bélanger-Gravel, A. and Germain, M. (2007) Determinants of repeated blood donation among new and experienced blood donors, *Transfusion*, 47, 1607–15.

Goldberg, J.H., Halpern-Felsher, B.L. and Millstein, S.G. (2002) Beyond invulnerability: the importance of benefits in adolescents' decision to drink alcohol, *Health Psychology*, 21, 477–84.

Hagger, M. and Chatzisarantis, N.L.D. (2005) First- and higher-order models of attitudes, normative influences, and perceived behavioural control in the theory of planned behaviour, *British Journal of Social Psychology*, 44, 513–35.

Hagger, M., Chatzisarantis, N. and Biddle, S. (2002) A meta-analytic review of the theories of reasoned action and planned behavior in physical activity: predictive validity and the contribution of additional variables, *Journal of Sport and Exercise Psychology*, 24, 3–32.

Hagger, M.S., Chatzisarantis, N., Biddle, S.J.H. and Orbell, S. (2001) Antecedents of children's physical activity intentions and behaviour: predictive validity and longitudinal effects, *Psychology and Health*, 16, 391–407.

Hardeman, W., Johnston, M., Johnston, D., Bonetti, D, Wareham, N.J. and Kinmonth, A.L. (2002) Application of the theory of planned behaviour in behaviour change interventions: a systematic review, *Psychology and Health*, 17, 123–58.

Hausenblas, H.A., Carron, A.V. and Mack, D.E. (1997) Application of the theories of reasoned action and planned behavior to exercise behavior: a metaanalysis, *Journal of Sport and Exercise Psychology*, 19, 36–51.

Head, K.J. and Noar, S.M. (2014) Facilitating progress in health behaviour theory development and modification: the reasoned action approach as a case study, *Health Psychology Review*, 8, 34–52.

Jemmott, J.B.I., Jemmott, L.S. and Fong, G.T. (1998) Abstinence and safer sex HIV risk-reduction interventions for African American adolescents, *Journal of the American Medical Association*, 279, 1529–36.

Johnston, K.L. and White, K.M. (2003) Binge-drinking: a test of the role of group norms in the theory of planned behaviour, *Psychology and Health*, 18, 63–77.

Jonas, K. and Doll, J. (1996) A critical evaluation of the Theory of Reasoned Action and the Theory of Planned Behavior, *Zeischrift fur Sozialpsychologie*, 27, 18–31.

Keer, M., Conner, M., Van den Putte, B. and Neijens, P. (2014) The temporal stability and predictive validity of affect-based and cognition-based intentions, *British Journal of Social Psychology*, 53, 315–27.

Kraft, P., Rise, J., Sutton, S. and Roysamb, E. (2005) Perceived difficulty in the theory of planned behaviour: perceived behavioural control or affective attitude? *British Journal of Social Psychology*, 44, 479–96.

Lawton, R., Conner, M. and McEachan, R. (2009) Desire or reason: predicting health behaviors from affective and cognitive attitudes, *Health Psychology*, 28, 56–65.

Lawton, R., Conner, M. and Parker, D. (2007) Beyond cognition: predicting health risk behaviors from instrumental and affective beliefs, *Health Psychology*, 26, 259–67.

Leach, M., Hennesy, M. and Fishbein, M. (2001) Perception of easy–difficult: attitude or self-efficacy? *Journal of Applied Social Psychology*, 31, 1–20.

Lechner, L., de Nooijer, J. and de Vries, H. (2004) Breast self-examination: longitudinal predictions of intention and subsequent behaviour, *European Journal of Cancer Prevention*, 13, 369–76.

Liska, A.E. (1984) A critical examination of the causal structure of the Fishbein/Ajzen attitude–behavior model, *Social Psychology Quarterly*, 47, 61–74.

Manning, M. (2009) The effects of subjective norms on behaviour in the theory of planned behaviour: a meta analysis, *British Journal of Social Psychology*, 48, 649–705.

Manstead, A.S.R. (2000) The role of moral norm in the attitude–behavior relation, in D.J. Terry and M.A. Hogg (eds.) *Attitudes, Behavior, and Social Context* (pp. 11–30). Mahwah, NJ: Erlbaum.

Manstead, A.S.R. and Parker, D. (1995) Evaluating and extending the Theory of Planned Behaviour, in W. Stroebe and M. Hewstone (eds.) *European Review of Social Psychology* (Vol. 6, pp. 69–95). Chichester: Wiley.

McEachan, R.R.C., Conner, M., Taylor, N.J. and Lawton, R.J. (2011) Prospective prediction of health-related behaviors with the Theory of Planned Behavior: a meta-analysis, *Health Psychology Review*, 5, 97–144.

McEachan, R.R.C., Lawton, R.J. and Conner, M. (submitted) A meta-analysis of prospective prediction of health-related behaviors with the multi-component Theory of Planned Behavior. Manuscript submitted for publication.

McMillan, B. and Conner, M. (2003) Applying an extended version of the theory of planned behavior to illicit drug use among students, *Journal of Applied Social Psychology*, 33, 1662–83.

Miniard, P.W. and Cohen, J.B. (1981) An examination of the Fishbein–Ajzen behavioural–intentions model's concepts and measures, *Journal of Experimental Social Psychology*, 17, 309–39.

Moan, I.S. and Rise, J. (2005) Quitting smoking: applying an extended version of the theory of planned behaviour to predict intention and behaviour, *Journal of Applied Biobehavioural Research*, 10, 39–68.

Morrison, D.M., Baker, S.A. and Gillmore, M.R. (1998) Condom use among high-risk heterosexual teens: alongitudinal analysis using the theory of reasoned action, *Psychology and Health*, 13, 207–22.

Mullen, P.D., Hersey, J.C. and Iverson, D.C. (1987) Health behavior models compared, *Social Science and Medicine*, 24, 973–83.

Murphy, W.G. and Brubaker, R.G. (1990) Effects of a brief theory-based intervention on the practice of testicular self-examination by high school males, *Journal of School Health*, 60, 459–62.

Norman, P., Armitage, C.J. and Quigley, C. (2007) The theory of planned behavior and binge drinking: assessing the impact of binge drinker prototypes, *Addictive Behaviors*, 32, 1753–68.

Norman, P., Conner, M. and Bell, R. (2000) The theory of planned behaviour and exercise: evidence for the moderating role of past behaviour, *British Journal of Health Psychology*, 5, 249–61.

Notani, A.S. (1998) Moderators of perceived behavioural control's predictiveness in the theory of planned behaviour: a meta-analysis, *Journal of Consumer Psychology*, 3, 207–22.

O'Keefe, D. (1990) *Persuasion*. London: Sage.

Osgood, C.E., Suci, G.J. and Tannenbaum, P.H. (1957) *The Measurement of Meaning*. Urbana, IL: University of Illinois Press.

Ouellette, J.A. and Wood, W. (1998) Habit and intention in everyday life: the multiple processes by which past behavior predicts future behavior, *Psychological Bulletin*, 124, 54–74.

Parker, D., Manstead, A.S.R. and Stradling, S.G. (1995) Extending the TPB: the role of personal norm, *British Journal of Social Psychology*, 34, 127–37.

Parker, D., Stradling, S.G. and Manstead, A.S.R. (1996) Modifying beliefs and attitudes to exceeding the speed limit: an intervention study based on the theory of planned behavior, *Journal of Applied Social Psychology*, 26, 1–19.

Peak, H. (1955) Attitude and motivation, in M.R. Jones (ed.) *Nebraska Symposium on Motivation* (Vol. 3, pp. 149–88). Lincoln, NE: University of Nebraska Press.

Perugini, M. and Bagozzi, R.P. (2003) The distinction between desires and intentions, *European Journal of Social Psychology*, 33, 1–15.

Rhodes, R. and Conner, M. (2010) Comparison of behavioral belief structures in the physical activity domain, *Journal of Applied Social Psychology*, 40, 2105–20.

Rhodes, R.E. and Courneya, K.S. (2003a) Investigating multiple components of attitude, subjective norm, and perceived control: an examination of the theory of planned behaviour in the exercise domain, *British Journal of Social Psychology*, 42, 129–46.

Rhodes, R.E. and Courneya, K.S. (2003b) Self-efficacy, controllability and intention in the theory of planned behavior: measurement redundancy or causal dependence, *Psychology and Health*, 18, 79–91.

Rhodes, R.E. and Courneya, K.S. (2005) Threshold assessment of attitude, subjective norm, and perceived behavioural control for predicting exercise intention and behaviour, *Psychology of Sport and Exercise*, 6, 349–61.

Rhodes, R.E. and Dickau, L. (2013) Moderators of the intention–behaviour relationship in the physical activity domain: a systematic review, *British Journal of Sports Medicine*, 47, 215–25.

Rhodes, R.E., Blanchard, C.M., Courneya, K.S. and Plotnikoff, R.C. (2009) Identifying belief-based targets for the promotion of leisure-time walking, *Health Education and Behavior*, 36, 2381–93.

Richard, R., Van der Pligt, J. and de Vries, N. (1996) Anticipated affect and behavioral choice, *Basic and Applied Social Psychology*, 18, 111–29.

Richetin, J., Conner, M. and Perugini, M. (2011) Not doing is not the opposite of doing: implications for attitudinal models of behavioral prediction, *Personality and Social Psychology Bulletin*, 37, 40–54.

Rise, J., Sheeran, P. and Hukkelberg, S. (2010) The role of self-identity in the theory of planned behavior: a meta-analysis, *Journal of Applied Social Psychology*, 40, 1085–1105.

Rivis, A. and Sheeran, P. (2003a) Descriptive norms as an additional predictor in the theory of planned behaviour: a meta-analysis, *Current Psychology*, 22, 218–33.

Rivis, A. and Sheeran, P. (2003b) Social influences and the theory of planned behaviour: evidence for a direct relationship between prototypes and young people's exercise behaviour, *Psychology and Health*, 18, 567–83.

Rivis, A., Sheeran, P. and Armitage, C.J. (2009) Expanding the affective and normative components of the theory of planned behavior: a meta-analysis of anticipated affect and moral norms, *Journal of Applied Social Psychology*, 39, 2985–3019.

Rodgers, W., Conner, M. and Murray, T. (2008) Distinguishing among perceived control, perceived difficulty and self-efficacy as determinants of intentions and behaviours, *British Journal of Social Psychology*, 47, 607–30.

Røysamb, E., Rise, J. and Kraft, P. (1997) On the structure and dimensionality of health-related behaviour in adolescents, *Psychology and Health*, 12, 437–52.

Rutter, D.R. (2000) Attendance and reattendance for breast cancer screening: a prospective 3-year test of the Theory of Planned Behaviour, *British Journal of Health Psychology*, 5, 1–13.

Rutter, D.R. and Bunce, D.J. (1989) The theory of reasoned action of Fishbein and Ajzen: a test of Towriss's amended procedure for measuring beliefs, *British Journal of Social Psychology*, 28, 39–46.

Rutter, D.R. and Quine, L. (2002) *Changing Health Behaviour: Intervention and Research with Social Cognition Models*. Buckingham: Open University Press.

Ryan, R., Sheldon, K.M., Kasser, T. and Deci, E.L. (1996) All goals are not created equal: an organismic perspective on the nature of goals and their regulation, in P.M. Gollwitzer and J.A. Bargh (eds.) *The Psychology of Action* (pp. 7–26). London: Guildford Press.

Sandberg, T. (2005) Anticipated regret and health behaviour. Unpublished PhD thesis, University of Leeds.

Sandberg, T. and Conner, M. (2008) Anticipated regret as an additional predictor in the theory of planned behaviour: a meta-analysis, *British Journal of Social Psychology*, 47, 589–606.

Sandberg, T. and Conner, M. (2009) A mere measurement effect for anticipated regret: impacts on cervical screening attendance, *British Journal of Social Psychology*, 48, 221–36.

Sandberg, T. and Conner, M. (2011) Using self-generated validity to promote exercise behaviour, *British Journal of Social Psychology*, 50, 769–83.

Sanderson, C.A. and Jemmott, J.B.I. (1996) Moderation and mediation of HIV-prevention interventions: relationship status, intentions, and condom use among college students, *Journal of Applied Social Psychology*, 26, 2076–99.

Sarver, V.T., Jr. (1983) Ajzen and Fishbein's 'theory of reasoned action': a critical assessment, *Journal for the Theory of Social Behaviour*, 13, 155–63.

Sheeran, P. (2002) Intention–behavior relations: a conceptual and empirical review, in W. Strobe and M. Hewstone (eds.) *European Review of Social Psychology* (Vol. 12, pp. 1–30). Chichester: Wiley.

Sheeran, P. and Abraham, C. (2003) Mediator of moderators: temporal stability of intention and the intention–behavior relationship, *Personality and Social Psychology Bulletin*, 29, 205–15.

Sheeran, P. and Orbell, S. (1999) Augmenting the theory of planned behavior: roles for anticipated regret and descriptive norms, *Journal of Applied Social Psychology*, 29, 2107–42.

Sheeran, P. and Taylor, S. (1999) Predicting intentions to use condoms: a metaanalysis and comparison of the theories of reasoned action and planned behavior, *Journal of Applied Social Psychology*, 29, 1624–75.

Sheeran, P., Maki, A., Montanaro, E., Bryan, A., Klein, W.M.P., Miles, E. *et al.* (submitted) The impact of changing attitudes, norms, and self-efficacy on health-related intentions and behavior: A meta-analysis. Manuscript submitted for publication.

Sheeran, P., Norman, P. and Orbell, S. (1999) Evidence that intentions based on attitudes better predict behaviour than intentions based on subjective norms, *European Journal of Social Psychology*, 29, 403–6.

Sheeran, P., Trafimow, D. and Armitage, C.J. (2003) Predicting behaviour from perceived behavioural control: tests of the accuracy assumption of the theory of planned behaviour, *British Journal of Social Psychology*, 42, 393–410.

Sheppard, B.H., Hartwick, J. and Warshaw, P.R. (1988) The theory of reasoned action: a meta-analysis of past research with recommendations for modifications and future research, *Journal of Consumer Research*, 15, 325–39.

Sniehotta, F.F., Presseau, J. and Araujo-Soares, V. (2014) Time to retire the theory of planned behaviour, *Health Psychology Review*, 8, 1–7.

Sparks, P. (1994) Attitudes towards food: applying, assessing and extending the 'theory of planned behaviour', in D.R. Rutter and L. Quine (eds.) *Social Psychology and Health: European Perspectives* (pp. 25–46). Aldershot: Avebury.

Sparks, P. (2013). The psychology of sustainability: attitudes, identities, actions and engaging with the welfare of others, in H.C. van Trijp (ed.) *Encouraging Sustainable Behavior: Psychology and the Environment* (pp. 169–84). London: Psychology Press.

Sparks, P. and Shepherd, R. (1992) Self-identity and the theory of planned behavior – assessing the role of identification with green consumerism, *Social Psychology Quarterly*, 55, 388–99.

Sparks, P., Guthrie, C.A. and Shepherd, R. (1997) The dimensional structure of the perceived behavioral control construct, *Journal of Applied Social Psychology*, 27, 418–38.

Sparks, P., Harris, P.R. and Lockwood, N. (2004) Predictors and predictive effects of ambivalence, *British Journal of Social Psychology*, 43, 371–83.

Sparks, P., Hedderley, P. and Shepherd, R. (1992) An investigation into the relationship between perceived control, attitude variability and the consumption of two common foods, *European Journal of Social Psychology*, 22, 55–71.

Steadman, L., Rutter, D.R. and Field, S. (2002) Individually elicited versus modal normative beliefs in predicting attendance at breast screening: examining the role of belief salience in the Theory of Planned Behaviour, *British Journal of Health Psychology*, 7, 317–30.

Strack, F. and Deutsch, R. (2004) Reflective and impulsive determinants of social behavior, *Personality and Social Psychology Review*, 8, 220–47.

Sutton, S. (1994) The past predicts the future: interpreting behaviour–behaviour relationships in social psychological models of health behaviour, in D.R. Rutter and L. Quine (eds.) *Social Psychology and Health: European Perspectives* (pp. 71–88). Aldershot: Avebury.

Sutton, S. (1998) Explaining and predicting intentions and behavior: how well are we doing? *Journal of Applied Social Psychology*, 28, 1318–39.

Sutton, S. (2002) Testing attitude–behaviour theories using non-experimental data: an examination of some hidden assumptions, *European Review of Social Psychology*, 13, 293–323.

Terry, D.J. and Hogg, M.A. (1996) Group norms and the attitude–behavior relationship: a role for group identification, *Personality and Social Psychology Bulletin*, 22, 776–93.

Terry, D.J., Hogg, M. and White, K.M. (1999) The theory of planned behaviour: self-identity, social identity and group norm, *British Journal of Social Psychology*, 28, 225–44.

Towriss, J.G. (1984) A new approach to the use of expectancy value models, *Journal of the Market Research Society*, 26, 63–75.

Trafimow, D. (1998) Attitudinal and normative processes in health behavior, *Psychology and Health*, 13, 307–17.

Trafimow, D. and Findlay, K. (1996) The importance of subjective norms for a minority of people, *Personality and Social Psychology Bulletin*, 22, 820–8.

Trafimow, D. and Fishbein, M. (1995) Do people really distinguish between behavioral and normative beliefs? *British Journal of Social Psychology*, 34, 257–66.

Trafimow, D. and Sheeran, P. (1998) Some tests of the distinction between cognitive and affective beliefs, *Journal of Experimental Social Psychology*, 34, 378–97.

Trafimow, D., Sheeran, P., Conner, M. and Findlay, K.A. (2002) Evidence that perceived behavioral control is a multidimensional construct: perceived control and perceived difficulty, *British Journal of Social Psychology*, 41, 101–21.

Triandis, H.C. (1977) *Interpersonal Behavior*. Monterey, CA: Brooks/Cole.

Tyson, M., Covey, J. and Rosenthal, H.E.S. (2014) Theory of Planned Behavior interventions for reducing heterosexual risk behaviors: a meta-analysis, *Health Psychology*, 33, 1454–67.

Van den Putte, B. (1991) On the theory of reasoned action. Unpublished doctoral dissertation, University of Amsterdam.

Van den Putte, B., Yzer, M., Willemsen, M.C. and de Bruijn, G.J. (2009) The effects of smoking self-identity and quitting self-identity on attempts to quit smoking, *Health Psychology*, 28, 535–44.

Van der Pligt, J. and de Vries, N.K. (1998) Belief importance in expectancy-value models of attitudes, *Journal of Applied Social Psychology*, 28, 1339–54.

Van der Pligt, J., de Vries, N.K., Manstead, A.S.R. and van Harreveld, F. (2000) The importance of being selective: weighing the role of attribute importance in attitudinal judgment, *Advances in Experimental Social Psychology*, 32, 135–200.

Verplanken, B. (2006) Beyond frequency: habit as mental construct, *British Journal of Social Psychology*, 45, 639–56.

Warshaw, P.R. and Davis, F.D. (1985) Disentangling behavioral intentions and behavioral expectations, *Journal of Experimental Social Psychology*, 21, 213–28.

Webb, T.L. and Sheeran, P. (2006) Does changing behavioral intentions engender behavior change? A meta-analysis of the experimental evidence, *Psychological Bulletin*, 132, 249–68.

White, K.M., Robinson, N.G., Young, R.M., Anderson, P.J., Hyde, M.K., Greenbank, S. *et al.* (2008) Testing an extended theory of planned behaviour to predict young people's sun safety in a high risk area, *British Journal of Health Psychology*, 13, 435–48.

Wilson, T.D., Dunn, D.S., Kraft, D. and Lisle, D.J. (1989) Introspection, attitude change, and attitude–behaviour consistency: the disruptive effects of explaining why we feel the way we do, in L. Berkowitz (ed.) *Advances in Experimental Social Psychology* (pp. 287–343). New York: Academic Press.

Zanna, M.P. and Rempel, J.K. (1988) Attitudes: a new look at an old concept, in D. Bar-Tal and A.W. Kruglanski (eds.) *The Social Psychology of Knowledge* (pp. 315–34). Cambridge: Cambridge University Press.

Chapter 6

The prototype/willingness model

Frederick X. Gibbons, Meg Gerrard, Michelle L. Stock and
Stephanie D. Finneran

1 General background

Alarmed by what was thought to be an unacceptably high rate of unplanned pregnancies in the
USA, the Institute of Medicine (IOM) commissioned a study in 1994 of factors associated with
sexual behaviour and pregnancy among US teens. The report, entitled *The Best Intentions* (IOM
1995), estimated that more than 80% of adolescent pregnancies in the USA were unintended. One
of the most publicized surveys in the report involved sexual decision-making among high school
students. When asked about the situations and decisions associated with their loss of virginity, over 75% of the sexually active teens said that their first sexual encounter 'just happened'
(SIECUS/Roper Poll 1994; cf. Winter 1988). In other words, this very important health behaviour
(and potentially life-changing event) was apparently neither planned, nor in many instances
even anticipated. One reason why this survey received so much attention is that it contradicted
what was the most popular theoretical view among health psychologists of health decision-
making, the expectancy-value perspective (EVP).

   The EVP maintains that health behaviour, like any other behaviour, is the result of a conscious decision-making process that is both planful and reasoned (Ajzen 1985; Fishbein and
Ajzen 2010). The IOM report added to what was a growing concern expressed by health and
social psychologists that this assumption of planning and reasoning does not always apply to
behaviours that are health-related – which can be impulsive and often have a significant affective component. In fact, this concern is now more widespread and is reflected in a recent issue
of the journal *Health Psychology Review* (see Conner 2014; Head and Noar 2014; Sniehotta *et al.*
2014). Many health researchers have taken issue with the fundamental underlying assumption
behind the EVP, which is that health decision-making is the result of a deliberative process
that involves consideration of behavioural options and assessment of presumed consequences

associated with those actions (i.e. the 'consequentialist' approach; Loewenstein *et al.* 2001). The result of this deliberation is an intention to act or not to act. This view does not presume these actions are necessarily *rational* (as EVP researchers have pointed out repeatedly; Ajzen and Fishbein 2000; Fishbein and Ajzen 2010; Ajzen 2011), but it does assume they are reasoned, and that is the crux of the concern (Gibbons *et al.* 2011).

This is not to say the EVP is without value. In fact, several meta-analyses have shown that EVP theories are effective at predicting reasoned or reasonable behaviours (Webb and Sheeran 2006). McEachan *et al.* (2011), for example, reported that studies conducted using the theory of planned behaviour (Ajzen 1985, 1991) did a better job of explaining health-promoting behaviours, such as physical activity and diet (24% and 21% respectively) than health-impairing behaviours, such as unprotected sex, drug use, and general risk behaviour (14% or 15%). As a result, over the last 10–15 years, several theories/models have been proposed with alternative perspectives on the decision-making process, including fuzzy trace theory (Reyna and Farley 2006), implementation intentions (Gollwitzer 1999; Gollwitzer and Sheeran 2006), and reflective–impulsive theory (Strack and Deutsch 2004). Some of these have focused on health behaviour, and are discussed in detail in this volume. This chapter concerns one of those theories, the prototype/willingness model, which was developed by Gibbons and Gerrard in the late 1990s, but continues to evolve with new data and new input.

1.1 Dual-processing approaches

As the expectancy-value perspective has lost favour among many in the health arena, interest in dual-processing approaches to health has increased significantly, especially in the last few years (Ames *et al.* 2013; Conroy *et al.* 2013; Wills *et al.* 2013; Fleming and Bartholow 2014; Lannoy *et al.* 2014). Much of this attention has been focused on *automatic* or *non-conscious* processing (Sheeran *et al.* 2013). A prime example of this is work examining the effect of impulse on eating behaviour (e.g. Nederkoorn *et al.* 2010), indicating that consumption of tasty but unhealthy (fatty, sweet) foods often reflects temptation that can overcome intentions or plans not to indulge. In fact, researchers in this area have provided a convincing argument to the effect that some health-relevant behaviours are automatic (or almost automatic) reactions to stimuli (alcohol, food, drugs) triggered by associations and neural connections outside of conscious awareness or control (Heatherton 2011; Heatherton and Wagner 2011). More generally, this body of work strongly suggests that much health behaviour, but definitely health risk more than health promotion, involves little premeditation or forethought; instead, it is an unintended reaction to situational factors. This contention forms the basis of the prototype/willingness model.

2 Description of the model

The prototype/willingness model (PWM) is a modified dual-processing model of health behaviour. Like other dual-processing theories, but unlike the expectancy-value perspective, it maintains that decision-making involves two different kinds of information processing, referred to variously in the literature as experiential/rational (Epstein and Pacini 1999), reflective/impulsive (Strack and Deutsch 2004), System I/System II (Evans 2008; Stanovich and Toplak 2012), or heuristic/systematic (Chaiken 1980; Chaiken and Ledgerwood 2012). We use the terms analytic

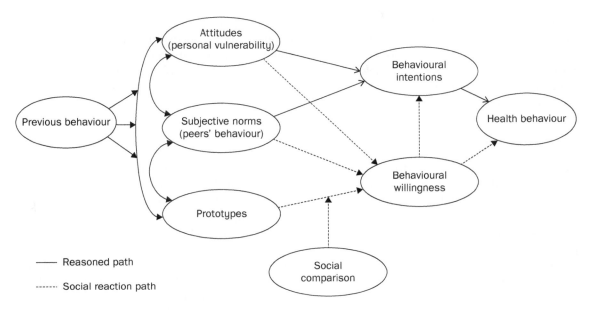

Figure 6.1 The prototype/willingness model (Gibbons *et al.* 2003)

and heuristic. The model was developed with the goal of augmenting (not replacing) the theories of reasoned action and planned behaviour (TRA/TPB), specifically with regard to the prediction of health behaviour, especially among adolescents. The two types of processing are operative in the two pathways to health behaviour described in the model (see Figure 6.1).

2.1 The reasoned pathway

The reasoned pathway involves analytic processing. It is the deliberative route to behaviour that is consistent with the expectancy-value perspective – even some very risky behaviours are the result of a consideration of options and expected outcomes associated with those behaviours. Elements of this route come directly from the theory of reasoned action, but with two modifications: (a) *attitudes* include conditional vulnerability (e.g. perceived personal risk, *if* one *were* to engage in the behaviour), and (b) *subjective norms* are descriptive more than injunctive (i.e. adolescents' perceptions of what others are doing, including friends and peers, role models such as actors and athletes, and, in some cases, parents; see further discussion below). The proximal antecedent to behaviour in this path is behavioural intention, which is defined as an intention (or plan) to engage in a particular behaviour. Outcomes for the reasoned path include health promotion (e.g. condom use), but also health risk behaviours (e.g. plans to get drunk or have casual sex).

2.2 The social reaction path

The social reaction path reflects a belief that certain behaviours are more reactive than reasoned – that is, a response to a particular situation or set of circumstances that may not have been sought or anticipated. Health-risk behaviours are a good example; but social reaction is typical of much adolescent behaviour, whether health-related or not. This path involves more heuristic process-ing. Relative to analytic processing, deliberation is truncated (especially consideration of con-sequences) and affect has more impact, cognition less impact. Images (e.g. prototypes) are influential; and, of course, heuristics play an important role. As Figure 6.1 indicates, both path-ways include attitudes and subjective norms as distal antecedents; however, the social reaction path also includes two constructs that are unique to the model.

2.3 Prototypes

Prototypes are the *images* (the two terms are used interchangeably here and in the model) that individuals have of the *type* of person who engages in the behaviour. They exist for both healthy and unhealthy behaviours: a 'fitness freak' vs. a 'couch potato', for example, or a typical drinker vs. a teetotaller. However, actions, especially risky actions are more salient and usually have more impact than inactions (cf. the 'feature positive effect'; Fazio *et al.* 1982), so high-risk prototypes (e.g. heavy drinkers) tend to show stronger relations with behaviour than low-risk prototypes (e.g. abstainers; Van Lettow *et al.* 2013). Prototypes include two primary dimensions: favourability (how positive is the individual's image) and similarity (how similar to the self does the individual think the prototype is). The more favourable the image and the more similar to the self it is thought to be, the more willing the person is to engage in the behaviour.

2.4 Behavioural willingness

Behavioural willingness is defined as an openness to risk opportunity. It captures the reactive aspect of behaviour, of which there is a considerable amount for adolescents and, more gen-erally, for actions that involve health risk (Reyna and Farley 2006; Webb and Sheeran 2006). Willingness is a recognition of capability: 'given certain circumstances, I might be willing to do X'. In this sense, it differs from an intention – it is not a plan of action or a goal state. Very few people plan on driving under the influence of alcohol or marijuana, for example, but many peo-ple are willing to do so (Flowers *et al.* 2008). When asked, they will acknowledge this – no inten-tions, but some willingness (Gibbons *et al.* 2006). Whether the behaviour occurs, then, is largely dependent on whether the risk opportunity materializes (Gibbons *et al.* 2004c).

Outcomes associated with the social reaction path typically have included risky health behav-iours, as one might expect; but there is no theoretical reason why that has to be the case and, in fact, there is no reason why the behaviour has to be negative. One might be willing to intervene in an altercation on the street, for example, and interveners do have an associated image. By the same token, most willingness-based behaviours are likely to involve some risk; but there have been studies indicating that positive behaviours, such as pro-environmental actions (Ohtomo and Ohnuma 2014) and organ donation (Hyde and White 2010, 2014) can be predicted effectively by the PWM (although the latter clearly has an element of premeditation). As long as the behaviour has a reactive component and an associated image, the PWM is potentially appropriate.

2.5 Process

The modification in the term 'modified dual processing' refers to the social reaction path and, specifically, the fact that although it includes several characteristics commonly associated with heuristic processing, it is also distinct in an important way. Willingness is influenced by factors such as affect (Gibbons *et al.* 2004a, 2012; Walsh *et al.* 2014) and social influence (Gibbons *et al.* 2004c), as well as heuristics – social images or prototypes (cf. Epstein and Pacini 1999), all of which are part of System I. Similarly, the thinking that precedes behavioural willingness is often truncated, especially consideration of consequences, which can be very brief. In fact, research suggests that behavioural willingness is associated with an avoidance of consideration of negative consequences (Stock *et al.* 2013). Such avoidance can lead to underestimation of personal risk, or 'optimistic bias' (Weinstein 1980), also a kind of heuristic (see below). But behavioural willingness is not an *automatic* response to risk opportunity, and while it can have an impulsive component, it also usually involves some cognition: 'What kind of person does this behaviour?', 'Am I like that type of person?' When individuals are asked about their willingness, various heuristics are instantiated, which then results in a determination, one that often ends up being a good predictor of behaviour, especially among adolescents (Andrews *et al.* 2008). In short, the social reaction pathway – and this is true for much health decision-making – relies heavily on heuristics, but this is a conscious more than an unconscious process and it is seldom automatic.

A final point with regard to process has to do with how prototypes 'work'. The PWM has its roots in social comparison theory, and an important assumption of the model is that images affect behavioural willingness through a *social comparison process* – self with the prototype. Thus, prototype influence is moderated by social comparison tendencies; those who are prone to compare (Gibbons and Buunk 1999) tend to be more affected by images, and so the link between prototype and behavioural willingness/behaviour is stronger for them (Gibbons and Gerrard 1995; Litt *et al.* in press).

2.6 Previous behaviour

One focus of the model is on behavioural change, and that is the primary reason why previous behaviour is included in the model; but it is there more as a control than an exogenous construct. Previous behaviour does have an impact on the three exogenous components of the model, but the relations are often non-recursive, and don't add a lot to the model theoretically (early behaviour may follow *or precede* development of an attitude, for example; Gerrard *et al.* 1996). Similarly, direct paths from previous behaviour to future behaviour emerge in many analyses of health behaviour (Ouellette and Wood 1998; de Bruijn *et al.* 2013), but they often reflect the influence of habit, and may not be of much theoretical interest. The PWM studies that have included previous behaviour typically have shown that elements of the model do mediate its relation with subsequent behaviour (Gerrard *et al.* 2006a; Dal Cin *et al.* 2009; Stock *et al.* 2011); but that depends to some extent on the type of behaviour and especially the age of the sample and the lag between measurements. Like most health behaviour models, the PWM is concerned with the cognitive and affective predictors of future behaviour whether or not they serve as mediators of the stability path from previous to future behaviour. Nonetheless, previous behaviour serves a useful purpose in assessments of behaviour change and is worth including in any health behaviour theory (Sheeran 2002).

3 Summary of research

A Google Scholar count indicated that the first two empirical articles introducing the PWM (Gibbons and Gerrard, 1995; Gibbons *et al.*, 1998) had received more than 700 citations; the two theoretical statements (the chapter by Gibbons *et al.* 2003; and Gerrard *et al.* 2008) had been cited over 400 times. The majority of these citations have occurred in the last five years, in part reflecting increasing interest in the applicability of the PWM to interventions (see below). In addition, two recent PWM meta-analyses have summarized studies prompted by the model (Van Lettow et al. in press; Todd et al. 2014); again, most of the studies included in these reviews were published within the last five years.

3.1 Meta-analyses

The study by Todd et al. (2014) provided an analysis of the general model, whereas that of Van Lettow et al. (in press) focused on a more specific issue – prototype similarity versus favourability. However, both meta-analyses reached essentially the same general conclusions: (a) constructs from the PWM, specifically prototypes and behavioural willingness, add significantly to the prediction of health behaviours; and (b) the model itself has utility and potential in terms of interventions.

3.1.1 Todd et al. (2014)

Todd et al. (2014) focused on studies examining the social reaction path – behavioural intention (BI), versus behavioural willingness (BW), and prototypes – and so they did not examine relations involving attitudes and subjective norms. Using several exclusion criteria (e.g. interventions that did not report cross-sectional relations; studies that looked at outcome rather than behaviour; and studies by authors who didn't respond to data requests in a timely fashion, or no longer had access to the data), they identified 81 studies examining 10 different health behaviours, including 21 interventions. In terms of overall model results, they found that prototype was a stronger predictor of BW than BI ($r = 0.34$, $k = 51$ and $r = 0.26$, $k = 40$, respectively), as the PWM would predict. Both BI and BW were correlated with behaviour ($r = 0.48$, $k = 35$ and $r = 0.44$, $k = 57$, respectively). In terms of behavioural prediction, BI accounted for 15.6% of the variance in outcome, while BW predicted an additional 4.9% and prototypes an additional 1.2%. Thus, the two PWM constructs increased the predictive power of BI from 15.6% to 21.7%. Although the additional 6.1% behavioural variance explained is not a large amount, the analysis included a number of studies with adults and/or behaviours that are likely to have been intentional if not habitual – smoking, for example, as well as exercise, vaccination, and social drinking. In fact, their analysis identified both of these factors, age/experience of the sample and type of behaviour, as significant moderators of relations in the PWM.

3.1.2 Van Lettow et al. (in press)

Van Lettow and colleagues' (in press) analysis included fewer articles than that of Todd et al., mostly because of their focus on prototype characteristics (also, their search ended almost a year earlier than Todd et al.). Their specific findings on prototype similarity versus favourability are discussed below. More generally, Van Lettow et al. concluded that: (a) health-risk prototypes are more strongly associated with outcomes than health-promotion prototypes; (b) prototypes (especially the similarity × favourability interaction) are related more strongly to behavioural willingness than behavioural intention; and (c) more research on the role of prototypes in interventions is needed.

3.2 Age and experience

The model was developed with adolescents in mind and that focus is still reflected in the research. Two prospective studies by Pomery et al. (2009, Study 1 and Study 2a) looked at the relative predictive power of BW versus BI from age 12 through 18 and found the anticipated pattern: controlling for previous substance use (Study 1) and then smoking behaviour (Study 2a), BW exceeded BI through age 16, at which point the substance use became more intentional (and more expected) for the next two waves. By age 18, the smoking behaviour had become more habitual and neither BW nor BI predicted significant amounts of variance; only previous behaviour was a predictor. However, a second study (2b) with non-smokers up to age 19 showed that subsequent *initiation* of smoking was predicted by BW. Consistent with these results, Todd and colleagues' analysis indicated that age was a significant moderator of the prototype → BW and BW → behaviour relations, leading them to conclude that, overall, the PWM worked significantly better for adolescents than either pre-adolescents or adults.

Age is correlated with behavioural experience, and both dimensions have been shown to moderate the relations between BW/BI and behaviour. Study 3 of Pomery *et al.* (2009) looked at a type of risk behaviour that is not health-related (skipping class), and found that when both BI and BW were included in the regression, BI predicted the behaviour for those students who had more semesters of classwork (i.e. more experience), whereas BW predicted the behaviour for those with fewer semesters. Along the same lines, Scott-Parker *et al.* (2013) examined risky driving (speeding) among young Australian drivers and found that BW to speed predicted subsequent speeding behaviour, whereas BI to follow the rules of the road did not. Presumably, that will change with age and experience (i.e. safety BI would exceed risk BW in predicting driving).

As a number of studies have indicated, among adolescents BW is often a better predictor than BI for risk behaviours such as substance use (e.g. smoking cigarettes: Hukkelberg and Dykstra 2009; Rivis *et al.* 2010; drug use: Litchfield and White 2006; Gibbons *et al.* 2010a; hookah use: Abedini *et al.* 2014; and drinking: Andrews *et al.* 2011a). One reason for this is that BW develops earlier than intentions, and, according to the model, is often a precursor for subsequent BI (the BW → BI path in the model; see discussion below). The age purview appears to be expanding, however, as an increasing number of researchers have used the model to examine adult behaviour (approximately 15% of the studies we reviewed for this chapter used samples that were over the age of 21; almost all of those studies were published within the last five years). Even for adults, behaviours that meet certain criteria should be candidates for PWM application: an identifiable related image, low prevalence (i.e. the behaviour is generally uncommon and/ or the individual has relatively little experience with it), and some element of risk, even if not physical or health related. Most likely the PWM will continue to be used primarily with adolescents, but more applications to adults are to be expected in the future.

3.3 Type of behaviour

Table 6.1 presents a list of the health behaviours that have been assessed frequently in PWM studies, together with one or two representative PWM studies for each behaviour. Todd and colleagues' list of 10 different health behaviours that had been examined in PWM studies included two that were health-promoting (i.e. exercise and flu vaccination) and two that had a risk and a protective component, sex (risky sex vs. condom use) and sun exposure (tanning vs. sunscreen use). The model did best in predicting substance use (e.g. drug use), as BI accounted for only 8.3% of the variance in behaviour, whereas BW accounted for an additional 20.2%; for sex, the figures were 16.9% for BI and 5.2% for BW. Todd *et al.* (2014) suggest these are behaviours with a significant social reaction component, which makes sense, as they are risky and often not

Table 6.1 Common health behaviours examined in PWM studies

Behaviour	References
Substance use – alcohol	Zimmermann and Sieverding (2010), Andrews *et al.* (2011b)
Substance use – tobacco	Gerrard *et al.* (2005b), Andrews *et al.* (2008)
Substance use – drugs	Dodge *et al.* (2013)
Driving	Rivis *et al.* (2011), Scott-Parker *et al.* (2013)
Sexual behaviour	Myklestad and Rise (2007)
Sun protection	Gibbons *et al.* (2005)
Exercise	Rivis and Sheeran (2003), Ouellette *et al.* (2005)

planned (IOM 1995). On the other hand, BW explained only 3.1% of the variance in cigarette use (vs. 24.1% for BI) and 1.4% of the variance in alcohol use (vs. 41.3% for BI). The model would suggest that these latter figures would vary considerably by age – as Pomery and colleagues' (2009) study indicated. For adolescents, roughly aged 13–17 years, BW should effectively predict tobacco and alcohol use, especially experimentation; after that age, the behaviour is more likely to become intentional. Some behaviours, however, are risky or rare enough that the image associated with them is pronounced and impactful, and they are less likely than drinking, smoking or UV exposure to become intentional or habitual even into adulthood; these behaviours include sexual 'cheating', drunk driving, and heavy drug use (crack, heroin, etc.), among others.

3.4 Health risk vs. health promotion

The initial focus of the model and the research it generated was on health risk behaviours and outcomes. One early exception to this was a study by Gerrard *et al.* (2002) that examined the effects of a healthy prototype, the (adolescent) non-drinker, as well as the more common unhealthy prototype (drinker) on adolescents' willingness to drink and their actual consumption (mean age 16.3 years at T1). Results indicated that the drinker image predicted drinking, mediated by BW to drink, as expected; but the non-drinker image had a more interesting pattern. There was a direct negative path from the abstainer image to drinking, and there was also an indirect path from the abstainer image to drinking through an image *contemplation* measure ('How often have you thought about this type of person?'). These results fit well with a dual-processing account: (a) non-drinkers had a favourable non-drinker image, and that image directly predicted their abstinence, suggesting *not drinking* was a goal for them; and (b) a favourable non-drinker image was associated with more image contemplation, which suggests more reasoned processing.

It is unlikely that a large percentage of 16- and 17-year olds have *not* drinking as a goal state; however, the fact that the non-drinker image does predict self-reported deliberation *and* less drinking is encouraging from an intervention perspective. In fact, that theme of promoting non-risk images can be seen in several interventions that were prompted by the results of Gerrard and colleagues' (2002) study (see below). Other healthy images that have been explored include condom users (e.g. Blanton *et al.* 2001; Mykelstad and Rise 2007, 2008), exercisers (Rivis and Sheeran 2003; Ouellette *et al.* 2005; Rivis *et al.* 2006; Hampson *et al.* 2007), healthy eaters (Gerrits *et al.* 2009, 2010; McCabe *et al.* 2015), sun (UV) protectors (Stock *et al.* 2009; Morris and

Swinbourne 2014), and, of course, alcohol and drug abstainers (Gerrard *et al.* 2002; Zimmerman and Sieverding 2011; Van Lettow *et al.* 2013).

Applying the PWM to healthy behaviours makes sense, and it is not difficult to envision the role that positive or healthy prototypes might play in this process. In terms of BW, *pro-social* willingness has been examined in several studies (e.g. blood donation, volunteerism), but the issue of 'healthy willingness' is a little more complex. For example, using condoms when a partner does not want to and serving as a designated driver are healthy behaviours that have an associated image and a willingness component. But there is also an element of resistance efficacy and/or planfulness, which suggests both paths of the PWM would be involved. Medical risks (and perhaps medical risk 'opportunities') with attendant images also potentially fit into the PWM domain. These images would include someone who chooses to undergo prophylactic mastectomy, or someone who enrols in a controversial or risky clinical trial (which may include pro-social as well as pro-health motives). Although these decisions are not *social* reactions, they all have images associated with them, as well as a degree of risk and some element of willingness. Some also have a reasoned component (e.g. the prophylactic mastectomy), and so illustrate both reasoned and reactive processing.

3.5 Behavioural willingness and behavioural intention: overview

The distinction between willingness and intention is central to the PWM and to its status as a dual-processing model. It also has been one of the more controversial aspects of the model. In this regard, proponents of the expectancy-value perspective have argued that intention to engage in a particular behaviour (BI), behavioural expectation (BE; i.e. perceived likelihood of engaging [Warshaw and Davis 1984; Armitage *et al.* in press]), and willingness (BW) to engage are all the same thing – that is, *readiness* to engage (Fishbein 2008; see also Fishbein and Ajzen 2010; Ajzen 2011). It is not clear if this readiness definition has replaced earlier definitions of BI, which were more instrumental in nature and consistently involved the concept of goal states (e.g. 'The amount of effort one is willing to exert to attain a goal' [Ajzen 1991], or 'Behavioural plans that...enable attainment of a behavioural goal' [Ajzen 1996]; cf. 'proximal goals' [Bandura 1997]). But, it does suggest less emphasis on instrumentality. Still, there are a number of health-relevant behaviours for which the distinctions among BI, BE, and BW are meaningful and potentially important, especially from an intervention or behavioural change perspective. One would certainly not argue that smoking for someone trying to quit, or eating fatty food for someone on a diet, or even unprotected sex for most teen-aged female virgins are goal states; but it is also inaccurate to suggest that for a dieter, plans to overeat, or expectations of overeating, or willingness to overeat are all the same thing – that is, some kind of readiness to consume. Do people ever say, or think, they are 'ready' to overeat or drive drunk?

In arguments against the construct and discriminant validity of BW, it has been pointed out that one of the first PWM papers (Gibbons *et al.* 1998) used what was termed a 'conditional intention' measure: 'imagine being with your boyfriend or girlfriend who wanted to have sex, but with no birth control available', followed by... 'how *likely* is it that you would...[have sex] [use withdrawal...]', etc. In fact, the third study in that 1998 paper did include the current BW wording 'how *willing* would you be to...' (p. 1173), as have all of our studies since the primary statement of the theory (Gibbons *et al.* 2003). Nonetheless, the point is well taken, and the issue is significant. We have argued elsewhere (Gibbons 2006) for the importance of viewing BI, BE, and BW as related but distinct constructs with independent predictive utility and relevance.[1] Conditional (or hypothetical) wording alone is not sufficient to assess social reaction effectively (see Section 5.2 for a discussion of BW measurement).

A related issue has to do with the conceptualization of the BW construct. A recent criticism of the PWM included the following description of the social reaction path: 'When people find themselves in situations that encourage certain behaviors, especially risk-taking behaviors such as smoking, it is not their preconceived intentions that determine their actions but rather their willingness to engage in the behaviors, i.e., their openness to the opportunity' (Ajzen 2011: 1121). This is not just a semantic issue, it is an important misunderstanding of the model and especially its dual-processing core. As mentioned earlier, the PWM was developed to augment the expectancy-value perspective; if we did, in fact, believe that risk BI does not predict risk behaviour – which would be a very difficult assertion to support – we would not have included the construct in the model. The BW construct does predict behaviour better than BI in some situations; but clearly, much health behaviour is reasoned and although the BI–behaviour correlation is often less than predicted, it is definitely robust and reliable (Ajzen 2014). We have consistently argued that for certain behaviours and populations, analyses that include *both* BW and BI are more likely to effectively predict health behaviour than BI alone. But for many other behaviours and many populations, BW is not relevant – asking an adult who has been drinking for 40 years whether he would be willing to have a cocktail at a friend's party most likely would elicit amusement more than self-reflection, and it would not produce an assessment that could predict above and beyond BI to drink.

3.6 Behavioural willingness and behavioural intention: survey studies

A number of survey studies have examined the BW/BI distinction, and most of those have been consistent with the PWM. Using data from the Family and Community Health Study (FACHS; $N = 889$ African American families), Gibbons *et al.* (2004c) found that parent substance use predicted their children's BI, and especially their BE to use substances (children of smokers have a long time to contemplate smoking and its consequences), but it did not predict BW to use. Social influence (i.e. perceived friends' use) and risk images, on the other hand, predicted both BW and BI, but the relations were stronger for BW (BW: $\beta = 0.41$ and 0.22, both $p < 0.001$; BI: $\beta = 0.07$ and 0.11, $p < 0.05$ and 0.001). As expected, BW was a stronger predictor of use than was BI ($\beta = 0.42$ vs. 0.22). The same BW pattern emerged at the next wave of data collection (Gibbons *et al.* 2010a); similar results were found in an intervention described below (Gerrard *et al.* 2006). In the Oregon Youth Substance Use Project (OYSUP), Andrews *et al.* (2011b) found relations among white adolescents that were very similar to those found with black adolescents in FACHS. For example, they reported that alcohol prototypes and descriptive norms at age 13–14 predicted initial levels of heavy drinking at age 16–17, but only through the social reactive path (i.e. drinking BW, not drinking BI). Finally, Litt *et al.* (2014) reported that among 'spring breakers' (college students), getting drunk – a fairly normative and, arguably, goal-oriented activity for this population – was better predicted by drinking BI, whereas 'real' risk behaviour, drinking until one actually passes out, was better predicted by drinking BW. This pattern is common among adults: there are many risk behaviours that are intentional up to a certain level; but people have their limits, and risk above that threshold can and often does become willingness based.

3.6.1 Behavioural willingness → behavioural intention

A contention of the PWM is that BW is often a precursor to BI – that is, it frequently 'evolves' into intention with age and/or experience (hence the BW → BI path in the model). We are not aware of any published analyses of the prospective relation between BW and subsequent BI, perhaps because this requires several waves of data, and also because most PWM studies have had behaviour or BW as outcomes (few PWM studies have looked at BI as an outcome). Consequently, we conducted those analyses for this chapter (see Table 6.2). Using FACHS substance use data, we regressed BI at W3 (age 15.5) and then at W4 (age 18.5) on previous BI at Step 1, and then entered previous BW (Step 2). As expected, BW predicted change in intentions to smoke and use drugs three years later. Unexpectedly, in two of the three sets of analyses, BW was a better predictor (albeit marginally) of future (next wave) BI than was current BI. The general pattern in these analyses was that BI predicted future BI well until BW was entered, at which point BI became a much weaker predictor of itself. It was only when predicting drug BI at W4 (age 18) from BI and BW at W3 (age 15) that current BI was a stronger predictor of future BI than was current BW. Although we would not characterize the PWM as a stage model – such a

Table 6.2 Substance use BW predicting change in substance use BI

Drugs				Smoking			
Criterion	Parameter	Beta	p-value	Criterion	Parameter	Beta	p-value
Wave 3				**Wave 4**			
BI				**BI**			
Block 1	W1 BI	−0.04	0.60	Block 1	W1 BI	0.17	0.063
	W2 BI	0.39	<0.0001		W2 BI	0.36	<0.0001
					W3 BI	0.31	<0.0001
Block 2	W1 BI	−0.06	0.427				
	W2 BI	0.22	0.008	Block 2	W1 BI	0.16	0.089
	W2 BW	0.61	<0.0001		W2 BI	0.35	<0.0001
					W3 BI	0.13	0.122
Wave 4					W3 BW	0.41	<0.0001
BI							
Block 1	W1 BI	−0.11	0.235				
	W2 BI	0.25	0.004				
	W3 BI	0.52	<0.0001				
Block 2	W1 BI	−0.12	0.182				
	W2 BI	0.25	0.004				
	W3 BI	0.39	<0.0001				
	W3 BW	0.30	<0.01				

Note: Mean age (years): Wave 1 = 10.5, Wave 2 = 12.5, Wave 3 = 15.5, Wave 4 = 18.5.

discussion is beyond the scope of this chapter – the fact that BW does predict BI is consistent with the belief that BI at an early age is often not very reliable, whereas BW is a better overall measure of a behavioural inclination for younger adolescents that will eventually evolve into BI for many of them. How BW transitions into BI, what factors (besides experience with the behaviour and risk opportunity) affect that transition, and how it can be interrupted or delayed, are important questions that deserve more attention.

3.7 Behavioural willingness and behavioural intention: experimental studies

Laboratory studies have examined the dual-process aspect of the PWM, and the difference between BW and BI in particular. Several of these studies examined a behaviour – casual sex – with a significant BW/BI distinction. Roberts *et al.* (2013) activated heuristic processing through priming (Bargh and Chartrand 1999). In the first study, single males' BI and BW for casual sex were assessed in a pre-test session (T1). They were then exposed, subliminally, either to photos of women posing provocatively in bikinis, or non-sexual control photos, and then their BI and BW were assessed again (T2). Females were also run (exposed to pictures of men in bathing suits), but in this study they reported little initial casual-sex BW at either wave. Based on their T1 BI self-reports, the males were divided into a 'no-BI' group (37% of the sample) and a 'some-BI' group (i.e. BI > zero; 63% of the sample), and then analyses were conducted on their T1 and T2 BI and BW. As expected, BW was greater than BI at T1; and, overall, T2 BW did not differ from T1 BW. It did differ for one group, however: the no-BI males reported a significant increase in BW from T1 to T2, even though their casual sex intentions remained the same. A second study replicated this effect for 'cheating' BW/BI, using supraliminal primes (again, provocative photos, this time interspersed with control photos). Once again, no-BI males reported a greater increase in BW after exposure to the prime than did the other three groups: no-BI individuals exposed to a control prime, or either of the some-BI groups. In contrast, the BI of this no-BI group was not affected by the sex-priming manipulation.

Differences in casual sex BW were also examined recently by Finneran *et al.* (2015), this time looking at relationship status as a moderator. Males were either socially excluded or not by other males in a game of *Cyberball* (Williams *et al.* 2012), and then their casual sex willingness and intentions were assessed (as they had been in pre-testing). Results indicated that males who were in a monogamous relationship had significantly lower casual sex BW after exclusion, whereas those who were single had significantly higher BW after exclusion. Once again, BI for casual sex was not affected by the social (exclusion) manipulation. The interpretation was that for the males with steady partners, the stress caused by the exclusion led to a desire for comfort and intimacy from their partner, and, therefore, less interest in 'cheating'. In contrast, those without a steady partner were more interested in ego- and mood-restoration after the rejection, and that could come from casual sex. Finally, in both the studies of Roberts *et al.* (2013) and Finneran *et al.* (2015), those males in a committed relationship reported lower casual sex BW than did the single males, as expected. However, in both instances, the committed men had significantly higher casual sex BW than BI. These effects were also replicated with women: (a) the BW/BI difference was significant for the monogamous women (although not as large as it was for the monogamous men), and (b) as with the men, the BW/BI difference was not as strong for the single women as it was for the monogamous women. We would expect that for the monogamous groups, BW would be a better predictor of cheating and relationship dissolution than would BI. More generally, we suspect the number of adults who are intending to cheat on their partner is lower than the number expecting they might do so, which, in turn, is smaller than the number who would be willing to do so under some circumstances.

3.8 Summary

Behavioural willingness and behavioural intention are clearly related, with correlations sometimes in the 0.60s. But there is now a considerable amount of evidence that supports the contention that they are different constructs; this research also identifies some circumstances and factors that distinguish between them. The high correlations reflect the fact that individuals often end up with the same conclusion about future behaviour, but how they get there, and whether they actually perform the behaviour, varies for the two constructs. One perspective on this comes from social judgement theory (Sherif and Hovland 1961): behavioural willingness indicates the boundaries of one's latitude of acceptance; given the right circumstances, the behaviour is likely to occur. Behavioural intention reflects the more central, or core element of that latitude. With age and experience, some boundary (i.e. BW-based) behaviours work their way to the core (become intentions), others drop out. Whether those boundary behaviours translate into action depends on the individual (their level of self-control, for example), but mostly the environment (e.g. risk opportunity, processing load). Finally, in the process of identifying factors that discriminate between BI and BW, this research has further demonstrated the utility of a dual-processing approach to the study of health behaviour, and illustrated its theoretical and translational value

4 Developments

4.1 Prototypes

4.1.1 Dimensions

An issue that has received considerable attention has to do with the two prototype dimensions. Both favourability and similarity are important aspects of the image; when both are high, BW is most likely; when they are low, it is least likely. Both of the recent meta-analyses of the PWM addressed this issue. Todd *et al.* (2014) reported that prototype (similarity and favourability combined) was correlated more highly with BW than BI ($r = 0.34$, $k = 51$ vs. $r = 0.26$, $k = 40$), as the model would suggest. They also reported that prototype similarity was more highly correlated with both BW and BI than favourability, although the difference was more pronounced for BI ($r = 0.47$, $k = 12$ vs. $r = 0.23$, $k = 15$) than for BW ($r = 0.41$, $k = 14$ vs. $r = 0.31$, $k = 17$). Van Lettow *et al.* (in press) also found that similarity generally explained more of the variance in behaviour than did favourability, and suggested this may reflect the importance of social identification with the prototype or the group it represents (cf. Rivis and Sheeran 2003). Undoubtedly, perceived similarity will influence BW/BI and behaviour. One important question is whether this predictive effect exists net the effect of previous behaviour. As others have suggested (Ajzen 2011), perceived similarity to an image is likely to be at least partly a reflection of past behaviour – in a deductive (self-perception) manner: 'I must be similar because I also do the behaviour'. Inclusion of past behaviour can't be determined from either meta-analysis. However, it is the case that a majority of studies that included similarity and favourability found that the similarity dimension was a stronger predictor for BI and BW. However, Van Lettow *et al.* (in press) also reported that studies that included similarity, favourability, and an *interaction* term (similarity × favourability) indicated that the interaction was a stronger predictor of behaviour ($r = 0.32, k = 12$) than was either similarity ($r = 0.27, k = 17$) or favourability ($r = 0.20, k = 38$). The same was true for BW, albeit with smaller samples (similarity × favourability: $r = 0.54$, $k = 4$; similarity: $r = 0.43, k = 5$; favourability: $r = 0.20, k = 14$).

Both elements of the prototype predict behaviour, but the combination of the two can provide additional information. In fact, the 'diagonals' are perhaps the most interesting group (i.e. those who are high in similarity but low in favourability or vice versa). Presumably, those in the latter category (low similarity but high favourability) are considering or about to consider starting the behaviour (analogous to 'pre-contemplators' or 'contemplators' in Prochaska and DiClemente's [1982] transtheoretical model). On the other hand, we would suspect that those in the high similarity/low favourability category may have relatively low self-esteem. More important, they clearly do not approve of the behaviour, and presumably are thinking (or concerned) they will end up engaging; or perhaps they already are engaging, and want to stop. Dalley and Buunk (2009), for example, found that, controlling for BMI, females were most likely to report trying to lose weight if they thought they were similar to the overweight prototype, but had a negative opinion of that image. More generally, it appears that image perception has significant potential for the design of future interventions. From an empirical perspective, we would encourage researchers to use both similarity and favourability whenever they can, and include main effects and interaction terms in their analyses.

4.1.2 Relations

Some studies have found evidence of a path from prototypes to BI. This is rare when both BW and BI are included in the analyses; usually, only the prototype → BW path is significant (e.g. Gerrard *et al.* 2006a; Pomery et al. 2009, Study 3). However, the prototype → BI relation is not inconsistent with the model. Health behaviour often is goal-based, and one goal can be acquisition of the image – exercising would be a good example of a healthy behaviour with an image that can act as a goal (Rivis and Sheeran 2003). But (normatively) negative images can also be goals, such as admission to a desired social group (e.g. 'dirts' or 'druggies'; see Sussman *et al.* 2007). In each case, the group has a recognizable negative image that can attract some.

Several studies have identified direct paths from prototypes to behaviour (e.g. Rivis and Sheeran 2003, 2013; Gerrard *et al.* 2005a; Oullette *et al.* 2005; van den Eijnden *et al.* 2006; Hampson *et al.* 2007; Norman *et al.* 2007; Dalley and Buunk 2009; Gerrits *et al.* 2009; Rivis *et al.* 2010, 2011; Teunissen *et al.* 2012). Most of them did not include BW or BI; however, a few have shown prototype influence circumventing both BW and BI (e.g. Araujo-Soares *et al.* 2013), which is an interesting finding with implications for the model. This could be evidence of impulsive responding, or perhaps some form of cue reactivity. The question is whether the cue is, in fact, the image or is the image just a proxy for the substance (or the behaviour, if it is sex)? Risk opportunity in the form of a cigarette, or joint, drink, etc., may instigate the behaviour for some individuals – those who are users, or perhaps adolescents who are low in self-regulation or self-control (Gerrard *et al.* 2006b). Similarly, seeing someone smoking a cigarette in a movie can activate neural responses of craving for those who engage in the behaviour (Wagner *et al.* 2011), which is one reason why these portrayals are very strong predictors of use (Dal Cin *et al.* 2009; Gibbons *et al.* 2010b). Advertising is also a strong stimulus to use (Wills *et al.* 2010), and ads usually include people; similarly, individuals who are known to drink, or smoke, or use drugs, or are sex symbols, can promote risky behaviour, but that's because of their association with the substance (or the behaviour in the case of sex). Clearly, there are elements of heuristic processing here (automaticity, associative responding) but the role of BW and prototypes is not as clear. It may very well be the case that a direct path from prototype to behaviour should be incorporated into the PWM. Before doing so, however, it would be important to explore the issue of image versus cue to see if the prototype does add to (or replace) the risk cue itself.

4.2 Subjective norms and attitudes

4.2.1 Norms

Some form of subjective norm construct can be found in almost all models of health behaviour, occasionally divided into two types: *descriptive* (perceptions of what others are doing) and *injunctive* (perceptions of what others want one to do). However, several studies have found that injunctive norms are less likely than descriptive norms to predict adolescent behaviour (Smith-McLallen and Fishbein 2008; Baumgartner *et al.* 2011; Hong *et al.* 2012), and so they are less commonly used now than before. Significant others establish subjective norms in the mind of the adolescent either by their own behaviour (descriptive norms) or their opinions of the adolescents' behaviour (injunctive norms) – or actually, the adolescents' *perceptions* of those behaviours and/or opinions. However, the two primary significant others for adolescents either consistently admonish against risk behaviour (parents), so there is little variance in the construct, or they don't care enough to try to influence the behaviours (peers) or express an opinion. In either case, these perceived social injunctions often don't have a lot of impact. When we asked a group of 18-year-olds whether they ever felt pressured to drink, 63% said never; only 9% said they did. When asked if they would give in to their boyfriend/girlfriend's pressure to have sex if they didn't want to, 63% said definitely not, while an additional 23% said probably not (Gibbons *et al.* 2004b). In short, injunctive norms have not typically explained enough variance in adolescent health risk behaviour to warrant inclusion in the PWM.

The two forms of subjective norms may also reflect another dual-processing distinction, however. Ohtomo and Hirose (2007) used the PWM to examine 'eco-friendly' and 'eco-unfriendly' behaviour (i.e. recycling, trash disposal) and found that prototype favourability and descriptive norms only predicted the eco-unfriendly behaviour, whereas injunctive norms only predicted the eco-friendly behaviour. The PWM describes paths from subjective norms to both BI and BW, but there is some reason to believe that may not be true for both types of norms. Engaging in a behaviour because you believe others want you to do it, whether it is healthy or unhealthy, requires some thought and reasoning (what do they want?, will this please them?); whereas doing a behaviour mostly for conformity reasons (i.e. the heuristic: 'everyone's doing it...') requires less reasoning and more reacting. Future research examining whether injunctive norms → BI whereas descriptive norms → BW would be worthwhile.

4.2.2 Attitudes

A similar dual-processing argument could be made for attitudes. Take perceived risk as an example: for adolescents and young adults, perceptions of danger (e.g. driving after consuming four or five drinks is dangerous) are usually higher than perceptions of personal risk, which often reflect some optimistic bias (e.g. 'I could have four or five drinks and drive home without a problem; I've done it before'). The former (perceived danger) should be more strongly related to BI, the latter (personal risk) more to BW. By the same token, attitudes comprise both cognitive and affective components (Edwards 1990; Eagly and Chaiken 1998; Lawton *et al.* 2009); the latter should be more strongly related to BW than are the former. More generally, it is likely that all constructs of the PWM (and other health behaviour models, for that matter) have some heuristic as well as analytic elements. Examining all of the PWM constructs from a dual-processing perspective is likely to prove fruitful and informative.

4.3 Intervention implications

A number of recent studies have been conducted with significant implications for behavioural interventions and preventive interventions. Before presenting the intervention work based on the PWM, we will discuss some of those intervention-relevant studies.

4.3.1 Perceived risk and dual-processing

Weinstein (1980, 1982) identified a form of heuristic processing, often seen in the health behaviour literature, that he called optimistic bias or unrealistic optimism. It is a perception that negative events (e.g. disease, unwanted pregnancy, car accident) are not likely to happen to the self – either in absolute terms ('it won't happen to me') or relative terms ('it is less likely to happen to me than other people'). One particular type of optimistic bias related to health risk is associated with experience. Weinstein (1982) coined the term 'absent-exempt' to refer to a perception that some people have that if they have been engaging in a risk behaviour for some time and nothing bad has happened, then they may be immune to the negative consequences. When asked, people often have difficulty articulating a reasonable (or, presumably, a reasoned) explanation for either the absent-exempt perception or for optimistic biases, but these biases do influence their behaviour. In this sense, they represent heuristic thinking (e.g. 'bad things don't happen to good people like me') and a limited consideration of actual risk. The absent-exempt heuristic has recently been applied to the study of sexual risk-taking in research that was based on the PWM.

In a series of three studies, Stock *et al.* (in press) showed that absent-exempt thinking is enhanced by (downward) social comparison with an individual who *has* experienced the associated risk (e.g. contracted a sexually transmitted disease, STD) even though they had not engaged in the risk behaviour very much at all ('if she "got caught" after just a couple of unprotected incidents, and I haven't after multiple incidents, then my immunity must be pronounced'). More important, this increase in absent-exempt thinking after the downward comparison was accompanied by a corresponding *increase* in BW to have casual sex among the already-at-risk individuals. The authors suggested this finding has important intervention implications, in part because public service announcements that include a theme along the lines of 'It only takes once!' are common (especially for sex). In other words, there is a real possibility of some iatrogenic effects within the group that is being targeted by the intervention – that is, increases in risk-taking among those who have been engaging in high risk without incident (so far).

There was also evidence of dual processing in this series of studies. First, although risk BW was affected (significantly increased) in all three studies, risk BI did not change in any of them. Second, in Study 3, reasoned processing was instantiated before the comparison opportunity and it wiped out the absent-exempt effect (i.e. the lowered risk perception and increased risk BW) completely. Most interesting, however, was the way that BI was affected. In one study, participants were asked about their BI to get tested for HIV infection. As expected, those high-risk participants who read about the infected, low-risk person (downward comparison target) reported reduced vulnerability to STDs and increased BW to have casual sex, but no change in risk BI. However, they also reported significantly *more BI to get tested for an STD*. In other words, the absent-exempt heuristic was associated with an increase in risk willingness, but this increase was not accompanied by a corresponding increase in risk intentions. Instead, it was accompanied by an increase in health promotion intentions – an example of reasoned action accompanying social reaction in the same individuals at the same time. It also is an example with intervention implications.

4.3.2 Reactance

Although not originally conceptualized from a dual-processing perspective, psychological reactance (Brehm 1966) as a cognitive response to perceived loss of freedom has elements of heuristic processing (Sherman *et al.* 2004; Rains and Turner 2007), and those elements are relevant to adolescent health behaviours and especially efforts to modify those behaviours. Several studies have documented a reactance response among adolescents who believed that their freedom to engage in a risky but popular behaviour, such as drug use or reckless driving, was being threatened by a parent, police officer, or public service announcement. The heuristics in play here include some version of 'you can't tell me what to do...' and 'if you're telling me not to do it, then it must be fun...', both of which can produce iatrogenic effects (e.g. Donaldson and Preston 1995; Werch and Owen 2002). In a series of four studies, Gibbons *et al.* (2014b) examined the hypothesis that reactance responses to behaviour change efforts would be more pronounced on BW measures than BI measures, and among high self-esteem individuals who have been engaging in risky behaviour (they tend to be most defensive about their risk behaviour; Gibbons *et al.* 1997; Gerrard *et al.* 2000). In their Study 1, Gibbons *et al.* (2014b) showed that an appearance-based intervention that has proven very effective at changing UV exposure cognitions and behaviour (Gibbons *et al.* 2005; Mahler *et al.* 2007; Stock *et al.* 2009) raised participants' BI to protect considerably, but it had no effect on their BW for exposure, which was high and remained so (when BW was reversed so that both BI and BW reflected protection, BI was much higher than BW). Study 2 also produced a strong intervention effect on BI for all participants. However, this time, high-risk highway workers (those who had engaged in high amounts of previous UV exposure) who were also high in self-esteem reported the most BW to engage in future unprotected sun exposure after the UV intervention. In contrast, these at-risk men did not differ from other participants in their BI to protect or their BW to let their *children* be exposed without protection – both of which should, presumably, reflect more analytic processing or reasoning.

Study 3 found the same pattern among college students with regard to an intervention (laboratory analog) pertaining to casual sex. Again, the participants were either high or low in self-esteem and in previous risk behaviour (four groups in a 2×2 design). The focal group – high self-esteem/high risk – reported more favourable risky-sex prototypes and more BW than did the other three groups (i.e. both low self-esteem groups and the high self-esteem/low risk group). Their BI, however, was no different. Study 4 replicated this pattern: more favourable risky-sex images and higher BW among the high-risk/high self-esteem participants, but no differences from the other groups in terms of their BI for casual sex. Finally, similar effects were reported in a survey study by Dodge *et al.* (2013), who examined BW and BI to use illegal performance-enhancing drugs (PEDs) among male college students. They invoked a heuristic they labelled as 'illegal is effective', reflecting a belief that PEDs that are illegal are likely to have a stronger effect on performance than those that are legal (there is also an element of reactance here as well). They found a fair amount of illegal PED use (75% of the 132 athletes reported some use). Path analyses indicated that BW to use in the future was predicted by favourable user prototypes, subjective norms, favourable PED attitudes, and endorsement of the illegal PED heuristic. Additionally, BI was predicted by norms and attitudes, but not by the heuristic, as the PWM would predict.

5 Operationalization of the model

5.1 Prototypes

People have fairly clear images of peers who engage in risky behaviours, even at an early age (9–10 years; Andrews *et al.* 2008, 2010), and so prototype measurement is straightforward. It will vary as a function of age of the sample, however. Prototypes are assessed on two dimensions: favourability and similarity. The most common method of favourability assessment involves adjective descriptors. When assessing favourability, it is best to avoid, as much as possible, an implication of stereotyping. For example, wording for adolescents (aged about 12–14) would be: '*We want to ask you about your images of people who do different behaviours. We're not talking about any particular person, and we are not saying these people are all alike. What we want to know is what YOU think these people are like. Please think about the type of person your age who _____. How much do you think each of these adjectives describes that type of person?*' This is followed by a list of adjectives, preferably a mix of positive and negative (e.g. smart, considerate, selfish, unpopular), with anchors 'not at all' to 'very much.' These descriptors are likely to vary somewhat in applicability from one behaviour to another (e.g. selfish may apply more to smokers than drinkers); however, item analyses have seldom turned up any meaningful differences in terms of relations with BW or behaviour. It is the *overall perception* of the image rather than its individual characteristics that is most important. Thus, for consistency, we recommend using the same basic list across behaviours, which allows for cross-behaviour comparisons. The similarity item is also usually assessed with a single, face-valid item: 'How similar to the type of person your age who [smokes] are you?'(e.g. Rivis *et al.* 2006). However, some researchers have assessed similarity by having participants evaluate themselves on the same adjectives as the prototype and then summing the self–other differences on each adjective (Aloise-Young *et al.* 1996). In addition, some researchers have also used an 'evaluation thermometer' (Haddock and Zanna 1994) when assessing both favourability (Norman *et al.* 2007) and similarity (Rivis *et al.* 2006). The thermometer typically adopts a 100-point scale (e.g. from 'extremely unfavourable' to 'extremely favourable').

5.2 Behavioural willingness

Assessment of BW includes a hypothetical scenario, for example: 'Imagine you're at a party sometime in the next [few months] and there are some drugs there you can have if you want' (Gerrard *et al.* 2012). This is usually preceded by some qualifier or disclaimer, such as: 'We're not suggesting you would ever be in this kind of situation, but try to imagine it happening'. Next, comes a question about how *willing* the respondent would be under these circumstances to do each of several behaviours that increase in risk (e.g. 'try some of the drugs', '...use enough to get high', '...buy some to use later'). Use of the subjunctive is important in order to avoid internal attributions (i.e. 'you didn't seek out the situation'). Also, we assume many adolescents are curious about risky behaviours, and although social influence is important, there is more to substance use or risky sex than an inability to 'just say no'. Behavioural willingness is different from resistance efficacy, and so implications of peer pressure should be avoided. Responses to the items are aggregated and used as a BW index. These prototype and BW measures have consistently produced valid and reliable indexes (alphas > 0.70; test–retest correlations > 0.50), even among children.

5.3 Behavioural intentions

Measurement of BI follows previous TRA and TPB guidelines with regard to specificity (Conner and Sparks, Chapter 5 this volume), including timeframe (same as BW): 'Do you intend to drink [plan on drinking] alcohol sometime in the next few months?' We recommend not using BE measures ('How likely is it...') interchangeably with BI measures (Gibbons 2006), though if distinguishing BI and BE is important, then, of course, both would be appropriate. Finally, if a goal of the research is to compare BW and BI, then comparability in terms of amount of behaviour would make sense: 'Do you intend to drink... [some alcohol] [a few drinks]...sometime in the next few months?'

5.4 Subjective norms and attitudes

Typically, participants are asked how many of their friends and peers engage in the behaviour, for example: 'How many of the kids at school or in the neighbourhood have tried a drink of alcohol (beer, wine, or hard liquor)?' and 'How many of your friends have tried a drink of alcohol?', with options ranging from 'none of them' to 'almost all of them' (Andrews *et al.* 2011b). Attitude items involve *conditional vulnerability*: respondents are told to imagine engaging in the behaviour and then indicate how likely they think it is that a negative outcome would occur: 'If you were to get tanned on a regular basis from being in the sun, what are your chances that you would develop skin cancer at some point in the future?' (from 'not at all likely' to 'very likely'; Walsh and Stock 2012).

6 PWM interventions

6.1 Intervention studies

As mentioned earlier, perceived risk is an important element in almost all health behaviour theories, and it is part of the expectancy-value perspective (EVP). Most interventions based on the EVP have focused on risk reasoning. In particular, they have attempted to encourage recipients to think about the dangers associated with specific risk behaviours in an effort to increase perceptions of vulnerability to the negative consequences of those behaviours. This approach to prevention is typically based on the assumption that informing people about potential health risks will decrease their intentions to engage in risk behaviours; or, if they are already engaging, increase their intentions to change those behaviours. An example of the shortcomings of this approach can be found in data on smoking behaviour after publication of the 1964 US Surgeon

General's Report on Smoking and Health. There was a steady increase in the percentage of Americans who believed that smoking caused lung cancer (from <40% to >70%) between the early 1950s, when the first evidence on smoking and cancer was made public, and the late 1960s, when the media had covered the report extensively (Pierce and Gilpin 2001). However, the percentage of smokers who quit following the report increased only by about 1% during this period (Gilpin and Pierce 2002). Findings such as these suggest that perceived risk (i.e. absolute risk perceptions) typically has only small effects on risk behaviour (Sheeran *et al.* 2014), and that knowing about the dangers, or actual risks, associated with a behaviour is frequently not sufficient to motivate behaviour change (Weinstein 1988; Fisher *et al.* 2006).

More than 50 studies have successfully manipulated various aspects of the PWM in efforts to test the malleability of prototypes or willingness, and/or the impact of these manipulations on subsequent behaviours. Some of these were extensive interventions like Click City® (Andrews *et al.* 2011a; see below), and some were smaller controlled experimental studies. The majority of the studies targeted tobacco and alcohol use, or UV exposure. However, there was a range of behaviours, including exercise (Ouellette *et al.* 2005), diet and sleeping (Werch *et al.* 2007; Steinhilber *et al.* 2012; Fuchs *et al.* 2013; McCabe *et al.* 2015), safe sex (Murry *et al.* 2011; Stock *et al.* 2013, in press), and marijuana use (Comello 2011). While most focused on risk prototypes and behaviours, a sizeable number appeared to be prompted by Gerrard *et al.* (2002) in showing that favourable images of people who engage in healthy behaviour can also motivate healthy changes (Comello 2011; Walsh *et al.* 2012; McCabe *et al.* 2015).

Our early research on adolescents assumed that many of them do not feel vulnerable to the potential negative consequences of a risk behaviour because they do not *intend* to engage in the behaviour. As the IOM report (1995) indicated, for example, many adolescents do not intend to have sexual intercourse, especially early in a relationship. But they eventually find themselves in circumstances in which they end up doing so. Because effective contraception and protection from STDs require planning, these adolescents often fail to protect themselves (Gerrard 1987). This combination of factors – low risk intentions, failure to feel vulnerable to negative consequences of unprotected sex, and being in risk-conducive situations – suggested a direction for intervention research – that is, studies that addressed the malleability of risk and non-risk prototypes and willingness, and also the effects of altering these components of the model on risk behaviour.

6.2 Manipulating prototypes

6.2.1 Risky sex

The first study that attempted to alter prototypes included a manipulation in which students were exposed to a persuasive communication on 'sexual behaviours and personality characteristics' (Blanton *et al.* 2001, Study 4; see also Todd and Mullan 2001). Students in the experimental group read a bogus newspaper article reporting the results of a personality survey indicating that people who do not use condoms are 'more selfish' and 'less responsible' than those who do use condoms. Students in the control condition read a message describing the typical person who does not vote as more selfish and less responsible than those who do. Relative to the control group, students in the condom condition reported less willingness to have sex without condoms after reading the message that emphasized the negative features of someone who has unprotected sex.

6.2.2 Prototype contemplation

Another paradigm employed a visualization/contemplation strategy in which participants were asked to write about their image of a person who does or does not engage in healthy behaviour. The first study using this method had participants write about the type of person who does or does not exercise regularly (Ouellette *et al.* 2005). Participants had little difficulty envisioning both prototypes, and wrote detailed descriptions of them. As expected, exerciser prototypes were much more favourable. More important, data from a one-month follow-up phone call (supposedly as part of an unrelated survey) revealed that those in the exerciser condition reported a significant increase in exercise in the interim while those in the non-exerciser condition reported a small decrease.

In an extension of Ouellette's visualization study, using terror management theory (Greenberg *et al.* 1997), Arndt *et al.* (2009) employed a mortality salience induction to address the question of *why* prototypes affect behaviour. Participants were randomly assigned to either a mortality salience condition in which they described the emotions that thoughts of their death would arouse, or a control condition about their emotions and thoughts associated with dental pain. They then visualized the prototypical exerciser or non-exerciser. Results showed that the combination of thinking about one's death and envisioning and contemplating the prototype of a regular exerciser increased the extent to which people derive a sense of self-worth from exercising, suggesting that it can also lead to increased commitment to exercising.

A series of brief interventions based on the PWM employed image-based messages to activate prototypes and future self-images. Werch *et al.* (2007), for example, randomly assigned participants to one of three conditions: (a) a meeting with a fitness specialist to develop a contract to target self-selected areas of behaviour change (e.g. exercise, diet, drinking); (b) a tailored one-on-one consultation using gain- and loss-framed messages to promote prototypes and self-images relevant to several health-promoting behaviours; and (c) a meeting with the fitness specialist to develop a contract and receive the image-based consultation. Results revealed significantly larger increases in healthy behaviours at the one-month follow-up in both conditions that included the consultation than the condition with just the contract. Thus, like Ouellette *et al.* (2005), this study demonstrated the efficacy of image-based interventions, but it also provided evidence of change in multiple behavioural areas as the result of a single brief intervention.

6.2.3 Risk salience

A series of sun-protection intervention studies have also been successful in altering prototypes of people who expose themselves to ultraviolet (UV) rays to get a tan. These studies employed a camera with a UV filter that produces a facial photograph that graphically depicts existing skin damage due to previous UV exposure (Fulton 1997; Mahler *et al.* 2007). The damage is not visible to the naked eye, but it is very common, even among younger adolescents, and is becoming more prevalent (Balk 2011). The goal of these studies was to use the UV photographs of participants' faces to make the damage they had already incurred salient and thereby change their images of tanning and tanners from something positive to something negative. In other words, the same (appearance) motivation behind the risk behaviour was used to motivate abandoning it. In the first of these studies, Gibbons *et al.* (2005) provided half the participants with their UV photos (the other half did not receive the photos), and then all participants were asked to consider prototypes of people who 'work on their tans'. There were immediate declines in prototype favourability and tanning willingness, whereas perceived vulnerability to skin damage increased. More important, these changes persisted over time, and mediated changes in tanning booth behaviour reported at three-week follow-up.

Two further recent studies of sun exposure extended this research by identifying important moderators of the impact of the UV photos. Walsh and Stock (2012) examined the effects of the UV camera intervention on men who are high in masculinity, a group that typically engages in low levels of health-promoting behaviours, including low levels of sun protection. As expected, masculinity moderated the effect of the UV photography, as the intervention was more effective at changing attitudes towards sun protection and increasing willingness to protect and intentions to undergo skin examinations for high-masculinity men than it was for low-masculinity men. Thus, it had a larger effect on the group most at risk. In a second study, the authors examined the effects of having women focus on their 'thoughts' or their 'feelings' when they viewed the UV photos in an effort to encourage heuristic or analytic processing about the risk (Walsh et al. 2014). As expected, focusing attention on cognitions rather than affect was beneficial – that is, the older women in the cognitive focus condition had lower sun risk willingness and higher perceived skin cancer vulnerability than those in the affective focus group. The results suggest that altering type of processing regarding risk can lead to a reduction in risk behaviour.

6.2.4 Conclusions

These intervention studies were successful in demonstrating that risk and non-risk prototypes are malleable. They also showed that there are a variety of ways to alter prototype favourability, and that reducing risk prototype favourability and increasing the favourability of non-risk prototypes can reduce willingness to engage in a variety of risk behaviours. Finally, as the model predicts, decreasing willingness mediates the impact of prototype change on behaviour change. It should be noted, however, that these studies were relatively small and most were conducted with college students; also, all of them relied on self-reports of behaviour change. These limitations have been addressed by interventions conducted on other populations, which were designed to test the efficacy of the model in changing a variety of behaviours in the field.

6.3 Behavioural interventions

Although there are few published interventions that have tested the entire PWM, a number of recent interventions have incorporated elements of the model and provided evidence of the efficacy of these different elements as components of interventions. What follows is a description of several published dual-process interventions that are based on the PWM, and then descriptions of some research (published and in progress) that has provided support for the efficacy of the model. In addition, Table 6.3 includes a list of representative PWM interventions.

6.3.1 The Strong African American Families Program (SAAF)

Studies based on the PWM have shown that parents can play a very active role in forming a base of risk and non-risk cognitions that affect a child's eventual behaviour by promoting unfavourable risk prototypes and decreasing willingness (Blanton et al. 1997; Gerrard et al. 1999; Ouellette et al. 1999; Gibbons et al. 2002). These findings, together with work by Brody and Ge (2001) on family process, led to the development of the SAAF Program. The SAAF is a family-centred preventive intervention designed to inhibit or delay the onset of alcohol use (Brody et al. 2004).

Table 6.3 Key intervention studies

Outcome	Target group	Intervention	Reference
Willingness to smoke	Middle school students	Click City®: tobacco	Andrews *et al.* (2014)
Willingness to smoke	Elementary and middle school students	Click City®: tobacco	Andrews *et al.* (2011a)
Early unprotected sex	African American children	SAAF (family-based intervention)	Murry *et al.* (2011)
Drinking	African American children	SAAF	Gerrard *et al.* (2006a)
Tanning booth use	College students	Salience of skin damage	Gibbons *et al.* (2005)
Sun protection	Outdoor workers	Salience of skin damage	Stock et al. (2009)
Exercise	College students	Prototype visualization/ contemplation	Ouellette *et al.* (2005)

Consistent with the PWM, and the dual-process focus, SAAF had two components. One, which was directed at the parents, targeted the reasoned path, by increasing communication of expectations with children about alcohol use. The second, more heuristic arm was directed at the children, and was designed to: (a) make their images of drinkers more negative, and (b) educate them on the differences between planned and reactive behaviour, while reducing their willingness to drink. The intervention was successful in decreasing the favourability of the children's images of the typical drinker, and their intentions and willingness to drink, while increasing self-reports of parent–child communication. More important, the intervention effect on alcohol consumption at 24-month follow-up was significant (Gerrard *et al.* 2006a). The intervention also replicated and extended earlier PWM studies by demonstrating the efficacy of combining a heuristic *and* an analytic approach to altering children's decision-making processes and behaviour. Specifically, the reasoned path from the intervention to drinking was mediated by changes in parenting and then intentions, whereas the social reaction path was mediated by changes in prototypes and willingness. Both paths (indirect effects) were significant, but the social reaction path was stronger, mostly because the BW → behaviour relation was stronger than the BI → behaviour relation. Importantly, however, a structural model that included *both* the reasoned and the social reaction paths provided a significantly better fit of the data than a model with either path alone.

6.3.2 Sun protection intervention for highway workers

Another intervention based on the PWM focused on an older, high-risk population – road maintenance workers (Stock *et al.* 2009). The intervention was similar to other UV-photo interventions (Mahler *et al.* 2007) in that participants were shown UV photographs of their faces and then listened to a brief (12-minute) educational video on UV risk (focusing on either skin cancer or photo-ageing). Each video also provided information about sunscreen use and skin protection (e.g. how much sunscreen to use, what level of SPF is best). In addition to assessing self-reported sun protective behaviours, as a measure of UV exposure, this study also assessed changes in skin tone as measured by a spectrophotometer, which provides an objective quantification of skin colour. As in the SAAF intervention, the total effect of the UV intervention at 14-month follow-up was significant and there were two significant paths to the outcome measures. There was a direct path from the intervention to changes in sun protection and skin colour, *and* an indirect path that was mediated by changes in risk cognitions suggested by the PWM (e.g. prototype-relevant – being tanned is attractive, and also perceived vulnerability to skin cancer). Thus, the study suggested, once again, that the most effective intervention for this high-risk population included both reasoned (educational) and heuristic approaches.

6.3.3 Click City®: tobacco

Another dual-process intervention based on the PWM is Click City®, a computer-based tobacco prevention programme for children (Andrews *et al.* 2011a, 2014). The programme is delivered to 10-year-olds via a series of linked computers that allow elementary school students to receive social norm information on their classmates' beliefs about tobacco use while engaging in a programme that targets willingness, intentions, and initiation of tobacco use. The first (short-term) study of the intervention (Andrews *et al.* 2011) documented changes in intentions and willingness to use tobacco from baseline to one-week follow-up. It also demonstrated that the intervention was most efficacious for students who were most at risk (i.e. those who had tried smoking at baseline or had a family member who smoked). Likewise, the long-term follow-up, which included a sixth-grade booster, and followed the students through the seventh grade, replicated these results, showing that students in the schools that participated in the Click City® programme (vs. schools that did not) showed smaller increases in the favourability of smoker prototypes, willingness, and intentions to smoke. Notably, this follow-up also replicated the finding that the intervention was most effective for high-risk adolescents.

6.4 Conclusion

In addition to these studies, we are aware of a number of ongoing dual-process interventions that are based in part or completely on the PWM. For example, Litt, Lewis, and colleagues at the University of Washington are conducting a series of studies, theoretically informed by the PWM, of personalized feedback interventions designed to reduce alcohol-related risky sexual behaviour.[2] The rapid rise of late in the number of intervention studies (65% have been published in the last four years), and the fact that 18 dual-process and/or PWM intervention grants are currently funded by the National Institutes of Health (NIH Reporter July 2014), suggests that researchers are increasingly acknowledging the efficacy of dual-process approaches to intervention research.

7 Future directions

There are a number of important issues that either have yet to be addressed, or are worthy of more empirical attention in the future. Below are some of those issues.

7.1 Social distancing

The healthy-image work mentioned earlier presents an interesting topic for future research that has a theoretical link to the roots of the PWM. In our first health prototype study, we looked at the extent to which smokers engage in 'social distancing' from the smoker prototype as part of their effort to quit smoking (Gibbons and Boney McCoy 1991). The term refers to a process that includes derogating the image, while looking for evidence of distinction from the self. It does predict successful cessation (Gibbons and Eggleston 1996; Gerrard *et al.* 2005b), which led us to consider how the process might unfold in the opposite direction: increasingly favourable and similar (to self) perceptions of the prototype leading to increased willingness to try the behaviour – which is, in essence, the basis of the PWM. Surprisingly, few studies have looked at the role of images in cessation efforts. An early cessation study found that a negative smoker image was a better predictor of quitting than was a positive *former smoker* image (Gibbons and Eggleston 1996). Similarly, Dalley and Buunk (2009) found that the overweight image was a stronger predictor of weight loss efforts than was the thin image. Finally, Piko *et al.* (2007) found that negative smoker prototypes were more motivating for non-smokers to avoid smoking than positive smoker prototypes were for smokers to start or continue smoking. These results are generally consistent with other approach/avoidance studies (Boyd *et al.* 2011), as well as research in the possible-self area (Quinlan *et al.* 2006), and suggest that the desire to stop being (or avoid becoming) a negative exemplar may be a stronger motivator than the desire to become a positive exemplar (see deviance regulation theory; Blanton and Christie 2003). These results also have implications for preventive and intervention efforts, and suggest that this issue is likely to be an area of interest for future PWM research.

7.2 Behavioural intention → behavioural willingness

As mentioned earlier, an important issue involves examining the evolution of BW into BI, a process that is common among adolescents. Less common, but still quite possible, is the inverse relation. Specifically, the empirical question is: 'How and why does BI *not* to engage in a risk behaviour turn into BW to do it?' Generally speaking, adolescents who do not have a clear intention to *avoid engaging* in unhealthy behaviours are at risk to do so – more so if they are willing to engage. But many adolescents do report intending to avoid a behaviour ('virginity pledges' being an example) and end up doing the behaviour nonetheless. Determining what factors promote 'pledge-breaking' like this, and the transition from negative intentions to positive willingness, would be interesting and informative.

7.3 Individual differences: *self-control*

Moderation of prototype effects (on BW and behaviour) by social comparison tendencies has been reported previously (Gibbons and Gerrard 1995; Litt *et al.* in press). Moderation of the BW/BI paths to behaviour has also been hypothesized, but received relatively little empirical attention. Gerrard *et al.* (2006b) examined the extent to which self-control moderated the relation between BW and behaviour. Interestingly, high and low self-control adolescents did not differ in amount of BW, but the relation between BW and subsequent behaviour, which was significant for both groups, was significantly stronger for those who were low in self-control (Wills *et al.* 2010). It would appear that although willingness to engage in risk is a part of growing up for many adolescents, whether they act on that BW depends not just on opportunity, but also on their temperament (e.g. level of self-control).

7.4 Individual differences: *genes*

As might be expected, given these relations involving self-control, there is also evidence of a biological substrate in social reaction. Analyses from the FACHS panel study of African American families (Gibbons *et al.* 2012) showed that the relation between stress (e.g. perceived racial discrimination) and risk cognitions (prototypes and BW) and then risk behaviour was significantly stronger for those adolescents with a specific genetic architecture, including two so-called 'risk' genes: the serotonin transporter (5HTTLPR) and the dopamine receptor (DRD4-7R). A follow-up showed the same moderated relations between discrimination and both self-control and anger (Gibbons *et al.* 2014a). In fact, in both cases the pattern provided evidence of *genetic sensitivity* to the environment: more risk for adolescents who had experienced a lot of discrimination, but significantly *less risk* for those who grew up in an environment that was relatively free of discrimination (for a discussion of genetic sensitivity, see Ellis *et al.* 2011). We expect to see more attention devoted to the examination of individual differences, including genetics, in assessments of the PWM and in interventions that are based on it.

7.5 Cross-cultural perspectives

Published studies using the PWM have emanated from more than 20 countries. After the USA, the most contributions have come from the UK and the Netherlands, which is not surprising given the interest and focus in these two countries on health psychology in general, and especially the health–social psychology hybrid – acceptance of which has been comparatively slow in the USA (Klein *et al.* 2014). Few studies have included cross-cultural analyses, but several have speculated on how elements of the model, mostly prototypes, might differ across different countries and cultures. Drinker prototypes, for example, are likely to be more favourable in the Netherlands than in the USA. But, the *opposite* is likely for the image of the adult who drives while drunk – negative in Europe and the USA, of course, but less negative in the USA. These differences reflect norms and prevalence of the different risk behaviours, so they don't have much theoretical importance, but they do have intervention implications. Few studies have looked at either the BW/BI distinction or differences in dual processing across cultures. Ohtomo *et al.* (2011) examined unhealthy eating in Japan and the Netherlands and concluded that this type of risk behaviour is more likely to be intentional in the Netherlands and more impulsive and willingness based in Japan. Although elements of the PWM are likely to vary from one culture to another, we are aware of no studies that have suggested the basic relations in the PWM differ significantly across countries. Nonetheless, we expect to see more research on this topic in the future.

7.6 Neural correlates

Previous studies on dual processing have shown increased activity in the limbic network during heuristic processing, as opposed to more prefrontal activity for analytic processing (e.g. Hampton and O'Doherty 2007; Lannoy *et al.* 2014). That being the case, one interesting hypothesis worth pursuing is that BW, or social reaction, is associated with neural activity in different areas of the brain than reasoned action, or BI. A related question is whether prototype stimuli also activate areas associated with heuristic processing, and whether that differs as a function of the type of prototype – healthy versus unhealthy, for example. Yet another interesting question is whether impulsive decisions *not* to engage in risk (see Carver and White's, 1994, discussion of BIS/BAS) also involve limbic activity.

7.7 Behavioural willingness and prototype development

Examining factors that affect the development of images and BW would have value from both an applied and theoretical perspective. We know that risk images can become clear and influential for children as young as 8 or 9 years, and we know that the media are an important source for them, especially movies and movie stars (Dal Cin *et al.* 2009; Gibbons *et al.* 2010b). Laboratory studies are currently underway looking at how movie portrayals affect images and which individual differences moderate that process. We also know that by age 13 or 14, adolescents can articulate the difference between intentions and willingness and the behaviours associated with each construct.[3] Further examination of this developmental process is called for. As mentioned earlier, the same is true for the study of factors that affect BW and prototypes and also those that can effect change in them. Finally, it should be noted that interventions that are based on the PWM face an ethical issue when they involve negative images or prototypes. Manipulations intended to exacerbate the image associated with certain groups (e.g. overweight individuals, smokers, alcoholics) can help stigmatize members of those groups. For this reason, we would encourage additional research efforts aimed at examining social distancing – looking for evidence of *distinction* between the self and the prototype – *without including derogation* of that prototype or exemplars of the group.

8 Conclusion

Interest in the PWM has increased within the last four or five years. We do not believe this is primarily attributable to disillusionment with the expectancy-value perspective. Rather, we see it as evidence of increasing acceptance of the dual-processing perspective upon which the PWM is based, along with enthusiasm for the utility of the perspective for explaining, predicting, and changing health behaviour. Although the basics of the PWM appear to have withstood empirical test (and scrutiny), there is a need for additional studies, especially experimental studies that examine the various components of the model and their relations with each other. We look forward to seeing the conclusions from these studies, and also the results from the different interventions and preventive interventions that are currently underway. This new information will allow us and other researchers to further develop and improve the model.

Notes

1. Studies based on the TRA or TPB have often used BI and BE measures interchangeably (Armitage and Conner 2001). Although we would agree that those two constructs are more similar to each other than they are to BW (Gibbons 2006), we believe there can be value in looking at them separately. In fact, in a recent study Armitage *et al.* (2015) showed that BE was a better predictor of alcohol consumption and weight loss than was BI, controlling for baseline measures of each.

2. NIH grants: R01AA020869 and R01AA021379.
3. We asked a group of 208 13- and 14-year-olds to define BW and BI, whether they thought the two constructs were the same or different, and if different, how they were different. Their definitions were generally consistent with those provided in the PWM: ~95% said they were two different constructs. Descriptions of the differences frequently (63%) mentioned something about planning ahead of time and social/situational influence (55%).

References

Abedini, S., MorowatiSharifabad, M.A., Chaleshgarkordasiabi, M. and Ghanbarnejad, A. (2014) Predictors of non-Hookah smoking among high school students based on Prototype/Willingness Model, *Health Promotion Perspectives*, 4 (1), 46–53.

Ajzen, I. (1985) From intentions to actions: a theory of planned behavior, in J. Kuhl and J. Beckmann (eds.) *Action Control: From Cognition to Behavior* (pp. 11–39). Heidelberg: Springer.

Ajzen, I. (1991) The theory of planned behavior, *Organizational Behavior and Human Decision Processes*, 50 (2), 179–211.

Ajzen, I. (1996) The social psychology of decision making, in E.T. Higgins and A.W. Kruglanski (eds.) *Social Psychology: Handbook of Basic Principles* (pp. 297–325). New York: Guilford Press.

Ajzen, I. (2011) The theory of planned behaviour: reactions and reflections, *Psychology and Health*, 26 (9), 1113–27.

Ajzen, I. (2014) The theory of planned behaviour is alive and well, and not ready to retire: a commentary on Sniehotta, Presseau, and Araujo-Soares, *Health Psychology Review*, 8, 1–7.

Ajzen, I. and Fishbein, M. (2000) Attitudes and the attitude–behavior relation: reasoned and automatic processes, *European Review of Social Psychology*, 11 (1), 1–33.

Aloise-Young, P.A., Hennigan, K.M. and Graham, J.W. (1996) Role of the self-image and smoker stereotype in smoking onset during early adolescence: a longitudinal study, *Health Psychology*, 15, 494–7.

Ames, S.L., Grenard, J.L. and Stacy, A.W. (2013) Dual process interaction model of HIV-risk behaviors among drug offenders, *AIDS and Behavior*, 17 (3), 914–25.

Andrews, J., Gordon, J., Hampson, S., Christiansen, S., Gunn, B., Slovic, P. *et al.* (2011a) Short-term efficacy of Click City® tobacco: changing etiological mechanisms related to the onset of tobacco use, *Prevention Science*, 12 (1), 89–102.

Andrews, J.A., Gordon, J.S., Hampson, S.H., Gunn, B., Christiansen, S.M. and Slovic, P. (2014) Long-term efficacy of Click City® tobacco: a school-based tobacco prevention program, *Nicotine and Tobacco Research*, 16 (1), 33–41.

Andrews, J.A., Hampson, S. and Peterson, M. (2011b) Early adolescent cognitions as predictors of heavy alcohol use in high school, *Addictive Behaviors*, 36 (5), 448–55.

Andrews, J.A., Hampson, S.E., Barckley, M., Gerrard, M. and Gibbons, F.X. (2008) The effect of early cognitions on cigarette and alcohol use during adolescence, *Psychology of Addictive Behaviors*, 22 (1), 96–106.

Andrews, J.A., Hampson, S.E., Greenwald, A.G., Gordon, J. and Widdop, C. (2010) Using the implicit association test to assess children's implicit attitudes toward smoking, *Journal of Applied Social Psychology*, 40 (9), 2387–2406.

Araujo-Soares, V.V., Rodrigues, A.A., Presseau, J.J. and Sniehotta, F.F. (2013) Adolescent sunscreen use in springtime: a prospective predictive study informed by a belief elicitation investigation, *Journal of Behavioral Medicine*, 36 (2), 109–23.

Armitage, C.J. and Conner, M. (2001) Efficacy of the theory of planned behaviour: a meta-analytic review, *British Journal of Social Psychology*, 40 (4), 471–99.

Armitage, C., Norman, P., Alganem, S. and Conner, M. (2015) Expectations are more predictive of behavior than behavioral intentions: evidence from two prospective studies. *Annals of Behavioral Medicine* [49, 239–46. DOI: 10.1007/s12160-014-9653-4].

Arndt, J., Cox, C.R., Goldenberg, J.L., Vess, M., Routledge, C., Cooper, D.P. *et al.* (2009) Blowing in the (social) wind: implications of extrinsic esteem contingencies for terror management and health, *Journal of Personality and Social Psychology*, 96 (6), 1191–1205.

Balk, S.J. (2011) Ultraviolet radiation: a hazard to children and adolescents, *Pediatrics*, 127 (3), e791–817.

Bandura, A. (1997) *Self-efficacy: The Exercise of Control*. New York: Freeman.

Bargh, J.A. and Chartrand, T.L. (1999) The unbearable automaticity of being, *American Psychologist*, 54 (7), 462–79.

Baumgartner, S.E., Valkenburg, P.M. and Peter, J. (2011) The influence of descriptive and injunctive peer norms on adolescents' risky sexual online behavior, *Cyberpsychology, Behavior, and Social Networking*, 14 (12), 753–8.

Blanton, H. and Christie, C. (2003) Deviance regulation: a theory of action and identity, *Review of General Psychology*, 7 (2), 115–49.

Blanton, H., Gibbons, F.X., Gerrard, M., Conger, K.J. and Smith, G.E. (1997) Role of family and peers in the development of prototypes associated with substance use, *Journal of Family Psychology*, 11 (3), 271–88.

Blanton, H., Vanden Eijnden, R.J.J., Buunk, B.P., Gibbons, F.X., Gerrard, M. and Bakker, A. (2001) Accentuate the negative: social images in the prediction and promotion of condom use, *Journal of Applied Social Psychology*, 31 (2), 274–95.

Boyd, R.L., Robinson, M.D. and Fetterman, A.K. (2011) Miller (1944) revisited: movement times in relation to approach and avoidance conflicts, *Journal of Experimental Social Psychology*, 47 (6), 1192–7.

Brehm, J.W. (1966) *A Theory of Psychological Reactance*. New York: Academic Press.

Brody, G.H. and Ge, X. (2001) Linking parenting processes and self-regulation to psychological functioning and alcohol use during early adolescence, *Journal of Family Psychology*, 15 (1), 82–94.

Brody, G.H., Murry, V.M., Gerrard, M., Gibbons, F.X., Molgaard, V., Wills, T.A. *et al.* (2004) The Strong African American Families Program: translating research into prevention programming, *Child Development*, 75 (3), 900–17.

Carver, C.S. and White, T.L. (1994) Behavioral inhibition, behavioral activation, and affective responses to impending reward and punishment: the BIS/BAS scales, *Journal of Personality and Social Psychology*, 67 (2), 319–33.

Chaiken, S. (1980) Heuristic versus systematic information processing and the use of source versus message cues in persuasion, *Journal of Personality and Social Psychology*, 39 (5), 752–66.

Chaiken, S. and Ledgerwood, A. (2012) A theory of heuristic and systematic information processing, in P.M. Van Lange, A.W. Kruglanski and E. Higgins (eds.) *Handbook of Theories of Social Pychology* (Vol. 1, pp. 246–66). Thousand Oaks, CA: Sage.

Comello, M.L.G. (2011) Characterizing drug non-users as distinctive in prevention messages: implications of optimal distinctiveness theory, *Health Communication*, 26 (4), 313–22.

Conner, M. (2014) Extending not retiring the theory of planned behaviour: a commentary on Sniehotta, Presseau and Araújo-Soares, *Health Psychology Review* [DOI: 10.1080/17437199.2014.899060].

Conroy, D.E., Maher, J.P., Elavsky, S., Hyde, A.L. and Doerksen, S.E. (2013) Sedentary behavior as a daily process regulated by habits and intentions, *Health Psychology*, 32 (11), 1149–57.

Dal Cin, S., Worth, K.A., Gerrard, M., Gibbons, F.X., Stoolmiller, M., Wills, T.A. *et al.* (2009) Watching and drinking: expectancies, prototypes, and friends' alcohol use mediate the effect of exposure to alcohol use in movies on adolescent drinking, *Health Psychology*, 28 (4), 473–83.

Dalley, S.E. and Buunk, A.P. (2009) 'Thinspiration' vs. 'fear of fat': using prototypes to predict frequent weight-loss dieting in females, *Appetite*, 52 (1), 217–21.

De Bruijn, G.J., Gardner, B., van Osch, L. and Sniehotta, F.F. (2013) Predicting automaticity in exercise behaviour: the role of perceived behavioural control, affect, intention, action planning, and behaviour, *International Journal of Behavioral Medicine*, 21 (5), 767–74.

Dodge, T., Stock, M. and Litt, D. (2013) Judgments about illegal performance enhancing substances: reasoned, reactive or both? *Journal of Health Psychology*, 18 (7), 962–71.

Donaldson, T. and Preston, L.E. (1995) The stakeholder theory of the corporation: concepts, evidence, and implications, *Academy of Management Review*, 20 (1), 65–91.

Eagly, A.H. and Chaiken, S. (1998) Attitude structure and function, in D.T Gilbert, S.T. Fiske and G. Lindzey (eds.) *The Handbook of Social Psychology* (4th edn., Vol. 1, pp. 269–322). New York: McGraw-Hill.

Edwards, K. (1990) The interplay of affect and cognition in attitude formation and change, *Journal of Personality and Social Psychology*, 59 (2), 202–16.

Ellis, B.J., Boyce, W.T., Belsky, J., Bakermans-Kranenburg, M.J. and Van Ijzendoorn, M.H. (2011) Differential susceptibility to the environment: an evolutionary–neurodevelopmental theory, *Development and Psychopathology*, 23 (1), 7–28.

Epstein, S. and Pacini, R. (1999) Some basic issues regarding dual-process theories from the perspective of cognitive-experiential self-theory, in S. Chaiken and Y. Trope (eds.) *Dual-process Theories in Social Psychology* (pp. 462–82). New York: Guilford Press.

Evans, J.T. (2008) Dual-processing accounts of reasoning, judgment, and social cognition, *Annual Review of Psychology*, 59, 255–78.

Fazio, R.H., Sherman, S.J. and Herr, P.M. (1982) The feature-positive effect in the self-perception process: does not doing matter as much as doing? *Journal of Personality and Social Psychology*, 42 (3), 404–11.

Finneran, S.D., Gibbons, F.X. and Gerrard, M. (2015) Social exclusion and casual sex willingness: the role of gender and relationship status. Manuscript in preparation.

Fishbein, M. (2008) A reasoned action approach to health promotion, *Medical Decision Making*, 28 (6), 834–44.

Fishbein, M. and Ajzen, I. (2010) *Predicting and Changing Behavior: The Reasoned Action Approach*. New York: Psychology Press.

Fisher, J.D., Fisher, W.A., Amico, K. and Harman, J.J. (2006) An information–motivation–behavioral skills model of adherence to antiretroviral therapy, *Health Psychology*, 25 (4), 462–73.

Fleming, K.A. and Bartholow, B.D. (2014) Alcohol cues, approach bias, and inhibitory control: applying a dual process model of addiction to alcohol sensitivity, *Psychology of Addictive Behaviors*, 28 (1), 85–96.

Flowers, N.T., Naimi, T.S., Brewer, R.D., Elder, R.W., Shults, R.A. and Jiles, R. (2008) Patterns of alcohol consumption and alcohol-impaired driving in the United States, *Alcoholism: Clinical and Experimental Research*, 32, 639–44.

Fuchs, T., Steinhilber, A. and Dohnke, B. (2013) Improving adolescents' eating behaviour by changing prototype perceptions: an intervention study based on the Prototype/Willingness-Model, *Psychology and Health*, 28, 95–6.

Fulton, J.E. (1997) Utilizing the ultraviolet (UV detect) camera to enhance the appearance of photo damage and other skin conditions, *Dermatologic Surgery*, 23, 163–9.

Gerrard, M. (1987) Sex, sex guilt, and contraceptive use revisited: the 1980s, *Journal of Personality and Social Psychology*, 52 (5), 975–80.

Gerrard, M., Gibbons, F.X. and Reis-Bergan, M. (2000) Self-esteem, self-serving health cognitions and health risk behavior, *Journal of Personality*, 68 (6), 1177–1201.

Gerrard, M., Gibbons, F.X., Benthin, A.C. and Hessling, R.M. (1996) A longitudinal study of the reciprocal nature of risk behaviors and cognitions in adolescents: what you do shapes what you think, and vice versa, *Health Psychology*, 15 (5), 344–54.

Gerrard, M., Gibbons, F.X., Brody, G.H., Murry, V.M., Cleveland, M.J. and Wills, T.A. (2006a) A theory-based dual-focus alcohol intervention for preadolescents: the Strong African American Families Program, *Psychology of Addictive Behaviors*, 20 (2), 185–95.

Gerrard, M., Gibbons, F.X., Houlihan, A.E., Stock, M.L. and Pomery, E.A. (2008) A dual process approach to health risk decision making: the prototype willingness model, *Developmental Review*, 28 (1), 29–61.

Gerrard, M., Gibbons, F.X., Lane, D.J. and Stock, M.L. (2005a) Smoking cessation: social comparison level predicts success for adult smokers, *Health Psychology*, 24, 623–9.

Gerrard, M., Gibbons, F.X., Reis-Bergan, M., Trudeau, L., Vande Lune, L.S. and Buunk, B. (2002) Inhibitory effects of drinker and nondrinker prototypes on adolescent alcohol consumption, *Health Psychology*, 21 (6), 601–9.

Gerrard, M., Gibbons, F.X., Stock, M.L., Houlihan, A.E. and Dykstra, J.L. (2006b) Temperament, self-regulation, and the prototype willingness model of adolescent health risk behavior, in D. de Ridder and J. de Wit (eds.) *Self-regulation in Health Behaviour* (pp. 97–117). Chichester: Wiley.

Gerrard, M., Gibbons, F.X., Stock, M.L., Vande Lune, L.S. and Cleveland, M.J. (2005b) Images of smokers and willingness to smoke among African American pre-adolescents: an application of the prototype/willingness model of adolescent health risk behavior to smoking initiation, *Journal of Pediatric Psychology*, 30 (4), 305–18.

Gerrard, M., Gibbons, F.X., Zhao, L., Russell, D.W. and Reis-Bergan, M. (1999) The effect of peers' alcohol consumption on parental influence: a cognitive mediational model, *Journal of Studies on Alcohol and Drugs*, 13, 32–44.

Gerrard, M., Stock, M.L., Roberts, M.E., Gibbons, F.X., O'Hara, R E., Weng, C.-Y. *et al.* (2012) Coping with racial discrimination: the role of substance use, *Psychology of Addictive Behaviors*, 26, 550–60.

Gerrits, J.H., de Ridder, D.T., de Wit, J.B. and Kuijer, R.G. (2009) Cool and independent or foolish and undisciplined? Adolescents' prototypes of (un)healthy eaters and their association with eating behaviour, *Appetite*, 53 (3), 407–13.

Gerrits, J.H., O'Hara, R.E., Piko, B.F., Gibbons, F.X., de Ridder, D.T., Keresztes, N. *et al.* (2010) Self-control, diet concerns and eater prototypes influence fatty foods consumption of adolescents in three countries, *Health Education Research*, 25 (6), 1031–40.

Gibbons, F.X. (2006) Proximal antecedents: intentions, expectations, and willingness as precursors of health behavior, in M. Gerrard and K. McCaul (eds.) *A Web-based Health Lexicon*. Bethesda, MD: National Cancer Institute [http://cancercontrol.cancer.gov/brp/constructs/intent-expect-willingness/index.html].

Gibbons, F.X., Abraham, W.T., Gerrard, M., Stock, M.L., Beach, S.R.H., Wills, T.A. *et al.* (2014a) Racial sensitivity: genetic architecture moderates reactions to perceived racial discrimination among African Americans. Manuscript submitted for publication.

Gibbons, F.X. and Boney McCoy, S. (1991) Self-esteem, similarity and reactions to active vs. passive downward comparison, *Journal of Personality and Social Psychology*, 60, 414–24.

Gibbons, F.X. and Buunk, B.P. (1999) Individual differences in social comparison: development of a scale of social comparison orientation, *Journal of Personality and Social Psychology*, 76 (1), 129–42.

Gibbons, F.X. and Eggleston, T.J. (1996) Smoker networks and the 'typical smoker': a prospective analysis of smoking cessation, *Health Psychology*, 15 (6), 469–77.

Gibbons, F.X. and Gerrard, M. (1995) Predicting young adults' health risk behavior, *Journal of Personality and Social Psychology*, 69 (3), 505–17.

Gibbons, F.X., Eggleston, T.J. and Benthin, A. (1997) Cognitive reactions to smoking relapse: the reciprocal relation of dissonance and self-esteem, *Journal of Personality and Social Psychology*, 72 (1), 184–95.

Gibbons, F.X., Etcheverry, P.E., Stock, M.L., Gerrard, M., Weng, C.Y., Kiviniemi, M. *et al.* (2010a) Exploring the link between racial discrimination and substance use: What mediates? What buffers? *Journal of Personality and Social Psychology*, 99 (5), 785–801.

Gibbons, F.X., Gerrard, M. and Lane, D.J. (2003) A social-reaction model of adolescent health risk, in J.M. Suls and K.A. Wallston (eds.) *Social Psychological Foundations of Health and Illness* (pp. 107–36). Oxford: Blackwell.

Gibbons, F.X., Gerrard, M., Blanton, H. and Russell, D.W. (1998) Reasoned action and social reaction: willingness and intention as independent predictors of health risk, *Journal of Personality and Social Psychology*, 74, 1164–81.

Gibbons, F.X., Gerrard, M., Cleveland, M.J., Wills, T.A. and Brody, G.H. (2004a) Perceived discrimination and substance use in African American parents and their children: a panel study, *Journal of Personality and Social Psychology*, 86 (4), 517–29.

Gibbons, F.X., Gerrard, M., Lane, D.J., Mahler, H.I.M. and Kulik, J.A. (2005) Using UV photography to reduce use of tanning booths: a test of cognitive mediation, *Health Psychology*, 24 (4), 358–63.

Gibbons, F.X., Gerrard, M., Pomery, E.A., (2004b) *Risk and Reactance: Applying Social-psychological Theory to the Study of Health Behavior*, in R.A. Wright, J. Greenberg and S.S. Brehm (eds.) *Motivational Analyses of Social Behavior* (pp. 149–66). Hillsdale, NJ: Erlbaum.

Gibbons, F.X., Gerrard, M., Reimer, R.A. and Pomery, E.A. (2006) Unintentional behavior: a subrational approach to health risk, in D.T.M. de Ridder and J.B.F. de Wit (eds.) *Self-regulation in Health Behavior* (pp. 45–70). Chichester: Wiley.

Gibbons, F.X., Gerrard, M., Vande Lune, L.S., Wills, T.A., Brody, G. and Conger, R.D. (2004c) Context and cognition: environmental risk, social influence, and adolescent substance use, *Personality and Social Psychology Bulletin*, 30, 1048–61.

Gibbons, F.X., Kingsbury, J.H., Gerrard, M. and Wills, T.A. (2011) Two ways of thinking about dual processing: a response to Hofmann, Friese and Wiers (2008), *Health Psychology Review*, 5 (2), 158–61.

Gibbons, F.X., Lane, D.J., Gerrard, M., Reis-Bergan, M., Lautrup, C.L., Pexa, N. *et al.* (2002) Comparison level preferences after performance: is downward comparison theory still useful? *Journal of Personality and Social Psychology*, 83 (4), 865–80.

Gibbons, F.X., Pomery, E.A., Gerrard, M., Sargent, J.D., Weng, C.-Y., Wills, T.A. *et al.* (2010b) Media as social influence: racial differences in the effects of peers and media on adolescent alcohol cognitions and consumption, *Psychology of Addictive Behaviors*, 24, 649–59.

Gibbons, F.X., Roberts, M.E., Gerrard, M., Li, Z., Beach, S.R.H., Simons, R.L. *et al.* (2012) The impact of stress on the life history strategies of African American adolescents: cognitions, genetic moderation, and the role of discrimination, *Developmental Psychology*, 48, 722–39.

Gibbons, F.X., Stock, M.L. and Gerrard, M. (2014b) Social reaction as reactance: a dual-processing perspective on health behavior change. Manuscript submitted for publication.

Gilpin, E.A. and Pierce, J.P. (2002) Demographic differences in patterns in the incidence of smoking cessation: United States 1950–1990, *Annals of Epidemiology*, 12 (3), 141–50.

Gollwitzer, P.M. (1999) Implementation intentions: strong effects of simple plans, *American Psychologist*, 54 (7), 493–503.

Gollwitzer, P.M. and Sheeran, P. (2006) Implementation intentions and goal achievement: a meta-analysis of effects and processes, in M.P. Zanna (ed.) *Advances in Experimental Social Psychology* (Vol. 38, pp. 69–119). San Diego, CA: Elsevier Academic Press.

Greenberg, J., Solomon, S. and Pyszczynski, T. (1997) Terror management theory of self-esteem and social behavior: empirical assessments and conceptual refinements, in M.P. Zanna (ed.) *Advances in Experimental Social Psychology* (Vol. 29, pp. 61–139). New York: Academic Press.

Haddock, G. and Zanna, M.P. (1994) Preferring housewives to feminists: categorization and the favorability of attitudes toward women, *Psychology of Women Quarterly*, 18, 25–52.

Hampson, S.E. (2008) Mechanisms by which childhood personality traits influence adult well-being, *Current Directions in Psychological Science*, 17, 264–8.

Hampson, S.E., Andrews, J.A., Peterson, M. and Duncan, S.C. (2007) A cognitive-behavioral mechanism leading to adolescent obesity, *Annals of Behavioral Medicine*, 34, 287–94.

Hampton, A.N. and O'Doherty, J.P. (2007) Decoding the neural substrates of reward-related decision making with functional MRI, *Proceedings of the National Academy of Sciences USA*, 104 (4), 1377–82.

Head, K.J. and Noar, S.M. (2014) Facilitating progress in health behaviour theory development and modification: the reasoned action approach as a case study, *Health Psychology Review*, 8, 34–52.

Heatherton, T.F. (2011) Neuroscience of self and self-regulation, *Annual Review of Psychology*, 62, 363–90.

Heatherton, T.F. and Wagner, D.D. (2011) Cognitive neuroscience of self-regulation failure, *Trends in Cognitive Sciences*, 15 (3), 132–9.

Hong, T., Rice, J. and Johnson, C. (2012) Ethnic group and temporal influences of social norms: smoking behavior among a panel of adolescents, *Journal of Communication*, 62 (1), 158–74.

Hukkelberg, S.S. and Dykstra, J.L. (2009) Using the prototype/willingness model to predict smoking behaviour among Norwegian adolescents, *Addictive Behaviors*, 34 (3), 270–6.

Hyde, M.K. and White, K.M. (2010) Are organ donation communication decisions reasoned or reactive? A test of the utility of an augmented theory of planned behaviour with the prototype/willingness model, *British Journal of Health Psychology*, 15 (2), 435–52.

Hyde, M.K. and White, K.M. (2014) Perceptions of organ donors and willingness to donate organs upon death: a test of the prototype/willingness model, *Death Studies*, 38 (7), 459–64.

Institute of Medicine (IOM) (1995) Personal and interpersonal determinants of contraceptive use, in S.S Brown and L. Eisenberg (eds.) *The Best Intentions: Unintended Pregnancy and the Well-being of Children and Families* (pp. 160–82). Washington, DC: National Academy Press.

Klein, W.P., Shepperd, J.A., Suls, J., Rothman, A.J. and Croyle, R.T. (2014) Realizing the promise of social psychology in improving public health, *Personality and Social Psychology Review*, 19 (1), 77–92.

Lannoy, S., Billieux, J. and Maurage, P. (2014) Beyond inhibition: a dual-process perspective to renew the exploration of binge drinking, *Frontiers in Human Neuroscience*, 8, 405.

Lawton, R., Conner, M. and McEachan, R. (2009) Desire or reason: predicting health behaviors from affective and cognitive attitudes, *Health Psychology*, 28 (1), 56–65.

Litchfield, R.A. and White, K.M. (2006) Young adults' willingness and intentions to use amphetamines: an application of the theory of reasoned action, *E-journal of Applied Psychology*, 2 (1), 1–9.

Litt, D.M., Lewis, M.A., Patrick, M.E., Rodriguez, L., Neighbors, C. and Kaysen, D.L. (2014) Spring break versus spring broken: predictive utility of spring break alcohol intentions and willingness at varying levels of extremity, *Prevention Science*, 15, 85–93.

Litt, D., Stock, M.L. and Gibbons, F.X. (in press) Adolescent alcohol use: social comparison orientation moderates the impact of friend and sibling behavior, *British Journal of Health Psychology* [DOI: 10.1111/bjhp.12118].

Loewenstein, G.F., Weber, E.U., Hsee, C.K. and Welch, N. (2001) Risk as feelings, *Psychological Bulletin*, 127 (2), 267–86.

Mahler, H.M., Kulik, J.A., Gerrard, M. and Gibbons, F.X. (2007) Long-term effects of appearance-based interventions on sun protection behaviors, *Health Psychology*, 26 (3), 350–60.

McCabe, S., Arndt, J., Goldenberg, J.L., Vess, M., Vail, K., Gibbons, F.X. *et al.* (2015) The effect of visualizing healthy eaters after mortality reminders increases nutritious grocery purchases: an integrative terror management and prototype willingness analysis, *Health Psychology* [34, 279–82. DOI: 10.1037/hea0000154].

McEachan, R.R.C., Conner, M., Taylor, N.J. and Lawton, R.J. (2011) Prospective prediction of health-related behaviours with the theory of planned behaviour: a meta-analysis, *Health Psychology Review*, 5 (2), 97–144.

Morris, K. and Swinbourne, A. (2014) Identifying prototypes associated with sun-related behaviours in North Queensland, *Australian Journal of Psychology*, 66 (4), 216–23.

Murry, V., Berkel, C., Chen, Y., Brody, G.H., Gibbons, F.X. and Gerrard, M. (2011) Intervention induced changes on parenting practices, youth self-pride and sexual norms to reduce HIV-related behaviors among rural African American youths, *Journal of Youth and Adolescence*, 40 (9), 1147–63.

Myklestad, I. and Rise, J. (2007) Predicting willingness to engage in unsafe sex and intention to perform sexual protective behaviors among adolescents, *Health Education and Behavior*, 34 (4), 686–99.

Myklestad, I. and Rise, J. (2008) Predicting intentions to perform protective sexual behaviours among Norwegian adolescents, *Sex Education*, 8, 107–24.

Nederkoorn, C., Houben, K., Hofmann, W., Roefs, A. and Jansen, A. (2010) Control yourself or just eat what you like? Weight gain over a year is predicted by an interactive effect of response inhibition and implicit preference for snack foods, *Health Psychology*, 29 (4), 389–93.

Norman, P., Armitage, C.J. and Quigley, C. (2007) The theory of planned behavior and binge drinking: assessing the impact of binge drinker prototypes, *Addictive Behaviors*, 32, 1753–68.

Ohtomo, S. and Hirose, Y. (2007) The dual-process of reactive and intentional decision-making involved in eco-friendly behavior, *Journal of Environmental Psychology*, 27, 117–25.

Ohtomo, S. and Ohnuma, S. (2014) Psychological interventional approach for reducing resource consumption: reducing plastic bag usage at supermarkets, *Resources, Conservation and Recycling*, 84, 57–65.

Ohtomo, S., Hirose, Y. and Midden, C.J.H. (2011) Cultural differences of a dual-motivation model on health risk behaviour, *Journal of Risk Research*, 14 (1), 85–96.

Ouellette, J.A. and Wood, W. (1998) Habit and intention in everyday life: the multiple processes by which past behavior predicts future behavior, *Psychological Bulletin*, 124 (1), 54–74.

Ouellette, J.A., Gerrard, M., Gibbons, F.X. and Reis-Bergan, M. (1999) Parents, peers, and prototypes: antecedents of adolescent alcohol expectancies, alcohol consumption, and alcohol-related life problems in rural youth, *Psychology of Addictive Behaviors*, 13 (3), 183–97.

Ouellette, J.A., Hessling, R., Gibbons, F.X., Reis-Bergan, M. and Gerrard, M. (2005) Using images to increase exercise behavior: prototypes vs. possible selves, *Personality and Social Psychology Bulletin*, 31 (5), 610–20.

Pierce, J.P. and Gilpin, E.A. (2001) News media coverage of smoking and health is associated with changes in population rates of smoking cessation but not initiation, *Tobacco Control*, 10 (2), 145–53.

Piko, B.F., Bak, J. and Gibbons, F.X. (2007) Prototype perception and smoking: are negative or positive social images more important in adolescence? *Addictive Behaviors*, 32 (8), 1728–32.

Pomery, E.A., Gibbons, F.X., Reis-Bergan, M. and Gerrard, M. (2009) From willingness to intention: experience moderates the shift from reactive to reasoned behavior, *Personality and Social Psychology Bulletin*, 35 (7), 894–908.

Prochaska, J.O. and DiClemente, C.C. (1982) Transtheoretical therapy: toward a more integrative model of change, *Psychotherapy: Theory, Research and Practice*, 19 (3), 276–88.

Quinlan, S.L., Jaccard, J. and Blanton, H. (2006) A decision theoretic and prototype conceptualization of possible selves: implications for the prediction of risk behavior, *Journal of Personality*, 74 (2), 599–630.

Rains, S.A. and Turner, M.M. (2007) Psychological reactance and persuasive health communication: a test and extension of the intertwined model, *Human Communication Research*, 33 (2), 241–69.

Reyna, V.F. and Farley, F. (2006) Risk and rationality in adolescent decision making: implications for theory, practice, and public policy, *Psychological Science in the Public Interest*, 7 (1), 1–44.

Rivis, A. and Sheeran, P. (2003) Social influences and the theory of planned behaviour: evidence for a direct relationship between prototypes and young people's exercise behaviour, *Psychology and Health*, 18 (5), 567–83.

Rivis, A. and Sheeran, P. (2013) Automatic risk behaviour: direct effects of binge drinker stereotypes on drinking behavior, *Health Psychology*, 32, 571–80.

Rivis, A., Abraham, C. and Snook, S. (2011) Understanding young and older male drivers' willingness to drive while intoxicated: the predictive utility of constructs specified by the theory of planned behaviour and the prototype–willingness model, *British Journal of Health Psychology*, 16 (2), 445–56.

Rivis, A., Sheeran, P. and Armitage, C.J. (2006) Augmenting the theory of planned behaviour with the prototype/willingness model: predictive validity of actor versus abstainer prototypes for adolescents' health-protective and health-risk intentions, *British Journal of Health Psychology*, 11 (3), 483–500.

Rivis, A., Sheeran, P. and Armitage, C.J. (2010) Explaining adolescents' cigarette smoking: a comparison of four modes of action control and test of the role of self-regulatory mode, *Psychology and Health*, 25 (8), 893–909.

Rivis, A., Sheeran, P. and Armitage, C. J. (2011) Intention versus identification as determinants of adolescents' health behaviours: evidence and correlates, *Psychology and Health*, 26, 1128–42.

Roberts, M.E., Gibbons, F.X., Kingsbury, J.H. and Gerrard, M. (2013) Not intending but somewhat willing: the influence of visual primes on risky sex decisions, *British Journal of Health Psychology*, 19 (3), 553–65.

Scott-Parker, B., Hyde, M.K., Watson, B. and King, M.J. (2013) Speeding by young novice drivers: what can personal characteristics and psychosocial theory add to our understanding? *Accident Analysis and Prevention*, 50, 242–50.

Sheeran, P. (2002) Intention–behavior relations: a conceptual and empirical review, *European Review of Social Psychology*, 12 (1), 1–36.

Sheeran, P., Gollwitzer, P.M. and Bargh, J.A. (2013) Nonconscious processes and health, *Health Psychology*, 32 (5), 460–73.

Sheeran, P., Harris P.R. and Epton, T. (2014) Does heightening risk appraisals change people's intentions and behavior? A meta-analysis of experimental studies, *Psychological Bulletin*, 140, 511–43.

Sherif, M. and Hovland, C.I. (1961) *Social Judgment: Assimilation and Contrast Efforts in Communication and Attitude Change.* New Haven, CT: Yale University Press.

Sherman, S.J., Crawford, M.T. and McConnell, A.R. (2004) Thinking about the future as a technique to reduce resistance to persuasion, in E. Knowles and J. Linn (eds.) *Resistance and Persuasion.* Mahwah, NJ: Erlbaum.

SIECUS/Roper Poll (1994) Cited in Haffner, D., Sexuality Issues and Contraceptive Use. Paper prepared for *the Institute of Medicine Committee on Unintended Pregnancy* (pp. 181). Washington, DC: National Academy Press.

Smith-McLallen, A. and Fishbein, M. (2008) Predictors of intentions to perform six cancer-related behaviours: roles for injunctive and descriptive norms, *Psychology, Health and Medicine*, 13 (4), 389–401.

Sniehotta, F.F., Presseau, J. and Araujo-Soares, V. (2014) Time to retire the theory of planned behaviour, *Health Psychology Review*, 8, 1–7.

Stanovich, K.E. and Toplak, M.E. (2012) Defining features versus incidental correlates of Type 1 and Type 2 processing, *Mind and Society*, 11 (1), 3–13.

Steinhilber, A., Bocker, C., Fuchs, T. and Dohnke, B. (2012) A cross-cultural analysis: eating behaviour of adolescents in Turkey and Germany. Poster presented at the 26th Conference of the European Health Psychology Society (EHPS), Prague, Czech Republic, 21–25 August.

Stock, M.L., Gerrard, M., Gibbons, F.X., Dykstra, J.L., Mahler, H.I., Walsh, L.A. *et al.* (2009) Sun protection intervention for highway workers: long-term efficacy of UV photography and skin cancer information on men's protective cognitions and behavior, *Annals of Behavioral Medicine*, 38 (3), 225–36.

Stock, M.L., Gibbons, F.X., Beekman, J. and Gerrard, M. (in press) It only takes once: the absent exempt heuristic and reactions to comparison-based sexual risk information, *Journal of Personality and Social Psychology*.

Stock, M.L., Gibbons, F.X., Walsh, L.A. and Gerrard, M. (2011) Racial identification, racial discrimination, and substance use vulnerability among African American young adults, *Personality and Social Psychology Bulletin*, 37 (10), 1349–61.

Stock, M.L., Litt, D.M., Arlt, V., Peterson, L.M. and Sommerville, J. (2013) The Prototype/Willingness model, academic versus health-risk information, and risk cognitions associated with nonmedical prescription stimulant use among college students, *British Journal of Health Psychology*, 18 (3), 490–507.

Strack, F. and Deutsch, R. (2004) Reflective and impulsive determinants of social behavior, *Personality and Social Psychology Review*, 8 (3), 220–47.

Sussman, S., Pokhrel, P., Ashmore, R.D. and Brown, B.B. (2007) Adolescent peer group identification and characteristics: a review of the literature, *Addictive Behaviors*, 32 (8), 1602–27.

Teunissen, H., Spijkerman, R., Larsen, H., Kremer, K., Kuntsche, E., Gibbons, F.X. *et al.* (2012) Stereotypic information about drinkers and students' observed alcohol intake: an experimental study on prototype–behavior relations in males and females in a naturalistic drinking context, *Drug and Alcohol Dependence*, 125, 301–6.

Todd, J. and Mullan, B. (2001) Using the theory of planned behavior and prototype willingness model to target binge drinking in female undergraduate university student, *Addictive Behavior*, 36 (10), 980–6.

Todd, J., Kothe, E., Mullan, B. and Monds, L. (2014) Reasoned versus reactive prediction of behavior: a meta-analysis of the prototype willingness model, *Health Psychology Review* [DOI: 10.1080/17437199.2014.922895].

Van Den Eijnden, R.J.J.M., Spijkerman, R. and Engels, R.C.M.E. (2006) Relative contribution of smoker prototypes in predicting smoking among adolescents: a comparison with factors from the theory of planned behavior, *European Addiction Research*, 12, 113–20.

Van Lettow, B., Vermunt, J.K., de Vries, H., Burdorf, A. and Van Empelen, P. (2013) Clustering of drinker prototype characteristics: what characterizes the typical drinker? *British Journal of Psychology*, 104 (3), 382–99.

Van Lettow, B., de Vries, H., Burdorf, A., & van Empelen, P. (in press) Quantifying the strength of the associations of prototype perceptions with behaviour, behavioural willingness and intentions: a meta-analysis (in press). *Health Psychology Review*.

Wagner, D.D., Dal Cin, S., Sargent, J.D., Kelley, W.M. and Heatherton, T.F. (2011) Spontaneous action representation in smokers when watching movie characters smoke, *Journal of Neuroscience*, 31 (3), 894–8.

Walsh, L.A. and Stock, M.L. (2012) UV photography, masculinity, and college men's sun protection cognitions, *Journal of Behavioral Medicine*, 35 (4), 431–42.

Walsh, L.A., Stock, M.L., Peterson, L.M. and Gerrard, M. (2014) Women's sun protection cognitions in response to UV photography: the role of age, cognition, and affect, *Journal of Behavioral Medicine*, 37 (3), 553–63.

Warshaw, P.R. and Davis, F.D. (1984) Self-understanding and the accuracy of behavioral expectations, *Personality and Social Psychology Bulletin*, 10, 111–18.

Webb, T.L. and Sheeran, P. (2006) Does changing behavioral intentions engender behavior change? A meta-analysis of the experimental evidence, *Psychological Bulletin*, 132 (2), 249–68.

Weinstein, N.D. (1980) Unrealistic optimism about future life events, *Journal of Personality and Social Psychology*, 39 (5), 806–20.

Weinstein, N.D. (1982) Unrealistic optimism about susceptibility to health problems, *Journal of Behavioral Medicine*, 5, 441–60.

Weinstein, N.D. (1988) The precaution adoption process, *Health Psychology*, 7 (4), 355–86.

Werch, C.E. and Owen, D.M. (2002) Iatrogenic effects of alcohol and drug prevention programs, *Journal of Studies on Alcohol and Drugs*, 63 (5), 581.

Werch, C.E.C., Bian, H., Moore, M. J., Ames, S., DiClemente, C.C. and Weiler, R.M. (2007) Brief multiple behavior interventions in a college student health care clinic, *Journal of Adolescent Health*, 41 (6), 577–85.

Williams, K.D., Yeager, D.S., Cheung, C.K. and Choi, W. (2012) *Cyberball 4.0* [software].

Wills, T.A., Bantum, E.O.C., Pokhrel, P., Maddock, J.E., Ainette, M.G., Morehouse, E. *et al.* (2013) A dual-process model of early substance use: tests in two diverse populations of adolescents, *Health Psychology*, 32 (5), 533.

Wills, T.A., Gibbons, F.X., Sargent, J.D., Gerrard, M., Lee, H.R. and Dal Cin, S. (2010) Good self-control moderates the effect of mass media on adolescent tobacco and alcohol use: tests with studies of children and adolescents, *Health Psychology*, 29 (5), 539–49.

Winter, L. (1988) The role of sexual self-concept in the use of contraceptives, *Family Planning Perspectives*, 20 (3), 123–7.

Zimmermann, F. and Sieverding, M. (2010) Young adults' social drinking as explained by an augmented theory of planned behaviour: the roles of prototypes, willingness, and gender, *British Journal of Health Psychology*, 15 (3), 561–81.

Zimmermann, F. and Sieverding, M. (2011) Young adults' images of abstaining and drinking: prototype dimensions, correlates and assessment methods, *Journal of Health Psychology*, 16 (3), 410–20.

Chapter 7

Social cognitive theory

Aleksandra Luszczynska and Ralf Schwarzer

1 General background

Social cognitive theory (SCT; Bandura 1986) has become a fundamental resource in clinical, educational, social, developmental, health, and personality psychology. It has been applied to such diverse areas as school achievement, emotional disorders, mental and physical health, career choice, and socio-political change. This chapter describes key constructs such as perceived self-efficacy and outcome expectancies, and it also refers to related constructs such as goals and socio-structural impediments and facilitators in the context of health behaviour change. Historically, SCT dates back to the 1970s when a paradigm shift took place from a focus on behaviour to a focus on cognitions. In 1977, Bandura published his landmark article on self-efficacy. In his 1986 book, *Social Foundations of Thought and Action: A Social Cognitive Theory* (see also Bandura 2000a, 2000b, 2001), he fully developed his social cognitive theory of human functioning, and this work has been crowned by *Self-Efficacy: The Exercise of Control* (Bandura 1997).

2 Description of the model

According to social cognitive theory, human motivation and action are extensively regulated by forethought. This anticipatory control mechanism involves expectations that might refer to outcomes of undertaking a specific action. The theory outlines a number of crucial factors that influence behaviour. The first factor is perceived self-efficacy, which is concerned with people's beliefs in their capabilities to perform a specific action required to attain a desired outcome. Outcome expectancies are the other core construct of SCT, which are concerned with people's beliefs about the possible consequences of their actions. In addition to these two cognitions, SCT also includes goals, perceived impediments and facilitators. These constructs are displayed in Figure 7.1, which illustrates their interplay throughout the behaviour change process.

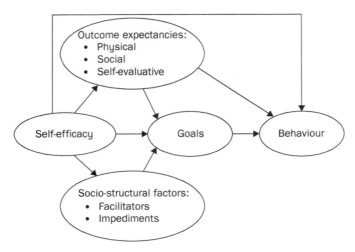

Figure 7.1 An illustration of social cognitive theory (Bandura 2000a)

2.1 Perceived self-efficacy

Perceived self-efficacy is concerned with individuals' beliefs in their capability to exercise control over challenging demands and their own functioning (Bandura 1997). In a unifying theory of behaviour change, Bandura hypothesized that expectations of self-efficacy are self-regulatory cognitions that determine whether instrumental actions will be initiated, how much effort will be expended, and how long it will be sustained in the face of obstacles and failures. Self-efficacy has an influence on preparing for action because self-related cognitions are a major ingredient in the motivation process. Self-efficacy levels can enhance or impede motivation and are also directly related to behaviour. Perceived self-efficacy represents the confidence that one can employ the skills necessary to resist temptation, cope with stress, and mobilize one's resources required to meet the situational demands. Self-efficacy beliefs affect the amount of effort to change risk behaviour and the persistence to continue striving in the face of barriers and setbacks that may undermine motivation. Self-efficacy is based on different sources (Bandura 1997). First, self-efficacy beliefs can be enhanced through personal accomplishment or mastery, as far as success is attributed internally and can be repeated. A second source is vicarious experience. When a 'model person' – that is, someone similar to the individual – successfully masters a difficult situation, social comparison processes can enhance self-efficacy beliefs. Third, verbal persuasion by others can also enhance self-efficacy beliefs (e.g. a health educator reassures a patient that she will definitely perform cancer screening properly due to her competence). The last source of influence is emotional arousal – that is, the person may experience no apprehension in a threatening situation, and as a result may feel capable of mastering the situation.

The four informational sources vary in strength and importance in the order presented here, with personal mastery being the strongest source of self-efficacy (see also Warner *et al.* 2011, 2014). Meta-analyses have examined sources of self-efficacy by comparing the effects of various intervention techniques upon self-efficacy for physical activity (Ashford *et al.* 2010; Williams and French 2011; French 2013). In particular, effective self-efficacy enhancement was observed in physical activity interventions that used vicarious experience, feedback referring to participant past performances or past performances of others (Ashford *et al.* 2010). Furthermore, such behaviour change techniques as 'action planning', 'providing an instruction', and 'reinforcing effort towards behaviour' were associated with significantly higher levels of both self-efficacy and physical activity (Williams and French 2011).

Self-efficacy is not the same as unrealistic optimism, as it is based on experience and does not lead to unreasonable risk-taking. Instead, it leads to venturesome behaviour that is within reach of one's capabilities. The essential distinction between self-efficacy and similar constructs such as self-esteem, self-concept, and sense of control has three aspects: (a) self-efficacy implies an internal attribution (a person is the cause of the action); (b) it is prospective, referring to future behaviours; and (c) it is an operative construct, which means that this cognition is proximal to the critical behaviour.

2.2 Outcome expectancies

While perceived self-efficacy refers to personal action control or agency, outcome expectancies pertain to the perception of possible consequences of one's action (Williams *et al.* 2005; Hankonen *et al.* 2013). Outcome expectancies can be organized along three dimensions: (a) area of consequences, (b) positive or negative consequences, and (c) short-term or long-term consequences. Areas of consequences can be split into three. *Physical outcome expectations*, such as expectations of discomfort or disease symptoms, refer to the anticipation of what will be experienced after behaviour change takes place. These include both the short- and long-term effects of behaviour change. For example, immediately after quitting smoking, an ex-smoker might observe a reduction of coughing (positive consequence) and a higher level of muscle tension (negative consequence). In the long run, an ex-smoker might expect lower susceptibility to respiratory infections (positive consequence) but an increased susceptibility to weight gain (negative consequence). *Social outcome expectancies* refer to anticipated social responses after behaviour change. Smokers might expect disapproval from friends who continue to smoke, or, positively, they might expect their family to congratulate them on quitting smoking. In the long run, ex-smokers might expect that they will increase their chances to find and maintain an attractive partner or a better job. *Self-evaluative outcome expectations* refer to the anticipation of affective experiences, such as being ashamed, being proud of oneself or satisfied, due to internal standards. This three-factor structure of outcome expectancies has received empirical support (see Dijkstra *et al.* 1997).

Expectancies about outcomes of personal actions and self-efficacy beliefs include the option to cope instrumentally with health threats by taking preventive action (Dijkstra *et al.* 1997). These action beliefs and personal resource beliefs reflect a functional optimism. Empirically, the distinction between them may be difficult to confirm because they often operate in tandem. In making judgements about health-related goals, people often unite personal agency with appropriate means. Perceived self-efficacy may include outcome expectancies because individuals believe that they can produce the responses necessary for desired outcomes. It might also be argued that outcome expectancies, or judgements about what will happen if an individual performs a certain action, assume that the person might be able to perform the action leading to these results. On the other hand, outcome expectancies and self-efficacy beliefs may diverge in certain situations. For example, many smokers may believe that quitting would lead to positive health outcomes, but at the same time do not feel confident in their ability to quit.

Both outcome expectancies and self-efficacy beliefs play influential roles in adopting new health behaviours, eliminating detrimental habits, and maintaining what has been achieved. These constructs are seen as direct predictors of behaviours. They also operate through indirect pathways, affecting goal setting and the perception of socio-structural factors.

2.3 Goals, socio-structural factors, and their relations to self-efficacy

In adopting a desired behaviour, individuals first form a *goal* and then attempt to execute the action. Goals serve as self-incentives and guides to health behaviours. According to SCT, a distinction can be made between distal goals and proximal goals. The latter regulate the amount of invested effort and guide action. Intentions, as defined in other social cognitive theories, are more similar to proximal goals than to distal goals (Bandura 1997). Terms such as 'I intend to' or 'I aim to' reflect goals. All major theories agree upon the proposition that goals or intentions should be as specific as possible in order to facilitate subsequent action (Bandura 1997; Gollwitzer 1999; Fishbein and Ajzen 2010), although the preferred terms differ between these theories. There is a continuum from distal to proximal goals, which have complementary regulative function, as well as a continuum from goal intentions to implementation intentions. Distal goals give purpose and general direction to actions, whereas proximal goals capture specific activities in the near future. In any case, goals (or intentions) are seen as key predictors of behaviour.

People would not set goals for themselves if they thought that the pursuit of such goals would have more disadvantages than advantages. Thus, outcome expectancies are seen as important determinants in the initial formation of intentions, but may be less important in the later phases of behaviour change. Self-efficacy, on the other hand, remains crucial, especially after the formation of an intention to adopt health behaviour when the task is to translate the intention into action and to self-regulate the goal pursuit process. According to SCT, forming a goal is a necessary but not sufficient condition; it is a precondition but does not ensure that an individual will actually pursue the goal (Bandura 2000a, 2000b).

Self-efficacy beliefs affect behaviours indirectly through their impact on goals. Self-efficacy, among other factors, influences what challenges people decide to meet and how high they set their goals. Persons with high self-efficacy in a specific domain select more challenging and ambitious goals. Optimistic self-beliefs about one's capability to exert control over one's actions influence how people respond to discrepancies between their personal goals and their performance. Compared with people with low optimistic self-beliefs, self-efficacious individuals invest more effort when the discrepancies are larger (see DeVellis and DeVellis 2000). High self-efficacy not only improves goal-setting, but leads to more persistence in pursuing the goal. Self-efficacy also promotes the effective use of cognitive resources, diagnosing and searching for solutions when obstacles arise (Maddux and Lewis 1995).

Goal-setting also depends on perceived socio-structural factors. These factors refer to the impediments (barriers) or opportunities that reside in living conditions, and health, political, economic or environmental systems (Bandura 1997). Optimistic self-beliefs about one's efficacy also control how people perceive opportunities and impediments. Self-efficacy influences whether individuals pay attention to opportunities or barriers in their life circumstances. Self-efficacious individuals who, for example, intend to exercise might focus on cues in their environment, such as hiking paths and cycling routes. Those who are less confident about their physical competence might focus instead on the lack of a gym in their neighbourhood. People with strong self-efficacy recognize that they are able to overcome obstacles, and focus on opportunities. They believe that they are able to exercise control, even if the environment provides constraints rather than opportunities (see Bandura 1997, 2000a, 2000b).

3 Summary of research

Many studies have included self-efficacy, outcome expectancies, goals, and impediments to assess their impact on the initiation and performance of health-related practices. But most of the research that claims to test SCT assesses only self-efficacy and outcome expectancies. There are also studies that merge SCT with other approaches, such as the transtheoretical model (TTM; Prochaska and DiClemente, 1983) or the theory of planned behaviour (TPB; Ajzen, 2002).

Table 7.1 provides details of a number of studies that have tested SCT components as predictors of health behaviours. Some authors seem to believe that SCT is equivalent to self-efficacy theory (SET), provoking repeated statements by Bandura (1997) that SCT is not a 'one-factor theory'. There are hundreds of studies that include perceived self-efficacy, but in the present context, we focus on some typical studies that shed light on the particular function that self-efficacy may have in predicting health behaviour change in combination with other SCT constructs.

3.1 Adherence to medication and rehabilitation

Adherence to medication requirements or suggested treatment is related to self-regulatory beliefs. Self-efficacy is related to adherence to treatments for different chronic health problems. Clark and Dodge (1999) reported that taking medicine as prescribed, getting adequate exercise, managing stress, and following a recommended diet were explained by self-efficacy beliefs measured 4 and 12 months earlier. Optimistic self-beliefs have also been shown to mediate the relation between emotional distress and adherence to a medical regimen and glycemic control in patients with diabetes (Stewart *et al.* 2003). Self-efficacy has been found to be associated with patients' compliance with blood glucose testing, diet, and exercise (Williams and Bond 2002). Patients with the highest rates of glucose testing were found to have high self-efficacy and high outcome expectancies. Those with high outcome expectancies, but low self-efficacy, did not have blood tests performed as often as recommended. Additionally, perceived family support was associated with diabetic self-care. However, when the effects of self-efficacy were controlled, social support no longer predicted compliance. Furthermore, compared with outcome expectancies and locus of control, self-efficacy is the strongest correlate of objectively measured adherence to diabetes regimens, indicated by levels of HbA1c (O'Hea *et al.* 2009). Randomized controlled trials conducted among patients with type 2 diabetes showed that interventions targeting self-efficacy through vicarious experience result in favourable changes in blood glucose control at follow-up (Campbell *et al.* 2013). Brief interventions targeting self-efficacy to adhere to continuous positive airway pressure (CPAP) treatment among patients with obstructive sleep apnoea resulted in significant changes in self-efficacy beliefs, a fourfold increase in the use of CPAP treatment, and a reduction of daytime sleepiness at two-month follow-up (Lai *et al.* 2014).

New treatments for HIV can improve immune status and decrease mortality, but nearly one-third of patients miss medication doses every five days (see Catz *et al.* 2000). This poor compliance

Table 7.1 Illustrative applications of social cognitive theory

Behaviours	SCT predictors	References
Adherence to medication and rehabilitation	Self-efficacy	Catz et al. (2000), Bosse et al. (2002)
	Self-efficacy, outcome expectancies	Williams and Bond (2002), O'Hea et al. (2009), Fleig et al. (2011)
Sexual risk behaviours	Self-efficacy	Trobst et al. (2002), Reid and Aiken (2011), Newcomb and Mustanski (2014)
	Self-efficacy, outcome expectancies	Dilorio et al. (2000a, 2000b, 2001), Semple et al. (2000)
Physical exercise	Self-efficacy	Strauss et al. (2001), Rodgers et al. (2009, 2013), Maddison et al. (2014)
	Self-efficacy, outcome expectancies	Rovniak et al. (2002)
	Self-efficacy, perceived impediments	Booth et al. (2000)
	Self-efficacy, outcome expectancies, goals, perceived facilitators	Dewar et al. (2013)
	Self-efficacy, environmental factors	Vorhees et al. (2011)
Nutrition and weight control	Self-efficacy	Savoca and Miller (2001), Dearden et al. (2002), Pinto et al. (2002b), Luszczynska and Haynes (2009), Ochsner et al. (2013)
	Self-efficacy, outcome expectancies	Anderson et al. (2000), Resnicow et al. (2000), Godinho et al. (2014)
	Self-efficacy, goals	Schnoll and Zimmerman (2001), Luszczynska et al. (2010)
	Self-efficacy, perceived impediments and facilitators	Van Duyn et al. (2001), King et al. (2010)
	Self-efficacy, goals, perceived facilitators	Szczepanska et al. (2013)
Detection behaviours	Self-efficacy	Luszczynska and Schwarzer (2003), Friedman et al. (2014)
	Self-efficacy, outcome expectancies	Kremers et al. (2000), Umeh and Rogan-Gibson (2001), Cormier et al. (2002), Schnoll et al. (2002), Luszczynska et al. (2012)
Addictive behaviours	Self-efficacy	Dijkstra and De Vries (2000), Shiffman et al. (2000), Christiansen et al. (2002), Gwaltney et al. (2002), Rosenberg et al. (2011), Mee (2014), Smit et al. (2014)
	Self-efficacy, outcome expectancies	Cohen and Fromme (2002), Willems et al. (2013)

may result partly from patients' experience of adverse side-effects, but it may also be due to a lack of self-regulatory skills. Studies on adherence in highly active antiretroviral therapy (HAART) provide consistent findings on the predictors of medication adherence. Non-compliance is known to be related to the complexity and adverse side-effects of treatment. Considering psychosocial factors, it is also related to lack of social support and lack of self-efficacy (Catz et al. 2000). Systematic reviews seeking the strongest predictors and correlates of adherence to combination antiretroviral therapy (cART) for people living with HIV indicated that adherence self-efficacy was the strongest predictor of adherence (*SMD* = 0.60; Langebeek *et al.* 2014). The associations between other correlates (e.g. concerns about cART, beliefs about the utility of cART, social support, and current substance use) and adherence were weaker (*SMD* < 0.40).

Recovery from disease or adaptation after surgery may be influenced by self-regulatory beliefs, such as self-efficacy. Longitudinal research showed that post-operative self-efficacy was predictive of recovery outcomes in osteoarthritis patients undergoing joint replacement (Magklara *et al.* 2014). Pre-operative self-efficacy, however, was not related to patients' recovery. Post-rehabilitation telephone support was found to promote physical activity maintenance by fostering physical-activity-specific self-efficacy beliefs among cardiac and orthopaedic rehabilitation patients (Fleig *et al.* 2013). Moreover, patients' confidence in their ability to resume life activities after severe injury followed by an amputation of a limb was among the most powerful psychosocial predictors of post-surgical adaptation. A study on patients after amputation or reconstruction of a leg showed that their recovery and adaptation two years after surgery was predicted not only by socio-economic status, but also by self-efficacy (Bosse *et al.* 2002). Woodgate and Brawley (2008) reviewed research on exercise and self-efficacy and concluded that most studies examined self-efficacy only during the intensive in-patient phase of cardiac rehabilitation, with little attention to long-term maintenance.

3.2 Sexual risk behaviours

Most of the studies on risky sexual behaviours have examined social cognitive predictors of condom use. Optimistic beliefs in one's capability to negotiate safer sex practices have emerged as the most important cognitive predictor of decreased odds of unprotected sex (cf. Newcomb and Mustanski 2014). Among women with casual partners, condom use at follow-up was best explained by self-efficacy, compared with other constructs from social cognitive theory, the theories of planned behaviour and reasoned action, and the information-motivation-behavioural skills model (Reid and Aiken 2011). Support for SCT has been provided in a study of sexually active college students (Dilorio *et al.* 2000a). Self-efficacy was directly related to condom use, but optimistic self-beliefs were also indirectly related to condom use, through the effect of self-efficacy on outcome expectancies. In line with theory, self-efficacy predicted emotional state (anxiety), but this state was unrelated to health protective behaviour. Among sexually active adolescents, those who expressed confidence in their ability to put on a condom and in being able to refuse intercourse with a sexual partner were more likely to use condoms consistently. In addition, holding favourable outcome expectancies, associated with condom use, predicted more protective behaviours (Dilorio *et al.* 2001). Recent systematic reviews have investigated the characteristics of sexual communication that may best explain adolescents' condom use (Widman *et al.* 2014). Communication referring to self-efficacy (compared with communication referring to fear/concerns or intentions to use condoms) was the strongest predictor of the use of condoms (Widman *et al.* 2014). Men with anonymous sexual partners have been found to have the lowest scores on self-efficacy and outcome expectancies regarding condom use, negotiation with their partners, and disclosure (see Semple *et al.* 2000). Unprotected anal intercourse was predicted by low outcome expectancies for safer sex negotiation. It was also related to low self-efficacy for condom use and for negotiation. Self-efficacy has also been found to discriminate high- and low-risk groups of drug addicts that differ in shared needle usage and sexual contacts (Trobst *et al.* 2002).

Outcome expectancies and self-efficacy might refer to the same area of skills necessary to achieve a specific goal. For example, regarding safe sexual behaviour, they might refer to communication skills. Self-efficacy includes the confidence in one's ability to communicate about safe sex practices, whereas expectancies may pertain to outcomes of safer sex communication. Both factors should be directly related to actual safe sex communication and practice (see Dilorio *et al.* 2000b). In a sample of students, communication self-efficacy was directly and indirectly (via expectancies about outcomes of communication) related to the frequency of talking about safe sex practices with a partner. Both social cognitive variables predicted actual condom use. These associations were stronger than the relation between safe sex communication and safe sex practice itself.

3.3 Physical exercise

Regular physical exercise depends on the optimistic self-belief of being able to perform the behaviour appropriately. Perceived self-efficacy has been found to be a major instigating force in forming intentions to exercise and in maintaining the practice for an extended period (Rovniak *et al.* 2002; Rodgers *et al.* 2009, 2013; Luszczynska *et al.* 2010; see also the review by Woodgate and Brawley 2008).

Studies using objective measures of physical activity, such as a motion detector/accelerometer monitoring physical activity over some period of time, have shown that self-efficacy is related to a high level of physical activity among 10- to 16-year-old adolescents (Strauss *et al.* 2001). Investigations testing the role of SCT components in the context of physical activity showed that only self-efficacy was directly associated with behaviour at 12-month follow-up, whereas outcome expectancies and social support were related to goals only indirectly, through self-efficacy (Dewar *et al.* 2013). Physical activity levels were estimated with accelerometers worn for seven days (Dewar *et al.* 2013). In a random sample of persons over 60 years, physical activity was found to be related to perceived environmental barriers (such as access to local facilities and finding footpaths for safe walking) and self-efficacy (see Booth *et al.* 2000).

Participation in regular physical activity has been identified as the key health behaviour in preventing chronic disease. Patients with ischaemic heart disease taking part in cardiac rehabilitation programmes who received a mobile phone and internet intervention aiming at an increase of self-efficacy and physical activity engaged in more frequent leisure-time physical activity at 24-week follow-up (Maddison *et al.* 2014). Importantly, the association between participation in the intervention (compared with taking part in a control group) and changes in physical activity were mediated by changes in self-efficacy levels (Maddison *et al.* 2014). In an intervention with older adults, an increase in beliefs about the ability to overcome barriers led to increased adherence to physical activity up to 12 months (Brassington *et al.* 2002).

A few studies have compared the predictive power of constructs derived from different theories. Dzewaltowski (1989) compared the predictive utility of the theory of reasoned action (TRA; for an overview, see Fishbein and Ajzen 2010) and SCT in the field of exercise motivation. The exercise behaviour of 328 students was recorded for seven weeks and then related to prior measures of different cognitive factors. Overall, the TRA variables did not account for any unique variance in exercise behaviour after controlling for self-efficacy, outcome expectations, and satisfaction with physical activity and its outcomes. Other studies using constructs from different theories also show that the effects of self-efficacy on physical activity are stronger than those of other psychosocial determinants (see Rovniak *et al.* 2002).

3.4 Nutrition and weight control

Aspects of diet and weight control can also be governed by self-efficacy beliefs (Luszczynska and Haynes 2009; Ochsner *et al.* 2013). In the context of weight control, it has been found that self-efficacy operates best in concert with general lifestyle changes, including physical exercise and the provision of social support. In relation to diet, nationally representative surveys of US adults on daily food intake have shown that self-efficacy is among the factors most consistently and strongly associated with higher consumption of fruit and vegetables (see Van Duyn *et al.* 2001). Nutrition self-efficacy was a proximal predictor of fruit and vegetable intake measured at one-year follow-up among adolescents who reduced their body weight (from overweight/ obese to normal range) (Sczepanska *et al.* 2013). In turn, goal intentions and facilitating factors (such as social support and availability of fruit and vegetables at home) were indirectly related to behaviour at one-year follow-up (Szczepanska *et al.* 2013). Self-efficacy has been shown to be a significant predictor of physical, social, and self-evaluative outcome expectancies regarding healthy nutrition (Anderson *et al.* 2000; Williams *et al.* 2005; Godinho *et al.* 2013; Hankonen *et al.* 2013). A study using an objective measure of nutrition behaviour, namely grocery receipts, demonstrated that the effect of self-efficacy on fat, fibre, fruit and vegetable intake was mediated by physical outcome expectations. Nutrition goal-setting was linked to higher dietary fibre self-efficacy and actual fibre intake. Compared with students who did not set a nutrition goal, goal-setters scored 15% higher in optimistic self-beliefs on dietary fibre intake and reported a 91% higher consumption of fibre (see Schnoll and Zimmerman 2001). In a similar study, self-efficacy to eat more fruit and vegetables as well outcome expectancies in terms of fruit and vegetable intake predicted a 24-hour recall of actual fruit and vegetables intake (Resnicow *et al.* 2000). Additionally, these fruit- and vegetable-specific predictors were inversely related to an unhealthy diet (i.e. high-fat cooking).

Studies predicting nutrition in patients with chronic or terminal diseases usually provide support for SCT. Besides knowledge about proper nutrition, dietary self-efficacy and perceived spousal support were associated with dietary behaviours among type 2 diabetes patients (Savoca and Miller 2001). Diabetes-related self-efficacy was strongly related to maintenance of diabetes self-care (diet, exercise, and glucose testing; see Bond 2002). The most powerful effects were observed when strong optimistic self-beliefs were combined with strong beliefs about outcomes (Bond 2002). Nutrition and exercise self-efficacy were also connected to the maintenance of diet and physical activity in breast cancer patients (Pinto *et al.* 2002b).

Self-efficacy has also been found to be a significant determinant of caregiver behaviour. Self-efficacious caregivers supplied their 6- to 18-month-old children with healthy foods and washed their children's hands more often (see Dearden *et al.* 2002). Improving medical students' knowledge as well as their nutrition self-efficacy might translate into better professional practice in future physicians. When consulting cardiovascular patients, medical students with higher nutrition self-efficacy addressed the topic of preventive nutrition more frequently (see Carson *et al.* 2002).

3.5 Detection behaviours

The role of SCT has also been analysed in the context of symptom detection behaviours. Research has employed breast self-examination (BSE) and cervical cancer screening as examples of detective health behaviour. Women with high confidence in their capability to perform BSE are more likely to engage in regular self-examination (Luszczynska and Schwarzer 2003).

Positive and negative outcome expectancies also influence intentions; perceived benefits and barriers of engaging in BSE have been found to predict intentions as well as concurrent BSE behaviour (Umeh and Rogan-Gibson 2001). Some studies have provided evidence that both outcome expectancies and perceived self-efficacy are the best joint predictors of engaging in regular cervical cancer screening (Luszczynska *et al.* 2012).

Research involving high-risk populations also provides support for SCT. A study on first-degree relatives of prostate cancer patients supports the role of self-efficacy for screening behaviours. Physician recommendation, knowledge, and risk estimation were only poor predictors, whereas self-efficacy beliefs and positive outcome expectancies were more closely linked to prostate cancer screening (Cormier *et al.* 2002). In another study of 50- to 60-year-old patients, participation in endoscopic colorectal cancer screening was examined. Self-efficacy, followed by individuals' beliefs about the outcome of participation, discriminated between those who participated in the screening and those who did not (Kremers *et al.* 2000). High self-efficacy regarding scheduling, preparation, and post-screening recovery was a key predictor of objectively measured participation in screening colonoscopy among patients suffering from inflammatory bowel disease (Friedman *et al.* 2014).

Cancer screening might be a first step on the way to change everyday health behaviours. However, people who enrol in a single cancer screening (e.g. lung cancer) do not necessarily have high self-efficacy regarding behaviours related to this cancer (e.g. regular screening, quitting smoking). Women who smoked heavily were asked to participate in lung cancer screening that involved sputum cytology, chest X-ray, bronchoscopy, and spiral computer tomography (Schnoll *et al.* 2002). Almost two-thirds of those who participated in screening were classified as having low self-efficacy regarding smoking cessation. A minority of the women (25%) reported high levels of negative outcome expectancies of quitting smoking, although most of them (76%) reported high positive outcome expectancies of quitting. Finally, only a very few women actually quit smoking after consultation with an oncologist. Despite relatively high expectations about quitting smoking, the participants were unable to change their smoking habits. Persons who undergo cancer screening and are probably aware of the high risk of the disease might still be unable to change their risk behaviours, because they possess low optimistic self-beliefs.

3.6 Addictive behaviours

Optimistic self-beliefs influence the process of changing addictive behaviours. Confidence to overcome barriers can predict quitting smoking attempts (Dijkstra and DeVries 2000). Nicotine abstinence of self-quitters depends on various demographic, physiological, cognitive, and social factors, but only a few factors are common predictors of maintaining abstinence. These include physiological factors such as lower nicotine dependence and longer duration of previous abstinence, and cognitive factors such as high perceived self-efficacy (see Ockene *et al.* 2000). Although intention to quit may play a role in changes of smoking behaviour, self-efficacy is the most potent predictor of successful quitting attempts (Smit *et al.* 2014). Self-efficacy measured during preparation to quit smoking discriminated between quitters, relapsers, and persistent smokers at six-week follow-up (Smit *et al.* 2014).

Various researchers have verified relationships between perceived self-efficacy and outcome expectancies in the context of addictive behaviors. Low levels of self-efficacy regarding smoking cessation were characteristic of smokers who used evidence-based smoking cessation aids (SCA; Willems *et al.* 2013). Self-efficacy regarding smoking cessation was negatively related with intention to use SCA, whereas expecting positive outcomes after the use of SCA was positively related to intention to use SCA (Willems *et al.* 2013). In a longitudinal study on substance use in young adults, Cohen and Fromme (2002) showed that self-efficacy, together with positive and negative outcome expectancies, predicted alcohol, marijuana, and other drug use, all measured at the same wave of data collection. Self-efficacy was also related to both positive and negative outcome expectancies. However, the SCT constructs did not predict behaviour measured one year later; the only significant determinant of substance use frequency was past behaviour measured one year earlier (Cohen and Fromme 2002). The minor role of negative outcome expectancies for behaviour change has been shown in cross-sectional studies on alcohol consumption. Heavily drinking students who drank alone expected more negative drinking consequences of reducing alcohol consumption than those who drank heavily in a social context or who did not drink heavily. Those who were most likely to develop alcohol dependence had the highest negative outcome expectancies. Again, the crucial role of self-efficacy was confirmed: heavy drinkers had lower self-efficacy than those who drank less or who drank only in social situations (Christiansen *et al.* 2002).

Confidence in one's ability to abstain from smoking might refer to particular environmental or affective contexts, such as feelings of irritation or sadness, socializing with smokers, or being in a bar or a restaurant. Gwaltney *et al.* (2002) found that lapse episodes within a four-week abstinence period were predicted by abstinence self-efficacy. Abstinence self-efficacy differentiated between the temptation episodes in which the former smoker was able to resist smoking and situations that resulted in lapses. In a study on lapses and relapses of smokers who attempted to quit, self-efficacy was measured daily to determine whether changes in optimistic self-beliefs precede lapses during the 25 days after quitting smoking (Shiffman *et al.* 2000). On days when both groups were abstinent, persons who never lapsed during the monitoring period reported higher daily self-efficacy than those who lapsed. Daily average self-efficacy over the lapse-to-relapse interval was lower among persons who relapsed than daily average post-lapse self-efficacy among those who did not. Self-efficacy after the lapse significantly predicted subsequent behaviour. Laboratory studies have revealed that efficacy beliefs about resisting smoking along with the affective response in a stressful social situation are associated with smoking urges (Niaura *et al.* 2002).

4 Developments

Over the years, the notion of self-efficacy has become so appealing to health psychologists that it has been incorporated into most health behaviour theories. Becker and Rosenstock (1987) integrated it into their health belief model, mainly by reinterpreting what used to be 'barriers' to action. Ajzen (1991) extended the theory of reasoned action to the theory of planned behaviour by adding a predictor labelled 'perceived behavioural control', which is seen to be synonymous with self-efficacy. In contrast, his long-time co-author Fishbein (2001) has simply incorporated self-efficacy (in the same sense as Bandura) into his own revision of their theory of reasoned action. In the context of US nationwide attempts to prevent HIV infections by promoting condom use, the leading health behaviour theorists, including Bandura and Fishbein, were asked to develop an integrated framework to guide research on this topic, which has then been called the 'integrated behaviour model' (IBM; Fishbein and Ajzen 2010). Along with attitude and perceived norm variables, the IBM includes two personal agency variables, self-efficacy and perceived control, which operate independently and are direct predictors of intention to perform the behaviour.

Self-efficacy has been also included in protection motivation theory (see Maddux and Lewis 1995). The theory most similar to SCT is the health action process approach (HAPA), with an elaboration of the goal pursuit phase (Schwarzer 2008). The HAPA includes self-efficacy, outcome expectancies, and intentions but has been designed to acknowledge in particular post-intentional processes. Thus, self-efficacy, planning, and action control are specified as more proximal predictors of actual behaviours to account for the initiation as well as maintenance of action (see Schwarzer and Luszczynska, Chapter 8 this volume).

These models and theories are described in more detail in other chapters of this book. Thus, 'self-efficacy models' are no longer really distinct from other approaches because the key construct that was originally developed within Bandura's social cognitive theory has subsequently proven to be an essential component of all major models.

4.1 Phase-specific self-efficacy

Owing to its popularity and unquestionable effects on human behaviour, researchers have proposed some further theoretical developments of the self-efficacy construct. Bandura (1997) suggested that self-efficacy should always refer to the particular task or specific behaviour that is being predicted. Other researchers suggest that it should be tailored to particular stages of behaviour change. Behaviour change can be described as a competent self-regulation process in which individuals monitor their responses to taxing situations, observe similar others facing similar demands, appraise their coping resources, create optimistic self-beliefs, plan a course of action, perform the critical action, and evaluate its outcome. Endorsing a process approach to behaviour change, Marlatt *et al.* (1995) proposed five categories of self-efficacy for corresponding phases of prevention (resistance and harm-reduction self-efficacy) and motivation development (action, coping, and recovery self-efficacy).

Resistance self-efficacy refers to the confidence in one's ability to avoid any substance use in the first place, which pertains to primary prevention. This implies resisting peer pressure to smoke, drink or take drugs. Young people who have low smoking resistance self-efficacy are more likely to engage in smoking behaviour (Mee 2014). Once a risk behaviour has been engaged in, the notion of resistance loses its significance. It is then of more importance to control further damage and to strengthen the belief that one is capable of minimizing the risk. *Harm-reduction self-efficacy* refers to one's confidence in being able to reduce the risk behaviour after having become involved with tobacco or drugs, which pertains to secondary prevention. This is particularly useful because most adolescents at least experiment with cigarettes and alcohol, which can be regarded as a normal stage in puberty when youngsters face developmental tasks, including self-regulation in tempting situations. Thus, the question is, how can a drug be curiously explored without becoming a gateway drug? The answer lies in the notion of harm-reduction self-efficacy. The individual must acquire not only the appropriate skills, but also the optimistic belief in control of the impending risk. High-drinking episodes occur less frequently among young people who have strong self-efficacy beliefs about their ability to employ harm reduction strategies, such as staying close by a trusted friend (Rosenberg *et al.* 2011).

The above two types of self-efficacy are related to prevention, whereas the following three are related to motivation development. This distinction, proposed by Marlatt *et al.* (1995), has been further developed to specify self-efficacy beliefs that are typical for particular phases of behaviour change (see Schwarzer and Luszczynska, Chapter 8 this volume). People initiate behaviour change when a critical situation arises. This requires that they firmly believe that they are capable of performing the action. *Pre-action self-efficacy* is an optimistic belief whereby an individual develops an intention to change. Coping self-efficacy or *maintenance self-efficacy* describes optimistic beliefs about one's capability to deal with barriers that arise during the maintenance period (see also Schwarzer and Renner 2000; Luszczynska and Sutton 2006; Higgins *et al.* 2014). *Recovery self-efficacy* pertains to one's conviction to get back on track after being derailed. The person trusts his or her competence to regain control after a setback or failure. Recovery self-efficacy is most functional when it comes to resuming an interrupted chain of action, whereas pre-action self-efficacy is most functional when facing a novel challenging demand (Scholz *et al.* 2005; Luszczynska *et al.* 2007a; Ochsner *et al.* 2013)

4.2 Affective outcome expectancies

Williams *et al.* (2005) have reviewed the role of outcome expectancies in physical activity, while the role of outcome expectancies in smoking (intention to quit smoking and quitting smoking) has been investigated extensively by Dijkstra *et al.* (1999). These authors emphasized the importance of self-evaluative outcome expectations – that is, being ashamed, current feelings of regret, being satisfied in the case of quitting, and regretting smoking if illness due to smoking was to occur. The stronger the self-evaluative outcome expectations, the greater the chances to quit smoking. Affective outcome expectancies may be the more salient ones when it comes to intention formation (Conner *et al.* 2011; Gellert *et al.* 2012). For example, emotional outcome expectancies may refer to anticipated regret ('If I do not use a condom tonight, then I will regret it tomorrow').

4.3 Environmental factors and predictors of cognitions

Besides self-efficacy and outcome expectancies, other more peripheral constructs of SCT have caught the attention of researchers. The theory includes a general hypothesis of reciprocity between the individual's cognitions, environment, and behaviour. Socio-structural factors, such as economic and educational conditions and socio-economic status, affect behaviours through their impact on people's cognitions (Bandura 1986). Most studies on health behaviours target the relations between cognitions and behaviour but there is also emerging interest in environmental factors (see Sallis *et al.* 2000; Dzewaltowski *et al.* 2002b). Environmental variables might influence psychosocial processes and subsequent behaviours. It has been suggested that there are four environmental factors that might affect health behaviours and cognitions: (a) feelings of connection between people in the environment; (b) feelings of autonomy in the environment that support taking control over one's own actions; (c) skill-building opportunities in the environment; and (d) healthy norms that refer to group norms in the environment, suggesting that a health behaviour is a normative one (see Dzewaltowski *et al.* 2002a, 2002b). These characteristics of the environment might be developed through influencing the behaviours and cognitions of leaders, educators or caregivers. The behaviours of educators or caregivers might, in turn,

Table 7.2 Components of social cognitive theory: examples of questionnaire items

Variable	Example question	Response scale
Self-efficacy: behaviour-specific	'I can use condoms even if I would have to negotiate it with my partner'	'Completely false' to 'Completely true' 1 – 2 – 3 – 4
Phase-specific self-efficacy: pre-action	'I can use condoms even if I have to develop a precise plan how to negotiate it with my partner'	
Phase-specific self-efficacy: maintenance	'I can use condoms even if I have to negotiate with my partner'	
Phase-specific self-efficacy: recovery	'I can return to using condoms even if I failed a few times to use it as planned'	
Outcome expectancies: physical	'If I use condoms I would avoid health problems (such as chlamydia)'	'Completely false' to 'Completely true' 1 – 2 – 3 – 4
Outcome expectancies: social	'If I use condoms my partner might be happy that I take care of him/her'	
Outcome expectancies: self-evaluative	'If I use condoms I would be proud of myself'	
Goals	'Starting tomorrow, I intend to use condoms during sexual intercourse'	'Completely false' to 'Completely true' 1 – 2 – 3 – 4
Socio-structural factors: impediments	'In my country, high-quality condoms are expensive'	'Completely false' to 'Completely true' 1 – 2 – 3 – 4
Socio-structural factors: facilitators	'In my town, one can easily buy condoms in public restrooms, drugstores or chemists'	

influence the cognitions and behaviours of their students or patients. When explaining physical activity, self-efficacy perceptions may operate in concert with the built environment and land use. For example, land use and neighbourhood accessibility of physical activity facilities predicted self-efficacy, which in turn was related to walking behaviour among urban adolescents (Voorhees *et al.* 2011).

5 Operationalization of the model

This section presents some general rules that researchers can use to develop their own measures of SCT constructs that pertain to their particular research context. All components of SCT are usually measured in a behaviour-specific way. Table 7.2 displays examples of the operationalization of the main SCT constructs. For brevity, we refer to one behaviour only: condom use.

5.1 Socio-cultural impediments and facilitators

To ensure a complete understanding of constructs, operational definitions are needed. In the area of socio-cultural impediments and facilitators, this remains a difficult task because a very broad range of possible factors might be of interest in studies based on SCT, including social support, social integration, ethnic group membership, education, knowledge, intelligence, affluence or poverty, and so on.

5.2 Goals

The definition of goals is easier since this is the same as the one for intentions. Typically, 5- or 7-point scales are used that have the structure 'I intend to do X within the next week (day, month, etc.)'. In line with other theories, the level of specificity is adjustable. One could say 'I intend to eat five portions of vegetables per day, starting tomorrow', or one could say 'I intend to eat a healthy diet in the near future'. Both are intentions or goals, varying in the level of specificity. It has to be noted that cognitions and behaviour should be measured at the same level of specificity to increase the prediction of behaviour (Fishbein and Ajzen 2010). Bandura (1997) mentions a continuum from proximal to distal goals. A distal goal could be something like a new year's resolution such as 'I intend to improve my diet over the course of next year', whereas a proximal one could be 'I intend to resist my temptation to consume unhealthy snacks today'. It is up to the researcher and the context of the study to select the most appropriate level. In any case, it is preferred to focus on behaviour instead of outcomes. Instead of 'to lose weight' (a distant goal), one may choose 'to eat less calorie-rich foods' (a proximal goal).

5.3 Self-efficacy

Self-efficacy should also be assessed in a behaviour-specific manner. For dietary self-efficacy, a typical wording might be: 'I am confident that I can... (perform an action), even if... (a barrier).' An example of a self-efficacy item is: 'I am confident that I can skip desserts even if my family continues to eat them in my presence'. This rule need not be applied rigidly, but might serve as a heuristic. (Bandura [2006] has written a comprehensive book chapter with detailed guidelines on the construction of various kinds of self-efficacy measures.)

As self-efficacy is the most often employed construct of the SCT, self-efficacy scales that are more or less adequate have been published for a wide range of health behaviours. Various psychometric instruments have been developed to assess self-efficacy for physical activities (see Motl *et al.* 2002; Rodgers *et al.* 2009). The scales are usually adjusted to the age and development of the respondents. For example, children are asked whether they would be physically active during their free time even if they could watch TV or play video games instead (see Motl *et al.* 2002).

Measures of self-efficacy for dietary behaviours address beliefs about the ability to perform a lifestyle change. These behaviours may be defined broadly (i.e. healthy food consumption) or more narrowly (i.e. fruit intake, salt avoidance, or consumption of high-fibre food). The measurement of dietary self-efficacy aims at statements that include control over the temptation to eat too much or to choose the wrong foods. Items can include particular foods, such as 'I am certain that I can eat five portions of fruits and vegetables per day', or can refer to self-regulatory efforts, such as 'I am confident that I can resist my craving for chocolate'. Some instruments target very specific components of nutrition, such as fat intake in specific populations. A scale to measure nutrition self-efficacy has been developed by Schwarzer and Renner (2000). The scale refers to barriers that arise while developing the motivation to initiate health behaviour change (e.g. 'How certain are you that you could overcome the following barriers?', 'I can manage to stick to healthful food, even if I have to rethink my entire way of nutrition'). The items also refer to the barriers that are specific for the maintenance period (e.g. 'I can manage to stick to healthful food, even if I do not receive a great deal of support from others when making my first attempts') (see also Godinho *et al.* 2014).

Compliance with a medical recommendation might refer to more than one health behaviour. Patients with diabetes or those having suffered a myocardial infarction are usually asked to comply with medication or to have blood glucose tests, but also to increase their physical activity and to change their diet. Therefore, self-efficacy scales that assess the ability to perform such behaviours in each regimen area have been developed (see Williams and Bond 2002).

5.4 Outcome expectancies

Outcome expectancies may also be assessed in a behaviour-specific manner. To simplify test construction, one can keep in mind that outcome expectancies are best worded with if–then statements. Thus, the semantic structure of outcome expectancies is: 'If…(a behaviour), then…(consequences)'. Measures of outcome expectancies may capture negative as well as positive consequences of action. For example, engaging in regular cervical cancer screening may result in feelings of embarrassment, but also in being glad that one takes control over one's own health (Luszczynska *et al.* 2012). In the study by Godinho *et al.* (2013), the positive outcome expectancy measure started with 'If I ate five portions of fruit and vegetables a day…' and was followed by four consequences that constitute the items of the scale: 'I would improve my health', 'I would feel satisfaction and pleasure', 'I would feel better', and 'I would prevent cardiovascular diseases'. In research on predictors of cervical cancer screening, the negative outcome expectancy measure started with 'If I took part in cervical cancer screening' and was followed by examples of consequences, such as 'I would feel embarrassed during the examination', 'I would feel discomfort', and 'I would find the examination unpleasant' (Luszczynska *et al.* 2012).

It is suggested to assess a variety of (a) barriers that might arise if an individual tries to change a behaviour, and (b) outcome expectancies, both positive and negative. Individuals face various social, personal, and environmental obstacles or barriers. For example, people have many reasons why they should quit smoking or why they find it better to continue. Therefore, questionnaire items should refer to multiple possible barriers and outcomes that are specific for a health behaviour.

A point of consideration is whether one wants to balance positive and negative outcome expectancies and whether to look at both sides of the coin: to behave and not to behave. The cognitions related to performing and not performing a behaviour may independently contribute to the prediction of intentions and behaviours (Richetin et al. 2011). Performing a behaviour and not performing a behaviour may have both positive and negative consequences.

6 Intervention studies

Hyde *et al.* (2008) conducted a systematic literature review on interventions to increase self-efficacy in the context of addiction behaviours. The majority of reviewed studies reported positive effects of interventions upon self-efficacy; those that assessed behaviour change reported a significant intervention effect (Hyde et al. 2008). Unfortunately, analyses showing that behaviour change is mediated by changes in self-efficacy are rarely reported (Hyde et al. 2008).

Systematic reviews of self-efficacy interventions suggest that their effects on physical activity may depend on the type of population and the techniques of self-efficacy enhancement. The effects of self-efficacy interventions on physical activity vary from small ($d = 0.14$; French et al. 2014) among older adults to moderate ($d = 0.50$) among obese adults (Olander et al. 2013). When interventions targeted community-dwelling adults aged 60 years or more, self-regulatory techniques such as setting behavioural goals, prompting self-monitoring of behaviour, and providing feedback on performance were associated with lower levels of both self-efficacy and physical activity (French et al. 2014). In contrast, a meta-analysis of the effects of interventions targeting physical activity in obese individuals showed that goal-setting, prompting self-monitoring, and providing feedback on performance were associated with higher levels of physical activity (Olander et al. 2013). Furthermore, prompting self-monitoring in obese adults was related to higher levels of self-efficacy.

Experimental studies on improving dietary self-efficacy as well as nutrition have been presented, for example, by Luszczynska et al. (2007b) and Kreausukon et al. (2012). Prestwich et al. (2014) conducted a meta-analysis on behaviour change techniques to improve dietary self-efficacy. Dietary self-efficacy was enhanced significantly by interventions that incorporated self-monitoring, provided performance feedback, prompted review of intentions, or provided contingent diet success rewards. The amount of intervention studies, in particular in the domains of physical exercise and dietary changes has become so large, that it is hard to summarize this research. For example, in 265 nutrition interventions published in the 1980s and 1990s, outcome expectancies or self-efficacy were used in about 90% of the studies: Contento et al. (2002) conclude from their review that changes in preferences or different attitudes seem to be of less importance than changes in self-efficacy or outcome expectancies. Changes in SCT constructs are more likely to produce changes in nutrition. Some examples of studies that report experimental manipulations of SCT constructs are displayed in Table 7.3.

Interventions might include strategies designed to increase participants' sense of mastery and ability to handle difficult situations that might arise during initiation or maintenance of a

Table 7.3 Examples of intervention studies that report experimental manipulations of specific SCT constructs

Behaviours	References
Adherence to medication and rehabilitation	Campbell et al. (2013), Lai et al. (2014)
Sexual risk behaviours	NIH (2001)
Physical exercise	Parent and Fortin (2000), Bock et al. (2001), Brassington et al. (2002), Dishman et al. (2004)
Nutrition and weight control	Carson et al. (2002), Baranowski et al. (2003), Luszczynska et al. (2007b), Kreausukon et al. (2012)
Detection behaviours	Luszczynska (2004)
Addictive behaviours	Dijkstra and De Vries (2000), Winkleby et al. (2001)
Oral self-care	Schwarzer et al. (2015)

health-enhancing behaviour. Another kind of treatment might be education about a behaviour and benefits of its adoption. Programmes based on SCT might lead to change in targeted theoretical outcomes, such as self-efficacy, outcome expectancies, or health behaviour change. In this section, we compare the effectiveness of interventions that use mastery experience and vicarious experience components. The short- and long-term effects of such interventions are then addressed.

6.1 Mastery and vicarious experience interventions enhancing SCT components

There are two main sources of perceived self-efficacy (see Bandura 1997; Warner *et al.* 2014). *Personal mastery experience*, such as practising a behaviour, is most effective for self-efficacy enhancement because it provides observable evidence for goal attainment. *Vicarious experience*, such as observing a model person who is able to perform a difficult behaviour, can also enhance self-efficacy.

Vicarious and mastery experience might be obtained by means of computerized interventions. For example, treatment of children might include multimedia games aimed at behaviour change. The education activities in the game might be designed to increase preferences for healthy behaviour, such as healthy food consumption (see Baranowski *et al.* 2003). Using multiple exposures, this approach has been found to increase mastery in asking for healthy foods at home and when eating out. It also increased skills for preparing healthy food by means of virtual recipes and virtual food preparation. A study on increased fruit and vegetable consumption showed that, compared with controls, pre-adolescents participating in such an intervention increased their consumption (see Baranowski *et al.* 2003).

Health behaviour change might be obtained by vicarious experience only, in which a person models a desirable health behaviour (example testimonial: 'I thought I could never quit smoking, but after I managed to stay away from cigarettes for one day, I realized that I am capable of doing better'). A study on patients after coronary artery bypass graft surgery showed that an intervention in which former patients exemplify the physically active lifestyles they lead after surgery can affect post-operative exercise (see Parent and Fortin 2000). Patients who received the intervention developed stronger self-efficacy than controls five days after surgery, and they reported more walking and stair climbing and a higher level of general activity. Four weeks after surgery, patients who participated in a modelling intervention reported a more active lifestyle.

Social cognitive theory identifies five components that might lead to the adoption of a health behaviour, especially risk reduction behaviour (Bandura 1997). These are: provision of information, mastery of self-protective skills, and self-efficacy for implementation of these skills, social competence, and social support for the adoption of precautious actions. Following these suggestions, Lawrence *et al.* (1997) developed an intervention that included HIV/AIDS education, teaching and rehearsing skills targeting social competence (negotiations with a partner, refusal), mastery of self-protective skills (condom application and increasing sterility of intravenous drug application), technical competence, generating a supportive climate among participants, and normalizing self-protective behaviours. The intervention targeted a high-risk population of incarcerated women, of whom approximately one-third were drug users, and almost a half were treated for sexually transmitted diseases. Most respondents reported a large number of lifetime sex partners. Incarcerated women had opportunities to meet their partners in private and to have sexual intercourse during their imprisonment. Women participating in the intervention reported higher self-efficacy and higher frequency of communication with their partners about condom use at follow-up. The participants also improved their condom application skills.

6.2 Short- and long-term effects of SCT-based interventions

Interventions designed to increase compliance with healthy nutrition, physical activity or cancer screening are not always successful in changing the long-term maintenance of a behaviour. Using SCT and the transtheoretical model, Pinto *et al.* (2002a) developed a fully automated counselling system, available by phone, aimed at promoting physical activity in sedentary adults. The intervention, available for six months, resulted in behaviour change during the availability of the counselling. Persons who received automatic information promoting moderate intensity of physical activity met more recommendations regarding activity than controls. They also reported significantly higher daily kilocalorie expenditure than controls, who received automatic information on nutrition. However, the results were not maintained six months after the first measurement. In a similar study, telephone-based exercise counselling was provided to sedentary older adults (Brassington *et al.* 2002). After 12 months of intervention, adherence to suggested physical activity increased. The increments in self-efficacy and fitness outcome expectancies were related to a more active lifestyle.

Individually tailored interventions based on SCT might affect behaviour more strongly and lead to better maintenance than non-tailored interventions. To increase physical activity, a typical treatment would aim to improve self-efficacy and address benefits and barriers to activity. In one study, self-help guidebooks, mailed three times to the participants, were tailored by targeting the deficiencies found in previous assessment responses in the participants' use of self-efficacy (see Bock *et al.* 2001). The respondents showed increased self-efficacy after the treatment and at six-month follow-up. Those who maintained physical activity at follow-up had higher self-efficacy beliefs at post-test and follow-up. Individuals who achieved the recommended levels of physical activity by the end of the intervention were more likely to maintain their physical activity level six months later.

Not all interventions lead to changes in the targeted health behaviours. Social cognitive constructs of a sense of community, self-efficacy, outcome expectancies, incentive value, policy control, and leadership competence guided a programme for students from low-income neighbourhoods. The intervention aimed to reduce alcohol and drug use. However, no decrease of alcohol consumption or use of tobacco and other psychoactive substances was observed after completion of the programme (Winkleby *et al.* 2001), even though the post-treatment measurement revealed increased levels of the social cognitive constructs. The lack of behaviour change might result from a lack of adjustment of the intervention to culture and developmental level. Other studies have demonstrated that culturally and developmentally tailored interventions based on SCT might bring short-term changes in behaviour. The changes might be not maintained, however. For example, treatment for reduction of HIV risk based on SCT, tailored for African-American pre-adolescents and young adolescents, affected condom use six months after the intervention. However, the rate of condom use decreased at 12-month follow up, and the differences became non-significant (see Stanton *et al.* 1996).

7 Future directions

The construct of perceived self-efficacy may be the most powerful single factor in predicting behaviour. However, self-efficacy is not the 'magic bullet' to solve all problems that can arise in health behaviour change. Also, peer pressure and social norms usually have predictive value, although some studies have found a negligible effect of perceived norms on nutrition behaviour and dieting (Field *et al.* 2001). Another determinant of behaviour, namely social support, also has potential as a resource factor. When people are encouraged to cope with a barrier ('I know that you are capable of overcoming this'), they may become persuaded to believe in their competence. Thus, support can raise self-efficacy, which has been studied under the term 'enabling effect' (Benight and Bandura 2004; Schwarzer and Knoll 2007). But the opposite causal direction is also possible: the 'support cultivation' effect. The degree to which social support operates, then, rests on one's self-efficacy to build, maintain, and mobilize social networks (Wills *et al.* 2000). Studies have included social support as an external resource factor in the social cognitive framework (Scholz *et al.* 2013; Ernsting *et al.* 2015).

An unresolved question regards the optimal degree of specificity of the self-efficacy construct. According to Bandura (1997), perceived self-efficacy should always be as situation-specific as possible. This specificity issue can even be further subdivided into a formal and a substantial facet. In a formal or temporal sense, Marlatt *et al.* (1995) conceptualized five kinds of self-efficacy that reflect different stages. In a substantial sense, one has to tailor the questions to the situation, such as smoking cessation or condom use. Although there is nothing wrong with more and more specificity, there still exist domain-specific and also general measures that can have considerable predictive value (Luszczynska *et al.* 2005). High specificity of self-efficacy enables the prediction of only a narrow range of behaviours such as dental flossing (Schwarzer *et al.* 2015). A general measure of self-efficacy provides the opportunity to assess self-efficacy in a parsimonious way, if the study deals with the adoption of a general lifestyle, general stress adaptation, well-being or overall compliance with a range of healthy practices.

Bandura (1997: 3) defines self-efficacy as 'belief in one's capabilities to organize and execute the courses of action'. Therefore, self-efficacy not only refers to beliefs about an individual's ability to execute a specific behaviour (e.g. 'I can eat healthy food'), but also to an individual's ability to regulate the behaviour change process (e.g. 'I can eat healthy food despite lack of support from my spouse'). Due to the continuous influence that self-efficacy has at different phases throughout this process, its measurement might be adjusted to the particular point in time when self-regulation is at stake, for example at the moment of initiation of healthy behaviour, at the moment of maintenance, or at the moment of recovery after a lapse (Ochsner *et al.* 2013). A fine-grained adjustment of the self-efficacy concept to various phases in the health behaviour change process might help to explain how and why individuals successfully adopt or maintain healthy lifestyles (see Schwarzer and Luszczynska, Chapter 8 this volume). Developing phase-specific self-efficacy skills by means of intervention could, for example, help to get those on their way who are still undecided about what to do. For them, enhancement of pre-action self-efficacy could be helpful. Therefore, future interventions should be tailored to the specific phase of the health behaviour change process.

Perceived self-efficacy should be somewhat overly optimistic to generate motivational energy but it should not exceed a certain limit where unrealistic optimism would lead to disappointment or harm. Many interventions have focused on risk communication to lower defensive optimism.

The idea is to allow people to understand how much they really are at risk, which should affect their behaviour (see Ruiter *et al.* 2001). Perception of risk or threat is usually seen as a facilitator for deciding to change a behaviour but mostly in the early stages of behaviour change – that is, when the motivation to change is developed (Renner and Schupp 2011). Therefore, treatments might combine different approaches, increasing both risk perception and self-efficacy, but they should be tailored to the advancement of the participants in the change process. If intention formation (developing the motivation) is the primary outcome of an intervention, then the treatment should aim at risk perception, outcome expectancies, and self-efficacy. If instead maintenance is to be analysed or promoted, self-efficacy (among others) is crucial for goal pursuit, whereas risk perception and outcome expectancies lose their importance.

In conclusion, a myriad of SCT-based research, published in last three decades, provides evidence for the validity of many of the SCT assumptions, across different populations, contexts, as well as study designs. In particular, self-efficacy emerges as a strong, proximal predictor of health behaviours. A further strength of SCT is its appeal to practitioners and policy-makers responsible for large-scale interventions. For example, SCT has been among the most frequently applied psychological theories in school-based obesity prevention (Safron *et al.* 2011). However, more systematic research evidence is needed to clarify and confirm the associations between *all* SCT components as well as to estimate their combined and synergistic effects on behaviour change and its maintenance.

References

Ajzen, I. (1991) The theory of planned behavior, *Organizational Behavior and Human Decision Processes*, 50, 179–211.

Ajzen, I. (2002) Perceived behavioral control, self-efficacy, locus of control, and the theory of planned behavior, *Journal of Applied Social Psychology*, 32, 665–83.

Anderson, E.S., Winett, R.A. and Wojcik, J.R. (2000) Social-cognitive determinants of nutrition behavior among supermarket food shoppers: a structural equation analysis, *Health Psychology*, 19, 479–86.

Ashford, S., Edmunds, J. and French, D.P. (2010) What is the best way to change self-efficacy to promote lifestyle and recreational physical activity? A systematic review with meta-analysis, *British Journal of Health Psychology*, 15, 265–88.

Bandura, A. (1977) Self-efficacy: toward a unifying theory of behavioral change, *Psychological Review*, 84, 191–215.

Bandura, A. (1986) *Social Foundations of Thought and Action: A Social Cognitive Theory*. Englewood Cliffs, NJ: Prentice-Hall.

Bandura, A. (1997) *Self-efficacy: The Exercise of Control*. New York: Freeman.

Bandura, A. (2000a) Cultivate self-efficacy for personal and organizational effectiveness, in E.A. Locke (ed.) *The Blackwell Handbook of Principles of Organizational Behavior* (pp. 120–36). Oxford: Blackwell.

Bandura, A. (2000b) Exercise of human agency through collective efficacy, *Current Directions of Psychological Science*, 9, 75–8.

Bandura, A. (2001) Social cognitive theory: an agentic perspective, *Annual Review of Psychology*, 52, 1–26.

Bandura, A. (2006) Guide for creating self-efficacy scales, in F. Pajares and T. Urdan (eds.) *Self-efficacy Beliefs of Adolescents* (pp. 307–38). Greenwich, CT: Information Age Publishing.

Baranowski, T., Baranowski, J., Cullen, K.W., Marsh, T., Islam, N., Zakerei, I. *et al.* (2003) Squire's Quest: dietary outcome evaluation of a multimedia game, *American Journal of Preventive Medicine*, 24, 52–61.

Becker, M.H. and Rosenstock, I.M. (1987) Comparing social learning theory and the health belief model, in W.B. Ward (ed.) *Advances in Health Education and Promotion* (Vol. 2, pp. 245–9). Greenwich, CT: JAI Press.

Benight, C.C. and Bandura, A. (2004) Social cognitive theory of posttraumatic recovery: the role of perceived self-efficacy, *Behaviour Research and Therapy*, 42, 1129–48.

Bock, B.C., Marcus, B.H., Pinto, B.M. and Forsyth, L.H. (2001) Maintenance of physical activity following an individualized motivationally tailored intervention, *Annals of Behavioral Medicine*, 23, 79–87.

Bond, M.J. (2002) The roles of self-efficacy, outcome expectancies and social support in the self-care behaviors of diabetics, *Psychology, Health and Medicine*, 7, 127–41.

Booth, M.L., Owen, N., Bauman, A., Clavisi, O. and Leslie, E. (2000) Social-cognitive and perceived environmental influences associated with physical activity in older Australians, *Preventive Medicine*, 31, 15–22.

Bosse, M.J., McKenzie, E.J., Kellam, J.F., Burgess, A.R., Webb, L.X., Swiontkowski, M.F. *et al.* (2002) An analysis of outcomes of reconstruction or amputation after leg-threatening injuries, *New England Journal of Medicine*, 347, 1924–31.

Brassington, G.S., Atienza, A.A., Perczek, R.E., DiLorenzo, T.M. and King, A.C. (2002) Intervention-related cognitive versus social mediators of exercise adherence in the elderly, *American Journal of Preventive Medicine*, 23, 80–6.

Campbell, T., Dunt, D., Fitzgerald, J.L. and Gordon, I. (2013) The impact of patient narratives on self-efficacy and self-care in Australians with type 2 diabetes: stage 1 results of a randomized trial, *Health Promotion International*, 28, 1–11.

Carson, J.A.S., Gilham, M.B., Kirk, L.M., Reddy, S.T. and Battles, J.B. (2002) Enhancing self-efficacy and patient care with cardiovascular nutrition education, *American Journal of Preventive Medicine*, 23, 296–302.

Catz, S.L., Kelly, J.A., Bogart, L.M., Benotsch, E.G. and McAuliffe, T.L. (2000) Patterns, correlates, and barriers to medication adherence among persons prescribed new treatments for HIV disease, *Health Psychology*, 19, 124–33.

Christiansen, M., Vik, P.W. and Jarchow, A. (2002) College student heavy drinking in social contexts versus alone, *Addictive Behaviors*, 27, 393–404.

Clark, M.M. and Dodge, J.A. (1999) Exploring self-efficacy as a predictor of disease management, *Health Education and Behaviour*, 26, 72–89.

Cohen, E.S. and Fromme, K. (2002) Differential determinants of young adult substance use and high risk sexual behavior, *Journal of Applied Social Psychology*, 32, 1124–50.

Conner, M., Rhodes, R.E., Morris, B., McEachan, R. and Lawton, R. (2011) Changing exercise through targeting affective or cognitive attitudes, *Psychology and Health*, 26, 133–49.

Contento, I.R., Randell, J.S. and Basch, C.E. (2002) Review and analysis of education measures used in nutrition education intervention research, *Journal of Nutrition Education and Behavior*, 34, 2–25.

Cormier, L., Kwan, L., Reid, K. and Litwin, M. (2002) Knowledge and beliefs among brothers and sons of men with prostate cancer, *Urology*, 59, 895–900.

Dearden, K.A., Quan Ie, N., Do, M., Marsh, D.R., Schroeder, D.G., Pachon, H. *et al.* (2002) What influences healthy behavior? Learning from caregivers of young children in Viet Nam, *Food and Nutrition Bulletin*, 23, 119–29.

DeVellis, B.M. and DeVellis, R.F. (2000) Self-efficacy and health, in A. Baum, T.A. Revenson and J.E. Singer (eds.) *Handbook of Health Psychology* (pp. 235–47). Mahwah, NJ: Erlbaum.

Dewar, D.L., Plotnikoff, R.C., Morgan, P.J., Okely, A.D., Costigan, S.A. and Lubans D.R. (2013) Testing social-cognitive theory to explain physical activity change in adolescent girls from low income communities, *Research Quarterly for Exercise and Sport*, 84, 483–91.

Dijkstra, A. and DeVries, H. (2000) Self-efficacy expectations with regard to different tasks in smoking cessations, *Psychology and Health*, 15, 501–11.

Dijkstra, A., Bakker, M. and DeVries, H. (1997) Subtypes within a precontemplating sample of smokers: a preliminary extension of the stages of change, *Addictive Behaviors*, 22, 327–37.

Dijkstra, A., DeVries, H., Kok, G. and Roijackers, J. (1999) Self-evaluation and motivation to change: social cognitive constructs in smoking cessation, *Psychology and Health*, 14, 747–59.

Dilorio, C., Dudley, W.N., Kelly, M., Soet, J.E., Mbwara, J. and Sharpe Potter, J. (2001) Social cognitive correlates of sexual experience and condom use among 13- through 15-year-old adolescents, *Journal of Adolescent Health*, 29, 208–16.

Dilorio, C., Dudley, W.N., Lehr, S. and Soet, J.E. (2000a) Correlates of safer sex communication among college students, *Journal of Advanced Nursing*, 32, 658–65.

Dilorio, C., Dudley, W.N., Soet, J., Watkins, J. and Maibach, E. (2000b) A social cognitive model for condom use among college students, *Nursing Research*, 49, 208–14.

Dishman, R.K., Motl, R.W., Saunders, R., Felton, G., Ward, D.S., Dowda, M. *et al.* (2004) Self-efficacy partially mediates the effects of a school-based physical-activity intervention among adolescent girls, *Preventive Medicine*, 38, 628–36.

Dzewaltowski, D.A. (1989) Toward a model of exercise motivation, *Journal of Sport and Exercise Psychology*, 11, 251–69.

Dzewaltowski, D.A., Estabrooks, P.A., Gyurcsik, N.C. and Johnston, J.A. (2002a) Promotion and physical activity through community development, in J.L. Van Raalte and B.W. Brewer (eds.) *Exploring Sport and Exercise Psychology* (2nd edn., pp. 209–33). Washington, DC: American Psychological Association.

Dzewaltowski, D.A., Estabrooks, P.A. and Johnston, J.A. (2002b) Healthy young places promoting nutrition and physical activity, *Health Education Research*, 17, 541–51.

Ernsting, A., Schneider, M., Knoll, N. and Schwarzer, R. (2015) The enabling effect of social support on vaccination uptake via self-efficacy and planning, *Psychology, Health and Medicine*, 20, 239–46.

Field, A.E., Camargo, C.A., Taylor, C.B., Berkey, C.S., Roberts, S.B. and Colditz, G.A. (2001) Peer–parent, and media influences on the development of weight concerns and frequent dieting among preadolescent and adolescent girls and boys, *Pediatrics*, 107, 54–60.

Fishbein, M. (2001) Sexually transmitted diseases: psychosocial aspects, in N.J. Smelser and P.B. Baltes (eds.) *The International Encyclopedia of the Social and Behavioral Sciences* (Vol. 21, pp. 14026–32). Oxford: Elsevier.

Fishbein, M. and Ajzen, I. (2010) *Predicting and Changing Behavior: The Reasoned Action Approach*. New York: Psychology Press.

Fleig, L., Lippke, S., Pomp, S. and Schwarzer, R. (2011) Exercise maintenance after rehabilitation: how experience can make a difference, *Psychology of Sport and Exercise*, 12, 293–9.

Fleig, L., Pomp, S., Schwarzer, R. and Lippke, S. (2013) Promoting exercise maintenance: how interventions with booster sessions improve long-term rehabilitation outcomes, *Rehabilitation Psychology*, 58, 323–33.

French, D.P. (2013) The role of self-efficacy in changing health-related behaviour: cause, effect or spurious association? *British Journal of Health Psychology*, 18, 237–43.

French, D.P., Olander, E., Ahisholm, A. and McSharry, J. (2014) Which behavior change techniques are most effective at increasing older adults' self-efficacy and physical activity behavior? A systematic review, *Annals of Behavioral Medicine*, 48, 225–34.

Friedman, S., Cheifetz, A.S., Farraye, F.A., Banks, P.A., Makrauer, F.L., Burakoff, R. *et al.* (2014) High self-efficacy predicts adherence to surveillance colonoscopy in inflammatory bowel disease, *Inflammatory Bowel Disease*, 20, 1602–10.

Gellert, P., Ziegelmann, J.P. and Schwarzer, R. (2012) Affective and health-related outcome expectancies for physical activity in older adults, *Psychology and Health*, 27, 816–28.

Godinho, C.A., Alvarez, M.J. and Lima, M.L. (2013) Formative research on HAPA model determinants for fruit and vegetable intake: target beliefs for audiences at different stages of change, *Health Education Research*, 28, 1014–28.

Godinho, C.A., Alvarez, M.J., Lima, M.L. and Schwarzer, R. (2014) Will is not enough: coping planning and action control as mediators in the prediction of fruit and vegetable intake, *British Journal of Health Psychology*, 19, 856–70.

Gollwitzer, P.M. (1999) Implementation intentions: strong effects of simple plans, *American Psychologist*, 54, 493–503.

Gwaltney, C.J., Shiffman, S., Paty, J.A., Liu, K.S., Kassel, J.D., Gnys, M. *et al.* (2002) Using self-efficacy judgements to predict characteristics of lapses to smoking, *Journal of Consulting and Clinical Psychology*, 70, 1140–9.

Hankonen, N., Absetz, P., Kinnunen, M., Haukkala, A. and Jallinoja, P. (2013) Toward identifying a broader range of social cognitive determinants of dietary intentions and behaviors, *Applied Psychology: Health and Well-Being*, 5, 118–35.

Higgins, T.J., Middleton, K.R., Winner, L. and Janelle, C.M. (2014) Physical activity interventions differentially affect exercise task and barrier self-efficacy: a meta-analysis, *Health Psychology*, 33, 891–903.

Hyde, J., Hankins, M., Deale, A. and Marteau, T.M. (2008) Interventions to increase self-efficacy in the context of addiction behaviours: a systematic literature review, *Journal of Health Psychology*, 13, 607–23.

King, D.K., Glasgow, R.E., Toobert, D.J., Strycker, L.A., Estabrooks, P.A., Osuna, D. *et al.* (2010) Self-efficacy, problem solving, and social-environmental support are associated with diabetes self-management behaviors, *Diabetes Care*, 33, 751–3.

Kreausukon, P., Gellert, P., Lippke, S. and Schwarzer, R. (2012) Planning and self-efficacy can increase fruit and vegetable consumption: a randomized controlled trial, *Journal of Behavioral Medicine*, 35, 443–51.

Kremers, S.P., Mesters, I., Pladdet, I.E., van den Borne, B. and Stockbrügger, R.W. (2000) Participation in a sigmoidoscopic colorectal cancer screening program: a pilot study, *Cancer Epidemiology, Biomarkers and Prevention*, 9, 1127–30.

Lai, A.Y., Fong, D.Y., Lam, J.C., Weaver, T.E. and Ip, M.S. (2014) The efficacy of a brief motivational enhancement education program on CPAP adherence in OSA: a randomized controlled trial, *Chest*, 146, 600–10.

Langebeek, N., Gisolf, E., Reiss, P., Vercoort, S., Hafsteinsdottir, T., Richter, C. *et al.* (2014) Predictors and correlates of adherence to combination antiretroviral therapy (cArt) for chronic HIV infection: a meta-analysis, *BMC Medicine*, 12, 48–82.

Lawrence, J.S., Eldridge, G.D., Shelby, M.C., Little, C.E., Brasfield, T.L. and O'Bannon, R.E., III (1997) HIV risk reduction for incarcerated women: a comparison of brief interventions based on two theoretical models, *Journal of Consulting and Clinical Psychology*, 65, 504–9.

Luszczynska, A. (2004) Change in breast self-examination behavior: effects of intervention on enhancing self-efficacy, *International Journal of Behavioral Medicine*, 11, 95–103.

Luszczynska, A. and Haynes, C. (2009) Changing nutrition, physical activity, and body weight among student nurses and midwifes: effects of a planning intervention and self-efficacy beliefs, *Journal of Health Psychology*, 14, 1075–84.

Luszczynska, A. and Schwarzer, R. (2003) Planning and self-efficacy in the adoption and maintenance of breast self-examination: a longitudinal study on self-regulatory cognitions, *Psychology and Health*, 18, 93–10.

Luszczynska, A. and Sutton, S. (2006) Physical activity after cardiac rehabilitation: evidence that different types of self-efficacy are important in maintainers and relapsers, *Rehabilitation Psychology*, 51, 314–21.

Luszczynska, A., Cao, D.S., Mallach, N., Pietron, K., Mazurkiewicz, M. and Schwarzer, R. (2010) Intentions, planning, and self-efficacy predict physical activity in Chinese and Polish adolescents: two moderated mediation analyses, *International Journal of Clinical and Health Psychology*, 10, 265–78.

Luszczynska, A., Durawa, A., Scholz, U. and Knoll, N. (2012) Empowerment beliefs and intention to uptake cervical cancer screening: three psychosocial mediating mechanisms, *Women and Health*, 52, 162–81.

Luszczynska, A., Gutiérrez-Doña, B. and Schwarzer, R. (2005) General self-efficacy in various domains of human functioning: evidence from five countries, *International Journal of Psychology*, 40, 80–9.

Luszczynska, A., Mazurkiewicz, M., Ziegelman, J.P. and Schwarzer, R. (2007a) Recovery self-efficacy and intention as predictors of running: a cross-lagged panel analysis over a two-year period, *Psychology of Sport and Exercise*, 8, 247–60.

Luszczynska, A., Tryburcy, M. and Schwarzer, R. (2007b) Improving fruit and vegetable consumption: a self-efficacy intervention compared with a combined self-efficacy and planning intervention, *Health Education Research*, 22, 630–8.

Maddison, R., Pfaeffli, L., Stewart, R., Kerr, A., Jiang, Y., Rawstorn, J. *et al.* (2014) The HEART mobile phone trial: the partial mediating effects of self-efficacy on physical activity amnong cardiac patents, *Frontiers in Public Health*, 27, 56.

Maddux, J.E. and Lewis, J. (1995) Self-efficacy and adjustment: basic principles and issues, in J.E. Maddux (ed.) *Self-efficacy, Adaptation, and Adjustment: Theory, Research, and Application* (pp. 37–68). New York: Plenum Press.

Magklara, E., Burton, C.R. and Morrison, V. (2014) Does self-efficacy influence recovery and well-being in osteoarthritis patients undergoing joint replacement: a systematic review, *Clinical Rehabilitation*, 28, 835–46.

Marlatt, G.A., Baer, J.S. and Quigley, L.A. (1995) Self-efficacy and addictive behavior, in A. Bandura (ed.) *Self-efficacy in Changing Societies* (pp. 289–315). New York: Cambridge University Press.

Mee, S. (2014) Self-efficacy: a mediator of smoking behaviour and depression among college students, *Pediatric Nursing*, 40, 9–15.

Motl, R.W., Dishman, R.K., Saundres, R.P., Dowda, M., Felton, G., Ward, D.S. *et al.* (2002) Examining social-cognitive determinants of intention and physical activity among Black and White adolescent girls using structural equation modelling, *Health Psychology*, 21, 459–67.

National Institute of Mental Health Multisite HIV Prevention Trial Group (2001) Social-cognitive theory mediators of behavior change in the National Institute of Mental Health Multisite HIV Prevention Trial, *Health Psychology*, 20, 369–76.

Newcomb, M.E. and Mustanski, B. (2014) Cognitive influences on sexual risk and risk appeals in men who have sex with men, *Health Psychology*, 33, 690–8.

Niaura, R., Shadel, W.G., Britt, D.M. and Abrams, D.B. (2002) Response to social stress, urge to smoke, and smoking cessation, *Addictive Behaviors*, 27, 241–50.

Ochsner, S., Scholz, U. and Hornung, R. (2013) Testing phase-specific self-efficacy beliefs in the context of dietary behaviour change, *Applied Psychology: Health and Well-Being*, 5, 99–117.

Ockene, J.K., Emmons, K.M., Mermelstein, R.J., Perkins, K.A., Bonollo, D.S., Voorhees, C.C. *et al.* (2000) Relapse and maintenance issues for smoking cessation, *Health Psychology*, 19, 17–31.

O'Hea, E.L., Moon, S., Grothe, K.B., Bordeaux, E., Bodenlos, J.S., Wallson, K. *et al.* (2009) The interaction of locus of control, self-efficacy, and outcome expectancy in the relation to HbA1c in medically underserved individuals with type 2 diabetes, *Journal of Behavioral Medicine*, 32, 106–17.

Olander, E.K., Fletcher, H., Williams, S., Atkinson, L., Turner, A. and French, D.P. (2013) What are the most effective techniques in changing obese individuals' physical activity self-efficacy and behaviour: a systematic review and meta-analysis, *International Journal of Behavioral Nutrition and Physical Activity*, 10, 29.

Parent, N. and Fortin, F. (2000) A randomized controlled trial of vicarious experience through peer support for male first-time cardiac surgery patients: impact on anxiety, self-efficacy expectation, and self-reported activity, *Heart and Lung*, 29, 389–400.

Pinto, B.M., Friedman, R., Marcus, B.H., Kelly, H., Tennstedt, S. and Gillman, M.W. (2002a) Effects of computer-based, telephone-counseling system on physical activity, *American Journal of Preventive Medicine*, 23, 113–20.

Pinto, B.M., Maruyama, N.C., Clark, M.M., Cruess, D.G., Park, E. and Roberts, M. (2002b) Motivation to modify lifestyle risk behaviors in women treated for breast cancer, *Mayo Clinic Proceedings*, 77, 122–9.

Prestwich, A., Kellar, I., Parker, R., MacRae, S., Learmonth, M., Sykes, B. *et al.* (2014) How can self-efficacy be increased? Meta-analysis of dietary interventions, *Health Psychology Review*, 8, 270–85.

Prochaska, J.O. and DiClemente, C.C. (1983) Stages and processes of self-change of smoking: toward an integrative model of change, *Journal of Consulting and Clinical Psychology*, 51, 390–5.

Reid, A.E. and Aiken, L.S. (2011) Integration of five health behavior models: common strengths and unique contributions to understanding condom use. *Psychology and Health*, 26, 1499–520.

Renner, B. and Schupp, H. (2011) The perception of health risks, in H. Friedman (ed.) *The Oxford Handbook of Health Psychology* (pp. 637–65). Oxford Library of Psychology. New York: Oxford University Press.

Resnicow, K., Wallace, D.S., Jackson, A., Digirolamo, A., Odom, E., Wang, T. *et al.* (2000) Dietary change through African American churches: baseline results and program description of the eat for life trial, *Journal of Cancer Education*, 15, 156–63.

Richetin, J., Conner, M. and Perugini, M. (2011) Not doing is not the opposite of doing: implications for attitudinal models of behavioral prediction, *Personality and Social Psychology Bulletin*, 37, 40–54.

Rodgers, W.M., Murray, T.C., Courneya, K.S., Bell, G.J. and Harber, V.J. (2009) The specificity of self-efficacy over the course of a progressive exercise program, *Applied Psychology: Health and Well-Being*, 1, 211–32.

Rodgers, W.M., Murray, T.C., Selzler, A.M. and Norman, P. (2013) Development and impact of exercise self-efficacy types during and after cardiac rehabilitation, *Rehabilitation Psychology*, 58, 178–84.

Rosenberg, H., Bonar, E.E., Hoffmann, E., Kryszak, E., Young, K.M., Kraus, S.W. *et al.* (2011) Assessing university students' self-efficacy to employ alcohol-related harm reduction strategies, *Journal of the American College Health*, 59, 736–42.

Rovniak, L.S., Anderson, E.S., Winett, R.A. and Stephens, R.S. (2002) Social cognitive determinants of physical activity in young adults: a prospective structural equation analysis, *Annals of Behavioral Medicine*, 24, 149–56.

Ruiter, R.A.C., Abraham, C. and Kok, G. (2001) Scary warnings and rational precautions: a review of the psychology of fear appeals, *Psychology and Health*, 16, 613–30.

Safron, M., Cislak, A., Gaspar, T. and Luszczynska, A. (2011) Effects of school-based interventions targeting obesity-related behaviors and body weight change: a systematic umbrella review, *Behavioral Medicine*, 37, 15–25.

Sallis, J.F., Prochaska, J.J. and Taylor, W.C. (2000) A review of correlates of physical activity and fitness in children and adolescents, *Medicine and Science in Sports and Exercise*, 32, 963–75.

Savoca, M. and Miller, C. (2001) Food selection and eating patterns: themes found among people with type-2 diabetes mellitus, *Journal of Nutrition Education*, 33, 224–33.

Schnoll, R. and Zimmerman, B.J. (2001) Self-regulation training enhances dietary self-efficacy and dietary fiber consumption, *Journal of the American Dietetic Association*, 101, 1006–11.

Schnoll, R.A., Miller, S.M., Unger, M., McAleer, C., Halbherr, T. and Bradley, P. (2002) Characteristics of female smokers attending a lung cancer screening program: a pilot study with implications for program development, *Lung Cancer*, 37, 257–65.

Scholz, U., Ochsner, S., Hornung, R. and Knoll, N. (2013) Does social support really help to eat a low-fat diet? Main effects and gender differences of received social support within the Health Action Process Approach, *Applied Psychology: Health and Well Being*, 5, 270–90.

Scholz, U., Sniehotta, F.F. and Schwarzer, R. (2005) Predicting physical exercise in cardiac rehabilitation: the role of phase-specific self-efficacy beliefs, *Journal of Sport and Exercise Psychology*, 27, 135–51.

Schwarzer, R. (2008) Modeling health behavior change: how to predict and modify the adoption and maintenance of health behaviors, *Applied Psychology: An International Review*, 57, 1–29.

Schwarzer, R. and Knoll, N. (2007) Functional roles of social support within the stress and coping process: a theoretical and empirical overview, *International Journal of Psychology*, 42, 243–52.

Schwarzer, R. and Renner, B. (2000) Social-cognitive predictors of health behavior: action self-efficacy and coping self-efficacy, *Health Psychology*, 19, 487–95.

Schwarzer, R., Antoniuk, A. and Gholami, M. (2015) A brief intervention changing oral self-care, self-efficacy, and self-monitoring, *British Journal of Health Psychology*, 20, 56–67.

Semple, S.J., Patterson, T.L. and Grant, I. (2000) Partner type and sexual risk behavior among HIV positive gay and bisexual men: social cognitive correlates, *AIDS Education and Prevention*, 12, 340–56.

Shiffman, S., Balabanis, M.H., Paty, J.A., Engberg, J., Gwaltney, C.J., Liu, K.S. *et al.* (2000) Dynamic effects of self-efficacy on smoking lapse and relapse, *Health Psychology*, 19, 315–23.

Smit, E.S., Hoving, C., Schelleman-Offermans, K., West, R. and de Vries, H. (2014) Predictors of successful and unsuccessful quit attempts among smokers motivated to quit, *Addictive Behaviors*, 39, 1318–24.

Stanton, B.F., Li, X., Ricardo, I., Galbraith, J., Feigelman, S. and Kaljee, L. (1996) A randomized, controlled trial of an AIDS prevention program for low-income African American youths, *Archives of Pediatrics and Adolescent Medicine*, 150, 363–72.

Stewart, S.M., Lee, P.W., Waller, D., Hughes, C.W., Low, L.C., Kennard, B.D. *et al.* (2003) A follow up study of adherence and glycemic control among Hong Kong youths with diabetes, *Journal of Pediatric Psychology*, 28, 67–79.

Strauss, R.S., Rodzilsky, D., Burack, G. and Colin, M. (2001) Psychosocial correlates of physical activity in healthy children, *Archives of Pediatrics and Adolescent Medicine*, 155, 897–902.

Szczepanska, K.W., Scholz, U., Liszewska, N. and Luszczynska, A. (2013) Social and cognitive predictors of fruit and vegetable intake among adolescents: the context of changes in body weight, *Journal of Health Psychology*, 18, 667–79.

Trobst, K.L., Herbst, J.H., Masters, H.L., III and Costa, P.T., Jr. (2002) Personality pathways to unsafe sex: personality, condom use and HIV risk behaviors, *Journal of Research in Personality*, 36, 117–33.

Umeh, K. and Rogan-Gibson, J. (2001) Perceptions of threat, benefits, and barriers in breast self-examination amongst asymptomatic women, *British Journal of Health Psychology*, 6, 361–72.

Van Duyn, M.A., Kristal, A.R., Dodd, K., Campbell, M.K., Subar, A.F., Stables, G. *et al.* (2001) Association of awareness, intrapersonal and interpersonal factors, and stage of dietary change with fruit and vegetable consumption: a national survey, *American Journal of Health Promotion*, 16, 69–78.

Voorhees, C.C., Yan, A.F., Clifton, K.J. and Wang, M.Q. (2011) Neighborhood environment, self-efficacy, and physical activity in urban adolescents, *American Journal of Health Behavior*, 35, 674–88.

Warner, L.M., Schüz, B., Knittle, K., Ziegelmann, J.P. and Wurm, S. (2011) Sources of perceived self-efficacy as predictors of physical activity in older adults, *Applied Psychology: Health and Well-Being*, 3, 172–92.

Warner, L.M., Schüz, B., Wolff, J.K., Parschau, L., Wurm, S. and Schwarzer, R. (2014) Sources of self-efficacy for physical activity, *Health Psychology*, 33, 1298–308.

Widman, L., Noar, S.M., Choukas-Bradley, S. and Francis, D.B. (2014) Adolescent sexual health communication and condom use: a meta-analysis, *Health Psychology*, 33, 1113–24.

Willems, R.A., Willemsen, M.C., Nagelhout, G.E. and de Vries, H. (2013) Understanding smokers' motivations to use evidence-based smoking cessation aids, *Nicotine and Tobacco Research*, 15, 167–76.

Williams, D.M., Anderson, E.S. and Winett, R.A. (2005) A review of the outcome expectancy construct in physical activity research, *Annals of Behavioral Medicine*, 29, 70–9.

Williams, K.E. and Bond, M.J. (2002) The roles of self-efficacy, outcome expectancies and social support in the self-care behaviors of diabetics, *Psychology, Health and Medicine*, 7, 127–41.

Williams, S.L. and French, D.P. (2011) What are the most effective intervention techniques for changing physical activity self-efficacy and physical activity behaviour – and are they the same? *Health Education Research*, 26, 308–22.

Wills, T.A., Gibbons, F.X., Gerrard, M. and Brody, G. (2000) Protection and vulnerability processes for early onset of substance use: a test among African-American children, *Health Psychology*, 19, 253–63.

Winkleby, M.A., Feighery, E.C., Altman, D.A., Kole, S. and Tencati, E. (2001) Engaging ethnically diverse teens in a substance use prevention advocacy program, *American Journal of Health Promotion*, 15, 433–6.

Woodgate, J. and Brawley, L.R. (2008) Self-efficacy for exercise in cardiac rehabilitation: review and recommendations, *Journal of Health Psychology*, 13, 366–87.

Chapter 8

Health action process approach

Ralf Schwarzer and Aleksandra Luszczynska

1 General background

Health behaviours may change continuously in a quantitative manner, but change can also be described in terms of qualitative stages. The health action process approach (HAPA; Schwarzer 2008) has been designed as a hybrid model with a stage layer as well as a continuum layer. It can be regarded as an extension and modification of social cognitive theory (SCT; Bandura 1986), but whereas SCT addresses all kinds of behaviour, HAPA has been explicitly developed to focus on health behaviour change. It was originally developed in 1988 (Schwarzer 1992), integrating the model of action phases (Heckhausen 1980) with SCT to understand the quantitative and qualitative processes of health behaviour change. It was designed to be an open architecture framework that is based on general principles rather than on specific testable hypotheses. Traditional continuum models such as the theory of planned behaviour have been criticized because they do not elaborate explicitly on the processes that occur after goals or behavioural intentions have been set. This lack of attention to post-intentional processes has been labelled the 'intention–behaviour gap' (Sheeran 2002). In contrast, the model of action phases (Rubicon model; Heckhausen 1980) makes a distinction between motivation and volition. In line with the Rubicon model, HAPA makes a distinction between (a) pre-intentional motivation processes that lead to a behavioural intention, and (b) post-intentional volition processes that lead to the actual health behaviour. Within the two phases, different patterns of social cognitive predictors emerge (see Figure 8.1). In the initial motivation phase, a person develops an intention to act. In this phase, risk perception is seen as a distal antecedent (e.g. 'I am at risk for cardiovascular disease'). Risk perception in itself is insufficient to enable a person to form an intention. Rather, it sets the stage for a contemplation process and further elaboration of thoughts about consequences and competencies. Similarly, positive outcome expectancies (e.g. 'If I exercise five times per week, I will reduce my cardiovascular risk') are chiefly seen as being important in the motivation phase, when a person balances the pros and cons of certain behavioural outcomes. Furthermore, one needs to believe in one's capability to perform a desired action (perceived self-efficacy; e.g. 'I am capable of adhering to my exercise schedule in spite of the temptation to watch TV'). Perceived self-efficacy operates in concert with positive outcome expectancies, both of which contribute to forming an intention. Both beliefs are needed for forming intentions to adopt health-enhancing behaviours or to refrain from refractory risk behaviours.

After a person develops an inclination towards a particular health behaviour, the behavioural intention has to be transformed into detailed instructions on how to perform the desired action. Once an action has been initiated, it has to be maintained. This is not achieved through a single act of will, but involves self-regulatory skills and strategies. Thus, the key influences in the post-intentional phase can be further broken down into more proximal factors, such as planning, action control, and maintenance/recovery self-efficacy. Other social cognition models have not explicitly addressed such post-intentional factors.

Research that is based on the continuum layer of HAPA employs path-analytic research designs when describing, explaining, and predicting health behaviours. When designing interventions, the stage layer is also considered to be useful. This is achieved through the identification of individuals who reside either at the motivational stage or the volitional stage. Then, each group becomes the target of a specific treatment that is tailored to this group. Moreover, it has been found useful to subdivide the volitional group further into those who already perform and those who only intend to perform. In the post-intentional pre-actional stage, individuals are labelled 'intenders,' whereas in the actional stage they are labelled 'actors.' Thus, a possible subdivision within the health behaviour change process yields three groups: pre-intenders, intenders, and actors. The term 'stage' in this context was chosen to allude to the stage theories, but not in the strict definition that includes irreversibility and invariance. The terms 'phase' or 'mindset' may be equally suitable for this distinction. The basic idea is that individuals pass through different qualitative mindsets on their way to behaviour change. Thus, interventions may be most efficient when tailored to these particular mindsets. For example, pre-intenders are supposed to benefit from confrontation with outcome expectancies and some level of risk communication. They need to learn that the new behaviour (e.g. becoming physically active) has positive outcomes (e.g. well-being, weight loss, fun) compared with the negative outcomes that accompany the current (sedentary) behaviour (e.g. developing an illness or being unattractive). In contrast, intenders should not benefit much from such health messages in the form of outcome expectancies because, after setting a goal, they have already moved beyond this mindset. Rather, they should benefit from planning to translate their intentions into action. Finally, actors do not need any treatment at all unless one wants to improve their relapse prevention skills and promote habit formation. Then, they should control their actions to be prepared for particular high-risk situations in which lapses are likely.

2 Description of the model

The HAPA consists of various constructs and mechanisms, as described in the following subsections (see Figure 8.1).

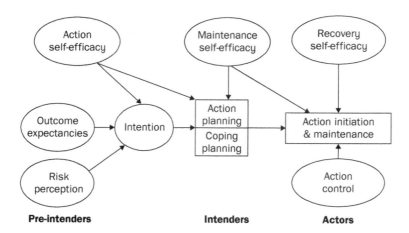

Figure 8.1 Diagram of the health action process approach (HAPA; Schwarzer 1992, 2008). Arrows represent causal paths; text at bottom of figure represents different phases of action. The terms *maintenance self-efficacy* and *coping self-efficacy* are used interchangeably

2.1 Constructs

2.1.1 Risk perception

At first glance, perceiving a health threat seems to be the most obvious prerequisite for the motivation to overcome a risk behaviour (e.g. smoking). However, general perceptions of risk (e.g. 'Smoking is dangerous') and personal perceptions of risk (e.g. 'I am at risk for lung cancer, because I am a smoker') often differ to a great extent. For example, individuals could be well informed about general aspects of certain risks and precautions (e.g. most smokers acknowledge that smoking can cause diseases), but, nevertheless, they might not feel personally vulnerable (Renner and Schupp 2011). However, risk perception is a distal antecedent in the health behaviour change process, and it need not necessarily exert a direct influence on intention formation.

2.1.2 Outcome expectancies

In addition to being aware of a health threat, people also need to understand the links between their actions and subsequent outcomes. These outcome expectancies can be the most influential beliefs in the motivation to change (Williams *et al.* 2005; Godinho *et al.*2013; Hankonen *et al.* 2013). The term 'outcome expectancies' is most common in SCT (Bandura 1986), whereas 'pros and cons' is used in the transtheoretical model, also called the stages of change model (Prochaska and DiClemente 1983), where they represent the decisional balance when people contemplate whether to adopt a novel behaviour or not. In the reasoned action approach (Fishbein and Ajzen 2010), the equivalent term is 'behavioural beliefs', which act as precursors of attitudes. The pros and cons represent positive and negative outcome expectancies. A smoker may find more good reasons to quit ('If I quit smoking, then my friend will like me much more') than reasons to continue smoking ('If I quit, I will become more tense and irritated'). This imbalance in favour of positive outcome expectancies will not lead directly to action, but it can help to generate the intention to quit. Outcome expectancies can also be understood as means–ends relationships, indicating that people know proper strategies to produce the desired effects. The perceived contingencies between actions and outcomes need not be explicitly worded; they can also be rather diffuse mental representations, loaded with emotions. Social cognition models are often misunderstood as rational models that deal with 'cold cognitions'. In contrast, health behaviour change, to a large degree, is an emotional process that turns into a cognitive one after people have been asked about their thoughts and feelings, thus making them aware of what is going on emotionally. An example of an emotional outcome expectancy is anticipated regret ('If I do not use a condom tonight, then I will regret it tomorrow').

2.1.3 Perceived self-efficacy

Perceived self-efficacy portrays individuals' beliefs in their capabilities to exercise control over challenging demands and over their own functioning. Perceived self-efficacy has been found to be important at all stages in the health behaviour change process (Bandura 1997), but it does not always constitute exactly the same construct. Its meaning depends on the particular situation of individuals who may be more or less advanced in the change process. In the domain of addictive behaviours, Marlatt *et al.* (1995) have proposed a distinction between action self-efficacy, coping self-efficacy, and recovery self-efficacy. The rationale for the distinction between several phase-specific self-efficacy beliefs is that during the course of health behaviour change, different tasks have to be mastered, and different self-efficacy beliefs are required to master these tasks successfully. For example, a person might be confident in his or her capability to be physically active in general (i.e. high action self-efficacy), but might not be very confident to resume physical activity after a setback (i.e. low recovery self-efficacy). In HAPA, three types of self-efficacy are distinguished: action self-efficacy, maintenance self-efficacy, and recovery self-efficacy.

Action self-efficacy (also called pre-action self-efficacy or task self-efficacy) refers to the first phase of the process, in which an individual does not yet act, but develops a motivation to do so. It is an optimistic belief during the pre-actional phase. Individuals high in action self-efficacy imagine success, anticipate potential outcomes of diverse strategies, and are more likely to initiate a new behaviour. Those with less self-efficacy imagine failure, harbour self-doubts, and tend to procrastinate.

Maintenance self-efficacy represents optimistic beliefs about one's capability to cope with barriers that arise during the maintenance period. (The equivalent term 'coping self-efficacy' has also been used in a different sense; therefore, the term 'maintenance self-efficacy' may be better.) A new health behaviour might turn out to be much more difficult to adhere to than expected, but a self-efficacious person responds confidently with better strategies, more effort, and prolonged persistence to overcome such hurdles. Once an action has been taken, individuals with high maintenance self-efficacy try harder and persist longer than those who are less self-efficacious.

Recovery self-efficacy addresses the experience of failure and recovery from setbacks. If a lapse occurs, individuals can fall prey to the 'abstinence violation effect' – that is, they attribute their lapse to internal, stable, and global causes, dramatize the event, and interpret it as a full-blown relapse (Marlatt *et al.* 1995). High self-efficacious individuals, however, avoid this effect by attributing the lapse to an external high-risk situation and by finding ways to control the damage and to restore hope. Recovery self-efficacy pertains to one's conviction to get back on track after being derailed. The person trusts his or her competence to regain control after a setback or failure and to reduce harm.

Whereas pre-action self-efficacy is instrumental in the motivation phase, the other two constructs pertain to the subsequent volitional phase and could, therefore, also be summarized under the heading of 'volitional self-efficacy'. There is a functional difference between these self-efficacy constructs, whereas their temporal sequence is less important. Different phase-specific self-efficacy beliefs may be harboured at the same point in time. The assumption is that they operate in a different manner. For example, action self-efficacy is most functional when facing a novel challenging demand, whereas recovery self-efficacy is most functional when it comes to resuming an interrupted chain of action.

This distinction between phase-specific self-efficacy beliefs has proven useful in various domains of behaviour change (Ochsner *et al.* 2013). Action self-efficacy tends to predict intentions, whereas maintenance self-efficacy tends to predict behaviours. Several authors (e.g. Rodgers *et al.* 2009) have found evidence for phase-specific self-efficacy beliefs in the domain of exercise behaviour (i.e. task self-efficacy, coping self-efficacy, and scheduling self-efficacy). Phase-specific self-efficacy has also been found to differ in the effects on various preventive health behaviours, such as breast self-examination (Luszczynska and Schwarzer 2003), dietary behaviours (Schwarzer and Renner 2000), and physical exercise (Scholz *et al.* 2005). For example, individuals who had recovered from a setback needed different self-beliefs than those who had maintained their levels of activity (Scholz *et al.* 2005).

2.1.4 Intention

In the process of motivation, intention has been regarded as a 'watershed' between an initial goal-setting phase (motivation) and a subsequent goal pursuit phase (volition). Although the construct of intention is indispensable in explaining health behaviour change, its predictive value is limited (Sheeran 2002). When trying to translate intentions into behaviour, individuals are faced with various obstacles, such as distractions, forgetting or conflicting bad habits. Godin and Kok (1996), who reviewed 19 studies, found a mean correlation of 0.46 between intention and health behaviour, such as exercise, screening attendance, and addictions. Abraham and Sheeran (2000) reported that behavioural intention measures account for a quarter of the variance in health behaviour measures. If not equipped with means to overcome these obstacles, motivation alone does not suffice to change behaviour. To overcome this limitation, further constructs are required that operate in concert with intention.

Planning

Intentions are more likely to be translated into action when people develop success scenarios and preparatory strategies for approaching a difficult task. Mental simulation helps to identify cues to action. Action plans may follow the SMART principles, which means that they should be specific (a narrow behaviour), measurable, assignable (who will perform), realistic, and time-related (when to perform the action). These are well-known principles that stem from the management-by-objectives literature (Doran 1981). The terms planning and implementation intentions have been used to address this phenomenon. To date, research has accumulated abundant evidence for the effectiveness of planning. Meta-analyses have summarized the effects of planning on health behaviours (Gollwitzer and Sheeran 2006; Amireault *et al.* 2013; Carraro and Gaudreau 2013; Kwasnicka *et al.* 2013). One means of planning is the anticipation of barriers and the generation of alternative behaviours to overcome them. This has been called 'coping planning' (Sniehotta *et al.* 2006b). People imagine scenarios that hinder them in performing their intended behaviour, and they develop one or more plans to cope with such a challenging situation. For example: 'If I plan to run on Sunday, but the weather does not permit it, I will go swimming instead', or 'If there is something exciting on TV tonight that I do not want to miss, I will reschedule my workout to the afternoon'. Coping planning might be a more effective self-regulatory strategy than mere action planning. After people contemplate the when, where, and how of action, they imagine possible barriers and generate coping strategies. Thus, coping planning comes on top of action planning. Planning is an alterable variable. It can be easily communicated to individuals with self-regulatory deficits. Randomized controlled trials have highlighted evidence in support of such planning interventions (for an overview, see Hagger and Luszczynska 2014).

2.1.5 Action control

While planning is a prospective strategy – that is, behavioural plans are made before the situation is encountered – action control is a concurrent self-regulatory strategy, where the ongoing behaviour is continuously evaluated with regard to a behavioural standard. Action control can comprise three facets: self-monitoring ('I consistently monitored when, where, and how long I exercise'), awareness of standards ('I have always been aware of my prescribed training programme'), and self-regulatory effort ('I took care to practise as much as I intended to').

2.2 Mechanisms and principles

The path model in Figure 8.1 illustrates the continuum layer of HAPA. This is a sequential mediator structure that can be tested by specifying corresponding structural equation models. However, empirical models cannot reflect exactly the same structure as the theoretical model because some constructs may be highly intercorrelated in some data sets and, due to multicollinearity, different results would emerge. For example, action planning and coping planning are sometimes highly intercorrelated and thus should not be used as distinct constructs but rather as indicators of a single latent variable. The same applies to the phase-specific self-efficacy constructs: in some data sets a latent variable 'volitional self-efficacy', with maintenance and recovery self-efficacy as its indicators fit the data better than separate constructs.

The other mechanism refers to the stage layer that seems to be appropriate for tailored intervention programmes. A segmentation of the participants into pre-intenders, intenders, and actors provides a basis to develop matching treatments that target the audience better than a one-size-fits-all approach.

HAPA can be briefly characterized by the following main principles:

- *Principle 1: Motivation and volition.* The health behaviour change process is divided into two phases. There is a switch of mindsets when people move from deliberation to action. First comes the motivation phase in which people develop their intentions. Afterwards, they enter the volitional phase.
- *Principle 2: Two volitional phases.* In the volitional phase, there are two groups of people: those who have not yet translated their intentions into action, and those who have. Thus, there are inactive as well as active persons in this phase. In other words, in the volitional phase one finds intenders as well as actors who are characterized by different psychological states. Thus, in addition to viewing health behaviour change as a continuous process, one can also create three categories of people with different mindsets,

depending on their current location within the course of behaviour change: pre-intenders, intenders, and actors. This segmentation serves to develop matching treatments.

- *Principle 3: Post-intentional planning.* Intenders who are in the volitional pre-actional stage are motivated to change, but they do not act because they might lack the correct skills to translate their intention into action. Planning is a key strategy at this point. It serves as an operative mediator between intentions and behaviour.
- *Principle 4: Two kinds of mental simulation.* Planning can be divided into action planning and coping planning. Action planning pertains to the when, where, and how of intended action. Coping planning includes the anticipation of barriers and the design of alternative actions that help to attain one's goal in spite of impediments.
- *Principle 5: Phase-specific self-efficacy.* Perceived self-efficacy is required throughout the entire process. However, the nature of self-efficacy differs from phase to phase. This is because there are different challenges as people progress from one phase to the next. Goal-setting, planning, initiation, action, and maintenance all pose challenges that are not of the same nature. Therefore, one can distinguish between action self-efficacy, maintenance self-efficacy, and recovery self-efficacy.

3 Summary of research

As the HAPA is not a directly testable set of hypotheses but rather an open architecture framework, one should not expect to find a single acid test of the entire model as displayed in Figure 8.1. Instead, researchers typically apply the main path analytic design of the model, using a subset of constructs – most frequently outcome expectancies, intention, planning, and self-efficacy – to study the predictors of intention and behaviour as well as the mediators that bridge the intention–behaviour gap. Risk perception, on the other hand, has been reported to be of negligible importance in some studies on physical exercise, smoking cessation, and nutrition (see below). All other elements of the model, however, have been found to be of substantial importance across a large body of research. Many studies have explicitly or implicitly used HAPA in a broad range of populations to explain and predict health-related behaviours. Examples of such studies include those on:

- *health-enhancing behaviours*, such as:
  - physical activity (Scholz *et al.* 2009a; Caudroit *et al.* 2011; Chiu *et al.* 2011; Parschau *et al.* 2012, 2013, 2014; Perrier *et al.* 2012; Barg *et al.* 2012; Ginis *et al.* 2013; Gellert *et al.* 2014; Kassavou *et al.* 2014; Lippke and Plotnikoff 2014);
  - healthy eating (Schwarzer *et al.* 2007; Renner *et al.* 2008; Scholz *et al.* 2009b; Richert *et al.* 2010; Wiedemann *et al.* 2012; Gholami *et al.* 2013; Lange *et al.* 2013; Szczepanska *et al.* 2013; Zhou *et al.* 2013; Godinho *et al.* 2014; Lhakhang *et al.* 2014b; Radtke *et al.* 2014);
  - food safety behaviour (Chow and Mullan 2010).
- *risk-reducing behaviours*, such as:
  - vaccination (Payaprom *et al.* 2011; Ernsting *et al.* 2013a);
  - condom use (Teng and Mak 2011; Carvalho *et al.* 2015);
  - smoking cessation (Radtke *et al.* 2011);
  - alcohol consumption (Murgraff *et al.* 2003);

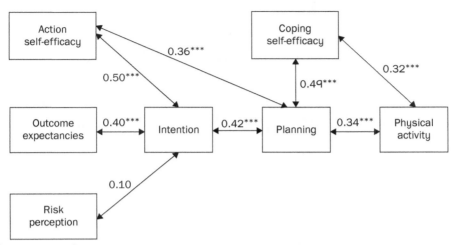

Figure 8.2 Meta-analytic population effect sizes (average weighted correlations) based on 11 studies on physical activity (Gholami 2014)

- *regular self-care*, such as:
  - oral self-care (Schüz *et al.* 2009; Dumitrescu *et al.* 2014; Schwarzer *et al.* 2015);
  - skin protection behaviour (Matterne *et al.* 2011; Craciun *et al.* 2012a); and
- *symptom detection behaviours*, such as:
  - skin self-examination (Auster *et al.* 2013);
  - breast self-examination (Luszczynska and Schwarzer 2003).

A meta-analysis of 11 studies on physical activity has yielded mean correlations as depicted in Figure 8.2 (Gholami 2014). Since not all studies make the distinction between action planning and coping planning, as well as further differentiate the self-efficacy construct, such meta-analyses have to focus on the smallest denominator of all the included studies. Also, action control is not always included, and even when it is, it is often constrained to the self-monitoring subset of this construct. Across the 11 studies, there are strong bivariate associations between the selected constructs (except for risk perception). Due to a lack of suitable studies on physical activity, no distinction could be made between action planning and coping planning, and action control and recovery self-efficacy are also missing.

Risk perception is considered to be a distal predictor of intentions, and it may have an influence early on when considering the behaviour but may no longer be relevant once outcome expectancies and self-efficacy have become the dominant proximal predictors of the intention. Although this is likely in the context of physical activity (and nutrition), it might be different in situations where the notion of a health risk is more imminent.

In most studies, structural equation modelling is employed to examine the longitudinal associations between the HAPA variables. Perceived risk, outcome expectancies, and pre-action self-efficacy are specified as predictors of intention. Intention and maintenance self-efficacy are specified as predictors of planning. Recovery self-efficacy and planning are specified as predictors of behaviour change. One such study was conducted in 166 Polish young adults (Schwarzer and Luszczynska 2008). As shown in Figure 8.3, all relations included in the model, except the

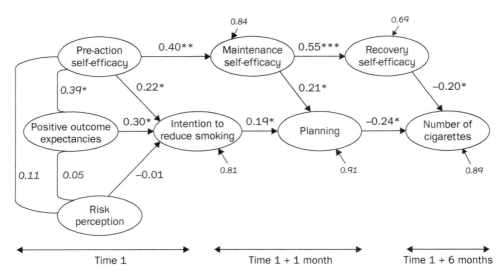

Figure 8.3 Longitudinal observation study to predict non-smoking in 166 Polish young adults (Schwarzer and Luszczynska 2008). Path coefficients are standardized parameter estimates (beta weights), large italics are correlations, small italics are residuals (unexplained variance)

path from risk perception to intention, were significant. Intention at Time 1 was predicted by stronger pre-action self-efficacy and more positive outcome expectancies, accounting for 19% of the variance. Planning at Time 2 was predicted by stronger maintenance self-efficacy and stronger intentions, accounting for 9% of the variance. Finally, lower levels of smoking at Time 3 were predicted by stronger recovery self-efficacy and planning measured six months earlier, accounting for 11% of the variance in the number of cigarettes smoked.

In cardiac rehabilitation, three phase-specific kinds of self-efficacy have been distinguished. Each demonstrated discriminant validity and were analysed regarding their predictions of intentions and behaviour. Individuals in the maintenance phase (actors who remained actors) were more likely to perform physical activities if they reported more maintenance self-efficacy than others. Study participants resuming their physical exercise after a health-related break were more successful if they had higher recovery self-efficacy than those who were active without a break (Scholz *et al.* 2005). Individuals in cardiac rehabilitation who had strong coping self-efficacy were more likely to maintain the recommended rehabilitation exercise at follow-up, whereas this type of self-efficacy did not help patients who had relapsed. Those who had experienced a setback in adhering to recommended exercise, but harboured strong recovery self-efficacy beliefs, were more likely to regain control after a relapse (Luszczynska and Sutton 2006).

Planning is proposed to serve as a mediator between intentions and behaviour, which means that levels of intention predict planning, and planning predicts behaviour, while the direct effect between intention and behaviour becomes negligible (e.g. Schwarzer *et al.* 2007). This has not only been shown in the general population (Scholz *et al.* 2008) but also in rehabilitation settings with inpatients (Reuter *et al.* 2010) and orthopaedic (Lippke *et al.* 2005; Fleig *et al.* 2013) and cardiac outpatients (Fleig *et al.* 2013) as well as in various countries. Not all HAPA studies have yielded such mediator effects of planning, but independent studies outside HAPA have confirmed that both

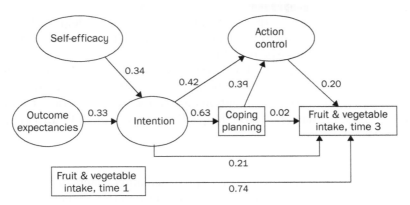

Figure 8.4 Simplified graph of serial mediation between intention and fruit and vegetable intake via planning and action control (Godinho et al. 2014). Path coefficients are standardized parameter estimates (beta weights)

action planning and coping planning are main candidates for bridging the intention–behaviour gap (for an overview, see Hagger and Luszczynska 2014). Planning (especially coping planning) has also been shown to independently predict behaviour change (Luszczynska 2006; Sniehotta *et al.* 2006b; Wiedemann *et al.* 2009, 2012; Conner *et al.* 2010; Pakpour *et al.* 2011; Amireault *et al.* 2013; Carraro and Gaudreau 2013; Kwasnicka *et al.* 2013).

Although planning is commonly regarded as a mediator between intention and action across a wide range of behaviours, this effect can vanish if other volitional constructs such as recovery self-efficacy or action control are included in the model. An example is the study by Godinho *et al.* (2014) on fruit and vegetable intake that included action control in the structural equation model (see Figure 8.4). Although planning was closely associated with intentions, its effect on behaviour was not a direct one but there was a serial mediation via action control. Moreover, in this study, as in some others, there was collinearity between action planning and coping planning. Depending on context, discriminant validity is sometimes missing. Thus, one can either collapse them into a single planning construct or neglect one of them.

4 Developments

The early draft of the HAPA (Schwarzer 1992) presented a quite straightforward and simple model of health behaviour. Subsequently, the HAPA has been extended by the addition and refinement of constructs. Planning has been subdivided into action planning and coping planning (Sniehotta *et al.* 2006b). The conceptualization of perceived self-efficacy has been adjusted to the point in time where it operates, resulting in pre-action self-efficacy, maintenance (or coping) self-efficacy, and recovery self-efficacy (Schwarzer and Renner 2000; Luszczynska and Schwarzer 2003; Ochsner *et al.* 2013). Action control has also been added at a later point in time (Sniehotta *et al.* 2005).

In recent years, researchers have expanded the HAPA further by exploring the inclusion of additional constructs such as social support, satisfaction, habits, and preparatory behaviours. Trait self-control has also been used within this framework (Hankonen *et al.* 2014). To account for interrelations between different health behaviours, some researchers have incorporated cross-behaviour cognitions, such as transfer from exercise to diet (Fleig *et al.* in press) and/or compensatory health cognitions (such as 'If I am a vegetarian, I don't need to exercise') (Ernsting *et al.* 2013b; Berli *et al.* 2014; Radtke *et al.* 2014).

As HAPA is an open framework, it allows for extensions by the inclusion of such additional constructs. For example, social support can be influential either in the motivational or in the volitional stage, making an impact on intentions as well as on behaviour (Chow and Mullan 2010; Scholz *et al.* 2013; Parschau *et al.* 2014; Reyes Fernández *et al.* 2014; Ernsting *et al.* 2015).

4.1 Preparatory behaviours

As researchers turn their attention towards more proximal antecedents of behaviour, instead of the intention–behaviour gap, it is the planning–behaviour gap that comes into focus. This gap can be overcome by specifying components of action control as well as preparatory acts that appear to be the most proximal antecedents of the target behaviour (Koring *et al.* 2013; Barz *et al.* 2014; Carvalho *et al.* 2015). Preparatory action is beyond cognitions and pertains to the behavioural domain that makes it a desirable secondary outcome of interventions. For example, signing up for an exercise course or selecting health foods when shopping can be useful intervention targets, although they are not the primary behavioural outcome.

When people intend and plan to perform higher levels of physical activity, they do not start on impulse without preparing. Preparation may be reflected by the acquisition of sports equipment as well as monitoring devices such as pedometers. Koring *et al.* (2013) conducted a longitudinal physical activity survey with university students who were offered a complementary pedometer. Collecting this free gift served as an indicator of preparatory behaviour. Collecting the pedometer was associated with higher levels of physical activity at follow-up. Outcome expectancies and self-efficacy predicted the likelihood to perform this preparatory behaviour.

In a study on condom use by Carvalho *et al.* (2015), planning was replaced by preparatory behaviours (buying and carrying condoms) to achieve a more proximal prediction of actual condom use. Self-reported actual condom use is an intimate and difficult behaviour and, as Carvalho *et al.*

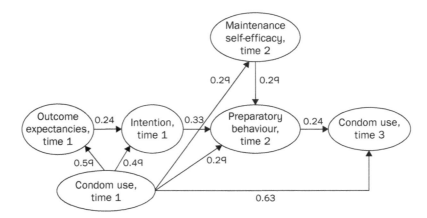

Figure 8.5 The role of preparatory behaviours and self-efficacy in predicting condom use (Carvalho *et al.* 2015). Path coefficients are standardized parameter estimates (beta weights)

discovered, is hard to assess and hard to predict. Prevention programmes that aim at preparatory behaviours constitute a small step in the right direction. In this study, preparatory behaviours were well predicted jointly by intentions, self-efficacy, and past behaviours, whereas actual behaviours were significantly, but less substantially, predicted by such preparations (see Figure 8.5).

5 Operationalization of the model

In this section, we provide example assessments for the HAPA constructs. In most research, no more than four items per construct are used. There is no recommended response format. One could use consistently 4-point, 5-point, 6-point or 7-point Likert scales.

5.1 Risk perception

Risk perception can be measured by items such as: 'How high do you rate the likelihood that you will ever get one of the following diseases, or that you will relapse to them: (a) cardiovascular disease (e.g. heart attack, stroke), (b) diseases of the musculoskeletal system (e.g. osteoarthritis)?' (with anchors of, for example, 'very low – low – high – very high'). Any other health risks can be added, especially if relevant to the individual sample included in the study (Fleig *et al.* 2011).

5.2 Outcome expectancies

Positive outcome expectancies (pros) and negative outcome expectancies (cons) can be assessed with the stem: 'If I engage in physical activity at least three [or two] times per week for 40 [or 20] minutes...' followed by pros and cons. Pros might be, for example: '...then I feel better afterwards', '...then I meet friendly people' or '...then my elasticity would increase'. Cons might be, for example: '...then every time would cost me a lot of money', '...then I would be financially burned' or '...then I would have to invest a lot of resources' (with anchors of, for example, 'not at all true – not true – true – completely true'). Examples of the assessment of outcome expectancies for dietary behaviours can be found in Godhino *et al.* (2013) and Hankonen *et al.* (2013).

5.3 Perceived self-efficacy

For self-efficacy, a semantic rule is: 'I am confident that I can... (perform an action), even if... (a barrier)'. An example of a self-efficacy item is: 'I am confident that I can skip desserts even if my family continues to eat them in my presence' (with anchors of, for example, 'not at all true – not true – true – completely true'). This semantic rule need not be applied rigidly, but might serve as a useful heuristic. For physical exercise, pre-action self-efficacy can be worded such: 'I am confident that I am able to practise at least moderate [vigorous] exercise [*this needs to be defined beforehand*] for at least [10, 20, 30, 40, etc.] minutes in one session without stopping'. Maintenance self-efficacy could be worded such: 'I am confident that I can continue to participate in this exercise programme for at least six weeks, even if...' [*here some barriers need to be defined, one for each item*]. Recovery self-efficacy could be worded: 'I am confident that I can resume my exercise programme after I have failed to be active for one [any time span] day/week even if it is hard for me [or any other barrier]'. Examples can be found in Arbour-Nicitopoulos *et al.* (2014). Bandura (2006) provides detailed guidelines on the construction of various kinds of self-efficacy measures (he also introduces a variety of possible response formats).

5.4 Planning

Action planning can be assessed with items addressing the when, where, and how of the activity. For example, the items in the rehabilitation study by Lippke *et al.* (2010) were worded: 'For the month after the rehabilitation, I have already planned...' (1) '...which physical activity I will perform (e.g. walking)', (2) '...where I will be physically active (e.g. in the park)', (3) '...on which days of the week I will be physically active', and (4) '...for how long I will be physically active'. Coping planning, on the other hand, can be measured with the item stem 'I have made a detailed plan regarding ...' and the items (1) '...what to do if something interferes with my plans', (2) '...how to cope with possible setbacks', (3) '...what to do in difficult situations in order to act according to my intentions', (4) '...which good opportunities for action to take', and (5) '...when I have to pay extra attention to prevent lapses'.

5.5 Action control

While planning is a prospective strategy – that is, behavioural plans are made before the situation is encountered – action control is a concurrent self-regulatory strategy, where the ongoing behaviour is continuously evaluated with regard to a behavioural standard. Action control has been assessed with a 6-item scale comprising three facets of the action control process (Sniehotta *et al.* 2005): self-monitoring (i.e. 'I consistently monitored myself whether I exercised frequently enough' and 'I consistently monitored when, where, and how long I exercised'), awareness of standards (i.e. 'I have always been aware of my prescribed training programme' and 'I often had my exercise intention on my mind'), and self-regulatory effort (i.e. 'I really tried hard to exercise regularly' and 'I took care to practise as much as I intended to').

5.6 Stage-based segmentation: pre-intenders, intenders, and actors

When using the continuum model for the prediction of behaviour, the HAPA constructs are specified as predictors and mediators in a path model (see Figure 8.1). When employing the stage variant to conduct an intervention study, a segmentation of the audience is performed. Stage theories employ algorithms for the staging procedure that can be regarded as a 'fast and frugal tree' with satisfactory validity (Lippke *et al.* 2009b, 2010). For a three-stage procedure, one needs several steps (see Figure 8.6). First, behaviour is assessed on the basis of a context-specific dichotomous criterion (yes = 'already active', no = 'not yet sufficiently active'). Those who meet the preselected criterion are defined as 'actors'. Those who don't are subject to the second step by asking them whether they intend to become active or not. If they do intend to do so, they are defined as 'intenders'; if they don't, they are 'non-intenders' (or 'pre-intenders'). Such straightforward diagnostic procedures may be too simple to account for response bias and temporal fluctuation. However, when subdividing large samples to assign stage-matched treatments, such a pragmatic procedure results in more homogeneous segments that allow for more effective interventions. As people proceed through an intervention, they change their mindsets

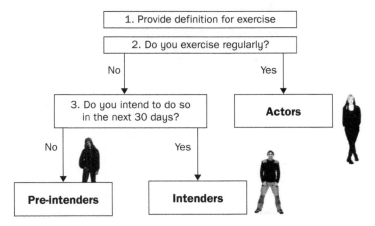

Figure 8.6 Example of a simple staging algorithm for physical exercise segmentation, yielding three subgroups as a basis for matched treatments

and accordingly their stage of change. Therefore, reassessments are needed to reassign participants to subsequent modules of a tailored intervention programme.

6 Intervention studies

In intervention studies, various behaviour change techniques (Michie *et al.* 2013) are applied to target participants' risk perceptions, outcome expectancies, and intentions in the motivational phase, whereas the self-regulatory components of self-efficacy, action planning, coping planning, and action control (self-monitoring) constitute the behavioural support to initiate and maintain the desired health behaviours. Motivational support targets intention formation as its primary outcome, whereas behavioural support targets action as its primary outcome, in line with the motivation and volition phases of the model. Most intervention studies concentrate on the mechanisms and constructs that characterize the continuum layer of HAPA. Few intervention studies make use of the stage layer (see below). As the main focus lies on the volition phase which makes HAPA distinct from other models, most studies target directly the initiation and maintenance of health behaviours, employing behaviour change techniques that are likely to serve this purpose such as goal-setting, planning, self-efficacy, feedback, and self-monitoring. Brief interventions of this kind provide participants with planning forms where they enter the when, where, and how of intended actions, and generate on top of this several coping plans, including imagined barriers and ways to overcome them. Moreover, they introduce role models by displaying testimonials of others who have coped well (for self-efficacy improvement). Additionally, daily diary forms or calendars are provided to allow for continuous self-monitoring (Gholami *et al.* 2013; Lhakhang *et al.* 2014a, 2014b; Schwarzer *et al.* 2015). As an example, Figure 8.7 displays one page from a leaflet that was part of a volitional 15-minute intervention on dental flossing in India (Lhakhang *et al.* 2014a).

There are a large number of mainly small-scale intervention studies more or less explicitly derived from HAPA. If an article reports a combination of coping planning, recovery self-efficacy

❖ Have you made a plan on flossing your teeth in addition to brushing them?
If so, please write here your most important plans regarding....

...**how often** to floss your teeth.	...**when to** floss and **how much time** to spend for flossing.	...**how to** use dental flossing.	How certain are you that you can follow these plans?			
Example: -X times a day.	Morning and before bed. At least 3 minutes each time.	Floss before brushing teeth.	❑ not at all	❑ hardly	❑ probably	☒ very certain
🖊			❑	❑	❑	❑
🖊			❑	❑	❑	❑
🖊			❑	❑	❑	❑

Remember the critical situations (such as forgetfulness) you have faced in the last two weeks when flossing your teeth and which you might face in the future. Please note in the table below your possible critical situations and coping strategies you use to cope with the help of the given example.

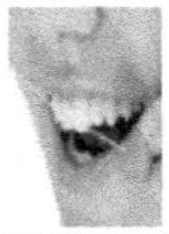

If I will face difficult situations that might prevent me from flossing... (which critical events) ⟹	...then I plan to overcome them by... (which strategies)	I am certain that I can follow these plans.			
Example: If i forget to floss...	...then I put the dental tape next to my tooth-brush.	❑ Not at all	❑ hardly	☒ probably	❑ Very certain
1.		❑	❑	❑	❑
2.		❑	❑	❑	❑
3.		❑	❑	❑	❑

Figure 8.7 Example page of a leaflet-based volitional intervention to promote dental flossing (Lhakhang *et al.*, 2014a). Participants generate action plans in the upper part, and coping plans in the lower part, and on the right-hand side, plan-specific self-efficacy is assessed

(or coping/maintenance self-efficacy), and action control (or self-monitoring), mediating between intervention and behavioural outcome, then it is considered an HAPA study, even if the model or its source is not mentioned. In other cases, where fewer of these constructs are investigated (e.g. planning and self-efficacy as mediators), it may not be clear whether the study has been derived from HAPA or not. As HAPA is an open-architecture framework, it also tends to inspire research that is not necessarily in line with the original model, and in many cases the published reports address only a narrow aspect that is in line with specific research questions, not providing a full account of the entire model that had informed the study. A meta-analysis on

HAPA-derived intervention studies is currently being conducted (Smith *et al.* 2013, 2014). In this review, authors found that there are many interventions on a narrow number of chronic-disease-related behaviours such as weight loss, and that the inconsistencies of terminology, definitions, and reporting make it hard to identify to what degree studies are really based on HAPA. So far, no quantitative details of this meta-analysis have been reported.

Large-scale HAPA projects have been conducted mainly on diet and exercise in the context of cardiovascular or diabetes risk reduction programmes, including:

- the Melbourne Diabetes Prevention Study (MDPS) (Dunbar *et al.* 2012; Davis-Lameloise *et al.* 2013);
- the German Railway metabolic syndrome prevention study (Fleig *et al.* 2010);
- the Greater Green Triangle (GGT) Diabetes Prevention Project (Laatikainen *et al.* 2007);
- the GOAL implementation study (Absetz *et al.* 2007, 2009);
- the Norfolk Diabetes Prevention Study (Murray *et al.* 2011);
- the Waste the Waist study (Gillison *et al.* 2012);
- the FaBA cardiac and orthopaedic rehabilitation study (Fleig *et al.* 2011, 2013, in press);
- the Berlin cardiac rehabilitation study (Sniehotta *et al.* 2005, 2006b);
- the Berlin Stays Fit study (older women fitness programme) (Evers *et al.* 2012);
- the Iranian Physical Activity Maintenance in Rehabilitation Project (Aliabad *et al.* 2014).

The nationwide LIFE! programme in Australia (http://www.lifeprogram.org.au) is an offspring of the MDPS and GGT, inspired by the Finnish GOAL implementation study. In these projects, the interventions typically consist of an initial individual session followed by a series of five or six structured group sessions of 1.5–2 hours in duration in groups of 6–15 participants that offer them skills, knowledge, support, and advice needed to make lifestyle changes to prevent metabolic syndrome or other cardiovascular conditions. The first few sessions are carried out at two-week intervals with the fifth or sixth sessions held six to eight months after the first one. Participants are encouraged to work towards adopting a healthy diet and active lifestyle to reduce their risk of developing the conditions. One session is co-facilitated by a physiotherapist, another by a dietitian. The sessions further address personal health goals, behavioral intentions, and outcome expectancies (e.g. the pros and cons of exercising and fruit and vegetable consumption). Action plans are further utilized to translate one's motivation to change behaviours into actions by providing participants with the self-regulatory skills needed for effective planning and action control. The sessions put particular emphasis on increasing skills to perform health behaviours by enhancing decisional balance, perceived self-efficacy, goal-setting, coping planning, and self-monitoring, the latter in the form of daily diaries that create a feedback loop, allowing comparison of one's accomplishments with one's intentions.

Many HAPA-derived interventions are in the areas of physical activity (e.g. Sniehotta *et al.* 2005, 2006b; Evers *et al.* 2012) and dietary changes (Luszczynska *et al.* 2007b; Kreausukon *et al.* 2012; Gholami *et al.* 2013; Lange *et al.* 2013; Lhakhang *et al.* 2014b), but some have addressed vaccination (Payaprom *et al.* 2011), smoking cessation (Radtke *et al.* 2011), skin cancer prevention by sunscreen use (Craciun *et al.* 2012a), breast self-examination (Luszczynska 2004), and oral self-care by dental flossing (Schüz *et al.* 2009; Gholami 2014; Lhakhang *et al.* 2014a; Schwarzer *et al.* 2015). Self-efficacy is required throughout the entire process of behaviour adoption and maintenance. The FaBA booster study found self-efficacy to be predictive of physical activity maintenance among cardiac and orthopaedic patients (Fleig *et al.* 2013). There is also evidence from rehabilitation samples on the changing nature of self-efficacy as people pass through different stages of change.

In an experimental trial to improve physical activity among orthopaedic patients, a volitional intervention worked only in study participants who were at a post-intentional stage, as hypothesized. Accordingly, planning was not beneficial for persons in the motivational stage (Lippke *et al.* 2004). This was replicated in an internet study that also demonstrated the specific mechanisms: the planning intervention facilitated change in the activity levels of the patients by means of intention and planning, but only in the case of intenders, not pre-intenders (Lippke *et al.* 2010). When exploring the effects of the planning intervention on actors, they seemed to benefit, but not as much as those who had not been active before (i.e. intenders). Such studies have confirmed that it is useful to distinguish the intention stage from the action stage. Pre-intenders first need to develop an intention before they benefit from a volitional intervention. Intenders benefit mainly from planning when adopting a new behaviour. In contrast, actors need relapse prevention that helps them to recover from setbacks, and, in case of a relapse, they need strategies for coping with them effectively.

Complex planning interventions promote sustained behaviour change after rehabilitation. Planning can be subdivided into action planning and coping planning, as has been evaluated in different samples of persons with chronic illness and disability who were supposed to improve their exercise levels. When addressing action planning and coping planning separately in interventions, different effects were found: persons in cardiac rehabilitation became more physically active when both kinds of planning were addressed in the intervention, as opposed to a mere action planning intervention (Sniehotta *et al.* 2005, 2006b). In another sample, at six months after cardiac rehabilitation, participants involved in a planning intervention consumed 13% less saturated fat than controls (Luszczynska *et al.* 2007a). In orthopaedic rehabilitation, a delayed effect of coping planning on behaviour demonstrated that coping planning seems to be of more importance for long-term maintenance: whereas behaviour adoption two weeks after rehabilitation was only correlated with action planning, coping planning came into play only four and 26 weeks later (Ziegelmann *et al.* 2006). In another study, action planning was found to be the mediator between intention and coping planning, and coping planning mediated the relationship between action planning and physical exercise (Ziegelmann and Lippke 2007). This was true for different age groups among rehabilitation participants with orthopaedic diagnoses.

In summary, an increasing number of HAPA-derived intervention studies, targeting various health behaviours in many countries, are being conducted. It is not always clear which ingredients of these studies are the most active ones because of the complex nature of the treatment packages. Identifying mediators between experimental conditions and target actions points to such active ingredients (Kreausukon *et al.* 2012; Lange *et al.* 2013; Lhakhang *et al.* 2014a).

6.1 Stage-specific analyses and matched interventions

The HAPA is designed as a sequence of two continuous self-regulatory processes, a goal-setting phase (motivation) and a goal-pursuit phase (volition). The second phase is subdivided into a pre-action phase and an action phase. One can superimpose these three phases on the continuum model as a second layer and regard phase as a moderator. This two-layer architecture allows one to switch between the continuum model and the stage model, depending on the research question. The stage layer is useful when designing stage-matched interventions (Lippke *et al.* 2004, 2010; Schüz *et al.* 2009; Craciun *et al.* 2012b; Parschau *et al.* 2012). For pre-intenders, one needs risk and resource communication, for example by addressing the pros and cons of the critical behaviour. Pre-intenders are supposed to benefit from confrontation with outcome expectancies and some level of risk communication. They need to learn that the new behaviour (e.g. becoming physically active) has positive outcomes (e.g. well-being, weight loss, fun) as opposed to the negative outcomes that accompany the current (sedentary) behaviour, such as developing an illness or being overweight. They also need to develop an optimistic belief that they are capable of performing the critical behaviour. In contrast, for intenders, planning treatments are helpful to support those who lack the necessary skills to translate their intentions into behaviour. Intenders should not benefit much from health messages in the form of outcome expectancies because, after setting a goal, they have already moved beyond this mindset. Rather, they should benefit from planning to translate their intentions into action. Finally, for actors, one needs to stabilize their newly adopted health behaviours by relapse prevention strategies. They should become ready to cope with particular high-risk situations. Interventions help them, if they so want, to change their routines (e.g. adopting, improving or altering a behaviour).

In general, interventions should not be designed in a purely rational manner, altering cognitions, because health behaviour change is also an emotional process that is analysed as a cognitive process only after people have been asked about their feelings. All the theoretical constructs are loaded with emotions in the first place. Thus, treatments need to focus on changes in emotions. The HAPA allows both the researcher and the practitioner to make a number of choices. Although it was initially inspired by distinguishing between a motivational and a volitional stage, and later extended to the distinction between pre-intenders, intenders, and actors, one need not necessarily group individuals according to such stages. For the purpose of stage-tailored interventions, however, usually two or three stage groups would be established. Stage-matched interventions require more preparation than one-size-fits-all interventions, and there are not many well-designed studies of this kind. In particular, one would need a complete match–mismatch research design to prove the appropriateness of a particular stage-matched treatment. Often such a design is not worthwhile, such as if pre-intenders can be motivated by a very brief (10 minutes) intervention to become intenders. After such a pre-treatment, all participants reside at the same stage and can benefit from an extended volitional intervention. This seems to be the case when it comes to the adoption of a simple behaviour such as dental flossing or hand washing (Zhou *et al.* 2013; Lhakhang *et al.* 2014a, 2014b). In contrast, when it involves refraining from refractory behaviours (e.g. smoking) and developing long-term adherence to health-enhancing behaviours (e.g. diet and exercise), a segmentation of the audience might be more fruitful in order to design stage-matched interventions. Research would benefit from more match–mismatch study designs (Dijkstra *et al.* 2006).

7 Future directions

7.1 Focus on more complex mechanisms

Although the universal mediator model (as in Figure 8.1) often works quite well when it comes to the description, explanation, and prediction of health behaviour change, there are also instances when it works less well. In particular, the relationships between intentions, planning, and behaviour do not always reflect a simple mediation model but might also depend on other factors. For example, the degree to which planning mediates between intentions and behaviour has been found to be higher in older than in younger persons (Renner *et al.* 2007; Scholz *et al.* 2007; Reuter *et al.* 2010; Gholami 2014). This represents a case of moderated mediation.

Mediation describes how something works, whereas moderation describes for whom something works. By comparing men and women, younger and older people, and those from different cultures, relevant moderators can be identified (Ziegelmann *et al.* 2006; Renner *et al.* 2007). When a mediator model has strong interrelations within one category of participants, but weak associations within another category, then this is a case of moderated mediation. The amount to which the mediator translates the effect of the independent variable on the dependent variable depends on the levels of a moderator variable. Perceived self-efficacy is one potential moderator of the degree to which planning has an effect on subsequent behaviours. It is expected to moderate the planning–behaviour relation because people harbouring self-doubts might fail to act upon their plans. For people with a high level of self-efficacy, planning might be more likely to facilitate goal achievement. Self-efficacious people feel more confident about translating their plans into actual behaviour. In other words, whether planning interventions (independent variable) actually affects behaviour (dependent variable) might depend on the individual's level of self-efficacy (moderator). In a study on physical activity, longitudinal data from an online survey were used to examine similar interrelationships (Lippke *et al.* 2009a). Only those persons who had a sufficiently high level of exercise self-efficacy acted upon their plans. In contrast, participants who were harbouring self-doubts failed to act upon their plans (see also Gutiérrez-Doña *et al.* 2009; Richert *et al.* 2010; Schwarzer *et al.* 2010; Luszczynska *et al.* 2011). Self-efficacy, planning, and action control, the key variables in the volitional phase, are candidates for a moderation effect (Soureti *et al.* 2012). Moreover, social support, habits, compensatory beliefs, trait self-control, conscientiousness, culture, age, and sex are good candidates for future research aimed at discovering more complex mechanisms.

The built-in moderator is, of course, stage of change. Remember that HAPA has two layers, a continuum layer and a stage layer. Depending on the research question, one might choose one or the other, or combine them. If one specifies stage as a moderator, then it implies that a mediation sequence (e.g. intention–planning–behaviour) works well at one stage but not so at a different stage.

7.2 Using modern information and communication technology

Public health promotion can benefit from information and communication technology (ICT)-based interventions such as text messaging and online courses (eHealth) as well as smartphone apps (mHealth) (Joseph *et al.* 2014). Technologies may offer strong support for health behaviour change. The availability of thousands of downloadable mHealth apps facilitates the adoption of devices to self-monitor health behaviours and conditions. This will allow users to track their goal-setting and goal-striving, changes in social cognitive variables, plans, and actual health behaviours. Information becomes easily accessible and interpretable. Web-linked devices offer a continuous environment for the access of text, image, audio, and other types of structured and semi-structured information. Built-in social media elements offer a wealth of social support options. Moreover, wearing sensors to assess physiological body responses (e.g. lifelogging) as well as tracking performance (e.g. accelerometers), coupled with powerful decision support techniques, provides a more dependable, information-rich profile of individuals as they pass through the behaviour change process. There is an overwhelming number of studies that have found advantages and limitations of web-based tailored interventions. For example, the advantages are that a large number of users can be reached at low cost and that behavioural change can be achieved after several years (Kohl *et al.* 2013; Schulz *et al.* 2014; Tang *et al.* 2014). Techniques such as email prompting to reuse the intervention platform have also been studied (Cremers *et al.* 2014). A limitation of online programmes is their high rate of attrition, as the ease of enrolment is matched by the ease of dropout (Eysenbach 2005).

Combining HAPA with ICT may optimize stratified behaviour interventions to enhance self-engagement and self-monitoring (Soureti *et al.* 2011; Lyons *et al.* 2014) because more frequent diagnostics allows the reclassification of individuals into concurrent stages, tailored for individual needs. A specific behaviour change model for internet interventions has been proposed (Ritterband *et al.* 2009) that is compatible with HAPA and other social cognitive models. This model states that environmental factors motivate the user, and the user characteristics affect website use, which, in turn, is influenced by digital support and website characteristics; behaviour then changes and is maintained through various mechanisms of change (e.g. HAPA). Plaete *et al.* (submitted) have developed a HAPA-based dynamic eHealth programme for the promotion of healthy lifestyles to be used in general practices. The intervention consists of three sessions for physical activity as well as fruit and vegetable intake, offered either on a website or tablet computers. Participants are guided to set goals, monitor their behaviour, receive tailored feedback, make action and coping plans, and increase their self-efficacy by modelling and problem-solving.

From an HAPA perspective, most of the eHealth and mHealth applications address individuals in the volition phase of health behaviour change. People do not sign up for online interventions or download smartphone apps if they don't have some level of motivation to change. Therefore, the three-stage approach described above usually does not apply to already motivated users of such ICT platforms. Users need behavioural support to overcome obstacles and maintain health behaviours after initiation. Here, a number of behaviour change techniques can be applied to support planning, action control, and maintenance self-efficacy.

The advanced technology allows for immediate feedback loops that keep users online, monitoring lapses as well as progress, and providing resource information that is individually tailored. Thus, what may be seen as a weakness of HAPA, its hybrid open architecture framework, may turn out to become a strength when technology allows for more fine-grained process characteristics to be included in the implementation of the model.

In conclusion, HAPA is becoming more appealing to health psychologists, after a great deal of research in the last decade has underscored the validity of its assumptions. Cumulative evidence shows that the shift from rather static motivation and attitude variables to more dynamic self-regulatory variables such as coping planning, maintenance self-efficacy, and action control is a promising step towards a better understanding of health behaviour change. The strength of the model lies in its focus on mediating mechanisms involving several volitional constructs. Future research should examine whether some of the putative mediators work better as moderators. In the past, more attention was paid to the continuum layer than to the stage layer. The latter is likely to come more to the fore as advanced technologies provide better opportunities for individual tailoring, instead of matching participants to only two or three stages.

References

Abraham, C. and Sheeran, P. (2000) Understanding and changing health behaviour: from health beliefs to self-regulation, in P. Norman, C. Abraham and M. Conner (eds.) *Understanding and Changing Health Behaviour* (pp. 3–24). Amsterdam: Harwood.

Absetz, P., Oldenburg, B., Hankonen, N., Valve, R., Heinonen, H., Nissinen, A. *et al.* (2009) Type 2 diabetes prevention in the real world: three-year results of the GOAL Lifestyle Implementation Trial, *Diabetes Care*, 32, 1418–20.

Absetz, P., Valve, R., Oldenburg, B., Heinonen, H., Nissinen, A., Fogelholm, M. *et al.* (2007) Type 2 diabetes prevention in the 'real world': one-year results of the GOAL Implementation Trial, *Diabetes Care*, 30, 2465–70.

Aliabad, H.O., Vafaeinasab, M., Morowatisharifabad, M.A., Afshani, S.A., Firoozabadi, M.G. and Forouzannia, S.K. (2014) Maintenance of physical activity and exercise capacity after rehabilitation in coronary heart disease: a randomized controlled trial, *Global Journal of Health Science*, 6 (6), 198–208.

Amireault, S., Godin, G. and Vézina-Im, L.-A. (2013) Determinants of physical activity maintenance: a systematic review and meta-analyses, *Health Psychology Review*, 7, 55–91.

Arbour-Nicitopoulos, K.P., Duncan, M., Remington, G., Cairney, J. and Faulkner, G.E. (2014) Development and reliability testing of a health action process approach inventory for physical activity participation among individuals with schizophrenia, *Frontiers in Psychiatry*, 5: 68.

Auster, J., Hurst, C., Neale, R.E., Youl, P., Whiteman, D.C., Baade, P. *et al.* (2013) Determinants of uptake of whole-body skin self-examination in older men, *Behavioral Medicine*, 39, 36–43.

Bandura, A. (1986) *Social Foundations of Thought and Action*. Englewood Cliffs, NJ: Prentice-Hall.

Bandura, A. (1997) *Self-efficacy: The Exercise of Control*. New York: Freeman.

Bandura, A. (2006) Guide for creating self-efficacy scales, in F. Pajares and T. Urdan (eds.) *Self-efficacy Beliefs of Adolescents* (pp. 307–38). Greenwich, CT: Information Age Publishing.

Barg, C.J., Latimer, A.E., Pomery, E.A., Rivers, S.E., Rench, T.A., Prapavessis, H. *et al.* (2012) Examining predictors of physical activity among inactive middle-aged women: an application of the health action process approach, *Psychology and Health*, 27, 829–45.

Barz, M., Parschau, L., Warner, L.M., Lange, D., Fleig, L., Knoll, N. *et al.* (2014) Planning and preparatory actions facilitate physical activity maintenance, *Psychology of Sport and Exercise*, 15, 516–20.

Berli, C., Loretini, P., Radtke, T., Hornung, R. and Scholz, U. (2014) Predicting physical activity in adolescents: the role of compensatory health beliefs within the Health Action Process Approach, *Psychology and Health*, 29, 458–74.

Carraro, N. and Gaudreau, P. (2013) Spontaneous and experimentally induced action planning and coping planning for physical activity: a meta-analysis, *Psychology of Sport and Exercise*, 14, 228–48.

Carvalho, T., Alvarez, M.J., Barz, M. and Schwarzer, R. (2015) Preparatory behavior for condom use among heterosexual young men: a longitudinal mediation model, *Health Education and Behavior*, 42, 92–9.

Caudroit, J., Stephan, Y. and Le Scanff, C. (2011) Social cognitive determinants of physical activity among retired older individuals: an application of the health action process approach, *British Journal of Health Psychology*, 16, 404–17.

Chiu, C.-Y., Lynch, R.T., Chan, F. and Berven, N.L. (2011) The Health Action Process Approach as a motivational model for physical activity self-management for people with multiple sclerosis: a path analysis, *Rehabilitation Psychology*, 56, 171–81.

Chow, S. and Mullan, B. (2010) Predicting food hygiene: an investigation of social factors and past behaviour in an extended model of the Health Action Process Approach, *Appetite*, 54, 126–33.

Conner, M., Sandberg, T. and Norman, P. (2010) Using action planning to promote exercise behavior, *Annals of Behavioral Medicine*, 40, 65–76.

Craciun, C., Schüz, N., Lippke, S. and Schwarzer, R. (2012a) A mediator model of sunscreen use: a longitudinal analysis of social-cognitive predictors and mediators, *International Journal of Behavioral Medicine*, 19, 65–72.

Craciun, C., Schüz, N., Lippke, S. and Schwarzer, R. (2012b) Enhancing planning strategies for sunscreen use at different stages of change, *Health Education Research*, 27, 857–67.

Cremers, H.P., Mercken, L., Crutzen, R., Willems, P., de Vries, H. and Oenema, A. (2014) Do email and mobile phone prompts simulate primary school children to reuse an internet-delivered smoking prevention intervention? *Journal of Medical Internet Research*, 16 (3): e86.

Davis-Lameloise, N., Hernan, A., Janus, E.D., Stewart, E., Carter, R., Bennett, C.M. et al. (2013) The Melbourne Diabetes Prevention Study (MDPS): study protocol for a randomized controlled trial, *Trials*, 14, 31.

Dijkstra, A., Conijn, B. and De Vries, H. (2006) A match–mismatch test of a stage model of behaviour change in tobacco smoking, *Addiction*, 101, 1035–43.

Doran, G.T. (1981) There's a S.M.A.R.T. way to write management's goals and objectives. *Management Review (AMA FORUM)*, 70 (11), 35–6.

Dumitrescu, A.L., Dogaru, B.C., Duta, C. and Manolescu, B.N. (2014) Testing five social-cognitive models to explain predictors of personal oral health behaviours and intention to improve them, *Oral Health Prevention Dentistry*, 12, 345–55.

Dunbar, J., Hernan, A., Janus, E., Davis-Lameloise, N., Asproloupos, D., O'Reilly, S. *et al.* (2012) Implementation salvage experiences from the Melbourne diabetes prevention study, *BMC Public Health*, 12: 806.

Ernsting, A., Gellert, P., Schneider, M. and Lippke, S. (201a) A mediator model to predict workplace influenza vaccination behaviour: an application of the health action process approach, *Psychology and Health*, 28, 579–92.

Ernsting, A., Schneider, M., Knoll, N. and Schwarzer, R. (2015) The enabling effect of social support on vaccination uptake via self-efficacy and planning, *Psychology, Health and Medicine*, 20, 239–46.

Ernsting, A., Schwarzer, R., Lippke, S. and Schneider, M. (2013b) 'I do not need a flu shot because I lead a healthy lifestyle': compensatory health beliefs make vaccination less likely, *Journal of Health Psychology*, 18, 825–36.

Evers, A., Klusmann, V., Schwarzer, R. and Heuser, I. (2012) Adherence to physical and mental activity interventions: coping plans as a mediator and prior adherence as a moderator, *British Journal of Health Psychology*, 17, 477–91.

Eysenbach, G. (2005) The law of attrition, *Journal of Medical Internet Research*, 7 (1), e11.

Fishbein, M. and Ajzen, I. (2010) *Predicting and Changing Behavior: The Reasoned Action Approach*. New York: Psychology Press.

Fleig, L., Küper, C., Schwarzer, R., Lippke, S. and Wiedemann, A.U. (in press) Cross-behavior associations and multiple behavior change: a longitudinal study on physical activity and fruit and vegetable intake, *Journal of Behavioral Medicine*.

Fleig, L., Lippke, S., Pomp, S. and Schwarzer, R. (2011) Exercise maintenance after rehabilitation: how experience can make a difference, *Psychology of Sport and Exercise*, 12, 293–9.

Fleig, L., Lippke, S., Wiedemann, A.U., Ziegelmann, J.P., Reuter, T. and Gravert, C. (2010) Förderung von körperlicher Aktivität im betrieblichen Kontext [Physical activity promotion in the workplace], *Zeitschrift für Gesundheitspsychologie*, 18 (2), 69–78.

Fleig, L., Pomp, S., Parschau, L., Barz, M., Lange, D., Schwarzer, R. *et al.* (2013) From intentions via planning and behavior to physical exercise habits, *Psychology of Sport and Exercise*, 14, 632–9.

Gellert, P., Ziegelmann, J.P., Krupka, S., Knoll, N. and Schwarzer, R. (2014) An age-tailored intervention sustains physical activity changes in older adults: a randomized controlled trial, *International Journal of Behavioral Medicine*, 21, 519–28.

Gholami, M. (2014) Self regulation and health behavior across the life span. Doctoral dissertation, Freie Universität Berlin [http://www.diss.fu-berlin.de/diss/servlets/MCRFileNodeServlet/FUDISS_derivate_000000015447/Dissertation_Maryam_Gholami_online_submission.pdf;jsessionid=B7C992882B27C8A262FCC10DD0AAAED2?hosts=].

Gholami, M., Lange, D., Luszczynska, A., Knoll, N. and Schwarzer, R. (2013) A dietary planning intervention increases fruit consumption in Iranian women, *Appetite*, 63, 1–6.

Gillison, F., Greaves, C.J., Stathi, A., Ramsay, R., Bennett, P., Taylor, G. *et al.* (2012) 'Waste the waist': the development of an intervention to promote changes in diet and physical activity for people with high cardiovascular risk, *British Journal of Health Psychology*, 17, 327–45.

Ginis, K.A., Tomasone, J.R., Latimer-Cheung, A.E., Arbour-Nicitopoulos, K.P., Bassett-Gunter, R.L. and Wolfe, D.L. (2013) Developing physical activity interventions for adults with spinal cord injury. Part 1: A comparison of social cognitions across actors, intenders, and nonintenders, *Rehabilitation Psychology*, 58, 299–306.

Godin, G. and Kok, G. (1996) The theory of planned behavior: a review of its applications to health-related behaviors, *American Journal of Health Promotion*, 11, 87–97.

Godinho, C.A., Alvarez, M.J. and Lima, M.L. (2013) Formative research on HAPA model determinants for fruit and vegetable intake: target beliefs for audiences at different stages of change, *Health Education Research*, 28, 1014–28.

Godinho, C.A., Alvarez, M.J., Lima, M.L. and Schwarzer, R. (2014) Will is not enough: coping planning and action control as mediators in the prediction of fruit and vegetable intake, *British Journal of Health Psychology*, 19, 856–70.

Gollwitzer, P.M. and Sheeran, P. (2006) Implementation intentions and goal achievement: a meta-analysis of effects and processes, *Advances in Experimental Social Psychology*, 38, 69–119.

Gutiérrez-Doña, B., Lippke, S., Renner, B., Kwon, S. and Schwarzer, R. (2009) How self-efficacy and planning predict dietary behaviors in Costa Rican and South Korean women: a moderated mediation analysis, *Applied Psychology: Health and Well-Being*, 1, 91–104.

Hagger, M.S. and Luszczynska, A. (2014) Implementation intention and action planning interventions in health contexts: state of the research and proposals for the way forward, *Applied Psychology: Health and Well-Being*, 6, 1–47.

Hankonen, N., Absetz, P., Kinnunen, M., Haukkala, A. and Jallinoja, P. (2013) Toward identifying a broader range of social cognitive determinants of dietary intentions and behaviors, *Applied Psychology: Health and Well-Being*, 5, 118–35.

Hankonen, N., Kinnunen, M., Absetz, P. and Jallinoja, P. (2014) Why do people high in self-control eat more healthily? Social cognitions as mediators, *Annals of Behavioral Medicine*, 47, 242–8.

Heckhausen, H. (1980) *Motivation und Handeln. Lehrbuch der Motivationspsychologie [Motivation and Action: Textbook of Motivation Psychology]*. Berlin: Springer.

Joseph, R.P., Durant, N.H., Benitez, T.J. and Pekmezi, D.W. (2014) Internet-based physical activity interventions, *American Journal of Lifestyle Medicine*, 8, 42–68.

Kassavou, A., Turner, A., Hamborg, T. and French, D.P. (2014) Predicting maintenance of attendance at walking groups: testing constructs from three leading maintenance theories, *Health Psychology*, 33, 752–6.

Kohl, L., Crutzen, R. and de Vries, N.K. (2013) Online prevention aimed at lifestyle behaviors: a systematic review of reviews, *Journal of Medical Internet Research*, 15 (7), e146.

Koring, M., Parschau, L., Lange, D., Fleig, L., Knoll, N. and Schwarzer, R. (2013) Preparing for physical activity: pedometer acquisition as a self-regulatory strategy, *Applied Psychology: Health and Well-Being*, 5, 136–47.

Kreausukon, P., Gellert, P., Lippke, S. and Schwarzer, R. (2012) Planning and self-efficacy can increase fruit and vegetable consumption: a randomized controlled trial, *Journal of Behavioral Medicine*, 35, 443–51.

Kwasnicka, D., Presseau, J., White, M. and Sniehotta, F.F. (2013) Does planning how to cope with anticipated barriers facilitate health-related behaviour change? A systematic review, *Health Psychology Review*, 7, 129–45.

Laatikainen, T., Dunbar, J.A., Chapman, A., Kilkkinen, A., Vartiainen, E., Heistaro, S. *et al.* (2007) Prevention of type 2 diabetes by lifestyle intervention in an Australian primary health care setting: Greater Green Triangle (GGT) Diabetes Prevention Project, *BMC Public Health*, 7, 249–56.

Lange, D., Richert, J., Koring, M., Knoll, N., Schwarzer, R. and Lippke, S. (2013) Self-regulation prompts can increase fruit consumption: a one-hour randomized controlled online trial, *Psychology and Health*, 28, 533–45.

Lhakhang, P., Gholami, M., Knoll, N. and Schwarzer, R. (in press) Comparing an educational with a self-regulatory intervention to adopt a dental flossing regimen, *Psychology, Health and Medicine*.

Lhakhang, P., Godinho, C., Knoll, N. and Schwarzer, R. (2014) A self-regulatory intervention increases fruit and vegetable intake: a comparison of two intervention sequences, *Appetite*, 82, 103–10.

Lippke, S. and Plotnikoff, R.C. (2014) Testing two principles of the Health Action Process Approach in individuals with type 2 diabetes, *Health Psychology*, 33, 77–84.

Lippke, S., Fleig, L., Pomp, S. and Schwarzer, R. (2010) Validity of a stage algorithm for physical activity in participants recruited from orthopedic and cardiac rehabilitation clinics, *Rehabilitation Psychology*, 55, 398–408.

Lippke, S., Wiedemann, A.U., Ziegelmann, J.P., Reuter, T. and Schwarzer, R. (2009a) Self-efficacy moderates the mediation of intentions into behavior via plans, *American Journal of Health Behavior*, 33, 521–9.

Lippke, S., Ziegelmann, J.P. and Schwarzer, R. (2004) Initiation and maintenance of physical exercise: stage-specific effects of a planning intervention, *Research in Sports Medicine*, 12, 221–40.

Lippke, S., Ziegelmann, J.P. and Schwarzer, R. (2005) Stage-specific adoption and maintenance of physical activity: testing a three-stage model, *Psychology of Sport and Exercise*, 6, 585–603.

Lippke, S., Ziegelmann, J.P., Schwarzer, R. and Velicer, W.F. (2009b) Validity of stage assessment in the adoption and maintenance of physical activity and fruit and vegetable consumption, *Health Psychology*, 28, 183–93.

Luszczynska, A. (2004) Change in breast self-examination behavior: effects of intervention on enhancing self-efficacy, *International Journal of Behavioral Medicine*, 11, 95–103.

Luszczynska, A. (2006) An implementation intentions intervention, the use of planning strategy, and physical activity after myocardial infarction, *Social Science and Medicine*, 62, 900–8.

Luszczynska, A. and Schwarzer, R. (2003) Planning and self-efficacy in the adoption and maintenance of breast self-examination: a longitudinal study on self-regulatory cognitions, *Psychology and Health*, 18, 93–108.

Luszczynska, A. and Sutton, S. (2006) Physical activity after cardiac rehabilitation: evidence that different types of self-efficacy are important in maintainers and relapsers, *Rehabilitation Psychology*, 51, 314–21.

Luszczynska, A., Scholz, U. and Sutton, S. (2007a) Planning to change diet: a randomized controlled trial of an implementation intentions training intervention to reduce saturated fat intake after myocardial infarction, *Journal of Psychosomatic Research*, 63, 491–7.

Luszczynska, A., Schwarzer, R., Lippke, S. and Mazurkiewicz, M. (2011) Self-efficacy as a moderator of the planning–behaviour relationship in interventions designed to promote physical activity, *Psychology and Health*, 26, 151–66.

Luszczynska, A., Tryburcy, M. and Schwarzer, R. (2007b) Improving fruit and vegetable consumption: a self-efficacy intervention compared to a combined self-efficacy and planning intervention, *Health Education Research*, 22, 630–8.

Lyons, E.J., Lewis, Z.H., Mayrsohn, B.G. and Rowland, J.L. (2014) Behavior change techniques implemented in electronic lifestyle activity monitors: a systematic content analysis, *Journal of Medical Internet Research*, 16, e192.

Marlatt, G.A., Baer, J.S. and Quigley, L.A. (1995) Self-efficacy and addictive behavior, in A. Bandura (ed.) *Self-efficacy in Changing Societies* (pp. 289–315). New York: Cambridge University Press.

Matterne, U., Diepgen, T.L. and Weisshaar, E. (2011) A longitudinal application of three health behaviour models in the context of skin protection behaviour in individuals with occupational skin disease, *Psychology and Health*, 26, 1188–207

Michie, S., Richardson, M., Johnston, M., Abraham, C., Francis, J., Hardeman, W. *et al.* (2013) The behavior change technique taxonomy (v1) of 93 hierarchically clustered techniques: building an international consensus for the reporting of behavior change interventions, *Annals of Behavioral Medicine*, 46, 81–95.

Murgraff, V., McDermott, M.R. and Walsh, J. (2003) Self-efficacy and behavioral enactment: the application of Schwarzer's Health Action Process Approach to the prediction of low-risk, single-occasion drinking, *Journal of Applied Social Psychology*, 33, 339–61.

Murray, N., Abadi, S., Blair, A., Dunk, M. and Sampson, M.J. (2011) The importance of type 2 diabetes prevention: the Norfolk Diabetes Prevention Study, *British Journal of Diabetes and Vascular Disease*, 11, 308–13.

Ochsner, S., Scholz, U. and Hornung, R. (2013) Testing phase-specific self-efficacy beliefs in the context of dietary behaviour change, *Applied Psychology: Health and Well-Being*, 5, 99–117.

Pakpour, A.H., Zeidi, I.M., Chatzisarantis, N., Molsted, S., Harrison, A.P. and Plotnikoff, R.C. (2011) Effects of action planning and coping planning within the theory of planned behaviour: a physical activity study of patients undergoing haemodialysis, *Psychology of Sport and Exercise*, 12, 609–14.

Parschau, L., Barz, M., Richert, J., Knoll, N., Lippke, S. and Schwarzer, R. (2014) Physical activity among adults with obesity: testing the Health Action Process Approach, *Rehabilitation Psychology*, 59, 42–9.

Parschau, L., Fleig, L., Koring, M., Lange, D., Knoll, N., Schwarzer, R. *et al.* (2013) Positive experience, self-efficacy, and action control predict physical activity changes: a moderated mediation analysis, *British Journal of Health Psychology*, 18, 395–406.

Parschau, L., Richert, J., Koring, M., Ernsting, A., Lippke, S. and Schwarzer, R. (2012) Changes in social-cognitive variables are associated with stage transitions in physical activity, *Health Education Research*, 27, 129–40.

Payaprom, Y., Bennett, P., Alabaster, E. and Tantipong, H. (2011) Using the Health Action Process Approach and implementation intention to increase flu vaccination uptake in high risk Thai individuals: a controlled before–after trial, *Health Psychology*, 30, 492–500.

Perrier, M.J., Sweet, S.N., Strachan, S.M. and Latimer-Cheung, A.E. (2012) 'I act, therefore I am': athletic identity and the health action process approach predict sport participation among individuals with acquired physical disabilities, *Psychology of Sport and Exercise*, 13, 713–20.

Plaete, J., De Bourdeaudhuij, I., Verloigne, M., Oenema, A. and Crombez, G. (submitted) The development of an eHealth intervention to promote physical activity and fruit and vegetable intake among adults who visit general practice. Manuscript submitted for publication.

Prochaska, J.O. and DiClemente, C.C. (1983) Stages and processes of self-change of smoking: toward an integrative model of change, *Journal of Consulting and Clinical Psychology*, 51, 390–5.

Radtke, T., Kaklamanou, D., Scholz, U., Hornung, R. and Armitage, C.J. (2014) Are diet-specific compensatory health beliefs predictive of dieting intentions and behaviour? *Appetite*, 76, 36–43.

Radtke, T., Scholz, U., Keller, R. and Hornung, R. (2011) Smoking is ok as long as I eat healthily: compensatory health beliefs and their role for intentions and smoking within the Health Action Process Approach, *Psychology and Health*, 27 (suppl. 2), 91–107.

Renner, B. and Schupp, H. (2011) The perception of health risks, iIn H. Friedman (ed.) *The Oxford Handbook of Health Psychology* (pp. 637–66). Oxford Library of Psychology, Part 4. New York: Oxford University Press.

Renner, B., Kwon, S., Yang, B.-H., Paik, K.-C., Kim, S.H., Roh, S. *et al.* (2008) Social-cognitive predictors of dietary behaviors in South Korean men and women, *International Journal of Behavioral Medicine*, 15, 4–13.

Renner, B., Spivak, Y., Kwon, S. and Schwarzer, R. (2007) Does age make a difference? Predicting physical activity of South Koreans, *Psychology and Aging*, 22, 482–93.

Reuter, T., Ziegelmann, J.P., Wiedemann, A.U., Lippke, S., Schüz, B. and Aiken, L.S. (2010) Planning bridges the intention–behaviour gap: age makes a difference and strategy use explains why, *Psychology and Health*, 25, 873–87.

Reyes Fernández, B., Montenegro-Montenegro, E., Knoll, N. and Schwarzer, R. (2014) Self-efficacy, action control, and social support explain physical activity changes among Costa Rican older adults, *Journal of Physical Activity and Health* [DOI: 10.1123/jpah.2013-0175].

Richert, J., Reuter, T., Wiedemann, A.U., Lippke, S., Ziegelmann, J. and Schwarzer, R. (2010) Differential effects of planning and self-efficacy on fruit and vegetable consumption, *Appetite*, 54, 611–14.

Ritterband, L.M., Thorndike, F.P., Cox, D.J., Kovatchev, B.P. and Gonder-Frederick, L.A. (2009) A behavior change model for internet interventions, *Annals of Behavioral Medicine*, 38, 18–27.

Rodgers, W.M., Murray, T.C., Courneya, K.S., Bell, G.J. and Harber, V.J. (2009) The specificity of self-efficacy over the course of a progressive exercise program, *Applied Psychology: Health and Well-Being*, 1, 211–32.

Scholz, U., Keller, R. and Perren, S. (2009a) Predicting behavioral intentions and physical exercise: a test of the health action process approach at the intrapersonal level, *Health Psychology*, 28, 702–8.

Scholz, U., Nagy, G., Göhner, W., Luszczynska, A. and Kliegel, M. (2009b) Changes in self-regulatory cognitions as predictors of changes in smoking and nutrition behaviour, *Psychology and Health*, 24, 545–61.

Scholz, U., Ochsner, S., Hornung, R. and Knoll, N. (2013) Does social support really help to eat a low-fat diet? Main effects and gender differences of received social support within the Health Action Process Approach, *Applied Psychology: Health and Well Being*, 5, 270–90.

Scholz, U., Schüz, B., Ziegelmann, J.P., Lippke, S. and Schwarzer, R. (2008) Beyond behavioural intentions: planning mediates between intentions and physical activity, *British Journal of Health Psychology*, 13, 479–94.

Scholz, U., Sniehotta, F.F. and Schwarzer, R. (2005) Predicting physical exercise in cardiac rehabilitation: the role of phase-specific self-efficacy beliefs, *Journal of Sport and Exercise Psychology*, 27, 135–51.

Scholz, U., Sniehotta, F.F., Burkert, S. and Schwarzer, R. (2007) Increasing physical exercise levels: age-specific benefits of planning, *Journal of Aging and Health*, 19, 851–66.

Schulz, D.N., Kremers, S.P., Vandelanotte, C., van Adrichem, M., Schneider, F., Candel, M. *et al.* (2014). Effects of a web-based tailored multiple-lifestyle intervention for adults: a two-year randomized controlled trial comparing sequential and simultaneous delivery modes, *Journal of Medical Internet Research*, 16 (1), e26.

Schüz, B., Sniehotta, F.F., Mallach, N., Wiedemann, A. and Schwarzer, R. (2009) Predicting transitions from pre-intentional, intentional and actional stages of change: adherence to oral self-care recommendations, *Health Education Research*, 24, 64–75.

Schwarzer, R. (1992) Self-efficacy in the adoption and maintenance of health behaviors: theoretical approaches and a new model, in R. Schwarzer (ed.) *Self-efficacy: Thought Control of Action* (pp. 217–43). Washington, DC: Hemisphere.

Schwarzer, R. (2008) Modeling health behavior change: how to predict and modify the adoption and maintenance of health behaviors, *Applied Psychology: An International Review*, 57, 1–29.

Schwarzer, R. and Luszczynska, A. (2008) How to overcome health-compromising behaviors: the health action process approach, *European Psychologist*, 2, 141–51.

Schwarzer, R. and Renner, B. (2000) Social-cognitive predictors of health behavior: action self-efficacy and coping self-efficacy, *Health Psychology*, 19, 487–95.

Schwarzer, R., Antoniuk, A. and Gholami, M. (2015) A brief intervention changing oral self-care, self-efficacy, and self-monitoring, *British Journal of Health Psychology*, 20, 56–67.

Schwarzer, R., Richert, J., Kreausukon, P., Remme, L., Wiedemann, A.U. and Reuter, T. (2010) Translating intentions into nutrition behaviors via planning requires self-efficacy: evidence from Thailand and Germany, *International Journal of Psychology*, 54, 260–8.

Schwarzer, R., Schüz, B., Ziegelmann, J.P., Lippke, S., Luszczynska, A. and Scholz, U. (2007) Adoption and maintenance of four health behaviors: theory-guided longitudinal studies on dental flossing, seat belt use, dietary behavior, and physical activity, *Annals of Behavioral Medicine*, 33, 156–66.

Sheeran, P. (2002) Intention–behavior relations: a conceptual and empirical review, *European Review of Social Psychology*, 12, 1–36.

Smith, J., Blockley, K., Murray, N., Greaves, C., Abraham, C. and Hooper, L. (2013) *A systematic review of intervention studies using Health Action Process Approach (HAPA) model components to target behaviours for preventing and managing chronic diseases.* PROSPERO International Prospective Register of Systematic Reviews, York University, UK.

Smith, J., Murray, N., Greaves, C., Hooper, L. and Abraham, C. (2014) *A systematic review of intervention studies using Health Action Process Approach (HAPA) model components to target behaviours for preventing and managing chronic diseases*, Presentation to the meeting of the European Health Psychology Society.

Sniehotta, F.F., Nagy, G., Scholz, U. and Schwarzer, R. (2006a) The role of action control in implementing intentions during the first weeks of behaviour change, *British Journal of Social Psychology*, 45, 87–106.

Sniehotta, F.F., Scholz, U. and Schwarzer, R. (2005) Bridging the intention–behaviour gap: planning, self-efficacy, and action control in the adoption and maintenance of physical exercise, *Psychology and Health*, 20, 143–60.

Sniehotta, F.F., Scholz, U. and Schwarzer, R. (2006b) Action plans and coping plans for physical exercise: a longitudinal intervention study in cardiac rehabilitation, *British Journal of Health Psychology*, 11, 23–37.

Soureti, A., Hurling, R., Van Mechelen, W., Cobain, M. and Chinapaw, M. (2012) Moderators of the mediated effect of intentions, planning, and saturated-fat intake in obese individuals, *Health Psychology*, 31, 371–9.

Soureti, A., Murray, P., Cobain, M., Chinapaw, M., van Mechelen, W. and Hurling, R. (2011) Exploratory study of web-based planning and mobile text reminders in an overweight population, *International Journal of Medical Internet Research*, 13 (4), e118.

Szczepanska, W.K., Scholz, U., Liszewska, N. and Luszczynska, A. (2013) Social and cognitive predictors of fruit and vegetable intake among adolescents: the context of changes in body weight, *Journal of Health Psychology*, 18, 667–9.

Tang, J., Abraham, C., Greaves, C. and Yates, T. (2014) Self-directed interventions to promote weight loss: a systematic review of reviews, *Journal of Medical Internet Research*, 16 (2), e58.

Teng, Y. and Mak, W.W.S. (2011) The role of planning and self-efficacy in condom use among men who have sex with men: an application of the Health Action Process Approach model, *Health Psychology*, 30, 119–28.

Wiedemann, A.U., Lippke, S. and Schwarzer, R. (2012) Multiple plans and memory performance: results of a randomized controlled trial targeting fruit and vegetable intake, *Journal of Behavioral Medicine*, 35, 387–92.

Wiedemann, A.U., Schüz, B., Sniehotta, F., Scholz, U. and Schwarzer, R. (2009) Disentangling the relation between intentions, planning, and behaviour: a moderated mediation analysis, *Psychology and Health*, 24, 67–79.

Williams, D.M., Anderson, E.S. and Winett, R.A. (2005) A review of the outcome expectancy construct in physical activity research, *Annals of Behavioral Medicine*, 29, 70–9.

Zhou, G., Gan, Y., Knoll, N. and Schwarzer, R. (2013) Proactive coping moderates the dietary intention–planning–behavior path, *Appetite*, 70, 127–33.

Ziegelmann, J.P. and Lippke, S. (2007) Planning and strategy use in health behavior change: a life span view, *International Journal of Behavioral Medicine*, 14, 30–9.

Ziegelmann, J.P., Lippke, S. and Schwarzer, R. (2006) Adoption and maintenance of physical activity: planning interventions in young, middle-aged, and older adults, *Psychology and Health*, 21, 145–63.

Chapter **9**

Stage theories

Stephen Sutton

1 General background

This chapter discusses two leading stage theories of health behaviour: the transtheoretical model (TTM; Prochaska and DiClemente 1983; Prochaska *et al.* 1992, 2008; Prochaska and Velicer 1997) and the precaution adoption process model (PAPM; Weinstein and Sandman 1992, 2002b; Weinstein *et al.* 2008). Other stage theories that should be mentioned, but are not discussed in this chapter, include: the health behaviour goal model (Gebhardt 1997; Maes and Gebhardt 2000); the Rubicon model, or model of action phases (Heckhausen 1991; Gollwitzer 1996); a four-stage model that forms the theoretical background to the work on implementation intentions (see Prestwich *et al.*, Chapter 10 this volume); the perspectives on change model (Borland *et al.* 2004); the AIDS risk reduction model (Catania *et al.* 1990); and theories of delay in seeking health care (Safer *et al.* 1979; Andersen *et al.* 1995; Scott *et al.* 2013). The health action process approach (HAPA; Schwarzer 2008; Schwarzer and Luszczynska, Chapter 8 this volume) is often classed as a stage model but to date it has been more frequently specified and tested as a continuum model (Sutton 2005, 2008a).

The chapter begins by presenting a hypothetical three-stage theory to explain the assumptions of stage theories and how they differ from continuum theories, and then discusses the TTM and the PAPM in turn.

1.1 A hypothetical three-stage theory

Figure 9.1 shows a hypothetical three-stage theory, in which the stages are assumed to be discrete. According to the theory, a person can move from Stage I to Stage III only via Stage II. The lower-case letters a–e are causal factors that are hypothesized to influence the stage transitions. Increases in factors a–c are assumed to increase the likelihood that the person will move from Stage I to Stage II; similarly, increases in factors c–e are held to increase the likelihood that a

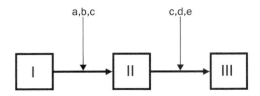

Figure 9.1 Hypothetical three-stage model

person in Stage II will move to Stage III. Thus, variables a–e are the independent variables and the transitions from one stage to the next are the dependent variables. In the simplest case, the latter can be treated as dichotomous: a person either stays in the same stage or moves to the next.

A key assumption of stage theories is that different factors are important at different stages. In this example, the set of factors that influence the transition from Stage I to Stage II, {a, b, c}, differs from the set of factors that influence the transition from Stage II to Stage III, {c, d, e}. Note that factor c influences both transitions. This is allowable, even if c has the same effect size for each of the two transitions, because the causal factors still differ as a set.

A more fully specified version of the theory would also specify the causal relationships among the explanatory factors that influence each transition. For example, for the first transition, one might specify that factors a, b, and c each have direct effects on the probability of stage movement but that a also has an indirect effect via b. This amounts to specifying a separate causal model for each transition.

A stage theory may be made more complex by incorporating additional stages and additional explanatory variables, and by allowing backward transitions and transitions to non-adjacent stages. However, even the simple three-stage theory outlined above has a more complex structure than most of the theories discussed in this book. A corollary of this complexity is that stage theories are also more difficult to test than other kinds of theories. More specifically, stage theories should be contrasted with continuum theories. *Continuum* theories specify a single prediction equation for behaviour; for example, the health belief model (Becker 1974; Abraham and Sheeran, Chapter 2 this volume) specifies that behaviour is influenced by perceived susceptibility, severity, benefits, and barriers. The difference in structure of these two types of theories has implications for how they are tested and used as the basis for health behaviour interventions. An intervention based on a continuum theory should target the determinants of behaviour that are specified by the theory, whereas for a stage theory, different interventions are required for people in different stages to encourage or help them to move to the next stage.

2 The transtheoretical model

2.1 Description of the model

The transtheoretical model (TTM) is the dominant stage model in health psychology and health promotion. It was developed in the 1980s by a group of researchers at the University of Rhode Island (hereafter referred to as the Rhode Island group). The model derived partly from an analysis of systems of psychotherapy but some of the first empirical applications were to smoking cessation (e.g. DiClemente and Prochaska 1982; Prochaska and DiClemente 1983). It has since been applied to a wide range of different health behaviours (Hall and Rossi 2008), although smoking remains the most popular application of the model. Although it is often referred to simply as the stages of change model, the TTM includes several different constructs: the *stages of change*, the *pros and cons of changing* (together known as *decisional balance*), *confidence and temptation*, and the *processes of change* (Table 9.1). The TTM was an attempt to integrate these different constructs drawn from different theories of behaviour change and systems of psychotherapy into a single coherent model, hence the name transtheoretical.

The stages of change provide the basic organizing structure. The most widely used version of the model specifies five stages: pre-contemplation, contemplation, preparation, action, and maintenance. (Some versions of the model also include a 'termination' stage in which the person has permanently adopted the new behaviour, but this has so far received little empirical attention.) The first three stages are pre-action stages and the last two stages are post-action stages (although preparation is sometimes defined partly in terms of behaviour change). People are assumed to move through the stages in sequence, but they may relapse from action or maintenance to an earlier stage. People may cycle through the stages several times before achieving long-term behaviour change.

The pros and cons are the perceived advantages and disadvantages of changing one's behaviour. They were originally derived from Janis and Mann's (1977) model of decision-making, although similar constructs occur in most theories of health behaviour. Note that applications to smoking cessation usually assess the pros and cons of smoking, which are assumed to be equivalent to the cons and pros of changing (quitting) respectively.

Confidence is similar to Bandura's (1986) construct of self-efficacy (see Luszczynska and Schwarzer, Chapter 7 this volume). It refers to the confidence that one can carry out the recommended behaviour across a range of potentially difficult situations. The related construct of temptation refers to the temptation to engage in the unhealthy behaviour across a range of difficult situations.

Finally, the processes of change are the covert and overt activities that people engage in to progress through the stages. The Rhode Island group has identified 10 such processes that appear to be common to a number of different behaviours: five experiential (or cognitive-affective) processes and five behavioural processes (Table 9.1).

In stage theories, the transitions between adjacent stages are the dependent variables, and the other constructs are variables that are assumed to influence these transitions – the independent variables. The processes of change, the pros and cons of changing, and confidence and temptation are all independent variables in this sense. Descriptions of the TTM to date have not specified the causal relationships among these variables. It is not clear, for example, whether the processes of change influence pros, cons, confidence and temptation, which in turn influence stage transitions; whether these variables have independent effects on stage transitions; or whether some other causal model is assumed to hold. It would be helpful if the Rhode Island group specified causal models for each of the four forward stage transitions and for remaining in the maintenance stage.

2.2 Summary of research

This section is organized by the four research designs that can be used to test predictions from stage theories (Weinstein *et al.* 1998b). These are: cross-sectional studies comparing people in different stages; examination of stage sequences; longitudinal prediction of stage transitions;

Table 9.1 The TTM constructs, adapted from Prochaska *et al.* (2008)

Construct	Description
Stages of change	
Pre-contemplation	Has no intention to take action within the next six months
Contemplation	Intends to take action within the next six months
Preparation	Intends to take action within the next 30 days and has taken some behavioural steps in this direction
Action	Changed overt behaviour for less than six months
Maintenance	Changed overt behaviour for more than 6 months
Termination	No temptation to relapse and 100% confidence
Decisional balance	
Pros	Benefits of changing
Cons	Costs of changing
Self-efficacy	
Confidence	Confidence that one can engage in the healthy behaviour across different challenging situations
Temptation	Temptation to engage in the unhealthy behaviour across different challenging situations
Processes of change	
Experiential processes	
Consciousness-raising	Finding and learning new facts, ideas, and tips that support the healthy behaviour change
Dramatic relief	Experiencing the negative emotions (fear, anxiety, worry) that accompany unhealthy behavioural risks
Self-re-evaluation	Realizing that the behaviour change is an important part of one's identity as a person
Environmental re-evaluation	Realizing the negative impact of the unhealthy behaviour or the positive impact of the healthy behaviour on one's proximal social and/or physical environment
Self-liberation	Making a firm commitment to change
Behavioural processes	
Helping relationships	Seeking and using social support for the healthy behaviour change
Counter-conditioning	Substitution of healthier alternative behaviours and cognitions for the unhealthy behaviour
Reinforcement management	Increasing the rewards for the positive behaviour change and decreasing the rewards of the unhealthy behaviour
Stimulus control	Removing reminders or cues to engage in the unhealthy behaviour and adding cues or reminders to engage in the healthy behaviour
Social liberation	Realizing that the social norms are changing in the direction of supporting the healthy behaviour change

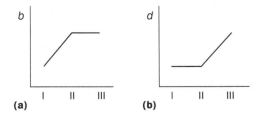

Figure 9.2 Two discontinuity patterns in a cross-sectional comparison of people in three different stages

and experimental studies of matched and mismatched interventions. The stronger research designs (i.e. longitudinal and experimental) have been used mainly in applications of the model to smoking cessation, physical activity, and dietary behaviours.

2.2.1 Cross-sectional studies

A very large number of studies of the TTM have used cross-sectional designs in which participants are classified into stages and compared on theoretically relevant variables (i.e. processes of change, pros and cons, confidence and temptation). Stage theories predict *discontinuity patterns* (Weinstein *et al.* 1998b; Kraft *et al.* 1999; Sutton 2000b). In our three-stage example, variable b would be predicted to be higher in Stage II than in Stage I but to show no difference between Stage II and Stage III, whereas variable d would be predicted to show no difference between Stage I and Stage II but to be higher in Stage III than in Stage II (Figure 9.2). This section focuses on meta-analyses of cross-sectional studies on the TTM (Rosen 2000; Marshall and Biddle 2001; Hall and Rossi 2008; Di Noia and Prochaska 2010a).

Rosen (2000) identified 34 studies, most of which were unpublished dissertations, that reported cross-sectional data on use of change processes by stage and included the action stage (because this is the stage in which behavioural processes are predicted to peak and cognitive-affective processes are predicted to decline). Although Rosen did not formally test for linearity and departure from linearity, he noted that:

> For most health problems, use of behavioral processes increased fairly linearly from precontemplation through action…[and] was typically constant or increased slightly between action and maintenance. Only for smoking did use of behavioral processes decline substantially between action and maintenance…Behavioral processes peaked during action or maintenance in 85% of all studies. (Rosen 2000: 596–7)

For smoking in particular, this is clear evidence of a discontinuity at the action stage. However, the decline in use of behavioural processes between action and maintenance is not informative about factors that facilitate this transition because it is implausible that *less* frequent use of behavioural processes would increase the likelihood of the transition. A more plausible explanation is that people in the maintenance stage need to use behavioural processes less frequently – that is, that the change in use is a consequence of the transition.

Rosen (2000) found that in less than half (41%) of studies did experiential processes peak in contemplation or preparation, as predicted by the TTM. This proportion varied by behaviour. Use of experiential processes peaked in contemplation or preparation in four of five studies of smoking. By contrast, use of these processes increased fairly linearly with stage of exercise adoption, peaking during action or maintenance in 11 of 12 studies. For other health behaviours, experiential processes were not consistently associated with any particular stage.

Rosen (2000) also noted that the steepest increase in use of all change processes typically occurred between the pre-contemplation and contemplation stages, particularly in the case of cognitive-affective processes. This could be interpreted as evidence for a discontinuity at the contemplation stage, although Rosen highlights the difficulty of interpreting this change in process use: 'Does this indicate that engagement in these processes motivates precontemplators to change their intentions? Or only that people who are already considering change are more likely to use cognitive-affective and behavioral processes of change?' (p. 603).

Rosen (2000) also reported some interesting findings for use of specific processes. For example, consciousness-raising was used most in the contemplation or preparation stages in 80% of studies on smoking and psychotherapy, but was used most in the action or maintenance stages in 88% of studies on substance abuse, exercise, and diet change; while reinforcement management was used most in the action or maintenance stage in nearly all studies of exercise, smoking, and psychotherapy, but was used most during contemplation or preparation in two-thirds of the studies on substance abuse and diet change.

The mainly linear patterns found by Rosen (2000), particularly for behavioural processes, do not provide strong support for a stage model. If differences in process use between adjacent stages are interpreted as causal effects of process use on stage transition, Rosen's findings suggest that interventions should encourage the use of behavioural processes *throughout the process of change* from pre-contemplation through action. As noted, the findings for experiential processes were more variable.

One problem with Rosen's (2000) analysis is that he combined studies that used different staging methods. Given the differences between the different methods, it would be preferable to combine only studies of a particular behaviour that used the same staging method.

Marshall and Biddle (2001) conducted a meta-analysis of applications of the TTM to physical activity and exercise. Unlike Rosen (2000), they excluded dissertations but they did include published conference abstracts. Effect sizes for comparisons of adjacent stages are shown in Table 9.2. All the effect sizes for self-efficacy were positive and significant; the effect size differed for different comparisons, although this was not tested formally. The effect sizes for the pros of changing were all positive and significant except for contemplation to preparation. The cons of changing showed significant decreases across successive stages. Effect sizes for the processes of change were based on fewer studies ($k = 5$) than for the other variables. For each of the behavioural processes, the largest effect was for the transition from pre-contemplation to contemplation and the smallest effect was for the transition from action to maintenance; the difference between action and maintenance was non-significant for four out of five processes. For the experiential processes, the largest effect again occurred between pre-contemplation and contemplation. Differences between action and maintenance were non-significant for four processes and significantly negative (i.e. showed a decrease) for the fifth (self-re-evaluation).

Do these results support a stage model? For pros and experiential processes, there is clear evidence for a discontinuity pattern. There is a steep increase between pre-contemplation and contemplation, little or no increase between contemplation and preparation, and an increase between preparation and action. For both behavioural and experiential processes, there is

Table 9.2 Mean sample-weighted corrected effect sizes (d_+) for differences between adjacent stages from the meta-analysis by Marshall and Biddle (2001)

Variable	k	PC vs. C	C vs. PR	PR vs. A	A vs. M
Self-efficacy	15–19	0.59*	0.36*	0.60*	0.72*
Pros	11–13	0.97*	0.01	0.24*	0.23*
Cons	11–13	−0.46*	−0.28*	−0.37*	−0.24*
Behavioural processes	5				
Counter-conditioning		0.74*	0.62*	0.62*	0.37*
Helping relationships		0.55*	0.10	0.44*	−0.05
Reinforcement management		0.97*	0.34	0.58*	0.03
Self-liberation		1.18*	0.41*	0.72*	0.04
Stimulus control		0.83*	0.15	0.49*	0.14
Experiential processes	5				
Consciousness-raising		0.93*	0.10	0.47*	0.04
Dramatic relief		0.65*	−0.18	0.27*	−0.07
Environmental re-evaluation		0.74*	−0.01	0.36*	−0.13
Social liberation		0.63*	0.19	0.32*	0.07
Self-re-evaluation		0.98*	0.01	0.57*	−0.15*

Note: k = number of independent samples; PC = pre-contemplation; C = contemplation; PR = preparation; A = action; M = maintenance.
* $p < 0.05$.

further evidence of discontinuity in that preparation to action is associated with an increase whereas action to maintenance is not.

Marshall and Biddle (2001) interpret their findings as mainly supportive of the TTM predictions. However, our interpretation of the findings in terms of discontinuity patterns leads to somewhat different conclusions. If we assume that a difference in process use between two adjacent stages reflects a causal effect of process use on the likelihood of making the transition, then Marshall and Biddle's findings suggest, for example, that pre-contemplators who use behavioural processes relatively frequently (compared with others in that stage) are more likely to move to the contemplation stage, but that people in the action stage who use behavioural processes relatively frequently (compared with others in that stage) are *not* more likely to move to the maintenance stage (with the possible exception of counter-conditioning). It is unlikely that the TTM would make these predictions. Similarly, the findings suggest that contemplators who make more frequent use of experiential processes are not more likely than others in the same stage to move to the preparation stage.

This highlights an important difference in the way in which the Rhode Island group interprets cross-sectional data on stage differences and the interpretation suggested by Weinstein

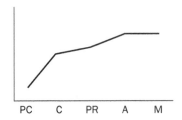

Figure 9.3 Hypothetical pattern of means across the five TTM stages. PC = pre-contemplation; C = contemplation; PR = preparation; A = action; M = maintenance

et al. (1998b) and Sutton (2000b). Consider Figure 9.3, which shows a hypothetical pattern of means across stages; assume that this represents the findings for behavioural processes. The Rhode Island group would interpret the relatively frequent use of behavioural processes among people in the action and maintenance stages as indicating that use of these processes is particularly important at these stages and therefore needs to be encouraged.

The alternative interpretation focuses on the *differences* between adjacent stages rather than the absolute levels. The steepest increase occurs between pre-contemplation and contemplation, suggesting that relatively frequent use of behavioural processes among those in the pre-contemplation stage may increase the likelihood that they move to the contemplation stage. Similarly, the lack of a difference in behavioural process use between action and maintenance could be interpreted as suggesting that relatively frequent use of behavioural processes is not beneficial in moving people to the maintenance stage. Of course, this alternative interpretation assumes a specific causal model in which behavioural process use is treated as a potential cause but not a consequence of the stage transition. Clearly, these two interpretations may have very different implications for intervention. The interpretation advocated here is consistent with the way that cross-sectional data on other theories of health behaviour are usually interpreted: the analysis focuses on the association between differences between individuals on one variable and differences between individuals on a second variable.

In their meta-analysis, Hall and Rossi (2008) calculated the difference in the mean scores for the pros and the difference in the mean scores for the cons across stages for each of 120 cross-sectional studies. More specifically, for the pros, the lowest mean in any stage from pre-contemplation to action was identified together with the highest mean in the subsequent stages. Similarly, for the cons, the highest mean in any stage from pre-contemplation to action was identified together with the lowest mean in the subsequent stages. The average effect sizes (standardized mean differences) across studies were 1.00 and 0.56 standard deviation units for the pros and the cons respectively, supporting Prochaska's (1994) strong and weak principles of behaviour change. There were differences in effect size across behaviours, with exercise, for example, showing the largest effect size for pros. Although Hall and Rossi (2008) regard their meta-analysis as a significant contribution to the field, it would be more useful to examine the pattern of means across stages with the aim of identifying discontinuities. Similar comments apply to the review by Di Noia and Prochaska (2010a) of decisional balance in studies of the TTM applied to dietary behaviour. As well as examining the maximum increases in the pros and the maximum decreases in the cons from pre-contemplation to action, they summarized the frequency of statistically significant stage differences, although they did not interpret the findings in terms of discontinuity patterns.

Following the practice of the Rhode Island group, many cross-sectional studies of the TTM report the results in terms of *T*-scores (standardized scores with a mean of 50 and a standard deviation of 10). This practice creates a problem when an investigator wishes to compare absolute levels of a variable across studies or to combine them in a meta-analysis (Sutton 2005). Primary studies of the TTM should therefore report stage means and standard deviations based on the raw scores.

2.2.2 Examination of stage sequences

Longitudinal data can be used to examine sequences of transitions through the stages. Many TTM studies have reported transition probabilities (the probability of moving from one stage to another or of staying in a particular stage). They include, for example: Martin *et al.* (1996), Velicer *et al.* (1996), Carbonari *et al.* (1999), Schumann *et al.* (2006), and Händel *et al.* (2009) for smoking cessation in adults; Guo *et al.* (2009b) for smoking acquisition and cessation in adolescents; Cardinal and Sachs (1995), Peterson and Aldana (1999), Cardinal *et al.* (2002), and Plotnikoff *et al.* (2001) for exercise/physical activity; De Vet *et al.* (2005b) for fruit intake; and Evers *et al.* (1998) for condom use. Some of these studies used latent transition analysis (LTA; Collins and Wugalter 1992) to test particular models; the others used a less formal approach. Some of these studies claimed support for the TTM, although it is not clear exactly what predictions the TTM would make.

A reasonable assumption for a stage model would state that, if a person moves at all, they should be more likely to move to an adjacent stage in the sequence than to more distant stages. However, stage models predict discontinuities in the transition probabilities. Put simply, moving to an adjacent stage should be much more likely than moving to a distant stage, and the probabilities of moving to each distant stage should be equally low. By contrast, a pattern in which the transition probabilities for a given stage declined steadily with increasing distance in both directions would be consistent with a pseudo-stage model (Weinstein *et al.* 1998b). If movement to other stages is equally likely, as in Guo *et al.* (2009b), this would be inconsistent with both a stage model and a pseudo-stage model.

Ideally, an empirical study should capture each stage movement. In practice, stage movements will be missed, especially if relatively long follow-up periods of several months are used, which makes it difficult to test predictions about patterns of stage transitions. In addition, the analysis of transition probabilities assumes that stage is measured validly and reliably; in other words, that observed changes in stage reflect true changes and not simply random measurement error.

A consistent finding in longitudinal studies of the TTM is that the initial pre-action stage of change predicts being in action or maintenance at follow-up: those in the preparation stage at baseline are more likely to be in action or maintenance at follow-up than those in contemplation, and those in contemplation at baseline are more likely to be in action or maintenance at follow-up than those in pre-contemplation at baseline. This is what the Rhode Island group calls a *stage effect* (e.g. Prochaska *et al.* 2004). However, on their own, stage effects do not provide strong evidence for a stage model because pseudo-stage models may yield similar effects. For example, continuous measures of intention predict future behaviour, and if such an intention measure is categorized into, say, three categories, one would expect to find a (pseudo)stage effect. Nevertheless, stage effects mean that stage measures may be useful in measuring progress towards smoking cessation. However, they may not be the best measures for this purpose (Farkas *et al.* 1996b; Pierce *et al.* 1998; Abrams *et al.* 2000; Sutton 2000a).

2.2.3 Longitudinal prediction of stage transitions

As well as examining stage sequences, longitudinal data can be used to test whether different theoretically relevant variables predict stage transitions among people in different baseline stages. The assumption is that such predictors represent causal factors that influence stage movement. Analyses of longitudinal data should be stratified by stage and should compare people who move to the next stage in the sequence with those who remain in a given stage with respect to baseline characteristics. A number of such studies have been published, in the domains of smoking cessation, physical activity, and dietary behaviours.

Herzog (2008) reviewed TTM-based studies of predictors of stage transitions in the domain of smoking cessation. He specified four inclusion criteria: baseline stages should be analysed individually; predictor variables must be assessed before stage transitions; a standard and current version of the TTM staging algorithm should be used; and the processes of change should be tested as predictors of stage progressions. Only two studies met these criteria (Herzog *et al.* 1999; Segan *et al.* 2004). Herzog noted that the authors of both these studies concluded that their results did not support the TTM. Herzog then reviewed a broader set of 11 studies and concluded that as a group they also failed to support the TTM (Prochaska *et al.* 1985; Wilcox *et al.* 1985; Perz *et al.* 1996; De Vries and Mudde 1998; Herzog *et al.* 1999; Velicer *et al.* 1999; Segan *et al.* 2002, 2004, 2006; Dijkstra *et al.* 2003; Hoving *et al.* 2006). Two studies of smoking cessation in adolescents (outside the scope of Herzog's review) also found little support for the TTM (Kleinjan *et al.* 2007; Guo *et al.* 2009a). For example, Kleinjan and colleagues found that none of the processes of change predicted movement from pre-contemplation to contemplation, only stimulus control predicted movement from contemplation to preparation, and only counter-conditioning predicted movement from preparation to action.

Two studies have reported predictors of stage transitions in the domain of physical activity. Plotnikoff *et al.* (2001) studied a population-based sample of Canadian adults over two consecutive six-month periods. None of the TTM variables predicted progression from pre-contemplation at time 1–2 but self-efficacy, pros, and behavioural processes significantly predicted progression from this stage at time 2–3. These same variables predicted forward transition from contemplation, over both time periods. None of the TTM variables predicted forward transition from preparation at time 1–2 but self-efficacy and (lower) cons predicted progression from this stage at time 2–3. Self-efficacy and behavioural processes predicted retention in the action/maintenance stage at time 1–2. Self-efficacy, pros, (lower) cons, experiential processes, and behavioural processes predicted retention in this stage at time 2–3.

In a study of people with diabetes, Plotnikoff *et al.* (2010) found that: higher pros of physical activity predicted progression from the pre-contemplation stage; none of the TTM variables predicted progression from the contemplation stage; higher self-efficacy predicted progression from the preparation stage; greater use of behavioural processes of change predicted movement from action to maintenance; and higher self-efficacy and higher pros predicted staying in the maintenance stage over a six-month period.

Finally, three studies investigated stage transitions for dietary behaviours. In a study of fruit consumption, De Vet *et al.* (2005a) showed that pros and self-efficacy predicted progression from pre-contemplation, self-efficacy predicted progression from contemplation, but cons did not predict stage transitions. Using the same dataset, de Vet *et al.* (2008a) found that both experiential and behavioural processes predicted progression from pre-contemplation, whereas only behavioural processes predicted progression from contemplation. In a different sample, de Vet *et al.* (2006) examined predictors of stage transitions over a one-week period for fruit, vegetable, and fish consumption. Pros and self-efficacy predicted progression from pre-contemplation for all three behaviours, but predictors from contemplation and preparation showed some differences across behaviours. Horwath *et al.* (2013) investigated fruit and vegetable consumption and found that, of the TTM variables (pros, cons, self-efficacy, processes of change), only one behavioural process (self-liberation) consistently predicted progression from the pre-contemplation stage. However, they used a p-value < 0.001, which makes it difficult to compare their findings with those from other studies. The study by Wright *et al.* (2009) on dietary fat intake appears relevant but their analysis did not focus on predictors of stage transitions from different baseline stages.

In most cases, the authors of the above studies concluded that their findings provided partial, moderate or mixed support for the TTM. However, the results are difficult to interpret because the Rhode Island group has not provided a clear statement of the TTM predictions.

Most of the studies reviewed in this section used relatively long follow-up periods (three months or more). Future studies should use shorter follow-up periods to minimize the likelihood that stage transitions will be missed (with the proviso that at least six months is required to detect the transition from action to maintenance). Researchers should also directly test whether the predictors of different stage transitions vary. For example, if pros significantly predict one stage transition but not another, a direct test may reveal that the two regression coefficients are not significantly different from each other. Similarly, if multiple time periods (or samples or behaviours) are included in the same study, direct tests should be used to test whether predictors of a given stage transition differ between different time periods/samples/behaviours.

2.2.4 Experimental studies

The strongest evidence for a stage theory would be to show consistently in randomized experimental studies that stage-matched interventions are more effective than stage-mismatched interventions in moving people to the next stage in the sequence. In our three-stage example, an intervention that was designed to increase variables a and b would be predicted to be more effective in moving people in Stage I to Stage II than an intervention designed to increase variables d and e; conversely, the second intervention should be more effective than the first for people in Stage II. Such evidence would be strengthened by showing that the interventions do indeed influence the target variables, and by mediation analyses yielding results consistent with the hypothesis that this was the mechanism through which the interventions had their effects on stage movement.

Seven studies to date have compared matched and mismatched interventions within the framework of the TTM or closely related models (Dijkstra *et al.* 1998a, 2006; Quinlan and McCaul 2000; Blissmer and McAuley 2002; Aveyard *et al.* 2006, 2009; De Vet *et al.* 2008b).[1] The studies by Aveyard *et al.* (2006, 2009) were not designed as match–mismatch studies but nevertheless report relevant findings. The five studies on smoking cessation (Dijkstra *et al.* 1998a, 2006; Quinlan and McCaul 2000; Aveyard *et al.* 2006, 2009) are considered first.

Dijkstra *et al.* (1998a) compared the effectiveness of individually tailored letters designed either to increase the pros of quitting and reduce the cons of quitting (outcome information) or to enhance self-efficacy, or both. Smokers were categorized into four stages of change: preparers (planning to quit within the next month); contemplators (planning to quit within the next six months); pre-contemplators (planning to quit within the next year or in the next five years); and immotives (planning to quit sometime in the future but not in the next five years, to smoke indefinitely but cut down, or to smoke indefinitely without cutting down). The sample size for the main analyses was 1100.

On the basis of two earlier cross-sectional studies (De Vries and Backbier 1994; Dijkstra *et al.* 1996), it was hypothesized that immotives would benefit most from outcome information only, preparers from self-efficacy enhancing information only, and the other two groups from both types of information. Thus, counterintuitively, pre-contemplators and contemplators were predicted to benefit from the same kind of information. A close examination of the cross-sectional studies reveals only partial empirical support for these hypotheses (Sutton 2000a). In the event, Dijkstra *et al.* (1998a) showed only weak evidence for a beneficial effect of stage-matched information. With respect to the likelihood of making a forward stage transition, assessed at 10-week follow-up, there were no significant differences between the three types of information among smokers in any of the four stages. However, preparers who received the self-efficacy-enhancing information only were significantly more likely to have quit smoking for seven days at follow-up than preparers in the outcome-information-only condition. Combining immotives and pre-contemplators, the percentage of smokers who made a forward stage transition did not differ significantly between those who received stage-matched and stage-mismatched information. Among contemplators and preparers combined, the percentage that made a forward stage transition and the percentage that quit for seven days were higher among those who received the stage-matched information than among those who received the stage-mismatched information, but these comparisons were marginally non-significant ($p < 0.10$). It is not clear why the researchers combined the stages in this way (immotives and pre-contemplators; contemplators and preparers), given the hypothesis of the study.

Quinlan and McCaul (2000) compared a stage-matched intervention, a stage-mismatched intervention, and an assessment-only condition in a sample of 92 college-age smokers in the pre-contemplation stage. The stage-matched intervention consisted of activities designed to encourage smokers to think more about quitting smoking. The stage-mismatched intervention consisted of action-oriented information and activities intended for smokers who are ready to quit smoking. Contrary to the hypothesis, at one month, a greater percentage of participants in the stage-mismatched condition (54%) had progressed to a later stage than in the stage-matched (30%) or assessment-only (35%) conditions; however, this difference was not significant. Significantly more smokers in the stage-mismatched condition tried to quit smoking than in the stage-matched condition.

Quinlan and McCaul (2000) suggest that a mismatched intervention may have different effects depending on whether it is matched to a later stage in the sequence (as in their own study) or to an earlier stage. For example, although it may not be detrimental for smokers in the pre-contemplation stage to receive an intervention designed for those in the preparation stage, it may be counterproductive to give preparers an intervention designed for pre-contemplators. Dijkstra and colleagues' (1998a) study provided very weak support for this hypothesis. Nevertheless, it may be worth testing in the future.

Aveyard *et al.* (2006) conducted a secondary analysis of data from a large ($n = 918$) pragmatic trial comparing the effect of two TTM-based interventions for pregnant women smokers with a control intervention that consisted of standard advice from a midwife and a self-help leaflet on stopping smoking. They argued that, because the leaflet was generally appropriate for women in the preparation stage, this intervention was stage-mismatched for women in the pre-contemplation and contemplation stages. They hypothesized that the relative benefit of the TTM-based interventions, which were stage-matched, would be greater for women in the pre-contemplation and contemplation stages. However, there were no significant interactions between intervention and baseline stage on stage progression or quitting smoking; if anything, it was the women in the preparation stage that benefited more from the TTM-based interventions.

Aveyard *et al.* (2009) conducted a similar analysis of data from another large trial ($n = 2471$) in smokers recruited through primary care and reported similar findings: no evidence that the effect of the TTM-based interventions compared with the control intervention differed for smokers in the preparation and pre-contemplation/contemplation stages. However, their content analysis of the manual used in the control condition suggested that it was to some extent stage-appropriate – that is, it encouraged the use of some processes of change that were appropriate for smokers in the early stages of change. This study cannot therefore be regarded as a strong test of the match–mismatch hypothesis.

Dijkstra *et al.* (2006) randomly assigned 481 smokers and ex-smokers to three different interventions (tailored letters) that were designed respectively to increase the positive outcome expectations for quitting (pros), decrease the negative outcome expectations for quitting (cons) or increase self-efficacy. The authors hypothesized that the pros information would be most effective in pre-contemplation and preparation, the cons information would be most effective in contemplation and preparation, and the efficacy information would be most effective in the action stage (although in their Introduction they also suggest that efficacy information would be effective in preparation).

Among smokers who were in the pre-contemplation stage at baseline, 34.1% of those who received information designed to increase the pros of quitting had moved to a later stage at two-month follow-up, compared with 18.9% among those who received information designed to reduce the cons of quitting, and 10.8% among those who received information designed to increase self-efficacy for quitting. By contrast, those who were in the contemplation stage at baseline benefited most from the cons information. Significant forward stage movement still occurred in the mismatched conditions but, without a no-information control condition, it is not possible to say whether the mismatched information was counter-productive.

The results for the preparation and action stages were less clear-cut. Smokers in the preparation stage appeared to benefit equally from the pros and the cons information; efficacy information was less effective, although the difference was not significant ($p = 0.101$). Participants in the action stage benefited more from efficacy information than from pros and cons information, although the difference was not significant at the conventional 0.05 level.

This study is the first to find clear evidence for positive matching effects in the domain of smoking cessation. However, it cannot be interpreted as evidence in support of the TTM because it used different stage definitions and a different staging algorithm (see Section 2.3) and omitted the processes of change (Sutton 2006).

In a study of physical activity, Blissmer and McAuley (2002) randomly assigned 288 university staff to four conditions, including: (a) stage-matched materials (personalized, stage-appropriate covering letter plus stage-matched manuals) delivered via campus mail on a monthly basis; and (b) stage-mismatched materials delivered in the same way. After 16 weeks, 40.4% of the matched group had progressed one or more stages compared with 31.8% of the mismatched group. This difference was in the predicted direction. The authors did not report a significance test, but secondary analysis showed that it did not approach significance at the 0.05 level: $\chi^2(2) = 0.91$, $p = 0.634$. A limitation of the study, which the authors acknowledge, is that 57% of participants were in the action or maintenance stage at baseline, and the short follow-up period would have prevented those who had recently entered the action stage from progressing to maintenance.

Finally, in a study of fruit intake, de Vet and colleagues (2008b) randomized pre-contemplators and contemplators to receive web-based tailored pre-contemplation, contemplation or action feedback. The feedback was delivered immediately after stage had been assessed. The content of the feedback was based on the research group's earlier findings. For example, the action feedback aimed to increase self-efficacy and the use of behavioural processes of change. Based on a sample of 524, no differences in stage progression were found between the three types of feedback. Among pre-contemplators, the percentages that had progressed to a more advanced stage one week after the feedback were 21%, 17%, and 22% for the pre-contemplation feedback, contemplation feedback, and action feedback respectively. Among contemplators, the corresponding percentages were 32%, 30%, and 38%.

Considered together, these studies of matched and mismatched interventions have provided little support for the TTM, although one study (Dijkstra *et al.* 2006) that used a related model found evidence that matched interventions were more effective than mismatched interventions for those in the early stages of change.

In his examination of the TTM applied to smoking cessation, Herzog (2008) argues that individually tailored interventions (such as those used by Dijkstra *et al.* 1998a, 2006 and De Vet *et al.* 2008b) are not stage based. This criterion is unnecessarily strict. It seems appropriate to consider an intervention to be stage-based if it aims to change variables that are hypothesized to influence movement to the next stage. A stage-based intervention may be tailored to the individual's values on these stage-specific variables or it may simply be targeted to the individual's stage such that everyone in that stage receives the same intervention (Armitage 2009). Both types of intervention are consistent with the rationale of a stage theory.

2.3 Developments

This section outlines several variants of the TTM. First, a group of researchers in the Netherlands has developed a version of the TTM and applied it in a number of studies of smoking cessation (e.g. Dijkstra *et al.* 1996, 1997, 1998a, 2003, 2006; De Vries and Mudde, 1998). The stage definitions in the Dutch version of the model differ from the most widely used TTM definitions in that the pre-action stages are defined purely in terms of intention: preparation is defined as planning to quit in the next month and contemplation as planning to quit in the next six months but not in the next month. In some studies, the group has subdivided the pre-contemplation stage (Dijkstra *et al.* 1998b; Dijkstra and De Vries 2001).

In the Dutch version of the TTM, the main factors hypothesized to influence stage transitions are self-efficacy and positive and negative outcome expectancies (the pros and cons of quitting), drawn from Bandura's (1986) social cognitive theory (see Luszczynska and Schwarzer, Chapter 7 this volume). These correspond respectively to confidence and the cons and pros of smoking in the TTM, although the latter are operationalized differently in the Dutch version. Processes of change are not emphasized in the Dutch version. In some studies, the set of independent variables has been expanded to include social influence, based on the attitude–social influence–efficacy (ASE) model (De Vries and Mudde 1998; De Vries *et al.* 1998). Research on the Dutch version of the TTM has included two experimental match–mismatch studies (Dijkstra *et al.* 1998a, 2006), which were discussed in Section 2.2.

Many studies have combined the stage of change construct from the TTM with constructs from other theories, most commonly the theory of planned behaviour (TPB; Ajzen 1991, 2006; Conner and Sparks, Chapter 5 this volume). In some cases, the stage measures or the analyses used were inconsistent with stage assumptions. For example, Honda and Gorin (2006) used TPB variables to predict physicians' stage of change to recommend colonoscopy where stage was assessed using a contemplation ladder; and Kosma *et al.* (2007) used stage of change as a mediator of the effects of TPB variables on physical activity. Other studies that have combined the TPB and TTM have treated the stages as potentially qualitatively distinct (e.g. Courneya *et al.* 2001; Armitage and Arden 2002; Armitage *et al.* 2004). For example, in a study of healthy eating, Armitage and Arden (2002) explored discontinuity patterns in TPB variables across stages of change and concluded that the findings were consistent with a pseudo-stage model. In a longitudinal study, Courneya *et al.* (2001) used the TPB variables as predictors of stage transitions in the exercise domain, although they compared stage progression, regression, and staying in the same stage rather than stage-to-stage transitions. There was some evidence for differential prediction. Subjective norm, for example, only predicted progression from the pre-contemplation stage. However, a single-item measure of intention emerged as a strong and consistent predictor across stages.

Several recent studies have combined the TTM with another social cognition model, protection motivation theory (PMT; Rogers and Prentice-Dunn 1997; Norman *et al.*, Chapter 3 this volume). For example, Lippke and Plotnikoff (2009) examined predictors of stage transitions in a longitudinal study on physical activity and found that threat appraisal (based on severity and vulnerability) did not predict any stage transitions, whereas coping appraisal (based on response efficacy and self-efficacy) predicted transitions from all stages. Unusually, they treated staying in contemplation, preparation and action, as well as maintenance, as a 'success'. In an experimental study, Prentice-Dunn *et al.* (2009) found that pre-contemplators and contemplators for sun protective behaviour were influenced by different kinds of information: the transition from pre-contemplation to contemplation was influenced by threat appraisal information, whereas the transition from contemplation to preparation was promoted by the combination of high threat and high coping information.

Given the conceptual and measurement problems with the TTM stage construct, it is doubtful whether combining the TTM with other theories is likely to be a fruitful avenue for future research.

2.4 Operationalization of the model

2.4.1 Stages of change

Two main methods have been used to measure stages of change: multi-dimensional questionnaires and staging algorithms or self-categorizations. In multi-dimensional questionnaires such as the University of Rhode Island Change Assessment (URICA; McConnaughy *et al.* 1983, 1989), each stage is measured by a set of questionnaire items, and scores are derived for each individual representing their position on each dimension. This approach has a number of problems, the most serious of which is that it allows people to score highly on more than one 'stage' (and many people do), which is inconsistent with the assumption of discrete stages (Sutton 2001). By contrast, a staging algorithm uses a small number of questionnaire items to allocate participants to stages in such a way that no individual can be in more than one stage. Self-categorizations are single-item measures in which participants are presented with a list of statements, each of which represents a stage, and are asked to select the one that best describes them. Although there are some differences between these two methods (e.g. self-categorizations are more transparent to the respondent than algorithms), they are similar in important ways (e.g. they both yield a categorical measure) and will be treated together in the remainder of this discussion (i.e. staging algorithm should be taken to mean staging algorithm or self-categorization).

The categorical approach has a number of advantages over multi-dimensional questionnaires: it is much simpler and the stages are clearly defined and mutually exclusive. Perhaps not surprisingly, the few studies that have compared the two approaches have found low concordance between them (e.g. Belding *et al.* 1996; Sfikaki 2001). The staging algorithm approach has been used in the vast majority of studies that have applied the TTM to smoking, exercise, and diet, whereas multi-dimensional questionnaires are more popular in applications of the model to alcohol and drug use and mental health problems.

Table 9.3 shows a staging algorithm for smoking that has been used in a large number of studies since it was first introduced by DiClemente *et al.* (1991). Pre-contemplation, contemplation, and preparation are defined in terms of current behaviour, intentions, and past behaviour (whether or not the person has made a 24-hour quit attempt in the past year), whereas action and maintenance are defined purely in terms of behaviour; ex-smokers' intentions are not taken into account.

Critics have pointed out a number of serious problems with this algorithm, some of which stem from the way that contemplation and preparation are defined (Pierce *et al.* 1996; Sutton 2000a; Etter and Sutton 2002; Borland *et al.* 2003). For example, according to this algorithm, a smoker cannot be in the preparation stage unless he or she has made a recent quit attempt. Thus, a smoker can never be 'prepared' for his or her first quit attempt (Sutton 1996b). Similarly, the subgroup of smokers in the contemplation stage who intend to quit in the next 30 days but have not made a quit attempt in the past year cannot move to the preparation stage. Thus, the stages are defined in such a way that some smokers cannot move directly to the next stage in the sequence (Sutton 2000a).

Farkas *et al.* (1996a) tabulated some of the different definitions used in the studies of smoking by the Rhode Island group between 1983 and 1991. Using data from a large sample of smokers from the California Tobacco Survey, they compared DiClemente and colleagues' (1991) staging algorithm with an earlier algorithm used by the Rhode Island group that classified smokers into pre-contemplation, contemplation, and relapse stages. The two algorithms produced markedly different stage distributions. Farkas *et al.* also showed that the earlier stage measure provided better prediction of cessation and quit attempts assessed at one- to two-year follow-up than the revised algorithm and that both schemes allocated smokers with very different probabilities of quitting to the same stage (see also Pierce *et al.* 1996).

Herzog and Blagg (2007) compared DiClemente and colleagues' (1991) staging algorithm with other questionnaire items and concluded that it systematically underestimated motivation to quit. For example, 45.5% of pre-contemplators indicated that they 'probably' or 'definitely' wanted to quit. Similarly, Aveyard *et al.* (2009) reported that only 22% of their pre-contemplators expressed no desire to stop smoking and for a quarter of them desire was strong or very strong.

Table 9.3 TTM measures for adult smoking (from http://www.uri.edu/research/cprc/measures.htm)

Stages of change
Are you currently a smoker?
- Yes, I currently smoke
- No, I quit within the last 6 months (ACTION STAGE)
- No, I quit more than 6 months ago (MAINTENANCE STAGE)
- No, I have never smoked (NON-SMOKER)

(For smokers only) In the last year, how many times have you quit smoking for at least 24 hours?
(For smokers only) Are you seriously thinking of quitting smoking?
- Yes, within the next 30 days (PREPARATION STAGE if they have one 24-hour quit attempt in the past year – refer to previous question...if no quit attempt, then CONTEMPLATION STAGE)
- Yes, within the next 6 months (CONTEMPLATION STAGE)
- No, not thinking of quitting (PRE-CONTEMPLATION STAGE)

Processes of change (Short Form)
The following experiences can affect the smoking habit of some people. Think of any similar experiences you may be currently having or have had in the last month. Then rate the FREQUENCY of this event on the following 5-point scale:

1 = Never
2 = Seldom
3 = Occasionally
4 = Often
5 = Repeatedly

1. When I am tempted to smoke I think about something else. ❑
2. I tell myself I can quit if I want to. ❑
3. I notice that non-smokers are asserting their rights. ❑
4. I recall information people have given me on the benefits of quitting smoking. ❑
5. I can expect to be rewarded by others if I don't smoke. ❑
6. I stop to think that smoking is polluting the environment. ❑
7. Warnings about the health hazards of smoking move me emotionally. ❑
8. I get upset when I think about my smoking. ❑
9. I remove things from my home or place of work that remind me of smoking. ❑
10. I have someone who listens when I need to talk about my smoking. ❑
11. I think about information from articles and ads about how to stop smoking. ❑
12. I consider the view that smoking can be harmful to the environment. ❑
13. I tell myself that if I try hard enough I can keep from smoking. ❑
14. I find society changing in ways that makes it easier for non-smokers. ❑
15. My need for cigarettes makes me feel disappointed in myself. ❑
16. I have someone I can count on when I'm having problems with smoking. ❑
17. I do something else instead of smoking when I need to relax. ❑
18. I react emotionally to warnings about smoking cigarettes. ❑
19. I keep things around my home or place of work that remind me not to smoke. ❑
20. I am rewarded by others if I don't smoke. ❑

Scoring:
Experiential Processes
      Consciousness-raising   4, 11
      Environmental re-evaluation   6, 12

(Continued)

Table 9.3 *Continued*

Self-re-evaluation	8, 15
Social liberation	3, 14
Dramatic relief	7, 18
Behavioural Processes	
Helping relationships	10, 16
Self-liberation	2, 13
Counter-conditioning	1, 17
Reinforcement management	5, 20
Stimulus control	9, 19

Self-efficacy/temptation (Short Form)
Listed below are situations that lead some people to smoke. We would like to know HOW TEMPTED you may be to smoke in each situation. Please answer the following questions using the following 5-point scale:

1 = Not at all tempted
2 = Not very tempted
3 = Moderately tempted
4 = Very tempted
5 = Extremely tempted

1. With friends at a party. ❑
2. When I first get up in the morning. ❑
3. When I am very anxious and stressed. ❑
4. Over coffee while talking and relaxing. ❑
5. When I feel I need a lift. ❑
6. When I am very angry about something or someone. ❑
7. With my spouse or close friend who is smoking. ❑
8. When I realize that I haven't smoked for a while. ❑
9. When things are not going my way and I am frustrated. ❑

Scoring:
Positive affect/social situation	1, 4, 7
Negative affect situation	3, 6, 9
Habitual/craving situation	2, 5, 8

Decisional balance (Short Form)
The following statements represent different opinions about smoking. Please rate HOW IMPORTANT each statement is to your decision to smoke according to the following 5-point scale:

1 = Not important
2 = Slightly important
3 = Moderately important
4 = Very important
5 = Extremely important

1. Smoking cigarettes relieves tension. ❑
2. I'm embarrassed to have to smoke. ❑
3. Smoking helps me concentrate and do better work. ❑
4. My cigarette smoking bothers other people. ❑
5. I am relaxed and therefore more pleasant when smoking. ❑
6. People think I'm foolish for ignoring the warnings about cigarette smoking. ❑

Table 9.3 *Continued*

Scoring:	
PROS	1, 3, 5
CONS	2, 4, 6

Note: It states on the website that 'All measures are copyright Cancer Prevention Research Center, 1991. Dr James O. Prochaska, Director of the CPRC, is pleased to extend his permission for you to use the Transtheoretical Model-based measures available on this website for research purposes only, provided that the appropriate citation is referenced.'

A variety of different staging algorithms have been used in the domain of exercise/physical activity (Bulley *et al.* 2007). Table 9.4 shows one that was used in nine studies in the Behaviour Change Consortium (Hellsten *et al.* 2008). Hellsten *et al.* report validation evidence for this algorithm using data from these nine studies by comparing stages on a range of physical activity measures, including self-report, objective, physiological, and fitness activity indicators. Their approach was to hypothesize stage differences occurring either between the preparation and action stages or between action and maintenance. For example, people in the action and maintenance stages were hypothesized to engage in more self-reported vigorous activity than people in the pre-action stages. Although Hellsten *et al.* interpret their findings as showing that the stage measure was 'behaviourally valid', the hypothesized stage differences were found in only 14 of 59 validity tests. (See Sutton [2008b] for a discussion of reliability and validity assessment for stage measures.)

Table 9.4 Staging algorithm for physical activity (from Nigg *et al.* 2005)

REGULAR PHYSICAL ACTIVITY: For physical activity to be regular it must be done for *30 minutes at a time* (or more) per day, and be done *at least* 4 days per week. For example, you could take a 30-minute brisk walk or ride a bicycle for 30 minutes. Physical activity includes such activities as walking briskly, biking, swimming, line dancing, and aerobics classes or any other activities where the exertion is similar to these activities. Your heart rate and/or breathing should increase, but there is no need to exhaust yourself. Please answer all questions with either 'Yes' or 'No'.

According to the definition above:
1. Do you currently engage in regular physical activity? Yes/No
2. Do you intend to engage in regular physical activity in the next 6 months? Yes/No
3. Do you intend to engage in regular physical activity in the next 30 days? Yes/No
4. Have you been regularly physically active in the past six months? Yes/No

SCORING

If item 1 = NO and item 2 = NO	Pre-contemplation
If item 1 = NO and item 2 = YES and item 3 = NO	Contemplation
If item 1 = NO and item 3 = YES	Preparation
If item 1 = YES and item 4 = NO	Action
If item 1 = YES and item 4 = YES	Maintenance

For dietary behaviours, a great variety of different stage measures have been used, partly reflecting the many different target behaviours in this domain (Spencer *et al.* 2007). As with physical activity, the standard approach is to define a criterion level, such as consuming five portions of fruit and vegetables per day, which is then referred to in the staging questions. This means that there may be people allocated to the pre-action stages who are engaging in the target behaviour though not at the level specified in the criterion. However, it seems implausible to treat someone who is consuming four portions of fruit and vegetables a day as being in a qualitatively different stage from a person who is consuming five.

Another problem, which applies to the great majority of staging algorithms, is that the time periods are arbitrary. For instance, action and maintenance are usually distinguished by whether or not the duration of behaviour change exceeds six months. Changing the time periods would lead to different stage distributions. The use of arbitrary time periods casts doubt on the assumption that the stages are qualitatively distinct – that is, that they are true stages rather than pseudo-stages (Sutton 1996a; Bandura 1997, 1998).

The staging algorithms listed on the Rhode Island group's website show inconsistencies across different health behaviours. For example, in the algorithm for adoption of mammography (Rakowski *et al.* 1992), action and maintenance are defined partly in terms of intentions (planning to have a mammogram in the coming year). Like DiClemente and colleagues' (1991) algorithm, this algorithm has logical flaws. For instance, it is possible for a woman to move directly from contemplation to maintenance simply by forming an intention, without passing through the action stage and without changing her behaviour.

2.4.2 TTM independent variables

Table 9.3 shows the measures of the other TTM variables for adult smoking as listed on the Rhode Island group's website. These are all the short-form measures; the long forms are also listed on the website.

Descriptions of the development of the long forms of measures can be found in Velicer *et al.* (1985) for decisional balance, DiClemente (1981), DiClemente *et al.* (1985), and Velicer *et al.* (1990) for confidence and temptation, and Prochaska *et al.* (1988) for the processes of change. Fava *et al.* (1995) outline the development of the short forms of these measures, except for confidence. In its studies of smoking cessation, the Rhode Island group has favoured the temptation measure over the confidence measure, because the scores tend to be highly (negatively) correlated and the temptation measure 'is more easily responded to by subjects in some of the stages' (Velicer *et al.* 1990: 273). However, Segan *et al.* (2006) have challenged the assumption that the two measures are interchangeable.

Compared with the long forms, the short-form measures are more suitable for use in studies that use telephone interviewing and in intervention studies involving repeated assessment. Using the short forms, all the constructs in the TTM can be measured with a total of 35 items. However, it is likely that the reliability of the short-form measures is lower than that of the long forms, and content validity may also be compromised because a construct may not be adequately represented by two or three items. For example, the short-form decisional balance scale does not include items about the health consequences of smoking, the financial costs, or the belief that smoking helps keep weight down.

The Rhode Island group's website lists measures of the TTM independent variables for exercise and some other health-related behaviours, although the full set of measures is not given for all the behaviours listed. Note that, for many behaviours, the confidence measure may be more appropriate than the temptation measure.

2.5 Intervention studies

The TTM implies that interventions should be matched to the participant's stage by targeting the variables that are assumed to influence the transition from that stage to the next. Such interventions should be more effective than generic interventions in which all participants are treated the same irrespective of their stage of change. Interventions based on the TTM have been developed for a range of different target behaviours, including condom use (Brown-Peterside *et al.* 2000), sun protective behaviours (Weinstock *et al.* 2002), smoking cessation (Prochaska *et al.* 1993), and multiple behaviours (Johnson *et al.* 2008). Some TTM-based interventions not only match materials to the participant's stage but also individually tailor the information on the basis of the other TTM variables.

A number of studies have compared TTM-based, stage-matched interventions with generic, non-matched interventions or no-intervention control conditions. Systematic reviews that have summarized the evidence on effectiveness are shown in Table 9.5. The reviews vary in their scope and in the conclusions they draw. A major limitation of these reviews is that they included studies that were not proper applications of the TTM. For an intervention to be labelled as TTM-based, it should (a) stratify participants by stage and (b) target the theory's independent variables (pros and cons, confidence and temptation, processes of change), focusing on different variables at different stages. Many of the studies included in the reviews did not meet this requirement. For example, the Newcastle exercise project (Harland *et al.* 1999; included in the reviews by van Sluijs *et al.* [2004], Bridle *et al.* [2005], and Spencer *et al.* [2006]) involved an intervention based on motivational interviewing and apparently did not stratify participants by stage of change or target the TTM's independent variables.

With the exception of Cahill *et al.* (2010), none of the reviews in Table 9.5 used meta-analysis to pool effect sizes and explore heterogeneity across studies. The field would benefit from a systematic review and meta-analysis of TTM-based intervention studies that meet the two criteria referred to above and that used stage transition or behaviour as outcomes.

Not surprisingly, the interventions that come closest to a strict application of the TTM are those developed by the Rhode Island group. The group's studies of TTM-based smoking cessation interventions have yielded mainly positive findings (e.g. Prochaska *et al.* 1993, 2001a, 2001b; Pallonen *et al.* 1998). By contrast, adaptations of these interventions evaluated by other research groups in the UK and Australia have yielded mainly null results (Aveyard *et al.* 1999, 2001, 2003; Borland *et al.* 2003; Lawrence *et al.* 2003).

Researchers who are planning trials of TTM-based interventions should consider including measures of the TTM independent variables and conducting process analyses to test whether the interventions influence the variables they target in particular stages and that forward stage movement can be explained by these variables. No such analyses have been published to date. Several studies have examined TTM variables as mediators of TTM-based interventions using behaviour (not stage transition) as the outcome (Napolitano *et al.* 2008; Di Noia and Prochaska 2010b; Papandonatos *et al.* 2012). Di Noia and Prochaska (2010b) examined stage as a potential mediating variable but the validity of this procedure is questionable because the measures of stage and behaviour were derived from the same set of items; in the TTM, stage is an outcome variable not a mediator.

Table 9.5 Systematic reviews of TTM-based interventions

Authors	Scope	k	Conclusions
Spencer et al. (2002)	Smoking cessation	22	'Interventions tailored to a smoker's stage were successful more often than non-tailored interventions in promoting forward stage movement'
Riemsma et al. (2003)	RCTs of smoking cessation interventions	23	'Limited evidence exists for the effectiveness of stage-based interventions in changing smoking behaviour'
Van Sluijs et al. (2004)	RCTs/CTs of lifestyle interventions in primary care	29	'The scientific evidence for the effect of stages-of-change-based lifestyle interventions in primary care is limited'
Bridle et al. (2005)	RCTs of health behaviour interventions	37	'Overall, these was limited evidence for the effectiveness of stage-based interventions as a basis for behavior change or for facilitating stage progression...'
Spencer et al. (2005)	Cancer screening behaviour	13	'Stage-based mammography interventions were supported'
Spencer et al. (2006)	Physical activity	32	'Results indicate preliminary support for the use of stage-matched exercise interventions'
Spencer et al. (2007)	Dietary behaviour and outcomes	25	'The evidence for using stage-based interventions is rated as suggestive in the areas of fruit and vegetable consumption and dietary fat reduction... evidence of the effectiveness of TTM-based interventions is not conclusive'
Salmela et al. (2009)	Dietary interventions in primary care in diabetes	5	'The existing data are insufficient for drawing conclusions on the benefits of the transtheoretical model'
Cahill et al. (2010)	RCTs of stage-based interventions for smoking cessation with minimum follow-up of six months	4	'...stage-based self-help interventions (expert systems and/or tailored materials) and individual counselling were neither more nor less effective than their non-stage-based equivalents...the additional value of adapting the intervention to the smoker's stage of change is uncertain'
Robinson and Vail (2012)	RCTs of smoking cessation interventions in adolescents	6	'Evidence exists for the effectiveness of stage-based interventions in promoting smoking cessation in adolescents'

Note: k = number of intervention studies included in review; RCTs = randomized controlled trials; CTs = controlled trials.

2.6 Future directions

The TTM has been very influential and has popularized the idea that behaviour change involves movement through a series of discrete stages. It has also stimulated the development of innovative interventions. However, the model cannot be recommended in its present form. Fundamental problems with the definition and measurement of the stages need to be resolved. Although a cursory glance at the huge literature on the TTM gives the impression of a large body of mainly positive findings, a closer examination reveals that there is remarkably little supportive evidence. It would be helpful if the Rhode Island group presented a fuller specification of the model that (a) stated which variables influence which stage transitions and (b) specified the causal relationships among the pros and cons, confidence and temptation, and processes of change. Predictions from the model should be tested using strong research designs: longitudinal studies of stage transitions with short time intervals and experimental studies of matched and mismatched interventions (Weinstein *et al.* 1998b). Studies of stage-matched interventions should examine whether the interventions influence the variables targeted in particular stages and whether forward stage transitions can be explained by these variables.

To date, the Rhode Island group has not responded to the detailed critiques of the TTM by Sutton (1996a, 2000a, 2001), Carey *et al.* (1999), Joseph *et al.* (1999), Rosen (2000), Littell and Girvin (2002), and Wilson and Schlam (2004). West's (2005) call for the TTM to be 'put to rest' prompted brief responses from the originators of the model (DiClemente 2005; Prochaska 2006). With the exception of Prochaska's (2010) brief comments on Herzog's (2008) paper, the Rhode Island group has not provided a critique of Weinstein and colleagues' (1998b) framework for the design and evaluation of stage theories. None of these responses adequately addressed the substantive issues raised.

3 The precaution adoption process model

3.1 Description of the model

The precaution adoption process model (PAPM) was originally developed to describe the process by which people come to adopt the precaution of testing their homes for radon (a naturally occurring carcinogenic gas). The model was first described by Weinstein (1988) but was subsequently revised. This section focuses on the revised version, which was first presented by Weinstein and Sandman (1992). The theory specifies seven discrete stages in the process of precaution adoption (Figure 9.4). In Stage 1, people are unaware of the health issue. People in Stage 2 are aware of the issue but they have never thought about adopting the precaution; they are not personally engaged by the issue. People who reach Stage 3 are undecided about whether or not to adopt the precaution. If they decide against adopting the precaution, they move into Stage 4; if they decide in favour, they move into Stage 5. Having reached Stage 5, people who act on their decision move to Stage 6. Finally, for some behaviours, a seventh stage (maintenance) may be appropriate.

The PAPM differs from the TTM in a number of ways (Figure 9.4). It has more stages: seven instead of five. Unlike the TTM, there is a stage (decided not to act) that is a side-path from the main sequence (although a person who reaches this stage may of course return to Stage 3 at some point and continue moving towards action). The decided to act stage is similar to the preparation stage in the TTM (at least when preparation is defined purely in terms of intentions or plans and not in terms of past behaviour). At first glance, deciding about acting appears to be similar to contemplation in the TTM. However, being undecided about doing something may not be the same as seriously thinking about doing something in the next six months. Weinstein and Sandman (1992) suggest that the contemplation stage may include both individuals who are

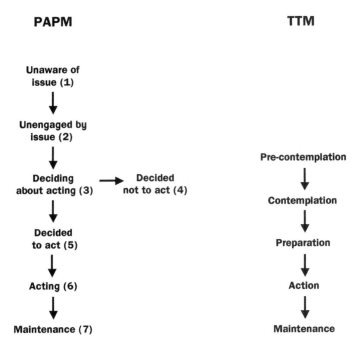

Figure 9.4 The PAPM compared with the TTM, from Weinstein and Sandman (2002a). (Only the acting/action and maintenance stages can be regarded as equivalent across the two models.)

undecided about action and those who have already decided to act. (Note that, unlike the TTM, none of the pre-action stages in the PAPM refers to specific time periods, which means that they are less arbitrary and perhaps more likely to represent genuine stages.) Finally, the PAPM in effect splits the TTM pre-contemplation stage into three stages (1, 2, and 4), which seem to represent important distinctions; in particular, it seems important to distinguish between (a) having never thought about adopting a precaution and (b) having thought about it and decided not to act.

Table 9.6 shows a transition matrix for the six-stage version of the PAPM (without the maintenance stage); allowable transitions are indicated by tick marks. The diagonal consists entirely of ticks, meaning that a person can stay in any of the stages indefinitely. For example, one person

Table 9.6 Stage transitions allowable under the PAPM

	1	2	3	4	5	6
1	✓	✓				
2		✓	✓			
3			✓	✓	✓	
4			✓	✓		
5			✓		✓	✓
6						✓

Note: The starting stage is the row and the destination stage is the column.

Table 9.7 Factors likely to determine progress between stages (from Weinstein *et al.* 2008)

Stage transition	Factor
Stage 1 to Stage 2	Media messages about the hazard and precaution
Stage 2 to Stage 3	Media messages about the hazard and precaution Communications from significant others Personal experience with hazard
Stage 3 to Stage 4 or Stage 5	Beliefs about hazard likelihood and severity Beliefs about personal susceptibility Beliefs about precaution effectiveness and difficulty Behaviours and recommendations of others Perceived social norms Fear and worry
Stage 5 to Stage 6	Time, effort, and resources needed to act Detailed 'how-to' information Reminders and other cues to action Assistance in carrying out action

may remain blissfully unaware of the health threat while another person may be constantly trying to decide what to do. Transitions above the diagonal represent forward movements. The ticks in this part of the matrix indicate the transitions illustrated in Figure 9.4, for example moving from being unaware about the issue to being aware but unengaged. Transitions in the upper diagonal that do not have a tick represent forward skips. Such skips may sometimes occur. For example, a person may make a decision to do something on the spur of the moment without having thought about it. Thus, they may move directly from Stage 2 to Stage 5, skipping Stage 3. It is possible to interpret this example in terms of the person moving rapidly through the intervening stage rather than skipping it completely. Conceptually, it is neater to proscribe skips and to assume that change follows the sequence postulated in Figure 9.4. In practice, it is difficult or impossible to distinguish between the two interpretations.

Transitions below the diagonal represent backward movements. Weinstein and Sandman (2002a: 71) state that: 'Movement backwards towards an earlier stage can ... occur, without necessarily going through all the intermediate stages, though obviously it is not possible to go from later stages to Stages 1 or 2.'

Table 9.7 shows the factors that are likely to influence key transitions in the PAPM. Weinstein *et al.* (2008) emphasize the importance of media messages in shifting people from Stage 1 to Stage 2. They also state that the factors that influence stage transitions may differ for different behaviours. Although the factors listed in Table 9.7 seem plausible, and there is a lot of indirect supporting evidence, there is as yet little direct evidence from the studies of the PAPM that have been conducted to date.

3.2 Summary of research

The PAPM has been applied to a range of different behaviours (Table 9.8). This section focuses on the longitudinal studies and an important experimental match–mismatch study on home

Table 9.8 Applications of the PAPM

Behaviour	Authors
Home radon testing	Weinstein and Sandman (1992); Weinstein et al. (1998a*)
Hepatitis B vaccine acceptance	Hammer (1998)
Osteoporosis prevention	Blalock (2007); Blalock et al. (1996, 2002*); Elliott et al. (2007); Sharp and Thombs (2003)
Using medications to treat osteoporosis	Mauck et al. (2002)
Mammography screening	Clemow et al. (2000); Costanza et al. (2009*)
Colorectal cancer screening	Costanza et al. (2005, 2007); Ferrer et al. (2011); Flight et al. (2012*); Sifri et al. (2010)
Prostate cancer screening	Costanza et al. (2011)
Sun protection	Crane et al. (2012*)
Meat consumption	Sniehotta et al. (2005)
Fruit consumption	De Vet et al. (2008c)
Dietary fibre consumption	Mohr et al. (2010)
Prevention of weight gain	Wammes et al. (2005)
Prevention of recreational water illnesses	McClain et al. (2005)

* Intervention studies.

radon testing. Other intervention studies, which did not involve a comparison of matched and mismatched interventions, are discussed in Section 3.4. First, however, we discuss Clemow and colleagues' (2000) cross-sectional study on mammography screening because it raises an important issue about the role of past behaviour.

Clemow et al. (2000) applied the PAPM in a cross-sectional study of a large sample ($n = 2507$) of women aged 50–80 years in Massachusetts whom they describe as 'under-utilizers' of mammography – that is, women who had never had a mammogram, or who had not had one in the 24 months prior to the survey, or who had had a mammogram in the previous 24 months but had not had one in the 24 months prior to the last mammogram. The staging algorithm they used differed from the recommended one (see Section 3.3). Participants were first classified into three groups with respect to their intention to have a mammogram in the next year or two: (a) definitely planning (Stage 5); (b) thinking about (Stage 3); and (c) not planning. (No respondent stated that they had never heard of a mammogram.) A second question was used to divide the not planning group into three stages: (a) never seriously considered getting a mammogram (Stage 2); (b) considered getting a mammogram, but decided against it (Stage 4); and (c) have thought about it but still undecided (Stage 3b).

Clemow et al. (2000) do not report a full comparison of adjacent stages, but their data show some evidence for discontinuity patterns. For example, compared with women in Stage 2, those in Stage 3 were significantly more likely to say that they worried 'a little' or 'a lot' about breast cancer. However, the two groups also differed with respect to the percentage that had had a prior mammogram (53.8% in Stage 3 vs. 11.6% in Stage 2). This is a potentially important confounding

Table 9.9 Stages of testing adoption and subsequent test orders (percent ordering a test) (from Weinstein and Sandman 1992)

Prior stage	Study I (n = 263)	Study II (n = 647)	Study III (n = 453)
Never thought about it	—[a]	2.0	5.3
Not needed	3.6	4.2	4.8
Undecided	3.3	12.9	3.5
Plan to test	26.2	23.6	28.2

[a] 'Never thought about it' was not given as a response option in this study.

factor. Ideally, such stage comparisons should control for past behaviour, for example by dividing the sample into those who had and those who had not had a previous mammogram. Such an analysis could also address the question of whether past behaviour is a moderator of stage transitions: the factors that influence a particular transition may differ depending on whether or not participants have prior experience of the behaviour.

Weinstein and Sandman (1992) briefly report results from three prospective studies of home radon testing that examined movement from the pre-action stages to the action stage (ordering a test). The staging algorithm used in these studies defined Stage 4 as 'test not needed', which may not be quite the same as 'decided not to test' in the recommended algorithm (see Section 3.3). The findings, which are summarized in Table 9.9, show that the percentage that subsequently ordered a test was much higher among those in the plan-to-test stage than among those in the other pre-action stages; differences between these other pre-action stages were relatively small. (Weinstein and Sandman [1992] note that the higher rate of testing by undecided participants in Study II may be a consequence of the rather aggressive intervention that occurred after their stage of testing had been assessed.) Although not tested formally, this is evidence not simply for what the Rhode Island group calls a *stage effect* (Prochaska *et al.* 2004) but for the predicted discontinuity pattern.

In the only other prospective study,[2] de Vet *et al.* (2008c) examined predictors of stage transitions for fruit consumption in a sample of 735 adults in the Netherlands. Data were collected in three waves (T0, T1, T2) with an interval of about one month between waves. At each wave, participants were allocated to stage using the following statements: (a) 'I have never thought about eating at least two servings of fruit each day' (unengaged stage); (b) 'I have thought about it, but I have not yet decided about eating at least two servings of fruit each day' (undecided stage); (c) 'I have decided not to eat at least two servings of fruit each day' (decided-not-to-act stage); (d) 'I have decided to start eating at least two servings of fruit each day' (decided-to-act stage); (e) 'I eat at least two servings of fruit each day' (acting stage). The unaware stage was not assessed.

Four different transitions were examined for two time periods, T0 to T1 and T1 to T2: Unengaged to Undecided; Undecided to Decided-not-to-act; Undecided to Decided-to-act; and Decided-to-Act to Acting. Different predictors were statistically significant for the different transitions (Table 9.10). The findings for the two time periods were not entirely consistent. The findings suggest, for example, that self-efficacy may be important for implementing a decision

Table 9.10 Statistically significant ($p < 0.05$) predictors of stage transitions (De Vet *et al.* 2008c)

T0 to T1	T1 to T2
Unengaged to Undecided	
Pros[a]	Pros[a]
Subjective norms[b]	
Undecided to Decided-not-to-act	
(Lower) Attitude[b]	
(Lower) Self-efficacy[b]	
Undecided to Decided-to-act	
Pros[a]	
Decided-to-act to Acting	
Attitude[b]	Attitude[b]
Self-efficacy[b]	Self-efficacy[b]

[a]Perceived importance of pros of fruit intake.
[b]With respect to eating at least two servings of fruit a day.

to act but may be less relevant for other forward transitions. Risk perceptions, participant's perception of their fruit intake, perceived importance of the cons of fruit intake, social support and modelling (behavioural norms) did not significantly predict any of the stage transitions. However, the focus on statistical significance may have exaggerated the apparent differences. For example, the effect sizes (odds ratios) for pros as a predictor of the Undecided to Decided-to-act transition were similar for the two periods (2.40 and 2.30 respectively), although only the former was statistically significant. Analyses should directly compare the effect of a particular predictor for different stage transitions and different time periods.

The staging algorithm assumes that those who were already eating at least two servings of fruit a day selected statement e as most applicable to them. Participants in the Decided-to-act stage reported a mean fruit intake of 224 g/day. Although this is less than two servings (250 g) a day, some participants in this stage may have been eating 250 g or more a day. To address this possible problem in future studies, it may be better to ask a question about fruit intake first and only to assess pre-action stage among participants who report eating less than two servings.

Weinstein *et al.* (1998a) reported an experimental study of the PAPM that compared matched and mismatched interventions. Participants (residents of Columbus, Ohio) first viewed a general informational video in their homes and were then staged by asking 'What are your thoughts about testing your home for radon?' in a telephone interview. The statements used for classifying people into Stages 2–5 were very similar to those in the recommended algorithm (see Section 3.3). The statement for the action stage was 'I have already completed a test, have a test in progress, or have purchased a test'. Stage 1 people, who had never heard about radon testing, had already been screened out of the study. Those people who were in either the *undecided* or the *decided to test* stage were randomly assigned to one of four experimental conditions and were sent the appropriate intervention materials and a questionnaire. A follow-up telephone interview was conducted 9–10 weeks after participants returned the questionnaire to find out whether they had purchased a radon test kit and, if not, to ascertain their final stage. (Weinstein *et al.* [1998a] note that buying a test kit is not equivalent to testing, but that they chose to use test kit purchase as the main outcome to avoid lengthening the follow-up period.)

The four experimental conditions were:

1. *High likelihood.* Participants in this condition received a five-minute video designed to convince them that they had a moderate to high chance of finding high radon levels in their homes. The covering letter mentioned that test kits could be ordered from the American Lung Association (ALA) but did not include an order form.
2. *Low effort.* The five-minute video sent to participants in this condition described how to select a kit type (including a specific recommendation), find and purchase a kit, and conduct a test. The procedure was described as simple and inexpensive. They were also sent a form to order test kits from the ALA.
3. *Combination.* Participants in this condition received a 10-minute video that simply combined the high-likelihood and low-effort videos and the same letter and order form as people in the low-effort condition.
4. *Control.* Participants in the control condition received a letter stating that their assistance in viewing a second video was not needed.

Manipulation checks showed that the high-likelihood intervention increased perceived radon risk and the low-effort intervention increased perceived ease of testing, as intended. The outcome results are shown in Table 9.11. The main outcome was the percentage of people who progressed *one or more* stages towards testing. This criterion (rather than forward movement of only a single stage) was chosen because people in the undecided stage who moved to the decided to test stage may have already possessed the information or skills required to progress further to the action stage. As predicted, both the stage × high-likelihood treatment interaction and the stage × low-effort treatment interaction were significant. The high-likelihood treatment was much more effective among undecided participants than among decided-to-act participants, and the low-effort treatment was more effective among the decided-to-act participants than among the undecided participants. This is clear evidence for the greater effectiveness of stage-matched over stage-mismatched interventions.

Table 9.11 Percentage of participants who progressed one or more stages toward testing (from Weinstein *et al.* 1998a)

Pre-intervention stage	Condition			
	Control	High-likelihood	Low-effort	Combination
Undecided	18.8 (138)	41.7 (144)	36.4 (130)	54.5 (139)
Decided-to-test	8.0 (339)	10.4 (338)	32.5 (329)	35.8 (345)

Note: The group size in each cell is shown in parentheses.

There was no evidence that the stage-mismatched interventions were counter-productive: they were still more effective than the control condition. The combination treatment was the most effective but, as Weinstein *et al.* (1998a) point out, it was approximately twice as long as each of its two components and therefore more expensive. However, it is possible that the high-likelihood video with an accompanying letter that included instructions on how to buy a test kit and an order form would be as effective as the combination treatment.

Weinstein *et al.* (1998a) is an exemplary study that provides a model for how stage theories can be tested experimentally.

3.3 Operationalization of the model

Table 9.12, from Weinstein and Sandman (2002b), gives a stage classification algorithm that would be suitable for any behaviour for which a maintenance stage is not applicable. These include behaviours that, if they are performed at all, are usually performed only once, for example having a predictive genetic test for inherited breast/ovarian cancer. Of course, virtually any behaviour can be repeated: a person may test their home for radon, then move house and test their new home for radon. If a significant proportion of people in the sample have adopted the precaution before, then it may be necessary to take past behaviour into account in the analysis and to reword the staging algorithm. Consider, for example, applying the model to participation in mammography screening. If the investigator is interested only in *first-time* attendance for screening, he or she could either select a sample of women who have recently reached the lower age limit for screening and use the algorithm in Table 9.12 to stage them, or select a sample of women who have never been screened and follow them over time until some of them have their first screen, using the algorithm to stage the sample on a number of occasions. Women who have had one mammogram could be allocated to stages with respect to having another mammogram. This would require modifications to the algorithm. Stage 1 would not be applicable for these women. And the statement used to classify women in Stage 2 could be reworded to something like 'I haven't thought about whether to have another mammogram'. (An alternative approach would be to classify women who have had repeated mammograms in accordance with the rec-ommended schedule as being in the maintenance stage. However, it would be difficult to know

Table 9.12 PAPM stage classification algorithm (from Weinstein and Sandman 2002b)

1. Have you ever heard about {home radon testing}?	
No	Stage 1
Yes [go to 2]	
2. Have you {tested your own house for radon}?	
Yes	Stage 6
No [go to 3]	
3. Which of the following best describes your thoughts about {testing your home}?	
I've never thought about {testing}	Stage 2
I'm undecided about {testing}	Stage 3
I've decided I don't want to {test}	Stage 4
I've decided I do want to {test}	Stage 5

Note: The words in curly brackets could be replaced with other precautions to develop a staging algorithm for these precautions.

how to classify women who have had more than one mammogram but whose pattern of attendance does not conform to the recommended schedule.)

The PAPM can also be applied to deliberate changes in ongoing behaviours such as the frequency of taking exercise or the amount of salt consumed per day. In this case, it is necessary to define a criterion level of behaviour, for example doing at least 30 minutes of moderate physical activity every day. Here it would be appropriate to specify a maintenance stage, possibly defined in terms of duration as in the TTM, for example having maintained at least 30 minutes of moderate physical activity a day for at least six months. However, as noted earlier, such time periods are arbitrary and do not have face validity as marking a transition between discrete stages.

Although not formally part of the PAPM, the factors likely to determine progress between stages (Table 9.7) need to be operationalized in applications of the model. Some of these are interventions (e.g. media messages and reminders). Others are beliefs about the hazard and the recommended action. In many cases, there exist standard or widely used measures for such beliefs that can found in other chapters in this book. For example, measures of beliefs about personal susceptibility and precaution effectiveness are given in Chapter 3 on protection motivation theory and perceived social norms in Chapter 5 on the theory of planned behaviour.

3.4 Intervention studies

Several intervention studies based on the PAPM have used simplified or otherwise modified versions of the model (e.g. Blalock *et al.* 2000, 2002; Costanza *et al.* 2009). This section focuses on intervention studies that are faithful to the PAPM – that is, they do not 'lump' or 'split' the stages and they use stage-matched interventions that are designed to move participants from one stage to the next.

Gielen and colleagues (2007) evaluated an intervention designed to increase parents' knowledge and behaviours related to child safety seats, smoke alarms, and poison storage. A total of 759 parents of young children were recruited in a paediatric emergency department and were randomly assigned to intervention or control. The intervention group received tailored, stage-based messages about the three child safety topics based on the PAPM. The control group received a generic report on other child health topics. A computer kiosk situated in the waiting room was used to generate and print the reports.

For each of the child safety topics, the authors specified a number of discrete behaviours, which they call 'behavioural profiles'. For example, for poison storage, the behaviours were: have a locked place; keep poisons in locked place; and return poisons to locked place after each use. For each behaviour there were six different PAPM stages (from unaware through to acting). The intervention reports were tailored to the behaviour and PAPM stage and were personalized with the child's name, gender, ethnicity, and age. The messages were designed to move parents to a higher stage within their behavioural profile or to the next behavioural profile if they were already in the highest stage.

At follow-up (2–4 weeks), the intervention group had significantly higher smoke alarm, poison storage, and total safety knowledge scores and were significantly more likely to be in a higher behavioural profile/stage for using child safety seats compared with the control group.

This study used an unmodified version of the PAPM. However, although Gielen *et al.* (2007) give an example of one of the messages, and Trifiletti *et al.* (2006) describe the development of the intervention materials, it is not clear which variables were being targeted to move participants from one stage to the next. Also, as the authors acknowledge, the study compared generic non-safety-related messages and tailored safety messages, so it is not informative about which components of the intervention were the active ingredients or whether tailoring was an essential aspect.

Flight and colleagues (2012) report an exploratory study conducted in Australia of a web-based intervention for bowel cancer screening (uptake of faecal occult blood tests or FOBTs). An interesting feature of this paper is the detailed specification of the tailored, stage-based intervention. The variables to be targeted in the intervention with the aim of moving participants to the next stage were drawn from the preventive health model (PHM; Vernon *et al.* 1997). They include salience and coherence of the screening behaviour, perceived susceptibility, response efficacy, and self-efficacy. Based on evidence from a single cross-sectional study, particular combinations of these variables were targeted in the stage-based intervention. For example, people who had never heard of FOBT received messages targeting salience/coherence and susceptibility, whereas those who had decided to use FOBT received messages that targeted response efficacy and self-efficacy. (Other PHM variables were targeted in the stage-based messages but the stage-specific variables were prioritized.)

Both web- and paper-based versions of the tailored intervention were developed and compared with a non-tailored intervention delivered through the same two modalities in a 2×2 design. There were no statistically significant effects on stage movement or screening uptake, but those who received the tailored web-based intervention showed greater increases in social influence and salience and coherence scores suggesting the potential for a positive effect.

Crane *et al.* (2012) evaluated the efficacy of a partially tailored intervention to promote sun protection of children by using clothing and hats and by avoiding sun exposure in the middle of the day. The study used the full seven-stage version of the PAPM. Action and maintenance were defined in terms of the frequency of the target behaviour. For example, for the use of clothing, one of the staging questions was, 'When your child is outside on sunny days in the summer between 11 in the morning and 3 in the afternoon, how often does your child wear clothes covering most of his/her arms and legs?' 'Half of the time or less' was defined as action and 'most/all of the time' was defined as maintenance, on the assumption that consistently performed behaviours would be more stable. Tailored newsletters and related sun protection resources were sent by mail to parents and children in the intervention group in the spring over three years; the control group received no intervention. The intervention was not individually tailored to the participant's stage. However, the sequencing of newsletters was based on the PAPM stage sequence. In each year, the first parent newsletter presented general information about skin cancer and its causes, in order to increase awareness of the issue. The second newsletter provided tailored information about risk factors specific to each child to personalize the threat. Later newsletters that year discussed the effectiveness of sun protection strategies and ways to overcome barriers.

Results are reported for the sample of 677 white, non-Hispanic children. In follow-up telephone interviews, the intervention group reported a higher PAPM stage and more frequent sun protective behaviours than the control group. The effects were small, and the authors suggest that the tailored newsletters could be used as part of a broader multi-component intervention.

These three studies show how the PAPM can be used to develop and evaluate interventions. However, there are insufficient studies to date to draw conclusions about the efficacy of PAPM-based interventions.

3.5 Future directions

The PAPM compares favourably with the TTM. The stages (particularly for the six-stage version, without the maintenance stage) have greater face validity than the TTM stages and make important distinctions that are not made by the TTM. Given the problems with the TTM, researchers and practitioners who are thinking of using the TTM should seriously consider the PAPM as an alternative.

Key tasks for future research are to specify the variables that are important for each of the stage transitions and to test whether they predict and influence these transitions. The factors listed in Table 9.7 provide a useful starting point, although they will need to be precisely operationalized in empirical studies. As noted in Section 3.1, Weinstein and Sandman (2002b) suggest that the factors that influence particular stage transitions may differ for different behaviours (in contrast to the TTM, which holds that stage transitions for many different behaviours are influenced by variables from the same limited set); however, they do not make any specific predictions about this. The model should be applied to a wider range of behaviours, including those that are relevant for novel threats where many people will fall into the early stages as well as those that are relevant for more established threats. It would be helpful if future studies of the PAPM used staging algorithms that were as similar as possible to the recommended version (Table 9.12) and sufficiently large sample sizes to avoid the need to collapse stages.

4 Concluding remarks

Stage theories are appealing because they seem to capture some of the complexities of the process of health behaviour change. However, the more complex structure of stage theories means that they are more difficult to test and to apply in practice than continuum theories like the TPB. Wherever possible, future studies should use strong research designs to test predictions from stage theories. It is remarkable that so few experimental studies of matched and mismatched interventions have been published to date. A prerequisite for such studies is that a stage theory is completely specified so that not only are the stages clearly defined, but the independent variables, and the causal relationships among them, are also clearly specified. To date, research on stage theories has been dominated by the TTM. However, partly in response to the problems that have been identified with this model, alternative stage theories are attracting attention, and this may benefit future research and practice in the field of health behaviour and health behaviour change.

Notes

1. A dissertation that reported a match–mismatch study based on the TTM was also identified (Laplante 2004). This is not discussed because the full text was not available. The abstract states that 'Stage-matched, stage-mismatched, and standard care interventions produced equivalent results in terms of adjacent stage progression...'. A study by Smith *et al.* (2007) was also excluded from the discussion in this section because it used a non-categorical measure of stage.
2. The study by Blalock (2007) is not included in this section because she collapsed the PAPM stages in her analysis.

References

Abrams, D.B., Herzog, T.A., Emmons, K.M. and Linnan, L. (2000) Stages of change versus addiction: a replication and extension, *Nicotine and Tobacco Research*, 2, 223–9.

Ajzen, I. (1991) The theory of planned behaviour, *Organizational Behavior and Human Decision Processes*, 50, 179–211.

Ajzen, I. (2006) The theory of planned behaviour [http://www.people.umass.edu/aizen/tbp.html, accessed 1 July 2014).

Andersen, B.L., Cacioppo, J.T. and Roberts, D.C. (1995) Delay in seeking a cancer diagnosis: delay stages and psychophysiological comparison processes, *British Journal of Social Psychology*, 34, 33–52.

Armitage, C.J. (2009) Is there utility in the transtheoretical model? *British Journal of Health Psychology*, 14, 195–210.

Armitage, C.J. and Arden, M.A. (2002) Exploring discontinuity patterns in the transtheoretical model: an application of the theory of planned behaviour, *British Journal of Health Psychology*, 7, 89–103.

Armitage, C.J., Sheeran, P., Conner, M. and Arden, M.A. (2004) Stages of change or changes of stage? Predicting transitions in transtheoretical model stages in relation to healthy food choice, *Journal of Consulting and Clinical Psychology*, 72, 491–9.

Aveyard, P., Cheng, K.K., Almond, J., Sherratt, E., Lancashire, R., Lawrence, T. *et al.* (1999) Cluster randomized controlled trial of expert system based on the transtheoretical ('stages of change') model for smoking prevention and cessation in schools, *British Medical Journal*, 319, 948–53.

Aveyard, P., Griffin, C., Lawrence, T. and Cheng, K.K. (2003) A controlled trial of an expert system and self-help manual intervention based on the stages of change versus standard self-help materials in smoking cessation, *Addiction*, 98, 345–54.

Aveyard, P., Lawrence, T., Cheng, K.K., Griffin, C., Croghan, E. and Johnson, C. (2006) A randomized controlled trial of smoking cessation for pregnant women to test the effect of a transtheoretical model-based intervention on movement in stage and interaction with baseline stage, *British Journal of Health Psychology*, 11, 263–78.

Aveyard, P., Massey, L., Parsons, A., Manaseki, S. and Griffin, C. (2009) The effect of transtheoretical model based interventions on smoking cessation, *Social Science and Medicine*, 68, 397–403.

Aveyard, P., Sherratt, E., Almond, J., Lawrence, T., Lancashire, R., Griffin, C. *et al.* (2001) The change-in-stage and updated smoking status results from a cluster-randomized trial of smoking prevention and cessation using the transtheoretical model among British adolescents, *Preventive Medicine*, 33, 313–24.

Bandura, A. (1986) *Social Foundations of Thought and Action: A Social Cognitive Theory*. New York: Prentice-Hall.

Bandura, A. (1997) The anatomy of stages, *American Journal of Health Promotion*, 12, 8–10.

Bandura, A. (1998) Health promotion from the perspective of social cognitive theory, *Psychology and Health*, 13, 623–49.

Becker, M.H. (ed.) (1974) *The Health Belief Model and Personal Health Behavior*. Thorofare, NJ: Slack.

Belding, M.A., Iguchi, M.Y. and Lamb, R.J. (1996) Stages of change in methadone maintenance: assessing the convergent validity of two measures, *Psychology of Addictive Behaviors*, 10, 157–66.

Blalock, S.J. (2007) Predictors of calcium intake patterns: a longitudinal analysis, *Health Psychology*, 26, 251–8.

Blalock, S.J., Currey, S.S., DeVellis, R.F., DeVellis, B.M., Giorgino, K.B., Anderson, J.J.B. *et al.* (2000) Effects of educational materials concerning osteoporosis on women's knowledge, beliefs, and behavior, *American Journal of Health Promotion*, 14, 161–9.

Blalock, S.J., DeVellis, B.M., Patterson, C.C., Campbell, M.K., Orenstein, D.R. and Dooley, M.A. (2002) Effects of an osteoporosis prevention program incorporating tailored education materials, *American Journal of Health Promotion*, 16, 146–56.

Blalock, S.J., DeVellis, R.F., Giorgino, K.B., DeVellis, B.M., Gold, D.T., Dooley, M.A. *et al.* (1996) Osteoporosis prevention in premenopausal women: using a stage model approach to examine the predictors of behaviour, *Health Psychology*, 15, 84–93.

Blissmer, B. and McAuley, E. (2002) Testing the requirements of stages of physical activity among adults: the comparative effectiveness of stage-matched, mismatched, standard care, and control interventions, *Annals of Behavioral Medicine*, 24, 181–9.

Borland, R., Balmford, J. and Hunt, D. (2004) The effectiveness of personally tailored computer-generated advice letters for smoking cessation, *Addiction*, 99, 369–77.

Borland, R., Balmford, J., Segan, C., Livingston, P. and Owen, N. (2003) The effectiveness of personalized smoking cessation strategies for callers to a Quitline service, *Addiction*, 98, 837–46.

Bridle, C., Riemsma, R.P., Pattenden, J., Sowden, A.J., Mather, L., Watt, I.S. *et al.* (2005) Systematic review of the effectiveness of health behavior interventions based on the transtheoretical model, *Psychology and Health*, 20, 283–301.

Brown-Peterside, P., Redding, C.A. and Leigh, R. (2000) Acceptability of a stage-matched expert system intervention to increase condom use among women at high risk of HIV infection in New York City, *AIDS Education and Prevention*, 12, 171–81.

Bulley, C., Donaghy, M. and Payne, A. (2007) A critical review of the validity of measuring stages of change in relation to exercise and moderate physical activity, *Critical Public Health*, 17, 17–30.

Cahill, K., Lancaster, T. and Green, N. (2010) Stage-based interventions for smoking cessation, *Cochrane Database of Systematic Reviews*, 11: CD004492.

Carbonari, J.P., DiClemente, C.C. and Sewell, K.B. (1999) Stage transitions and the transtheoretical 'stages of change' model of smoking cessation, *Swiss Journal of Psychology*, 58, 134–44.

Cardinal, B.J. and Sachs, M.L. (1995) Prospective analysis of stage-of-exercise movement following mail-delivered, self-instructional exercise packets, *American Journal of Health Promotion*, 9, 430–2.

Cardinal, B.J., Jacques, K.M. and Levy, S.S. (2002) Evaluation of a university course aimed at promoting exercise behaviour, *Journal of Sports Medicine and Physical Fitness*, 42, 113–19.

Carey, K.B., Purnine, D.M., Maisto, S.A. and Carey, M.P. (1999) Assessing readiness to change substance abuse: a critical review of instruments, *Clinical Psychology Science and Practice*, 6, 245–66.

Catania, J.A., Kegeles, S.M. and Coates, T.J. (1990) Towards an understanding of risk behavior: an AIDS risk reduction model (ARRM), *Health Education Quarterly*, 17, 53–72.

Clemow, L., Costanza, M.E., Haddad, W.P., Luckmann, R., White, M.J. and Klaus D. (2000) Underutilizers of mammography screening today: characteristics of women planning, undecided about, and not planning a mammogram, *Annals of Behavioral Medicine*, 22, 80–8.

Collins, L.M. and Wugalter, S.E. (1992) Latent class models for stage-sequential dynamic latent variables, *Multivariate Behavioral Research*, 27, 131–57.

Costanza, M.E., Luckmann, R., Rosal, M., White, M.J., LaPelle, N., Partin, M. *et al.* (2011) Helping men make an informed decision about prostate cancer screening: a pilot study of telephone counseling, *Patient Education and Counseling*, 82, 193–200.

Costanza, M.E., Luckmann, R., Stoddard, A.M., Avrunin, J.S., White, M.J., Stark, J.R. *et al.* (2005) Applying a stage model of behavior change to colon cancer screening, *Preventive Medicine*, 41, 707–19.

Costanza, M.E., Luckmann, R., Stoddard, A.M., White, M.J., Stark, J.R., Avrunin, J.S. *et al.* (2007) Using tailored telephone counseling to accelerate the adoption of colorectal cancer screening, *Cancer Detection and Prevention*, 31, 191–8.

Costanza, M.E., Luckmann, R., White, M.J., Rosal, M.C., LaPelle, N. and Cranos, C. (2009) Moving mammogram-reluctant women to screening: a pilot study, *Annals of Behavioral Medicine*, 37, 343–9.

Courneya, K.S., Plotnikoff, R.C., Hotz, S.B. and Birkett, N.J. (2001) Predicting exercise stage transitions over two consecutive 6-month periods: a test of the theory of planned behaviour in a population-based sample, *British Journal of Health Psychology*, 6, 135–50.

Crane, L.A., Asdigian, N.L., Barón, A.E., Aalborg, J., Marcus, A.C., Mokrohisky, S.T. *et al.* (2012) Mailed intervention to promote sun protection of children: a randomized controlled trial, *American Journal of Preventive Medicine*, 43, 399–410.

De Vet, E., de Nooijer, J., de Vries, N.K. and Brug, J. (2005a) Determinants of forward stage transition from precontemplation and contemplation for fruit consumption, *American Journal of Health Promotion*, 19, 278–85.

De Vet, E., de Nooijer, J., de Vries, N.K. and Brug, J. (2005b) Stages of change in fruit intake: a longitudinal examination of stability, stage transitions and transition profiles, *Psychology and Health*, 20, 415–28.

De Vet, E., de Nooijer, J., de Vries, N.K. and Brug, J. (2006) The transtheoretical model for fruit, vegetable and fish consumption: associations between intakes, stages of change and stage transition determinants, *International Journal of Behavioral Nutrition and Physical Activity*, 3, 13.

De Vet, E., de Nooijer, J., de Vries, N.K. and Brug, J. (2008a) Do the transtheoretical processes of change predict transitions in stages of change for fruit intake? *Health Education and Behavior*, 35, 603–18.

De Vet, E., de Nooijer, J., de Vries, N.K. and Brug, J. (2008b) Testing the transtheoretical model for fruit intake: comparing web-based tailored stage-matched and stage-mismatched feedback, *Health Education Research*, 23, 218–27.

De Vet, E., de Nooijer, J., Oenema, A., de Vries, N.K. and Brug, J. (2008c) Predictors of stage transitions in the precaution adoption process model, *American Journal of Health Promotion*, 22, 282–90.

De Vries, H. and Backbier, E. (1994) Self-efficacy as an important determinant of quitting among pregnant women who smoke: the Ø-pattern, *Preventive Medicine*, 23, 166–74.

De Vries, H. and Mudde, A.N. (1998) Predicting stage transitions for smoking cessation applying the attitude-social influence-efficacy model, *Psychology and Health*, 13, 369–85.

De Vries, H., Mudde, A.N., Dijkstra, A. and Willemsen, M.C. (1998) Differential beliefs, perceived social influences, and self-efficacy expectations among smokers in various motivational phases, *Preventive Medicine*, 27, 681–9.

DiClemente, C.C. (1981) Self-efficacy and smoking cessation maintenance: a preliminary report, *Cognitive Therapy and Research*, 5, 175–87.

DiClemente, C.C. (2005) A premature obituary for the transtheoretical model: a response to West (2005), *Addiction*, 100, 1046–8.

DiClemente, C.C. and Prochaska, J.O. (1982) Self-change and therapy change of smoking behavior: a comparison of processes of change in cessation and maintenance, *Addictive Behaviors*, 7, 133–42.

DiClemente, C.C., Prochaska, J.O., Fairhurst, S.K., Velicer, W.F., Velasquez, M.M. and Rossi, J.S. (1991) The process of smoking cessation: an analysis of precontemplation, contemplation, and preparation stages of change, *Journal of Consulting and Clinical Psychology*, 59, 295–304.

DiClemente, C.C., Prochaska, J.O. and Gibertini, M. (1985) Self-efficacy and the stages of self-change of smoking, *Cognitive Therapy and Research*, 9, 181–200.

Dijkstra, A. and De Vries, H. (2001) Do self-help interventions in health education lead to cognitive changes, and do cognitive changes lead to behavioural change? *British Journal of Health Psychology*, 6, 121–34.

Dijkstra, A., Bakker, M. and De Vries, H. (1997) Subtypes within a sample of precontemplating smokers: a preliminary extension of the stages of change, *Addictive Behaviors*, 22, 327–37.

Dijkstra, A., Conijn, B. and De Vries, H. (2006) A match–mismatch test of a stage model of behaviour change in tobacco smoking, *Addiction*, 101, 1035–43.

Dijkstra, A., De Vries, H. and Bakker, M. (1996) Pros and cons of quitting, self-efficacy, and the stages of change in smoking cessation, *Journal of Consulting and Clinical Psychology*, 64, 758–63.

Dijkstra, A., De Vries, H., Roijackers, J. and van Breukelen, G. (1998a) Tailored interventions to communicate stage-matched information to smokers in different motivational stages, *Journal of Consulting and Clinical Psychology*, 66, 549–57.

Dijkstra, A., De Vries, H., Roijackers, J. and van Breukelen, G. (1998b) Tailoring information to enhance quitting in smokers with low motivation to quit: three basic efficacy questions, *Health Psychology*, 17, 513–19.

Dijkstra, A., Tromp, D. and Conijn, B. (2003) Stage-specific psychological determinants of stage transition, *British Journal of Health Psychology*, 8, 423–37.

Di Noia, J. and Prochaska, J.O. (2010a) Dietary stages of change and decisional balance: a meta-analytic review, *American Journal of Health Behavior*, 34, 618–32.

Di Noia, J. and Prochaska, J.O. (2010b) Mediating variables in a transtheoretical model dietary intervention program, *Health Education and Behavior*, 37, 753–62.

Elliott, J.O., Seals, B.F. and Jacobson, M.P. (2007) Use of the precaution adoption process model to examine predictors of osteoprotective behaviour in epilepsy, *Seizure*, 16, 424–37.

Etter, J.-F. and Sutton, S. (2002) Assessing 'stage of change' in current and former smokers, *Addiction*, 97, 1171–82.

Evers, K.E., Harlow, L.L., Redding, C.A. and LaForge, R.G. (1998) Longitudinal changes in stages of change for condom use in women, *American Journal of Health Promotion*, 13, 19–25.

Farkas, A.J., Pierce, J.P., Gilpin, E.A., Zhu, S.-H., Rosbrook, B., Berry, C. *et al.* (1996a) Is stage-of-change a useful measure of the likelihood of smoking cessation? *Annals of Behavioral Medicine*, 18, 79–86

Farkas, A.J., Pierce, J.P., Zhu, S.-H., Rosbrook, B., Gilpin, E.A., Berry, C. *et al.* (1996b) Addiction versus stages of change models in predicting smoking cessation, *Addiction*, 91, 1271–80.

Fava, J.L., Velicer, W.F. and Prochaska, J.O. (1995) Applying the transtheoretical model to a representative sample of smokers, *Addictive Behaviors*, 20, 189–203.

Ferrer, R.A., Hall, K.L., Portnoy, D.B., Ling, B., Han, P.K.J. and Klein, W.M.P. (2011) Relationships among health perceptions vary depending on stage of readiness for colorectal cancer screening, *Health Psychology*, 30, 525–35.

Flight, I.H., Wilson, C.J., Zajac, I.T., Hart, E. and McGillivray, J.A. (2012) Decision support and the effectiveness of web-based delivery and information tailoring for bowel cancer screening: an exploratory study, *JMIR Research Protocols*, 1 (2), e12.

Gebhardt, W.A. (1997) Health behaviour goal model: towards a theoretical framework for health behaviour change. Unpublished doctoral dissertation, Leiden University.

Gielen, A.C., McKenzie, L.B., McDonald, E.M., Shields, W.C., Wang, M.-C., Cheng, Y.-J. *et al.* (2007) Using a computer kiosk to promote child safety: results of a randomized, controlled trial in an urban pediatric emergency department, *Pediatrics*, 120, 330–9.

Gollwitzer, P.M. (1996) The volitional benefits of planning, in P.M. Gollwitzer and J.A. Bargh (eds.) *The Psychology of Action: Linking Cognition and Motivation to Behavior* (pp. 287–312). New York: Guilford Press.

Guo, B., Aveyard, P., Fielding, A. and Sutton, S. (2009a) Do the transtheoretical model processes of change, decisional balance and temptation predict stage movement? Evidence from smoking cessation in adolescents, *Addiction*, 104, 828–38.

Guo, B., Aveyard, P., Fielding, A. and Sutton, S. (2009b) Using latent class and latent transition analysis to examine the transtheoretical model staging algorithm and sequential stage transition in adolescent smoking, *Substance Use and Misuse*, 44, 2028–42.

Hall, K.L. and Rossi, J.S. (2008) Meta-analytic examination of the strong and weak principles across 48 behaviors, *Preventive Medicine*, 46, 266–74.

Hammer, G.P. (1998) Factors associated with hepatitis B vaccine acceptance among nursing home workers, *Dissertation Abstracts International*, 59 (1-B): 0182.

Händel, G., Hannöver, W., Röske, K., Thyrian, J.R., Rumpf, H.-J., John, U. *et al.* (2009) Naturalistic changes in the readiness of postpartum women to quit smoking, *Drug and Alcohol Dependence*, 101, 196–201.

Harland, J., White, M., Drinkwater, C., Cinn, D., Farr, L. and Howel, D. (1999) The Newcastle exercise project: a randomised controlled trial of methods to promote physical activity in primary care, *British Medical Journal*, 319, 828–32.

Heckhausen, H. (1991) *Motivation and Action*. New York: Springer.

Hellsten, L.-A., Nigg, C., Norman, G., Burbank, P., Braun, L., Breger, R. *et al.* (2008) Accumulation of behavioral validation evidence for physical activity stage of change, *Health Psychology*, 27 (suppl.), S43–S53.

Herzog, T.A. (2008) Analyzing the transtheoretical model using the framework of Weinstein, Rothman, and Sutton (1998): the example of smoking cessation, *Health Psychology*, 27, 548–56.

Herzog, T.A. and Blagg, C.O. (2007) Are most precontemplators contemplating smoking cessation? Assessing the validity of the stages of change, *Health Psychology*, 26, 222–31.

Herzog, T.A., Abrams, D.B., Emmons, K.M., Linnan, L. and Shadel, W.G. (1999) Do processes of change predict smoking stage movements? A prospective analysis of the transtheoretical model, *Health Psychology*, 18, 369–75.

Honda, K. and Gorin, S.S. (2006) A model of stage of change to recommend colonoscopy among urban primary care physicians, *Health Psychology*, 25, 65–73.

Horwath, C.C., Schembre, S.M., Motl, R.W., Dishman, R.K. and Nigg, C.R. (2013) Does the transtheoretical model of behavior change provide a useful basis for interventions to promote fruit and vegetable consumption? *American Journal of Health Promotion*, 27, 351–7.

Hoving, E.F., Mudde, A.N. and de Vries, H. (2006) Smoking and the Ø pattern: predictors of transitions through the stages of change, *Health Education Research*, 21, 305–14.

Janis, I.L. and Mann, L. (1977) *Decision Making: A Psychological Analysis of Conflict, Choice and Commitment.* New York: Free Press.

Johnson, S.S., Paiva, A.L., Cummins, C.O., Johnson, J.L., Dyment, S.J., Wright, J.A. *et al.* (2008) Transtheoretical model-based multiple behaviour intervention for weight management: effectiveness on a population basis, *Preventive Medicine*, 46, 238–46.

Joseph, J., Breslin, C. and Skinner, H. (1999) Critical perspectives on the transtheoretical model and stages of change, in J.A. Tucker, D.M. Donovan and G.A. Marlatt (eds.) *Changing Addictive Behavior: Bridging Clinical and Public Health Strategies* (pp. 160–90). New York: Guilford Press.

Kleinjan, M., Brug, J., van den Eijnden, R.J.J.M., Vermulst, A.A., van Zundert, R.M.P. and Engels, R.C.M.E. (2007) Associations between the transtheoretical processes of change, nicotine dependence and adolescent smokers' transition through the stages of change, *Addiction*, 103, 331–8.

Kosma, M., Ellis, R., Cardinal, B.J., Bauer, J.J. and McCubbin, J.A. (2007) The mediating role of intention and stages of change in physical activity among adults with physical disabilities: an integrative framework, *Journal of Sport and Exercise Psychology*, 29, 21–38.

Kraft, P., Sutton, S.R. and Reynolds, H.M. (1999) The transtheoretical model of behaviour change: are the stages qualitatively different? *Psychology and Health*, 14, 433–50.

Laplante, M.-C. (2004) The effects of stage-matched, stage-mismatched, and standard care interventions on physical activity behaviour, stage transition, and hypothesized mediators of change: test of a stage model, *Dissertation Abstracts International: Section B: The Sciences and Engineering*, 64.

Lawrence, T., Aveyard, P., Evans, O. and Cheng, K.K. (2003) A cluster randomised controlled trial of smoking cessation in pregnant women comparing interventions based on the transtheoretical (stages of change) model to standard care, *Tobacco Control*, 12, 168–77.

Lippke, S. and Plotnikoff, R.C. (2009) The protection motivation theory within the stages of the transtheoretical model – stage-specific interplay of variables and prediction of exercise stage transitions, *British Journal of Health Psychology*, 14, 211–29.

Littell, J.H. and Girvin, H. (2002) Stages of change: a critique, *Behavior Modification*, 26, 223–73.

Maes, S. and Gebhardt, W. (2000) Self-regulation and health behavior: the health behavior goal model, in M. Boekaerts, P.R. Pintrich and M. Zeidner (eds.) *Handbook of Self-regulation: Theory, Research and Applications* (pp. 343–68). San Diego, CA: Academic Press.

Marshall, S.J. and Biddle, S.J.H. (2001) The transtheoretical model of behavior change: a meta-analysis of applications to physical activity and exercise, *Annals of Behavioral Medicine*, 23, 229–46.

Martin, R.A., Velicer, W.F. and Fava, J.L. (1996) Latent transition analysis to the stages of change for smoking cessation, *Addictive Behaviors*, 21, 67–80.

Mauck, K.F., Cuddihy, M.T., Trousdale, R.T., Pond, G.R., Pankratz, V.S. and Melton, L.J., III (2002) The decision to accept treatment for osteoporosis following hip fracture: exploring the woman's perspective using a stage-of-change model, *Osteoporosis International*, 13, 560–4.

McClain, J., Bernhardt, J.M. and Beach, M.J. (2005) Assessing parents' perception of children's risk for recreational water illnesses, *Emerging Infectious Diseases*, 11, 670–6.

McConnaughy, E.A., DiClemente, C. C., Prochaska, J. O. and Velicer, W. F. (1989) Stages of change in psychotherapy: a follow-up report. *Psychotherapy*, 4, 494-503.

McConnaughy, E.A., Prochaska, J.O. and Velicer, W.F. (1983) Stages of change in psychotherapy: measurement and sample profiles, *Psychotherapy: Theory, Research and Practice*, 20, 368–75.

Mohr, P., Quinn, S., Morell, M. and Topping, D. (2010) Engagement with dietary fibre and receptiveness to resistant starch in Australia, *Public Health Nutrition*, 13, 1915–22.

Napolitano, M.A., Papandonatos, G.D., Lewis, B.A., Whiteley, J.A., Williams, D.M., King, A.C. *et al.* (2008) Mediators of physical activity behavior change: a multivariate approach, *Health Psychology*, 27, 409–18.

Nigg, C., Hellsten, L., Norman, G., Burbank, P., Braun, L., Breger, R. *et al.* (2005) Physical activity staging distribution: establishing a heuristic using multiple studies, *Annals of Behavioral Medicine*, 29 (suppl.), 35–45.

Pallonen, U.E., Velicer, W.F., Prochaska, J.O., Rossi, J.S., Bellis, J.M., Tsoh, J.Y. *et al.* (1998) Computer-based smoking cessation interventions in adolescents: description, feasibility, and six-month follow-up findings, *Substance Use and Misuse*, 33, 935–65.

Papandonatos, G.D., Williams, D.M., Jennings, E.G., Napolitano, M.A., Bock, B.C., Dunsiger, S. *et al.* (2012) Mediators of physical activity behavior change: findings from a 12-month randomized controlled trial, *Health Psychology*, 31, 512–20.

Perz, C.A., DiClemente, C.C. and Carbonari, J.P. (1996) Doing the right thing at the right time? The interaction of stages and processes of change in successful smoking cessation, *Health Psychology*, 15, 462–8.

Peterson, T.R. and Aldana, S.G. (1999) Improving exercise behavior: an application of the stages of change model in a worksite setting, *American Journal of Health Promotion*, 13, 229–32.

Pierce, J.P., Farkas, A.J. and Gilpin, E.A. (1998) Beyond stages of change: the quitting continuum measures progress towards successful smoking cessation, *Addiction*, 93, 277–86.

Pierce, J.P., Farkas, A., Zhu, S.-H., Berry, C. and Kaplan, R.M. (1996) Should the stage of change model be challenged? *Addiction*, 91, 1290–2.

Plotnikoff, R.C., Hotz, S.B., Birkett, N.J. and Courneya, K.S. (2001) Exercise and the transtheoretical model: a longitudinal test of a population sample, *Preventive Medicine*, 33, 441–52.

Plotnikoff, R.C., Lippke, S., Johnson, S.T. and Courneya, K.S. (2010) Physical activity and stages of change: a longitudinal test in types 1 and 2 diabetes samples, *Annals of Behavioral Medicine*, 40, 138–49.

Prentice-Dunn, S., McMath, B.F. and Cramer, R.J. (2009) Protection motivation theory and stages of change in sun protective behavior, *Journal of Health Psychology*, 14, 297–305.

Prochaska, J.O. (1994) Strong and weak principles for progressing from precontemplation to action on the basis of twelve problem behaviors, *Health Psychology*, 13, 47–51.

Prochaska, J.O. (2006) Moving beyond the transtheoretical model, *Addiction*, 101, 768–73.

Prochaska, J.O. (2010) Herzog's (2008) criteria for evaluating TTM [Letter to the Editor], *Health Psychology*, 29, 102.

Prochaska, J.O. and DiClemente, C.C. (1983) Stages and processes of self-change of smoking: toward an integrative model of change, *Journal of Consulting and Clinical Psychology*, 51, 390–5.

Prochaska, J.O. and Velicer, W.F. (1997) The transtheoretical model of health behavior change, *American Journal of Health Promotion*, 12, 38–48.

Prochaska, J.O., DiClemente, C.C. and Norcross, J.C. (1992) In search of how people change: applications to addictive behaviors, *American Psychologist*, 47, 1102–14.

Prochaska, J.O., DiClemente, C.C., Velicer, W.F., Ginpil, S. and Norcross, J.C. (1985) Predicting change in smoking status for self-changers, *Addictive Behaviors*, 10, 395–406.

Prochaska, J.O., DiClemente, C.C., Velicer, W.F. and Rossi, J.S. (1993) Standardized, individualized, interactive, and personalized self-help programs for smoking cessation, *Health Psychology*, 12, 399–405.

Prochaska, J.O., Redding, C.A. and Evers, K.E. (2008) The transtheoretical model and stages of change, in K. Glanz, B.K. Rimer and K. Viswanath (eds.) *Health Behavior and Health Education: Theory, Research, and Practice* (4th edn., pp. 97–121). San Francisco, CA: Jossey-Bass.

Prochaska, J.O., Velicer, W.F., DiClemente, C.C. and Fava, J.L. (1988) Measuring the processes of change: applications to the cessation of smoking, *Journal of Consulting and Clinical Psychology*, 56, 520–8.

Prochaska, J.O., Velicer, W.F., Fava, J.L., Rossi, J.S. and Tsoh, J.Y. (2001a) Evaluating a population-based recruitment approach and a stage-based expert system intervention for smoking cessation, *Addictive Behaviors*, 26, 583–602.

Prochaska, J.O., Velicer, W.F., Fava, J.L., Ruggiero, L., Laforge, R.G., Rossi, J.S. *et al.* (2001b) Counselor and stimulus control enhancements of a stage-matched expert system intervention for smokers in a managed care setting, *Preventive Medicine*, 32, 23–32.

Prochaska, J.O., Velicer, W.F., Prochaska, J.M. and Johnson J.L. (2004) Size, consistency, and stability of stage effects for smoking cessation, *Addictive Behaviors*, 29, 207–13.

Quinlan, K.B. and McCaul, K.D. (2000) Matched and mismatched interventions with young adult smokers: testing a stage theory, *Health Psychology*, 19, 165–71.

Rakowski, W., Dube, C.E., Marcus, B.H., Prochaska, J.O., Velicer, W.F. and Abrams, D.B. (1992) Assessing elements of women's decisions about mammography, *Health Psychology*, 11, 111–18.

Riemsma, R.P., Pattenden, J., Bridle, C., Sowden, A.J., Mather, L., Watt, I.S. *et al.* (2003) Systematic review of the effectiveness of stage based interventions to promote smoking cessation, *British Medical Journal*, 326, 1175–7.

Robinson, L.M. and Vail, S.R. (2012) An integrative review of adolescent smoking cessation using the transtheoretical model of change, *Journal of Pediatric Health Care*, 26, 336–45.

Rogers, R.W. and Prentice-Dunn, S. (1997) Protection motivation theory, in D. Gochman (ed.) *Handbook of Health Behavior Research: Vol. 1 Determinants of Heath Behavior: Personal and Social* (pp. 113–32). New York: Plenum Press.

Rosen, C.S. (2000) Is the sequencing of change processes by stage consistent across health problems? A meta-analysis, *Health Psychology*, 19, 593–604.

Safer, M.A., Tharps, Q., Jackson, T. and Leventhal, H. (1979) Determinants of three stages of delay in seeking care at a medical clinic, *Medical Care*, 17, 11–29.

Salmela, S., Poskiparta, M., Kasila, K., Vähäsarja, K. and Vanhala, M. (2009) Transtheoretical model-based dietary interventions in primary care: a review of the evidence in diabetes, *Health Education Research*, 24, 237–52.

Schumann, A., John, U., Rumpf, H.-J., Hapke, U. and Meyer, C. (2006) Changes in the 'stages of change' as outcome measures of a smoking cessation intervention: a randomized controlled trial, *Preventive Medicine*, 43, 101–6.

Schwarzer, R. (2008) Modeling health behavior change: how to predict and modify the adoption and maintenance of health behaviours, *Applied Psychology: An International Review*, 57, 1–29.

Scott, S.E., Walter, F.M., Webster, A., Sutton, S. and Emery, J. (2013) The model of pathways to treatment: conceptualization and integration with existing theory, *British Journal of Health Psychology*, 18, 45–64.

Segan, C.J., Borland, R. and Greenwood, K.M. (2002) Do transtheoretical model measures predict the transition from preparation to action in smoking cessation? *Psychology and Health*, 17, 417–35.

Segan, C.J., Borland, R. and Greenwood, K.M. (2004) What is the right thing at the right time? Interactions between stages and processes of change among smokers who make a quit attempt, *Health Psychology*, 23, 86–93.

Segan, C.J., Borland, R. and Greenwood, K.M. (2006) Can transtheoretical model measures predict relapse from the action stage of change among exsmokers who quit after calling a quitline? *Addictive Behaviors*, 13, 414–28.

Sfikaki, M. (2001) Comparison of methods for assessing stage of change among heroin addicts in treatment: evaluation of a Greek sample. Unpublished master's thesis, University of London.

Sharp, K. and Thombs, D.L. (2003) A cluster analytic study of osteoprotective behavior in undergraduates, *American Journal of Health Behavior*, 27, 364–72.

Sifri, R., Rosenthal, M., Hyslop, T., Andrel, A., Wender, R., Vernon, S.W. *et al.* (2010) Factors associated with colorectal cancer screening decision stage, *Preventive Medicine*, 51, 329–31.

Smith, S.L., Kloss, J.D., Kniele, K. and Anderson, S.S. (2007) A comparison of writing exercises to motivate young women to practise self-examinations, *British Journal of Health Psychology*, 2, 111–23.

Sniehotta, F.F., Luszczynska, A., Scholz, U. and Lippke, S. (2005) Discontinuity patterns in stages of the precaution adoption process model: meat consumption during a livestock epidemic, *British Journal of Health Psychology*, 10, 221–35.

Spencer, L., Adams, T.B., Malone, S., Roy, L. and Yost, E. (2006) Applying the transtheoretical model to exercise: a systematic and comprehensive review of the literature, *Health Promotion Practice*, 7, 428–43.

Spencer, L., Pagell, F. and Adams, T. (2005) Applying the transtheoretical model to cancer screening behavior, *American Journal of Health Behavior*, 29, 36–56.

Spencer, L., Pagell, F., Hallion, M.E. and Adams, T.B. (2002) Applying the transtheoretical model to tobacco cessation and prevention: a review of the literature, *American Journal of Health Promotion*, 17, 7–71.

Spencer, L., Wharton, C., Moyle, S. and Adams, T. (2007) The transtheoretical model as applied to dietary behaviour and outcomes, *Nutrition Research Reviews*, 20, 46–73.

Sutton, S. (2000a) A critical review of the transtheoretical model applied to smoking cessation, in P. Norman, C. Abraham and M. Conner (eds.) *Understanding and Changing Health Behaviour: From Health Beliefs to Self-regulation* (pp. 207–25). Reading: Harwood Academic.

Sutton, S. (2000b) Interpreting cross-sectional data on stages of change, *Psychology and Health*, 15, 163–71.

Sutton, S. (2001) Back to the drawing board? A review of applications of the transtheoretical model to substance use, *Addiction*, 96, 175–86.

Sutton, S. (2005) Stage theories of health behaviour, in M. Conner and P. Norman (eds.) *Predicting Health Behaviour: Research and Practice with Social Cognition Models* (2nd edn., pp. 223–75). Maidenhead: Open University Press.

Sutton, S. (2006) Needed: more match–mismatch studies of well-specified stage theories: a commentary on Dijkstra *et al.* (2006), *Addiction*, 101, 915.

Sutton, S. (2008a) How does the Health Action Process Approach (HAPA) bridge the intention–behavior gap? An examination of the model's causal structure, *Applied Psychology: An International Review*, 57, 66–74.

Sutton, S. (2008b) *Stages.* US National Cancer Institute website on Health Behavior Constructs: Theory, Measurement and Research [http://cancercontrol.cancer.gov/brp/constructs/stages/stages.pdf, accessed 1 July 2014].

Sutton, S.R. (1996a) Can 'stages of change' provide guidance in the treatment of addictions? A critical examination of Prochaska and DiClemente's model, in G. Edwards and C. Dare (eds.) *Psychotherapy, Psychological Treatments and the Addictions* (pp. 189–205). Cambridge: Cambridge University Press.

Sutton, S.R. (1996b) Further support for the stages of change model? *Addiction*, 91, 1287–9.

Trifiletti, L.B., Shields, W.C., McDonald, E.M., Walker, A.R. and Gielen, A.C. (2006) Development of injury prevention materials for people with low literacy skills, *Patient Education and Counseling*, 64, 119–27.

Van Sluijs, E.M.F., van Poppel, M.N.M. and van Mechelen, W. (2004) Stage-based lifestyle interventions in primary care: are they effective? *American Journal of Preventive Medicine*, 26, 330–43.

Velicer, W.F., DiClemente, C.C., Prochaska, J.O. and Brandenburg, N. (1985) Decisional balance measure for assessing and predicting smoking status, *Journal of Personality and Social Psychology*, 48, 1279–89.

Velicer, W.F., DiClemente, C.C., Rossi, J.R. and Prochaska, J.O. (1990) Relapse situations and self-efficacy: an integrative model, *Addictive Behaviors*, 15, 271–83.

Velicer, W.F., Martin, R.A. and Collins, L.M. (1996) Latent transition analysis for longitudinal data, *Addiction*, 91 (suppl.), S197–S209.

Velicer, W.F., Norman, G.J., Fava, J.L. and Prochaska, J.O. (1999) Testing 40 predictions from the transtheoretical model, *Addictive Behaviors*, 24, 455–69.

Vernon, S.W., Myers, R.E. and Tilley, B.C. (1997) Development and validation of an instrument to measure factors related to colorectal cancer screening adherence, *Cancer Epidemiology, Biomarkers and Prevention*, 6, 825–32.

Wammes, B., Kremers, S., Breedveld, B. and Brug, J. (2005) Correlates of motivation to prevent weight gain: a cross sectional survey, *International Journal of Behavioral Nutrition and Physical Activity*, 2, 1.

Weinstein, N.D. (1988) The precaution adoption process, *Health Psychology*, 7, 355–86.

Weinstein, N.D. and Sandman, P.M. (1992) A model of the precaution adoption process: evidence from home radon testing, *Health Psychology*, 11, 170–80.

Weinstein, N.D. and Sandman, P.M. (2002a) Reducing the risks of exposure to radon gas: an application of the precaution adoption process model, in D. Rutter and L. Quine (eds.) *Changing Health Behaviour: Intervention and Research with Social Cognition Models* (pp. 66–86). Buckingham: Open University Press.

Weinstein, N.D. and Sandman, P.M. (2002b) The precaution adoption process model, in K. Glanz, B.K. Rimer and F.M. Lewis (eds.) *Health Behavior and Health Education: Theory, Research, and Practice* (3rd edn., pp. 121–43). San Francisco, CA: Jossey-Bass.

Weinstein, N.D., Lyon, J.E., Sandman, P.M. and Cuite, C.L. (1998a) Experimental evidence for stages of health behavior change: the precaution adoption process model applied to home radon testing, *Health Psychology*, 17, 445–53.

Weinstein, N.D., Rothman, A.J. and Sutton, S.R. (1998b) Stage theories of health behavior: conceptual and methodological issues, *Health Psychology*, 17, 290–9.

Weinstein, N.D., Sandman, P.M. and Blalock, S. (2008) The precaution adoption process model, in K. Glanz, B.K. Rimer and K. Viswanath (eds.) *Health Behavior and Health Education: Theory, Research, and Practice* (4th edn., pp. 123–47). San Francisco, CA: Jossey-Bass.

Weinstock, M.A., Rossi, J.S., Redding, C.A. and Maddock, J.E. (2002) Randomized controlled community trial of the efficacy of a multicomponent stage-matched intervention to increase sun protection among beachgoers, *Preventive Medicine*, 35, 584–92.

West, R. (2005) Time for a change: putting the transtheoretical (stages of change) model to rest, *Addiction*, 100, 1036–9.

Wilcox, N.S., Prochaska, J.O., Velicer, W.F. and DiClemente, C.C. (1985) Subject characteristics as predictors of self-change in smoking, *Addictive Behaviors*, 10, 407–12.

Wilson, G.T. and Schlam, T.R. (2004) The transtheoretical model and motivational interviewing in the treatment of eating and weight disorders, *Clinical Psychology Review*, 24, 361–78.

Wright, J.A., Velicer, W.F. and Prochaska, J.O. (2009) Testing the predictive power of the transtheoretical model of behavior change applied to dietary fat intake, *Health Education Research*, 24, 224–36.

Chapter 10

Implementation intentions

Andrew Prestwich, Paschal Sheeran, Thomas L. Webb and Peter M. Gollwitzer

1 General background

1.1 The intention–behaviour relation

Several theories that have been used extensively to predict health behaviours construe a person's *intention* to act as the most immediate and important predictor of subsequent action, such as the theory of planned behaviour (TPB; Ajzen 1991; Conner and Sparks, Chapter 5 this volume) and protection motivation theory (PMT; Rogers 1983; Norman *et al.*, Chapter 3 this volume). Intentions can be defined as the instructions that people give themselves to perform particular behaviours or to achieve certain goals (Triandis 1980), and are characteristically measured by items of the form 'I intend to do/achieve X'. Intentions are the culmination of the decision-making process; they signal the end of deliberation about a behaviour and capture the standard of performance that a person has set themselves, their commitment to the performance, and the amount of time and effort that will be expended during action (Gollwitzer 1990; Ajzen 1991). Given the centrality of the concept of intention to models of health behaviour, it is important to ask how well intentions predict behaviour.

Sheeran (2002) approached this question by conducting a meta-analysis of meta-analyses of prospective tests of the intention–behaviour relation. Across 422 studies involving 82,107 participants, intentions accounted for an average of 28% of the variance in behaviour. This is a 'large' effect size according to Cohen's (1992) power primer, and suggests that intentions are 'good' predictors of behaviour. However, Sheeran's (2002) meta-analysis does not address whether *changes* in intentions predict *changes* in behaviour. To answer this question, Webb and Sheeran (2006) performed a meta-analysis of 47 experimental studies that demonstrated that a medium-to-large-sized change in intentions led to a small-to-medium-sized change in behaviour. This suggests that intentions do influence behaviour, but that intentional control of behaviour is more limited than previous meta-analyses of correlational studies have suggested.

To investigate the sources of consistency and discrepancy between intention and behaviour, Orbell and Sheeran (1998) decomposed the intention–behaviour relation into a 2 (intention:

to act vs. not to act) × 2 (behaviour: acted vs. did not act) matrix (see also McBroom and Reid 1992). This decomposition revealed that intention–behaviour consistency is attributable to participants with positive intentions who subsequently act (termed 'inclined actors') and to participants with negative intentions who do not act ('disinclined abstainers'). Discrepancies between intentions and behaviour, on the other hand, can be attributed to participants with positive intentions who do not act ('inclined abstainers') and participants with negative intentions who ultimately perform the behaviour ('disinclined actors'). Orbell and Sheeran (1998) found that inclined abstainers – rather than disinclined actors – are principally responsible for the intention–behaviour 'gap'. Sheeran (2002) confirmed this conclusion in a review of health behaviours. Across studies of exercise, condom use, and cancer screening, the median proportion of participants with positive intentions who did not perform the behaviour was 47%, whereas the median proportion of participants with negative intentions who acted was only 7% (see also Rhodes and De Bruijn 2013). These findings indicate that approximately half of people with positive intentions to engage in health behaviours do not successfully translate those intentions into action.

1.2 Explaining intention–behaviour discrepancies

Why is it so difficult for people to enact their intentions? We suspect that three processes underlie intention–behaviour discrepancies. The first process is *intention viability*, which refers to the idea that it is impossible for most decisions to find expression in the absence of particular abilities, resources or opportunities. That is, a behavioural intention can only be realized if the person possesses actual control over the behaviour (Ajzen 1991). Consistent with this idea, Webb and Sheeran's (2006) review found that intentions have less impact on behaviour when participants lack control over the behaviour.

The second process that is relevant to discriminating between disinclined actors and inclined abstainers concerns *intention activation*. The activation level of an intention refers to the extent to which contextual demands alter the salience, direction or intensity of a focal intention relative to other intentions. To see the importance of situational demands on cognitive and motivational resources, consider that, for any particular time and context that a researcher chooses to specify in a measure of intention (e.g. 'Do you intend to exercise at the gym twice in the next week?'), research participants are likely to have multiple, and often conflicting, goals pertaining to the same point in time (e.g. 'Every evening this week is going to be spent writing that report for work') and context ('I must ask Ian and Sarah about their trip to Reykjavik when I see them at the gym'). Moreover, accumulated evidence indicates that situational features can activate goals and influence behaviour in a manner that operates outside people's conscious awareness (e.g. Bargh *et al.* 2001; Aarts *et al.* 2004; Custers and Aarts 2010). Relatedly, when particular goals involve short-term affective costs (e.g. forgoing a tempting dessert) or require mobilization of effort (e.g. bringing a change of clothes to work), then people may be especially vulnerable to more enjoyable or pressing alternatives. Thus, the relative activation level of any particular goal intention may be reduced by the situational activation of alternative goal representations.

Diminution of the activation level of a focal intention can have two important consequences – *prospective memory failure* and *goal reprioritization*. Prospective memory failure occurs when people forget to perform the behaviour. Empirical support for this explanation of intention–behaviour discrepancies comes from retrospective reports by inclined abstainers. For example, Orbell *et al.* (1997) found that 70% of participants who intended to perform a breast self-examination but did not do so offered 'forgetting' as their reason for non-performance (see also Milne *et al.* 2002). Goal reprioritization occurs when an intention fails to attract sufficient activation to permit its realization and is postponed or abandoned (at least temporarily). Consistent with this idea, Milne *et al.* (2002) found that 45% of participants who failed to enact their intention to exercise said that they were 'too busy', while Abraham *et al.* (1999) found that intentions to use a condom were not enacted because the goal of having sex was more important at the time than was the goal of protecting oneself against HIV/AIDS. Similarly, numerous studies attest to the lack of salience of pregnancy prevention *in situ* (reflected in statements such as 'I could not be bothered at the time' or 'We were carried away in the heat of the moment') as explanations of contraceptive non-use (for a review, see Sheeran *et al.* 1991).

The third process that can help to explain the intention–behaviour gap concerns *intention elaboration*. Thus, people may fail to engage in, or to elaborate in sufficient detail, an analysis of the particular responses and contextual opportunities that would permit realization of their intention. Most of the behaviours of interest to health psychologists are goals that can be achieved by performing a variety of behaviours (e.g. the goal or outcome 'losing weight' can be achieved by exercise, making changes to diet or both; cf. Bagozzi and Kimmel 1995). Equivalently, behavioural categories such as exercising or dieting may be indexed by a variety of specific actions (Abraham and Sheeran 2004; for an empirical example, see Sewacj *et al.* 1980). Moreover, health behaviours may involve complex action sequences wherein the failure to initiate relevant preparatory behaviours is likely to undermine goal pursuit. For example, the intention to use a condom might only be realized if the person has (a) bought, stored or carried condoms, (b) suggested using one to a sexual partner, and (c) thought of ways of overcoming a partner's reluctance to use a condom (Abraham *et al.* 1998; Sheeran *et al.* 1999). Understanding that health goals involve hierarchies of single acts undertaken in specific situational contexts clarifies how important it is to identify both the means (responses) and the context (internal or external cues) that will permit intention realization – especially in the case of behaviours that involve deadlines or windows of opportunity (e.g. a health check appointment). In the absence of such elaboration, the person is likely to miss opportunities to act, or not know how to act even if an opportunity presents itself.

1.3 Theoretical background to implementation intentions

Forming implementation intentions has been proposed as an effective tool for handling problems with sub-optimal elaboration of goal intentions, viability, activation or contextual threats (Gollwitzer 1993, 1996, 1999; Gollwitzer and Schaal 1998; Gollwitzer *et al.* 2005; Gollwitzer and Sheeran 2006; see Section 2.2). The theoretical background to the implementation intention construct is the model of action phases (MAP; Heckhausen and Gollwitzer 1987; Gollwitzer 1990). The MAP is a framework for understanding goal achievement that is based on the distinction between the motivational issue of goal-setting (intention formation) and the volitional issue of goal-striving (intention realization). The model assumes that the principles that govern intention formation and intention realization are qualitatively different. Whereas intention formation is guided by people's beliefs about the desirability and feasibility of particular courses of action, intention realization is guided by conscious and unconscious processes that promote the initiation and effective pursuit of the goal. The distinction between intention formation and intention realization is important because it clarifies the distinctiveness of the concept of implementation intentions. Social cognition models such as the TPB and PMT focus on the motivational phase of action. The primary concern of these theories is the specific types of feasibility and desirability considerations that determine intention formation – little attention is paid to how intentions are translated into action (Oettingen and Gollwitzer 2001; Sheeran 2002). Research on implementation intentions, on the other hand, provides an explicit theoretical analysis of processes that govern the enactment of intentions.

2 Description of the model

2.1 The nature of implementation intentions

Implementation intentions are if–then plans that connect good opportunities to act with cognitive or behavioural responses that are likely to be effective in accomplishing one's goals. Whereas behavioural or goal intentions specify what one wants to do or achieve (i.e. 'I intend to do/achieve X'), implementation intentions specify the response that one will perform in the service of goal achievement and the opportunity in which one will enact it (i.e. 'If opportunity Y occurs, then I will initiate goal-directed response Z!'). Implementation intentions are subordinate to goal intentions because, whereas a goal intention indicates *what* one will do, an implementation intention specifies the *when*, *where*, and *how* of what one will do.

To form an implementation intention, the person must first identify a response that will lead to goal attainment, and second, anticipate a suitable opportunity to initiate that response. For example, in order to enact the goal intention to exercise, the person might specify the behaviour 'go jogging for 20 minutes' and specify a suitable opportunity as 'tomorrow morning before work'. Implementation intention formation is, therefore, the mental act of linking the anticipated opportunity with a suitable goal-directed response. This process involves a conscious act of willing that results in an association being forged between the mental representation of the specified opportunity and the means of attaining the focal goal (i.e. cognitive or behavioural responses).

Goal and implementation intentions can therefore be differentiated both in terms of structure (goal intentions specify *what* one will do, while implementation intentions are if–then statements that *plan out in advance how this is to be executed*), and in terms of their impact on goal attainment. Evidence suggests that forming implementation intentions substantially increases the likelihood that goal intentions will be translated into action (for a review, see Gollwitzer and Sheeran 2006). In addition, studies of the neural processes involved in goal-striving also support a distinction between goal and implementation intentions (Gilbert *et al.* 2009; Hallam *et al.* submitted).

2.2 Implementation intentions and overcoming volitional problems in goal pursuit

When people have only formed goal intentions, they may encounter volitional problems that undermine goal pursuit and give rise to inclined abstainers rather than inclined actors. However, evidence suggests that these problems can be overcome by the psychological processes engendered by implementation intentions. Forming an implementation intention promotes goal achievement because the person is perceptually ready to encounter the cues specified in the if-component of the plan, and because these cues evoke the specified response swiftly and without the need for conscious awareness or effort. These benefits help to overcome volitional problems related to intentions that are not elaborated, not viable, not activated or thwarted by contextual threats.

2.2.1 Problems of intention elaboration

Forming an implementation intention helps to manage the problem of poorly elaborated goal intentions because if–then plans specify the response that one will perform in the service of the goal and the opportunity in which one will perform it. Whereas the person who has only formed a goal intention still has to identify the specific response(s) that will be effective in achieving their goal *and* identify a good opportunity in which to enact it, all of this work is finished when the person has formed an implementation intention: the plan specifies the response and opportunity in advance. This means that good opportunities to initiate a response that leads to goal attainment are recognized swiftly and precisely, rather than missed. Moreover, encountering a good opportunity instigates specific responses in a more immediate and less effortful fashion instead of generating deliberation about what one should do and/or the need to energize oneself to perform it.

2.2.2 Problems of intention viability

Forming an implementation intention can also help to deal with problems related to the viability of intentions – namely, that intentions may only translate into action if the person has the required abilities, resources or opportunities. If–then planning overcomes problems of unviable intentions because the person has to devote thought in advance to when, where, and how they will strive for the goal, and hence is more likely to anticipate and account for potential difficulties. Moreover, implementation intentions can be used to boost self-efficacy directly in order to overcome problems of intention viability. For instance, Bayer and Gollwitzer (2007) demonstrated that specifying a self-efficacy-enhancing response in an if–then plan ('And if I start a new task, then I will tell myself: I can solve this task!') was effective in promoting the realization of intentions to perform well in a mathematics test.

2.2.3 Problems of intention activation

Implementation intentions also help to circumvent problems associated with the activation level of the superordinate goal intention. This is because if–then plans delegate control of responses to specified cues that serve to elicit these responses directly. This contrasts with the predicament of the person who has only formed goal intentions and who must maintain the activation level of the intention in the face of multiple and often competing goals (and is vulnerable to prospective memory failure and goal reprioritization). Although research indicates that constructs such as anticipated regret and temporal stability of intention (for reviews, see Sheeran 2002; Cooke and Sheeran 2004) moderate the intention–behaviour relation, studies to date suggest little that the person could *deliberately* or strategically do to maintain the activation level of his or her intention (over and above cognitive rehearsal of that self-instruction and/or deployment of mnemonic devices such as diaries or knotted handkerchiefs). Forming implementation intentions is, therefore, a helpful intervention in this regard.

2.2.4 Problems of contextual threats

Recent research has explicitly tested whether implementation intentions can be used to help people overcome contextual threats, such as priming of goals that are antithetical to focal goal pursuit, the presence of attractive distractions, and detrimental self-states such as anxiety. Gollwitzer *et al.* (2011) tested whether implementation intentions can protect against the effect of priming goals that are antithetical to the focal goal. Across three studies, Gollwitzer *et al.* demonstrated that forming an implementation intention countered the effects of priming participants with slowness (Study 1), cooperation (Study 2), and moving fast (Study 3). Thus, implementation intentions may be used to offset the impact of cues that activate task-inhibiting or alternative goals – the strategic automaticity of if–then plans can overcome the automatic activation of antithetical goals (see also Webb *et al.* 2012).

Gollwitzer and Schaal (1998) showed implementation intentions could overcome the impact of attractive distractions on the time taken to solve boring arithmetic problems. Similar findings were obtained by Wieber *et al.* (2011), who demonstrated that, compared with forming intentions ('I will ignore distractions!'), forming implementation intentions ('If a distraction comes up, then I will ignore it') helped schoolchildren aged 5–8 years to deal with moderately or highly attractive distractions.

In summary, there is good evidence that forming implementation intentions helps to overcome contextual threats to intention activation that may undermine the realization of goal intentions. If–then plans prove useful (a) whether the threat is within or outside conscious awareness, and (b) whether the threat resides in the environment or is an internal self-state.

2.3 Operation of implementation intentions

Two processes are thought to explain the efficacy of forming if–then plans in improving the likelihood of goal attainment compared with only forming a respective goal intention (Gollwitzer 1993, 1996, 1999; Gollwitzer and Sheeran 2006). First, forming implementation intentions helps people to identify good opportunities to act. This is supported by demonstrations that forming implementation intentions increases the accessibility of cues (specified in the *if*-component of the plan) and that detection of, and attention to, the critical cue is thereby facilitated (Aarts *et al.* 1999; Webb and Sheeran 2004, 2007, 2008). Second, forming implementation intentions helps to automate the execution of the goal-directed response (specified in the *then*-component of the plan). This idea is supported by demonstrations that the initiation of responses in the presence of the critical cue are more automatic following the formation of implementation intentions, with responses being initiated more immediately, efficiently, and without the need for conscious awareness (Gollwitzer and Brandstätter 1997; Brandstätter *et al.* 2001; Lengfelder and Gollwitzer 2001; Webb and Sheeran 2004, 2007, 2008; Sheeran *et al.* 2005; Wieber and Sassenberg 2006; Bayer *et al.* 2009). The mere formation of a goal intention is not sufficient to produce these effects – the person still has to identify appropriate opportunities and goal-directed responses and then mobilize the self to act. Action control in this mode is, therefore, slower by comparison and requires conscious attention and effort.

2.3.1 Identification of the critical opportunity

Specifying a good opportunity to act in the if-component of an implementation intention means that the mental representation of the cues that comprise this opportunity become highly accessible. This heightened accessibility enhances information processing related to the specified cue with the result that it becomes easier to detect and attend to. Aarts *et al.* (1999) obtained evidence that forming implementation intentions heightens the accessibility of the specified cues in an experiment that asked one-half of participants to form an implementation intention about how they would later collect a coupon from a nearby room; the other half of participants (controls) formed an irrelevant implementation intention about how they would spend the coupon. All of the participants then took part in an ostensibly unrelated word recognition task (their task was to indicate as quickly and accurately as possible whether or not letter strings were words or non-words). Among the letter strings presented were words related to the location of the room where the coupon should be collected (e.g. 'corridor', 'swing-door').

Consistent with predictions, participants who formed if–then plans responded faster to words related to the cues representing the opportunity for action (e.g. 'corridor'), suggesting that the mental representation of the anticipated opportunity was rendered more accessible. Importantly, only 50% of participants in the control condition (who planned when they would spend, rather than collect, the coupon) collected a coupon, whereas 80% of participants who formed implementation intentions did so. Thus, implementation intentions affected both cue accessibility and goal achievement. Further analyses indicated that the accessibility of cues mediated (i.e. explained) the impact of forming implementation intentions on goal achievement.

Heightened accessibility should also mean that the specified cues attract and focus attention even though the person is occupied by other concerns. Achtziger *et al.* (2012, Study 1) tested this idea using a dichotic listening task. Findings indicated that the critical cues earlier specified in an implementation intention were highly disruptive, when presented in one ear, for attention to the focal tasks (switching off a light and repeating words in the other ear). Thus, words related to the critical opportunity grabbed participants' attention even though participants were supposed to be concentrating on demanding other tasks. These findings suggest that even though people may be wrapped up in their thoughts, emotions or activities that have nothing to do with an underlying goal intention, the critical opportunity specified in an if–then plan will penetrate current preoccupations and capture attention (see also Webb and Sheeran 2004).

2.3.2 Execution of the goal-directed response

Webb and Sheeran (2008, Study 2) tested the importance of the accessibility of cues and the strength of cue–behaviour links in mediating action control by implementation intentions. The study replicated the key features of the coupon collection paradigm used by Aarts *et al.* (1999); the main innovation was using a sequential priming procedure in the lexical decision task. Participants had to respond, as quickly as possible, to a target to indicate whether it was a word using a button box. The target was preceded by a masked priming word (related to the location of the coupon [e.g. 'corridor', 'right'] or matched neutral words). The target words were the specified behaviour ('collect'), an unrelated behaviour ('confirm'), the location words (cues), and filler words. In this way, it was possible to determine the impact of implementation intentions on both cue accessibility (response latencies to *neutral prime-location cue* targets) and the strength of cue–behaviour links (response latencies to *location prime-specified behaviour* targets) and all other prime–target combinations.

Findings showed that participants who formed implementation intentions were significantly more likely to collect the coupon than were participants who only formed goal intentions (64% vs. 39%). Moreover, both heightened accessibility of the specified opportunity and strong cue–response links mediated the impact of if–then plans on coupon collection. These findings support theoretical predictions about the processes underlying action control by implementation intention (Gollwitzer 1993), and provide good evidence that enhanced identification of critical cues and automated execution of responses are the mechanisms by which implementation intentions promote goal achievement.

A study by Papies *et al.* (2009) suggests that the process underlying implementation intention effects may not be merely associative. Requiring participants to visit the experimenter via the cafeteria (see Aarts *et al.* 1999), participants had to (1) form an implementation intention to go to the experimenter via the cafeteria, (2) complete an associative learning task to link the cue with the behaviour, or (3) complete an unrelated associative learning task (control condition). Rates of goal completion were similar across the implementation intention and associative learning conditions (and superior to the control group). However, when participants returned one week later and were provided with the same goal (without further implementation intention or associative learning manipulations), the implementation intention group outperformed those in both the associative learning and control groups. This suggests that the mechanisms underlying implementation intentions go beyond mere cue–behaviour association, with the authors speculating that forming implementation intentions leads to richer mental representations of goal-directed actions, which increase the likelihood that they are activated even after a delay.

2.3.3 Features of automaticity

Forming an implementation intention involves a strategic abdication of action control to the extent that the person specifies that they will perform a particular goal-directed response (in the *then*-component of a plan), at the moment specified in the *if*-component of the plan. Forming implementation intentions thus delegates control of the intended response from the self to specified cues that directly elicit the response (see Gollwitzer and Sheeran 2006). Nothing more needs to be done to ensure initiation of the intended response except encounter the specified opportunity. The consequence is that the execution of a response specified in an implementation intention exhibits features of *automatic* processes. According to Bargh (1992, 1994), key features of automatic processes are immediacy, efficiency, and lack of awareness (see also Moors and De Houwer 2006). Automaticity characterizes highly over-learned activities such as driving a car or typing. For example, drivers respond quickly to changes in the flow of traffic or road conditions. They can hold a conversation with a passenger despite the demands while they are driving at the same time (supporting the idea that driving is efficient in terms of cognitive resources). Drivers need devote little attention to the process of driving itself; they need only be aware of other traffic and their conversation partner. So what evidence is there that action control by implementation intentions exhibits features of automatic processes?

The *immediacy* of implementation intention effects is supported by several studies that have employed speed of responding as the dependent variable. For example, Webb and Sheeran (2004, Study 3) used a reaction time task to compare whether forming an implementation intention to respond especially quickly to a critical stimulus (in this case, the number 3) led to faster responses compared with merely holding equivalent goal intentions. Findings indicated that participants who formed if–then plans responded faster to the critical stimulus compared with both non-critical stimuli and participants who only formed goal intentions (see also Parks-Stamm *et al.* 2007). A field study by Orbell and Sheeran (2000) afforded a similar conclusion. Patients undergoing joint replacement surgery were asked to form implementation intentions about resuming functional activities upon their discharge from hospital. Despite equivalent goal intentions to resume the activities, three months later patients who formed implementation intentions initiated 18 of 32 activities sooner than did patients who had not formed if–then plans. Participants who formed implementation intentions were functionally active two and a half weeks sooner, on average, than were controls. Finally, Gollwitzer and Brandstätter (1997, Study 3) reported that participants who formed implementation intentions were quicker to make counter-arguments to racist remarks than participants who only formed goal intentions. Taken together, the evidence suggests that participants who form if–then plans are quicker to seize the opportunities to act than those who form goal intentions alone.

The *efficiency* of implementation intention effects is supported by studies that manipulated cognitive load either through selection of the sample (e.g. schizophrenic patients, heroin addicts under withdrawal) or by using a dual-task paradigm in experiments with college students (Brandstätter *et al.* 2001; Lengfelder and Gollwitzer 2001). For example, Brandstätter *et al.* (2001, Study 2) found that forming implementation intentions benefited task performance for schizophrenic patients just as much as for matched controls, even though schizophrenics are likely to have been preoccupied by unwanted thoughts. Similarly, forming an implementation intention to compose a curriculum vitae increased the likelihood of completing the task by the deadline regardless of whether or not addicts were still experiencing symptoms of opiate withdrawal (Brandstätter *et al.* 2001, Study 1). Two further studies manipulated the amount of mental load that participants experienced by having them perform two tasks at once (Brandstätter *et al.* 2001). Consistent with the idea that implementation intentions do not require much in the way of cognitive resources, enacting planned responses did not compromise performance on a secondary task (Study 3) and did not show evidence of task interference even when the task was very difficult (Study 4).

Efficiency is usually construed in terms of the cognitive demands that are placed on participants at the time of acting (e.g. Bargh 1992). However, Webb and Sheeran (2003) examined how effective implementation intentions were in promoting goal achievement when people's overall capacity for self-control (i.e. 'willpower') was diminished by prior exertion of self-control. Their study drew upon Baumeister and colleagues' research on 'ego-depletion' (e.g. Baumeister *et al.* 1998; for reviews, see Muraven and Baumeister 2000; Hagger *et al.* 2010). Ego-depletion refers to the temporary depletion of self-regulatory capacity brought about by an initial act of self-control. Webb and Sheeran (2003, Study 2) induced ego-depletion by asking participants to perform a dual balance-and-maths task that required considerable self-control (or not). Participants then either formed or did not form an implementation intention in relation to a subsequent Stroop colour-naming task. Consistent with previous research, ego-depleted participants performed worse on the Stroop task than did non-depleted controls. However, ego-depletion did not influence responses when participants had formed implementation intentions. Participants who formed if–then plans were as fast and accurate in their Stroop performance as were participants who had not been ego-depleted. These findings are consistent with the idea that implementation intentions are 'efficient' in that they do not draw on potentially limited self-regulatory resources. Even when participants' capacity for self-control was substantially diminished, forming an implementation intention still benefited task performance.

Two aspects of *lack of awareness* have been investigated with respect to the operation of implementation intentions, one related to the anticipated opportunity and the other related to the underlying goal intention. Bayer *et al.* (2009) obtained evidence that awareness of the specified cue is not required for implementation intention effects. In a first study, Bayer *et al.* used a retaliation paradigm wherein participants who had been insulted by an experimenter during an initial study were encouraged to form a goal intention to complain to the rude experimenter. In addition, a subset of participants formed implementation intentions (e.g. 'As soon as I see this person again, I'll tell her what an unfriendly person she is!'). In a second (ostensibly unrelated) study, participants had to read a series of adjectives used to describe people as quickly as possible. However, 100 ms before each adjective, either the face of the unfriendly experimenter or a neutral face was presented subliminally (participants were not consciously aware of the presentation because the face was pattern masked and appeared for only 10 ms). Findings indicated that participants who formed implementation intentions to tell the unfriendly experimenter what they thought of her were slower to respond to positive adjectives and faster to respond to negative adjectives following subliminal presentation of a picture of the unfriendly experimenter compared with the neutral face. These findings were not obtained among participants who only formed goal intentions or a second control group who had not been insulted. Thus, awareness of the critical cue is not needed for that specified opportunity directly to elicit cognitive responses that are consistent with the intended action.

Sheeran *et al.* (2005, Study 2) examined whether participants need be consciously aware of the goal underlying implementation intentions. Participants were given the goal to solve a series of puzzles as accurately as possible and they formed either an implementation intention to solve the puzzles quickly (relevant implementation intention condition) or they formed an irrelevant implementation intention. In addition, the goal to respond quickly was primed outside participants' awareness (using a word-recognition task that contained words related to being quick such as 'fast' and 'rapid'; cf. Bargh *et al.* 2001), or a neutral goal was primed. Debriefing indicated that participants were not aware of the activation of the goal to respond quickly. However, despite this lack of awareness of the respective goal, implementation intention effects were contingent upon activation of the goal to respond quickly. Specifically, solution times were fastest when participants had been primed with the goal to respond quickly and had formed a relevant implementation intention. Participants did not have to be consciously aware of the superordinate goal intention for implementation intentions to affect performance.

2.3.4 Alternative mechanisms

Although accumulating evidence points to the importance of cognitive processes such as heightened cue accessibility and strong cue–response links as mediators of the effect of forming implementation intentions on goal attainment, it is important to consider alternative explanations for the beneficial effects of if–then planning. Social cognition models such as the TPB (Conner and Sparks, Chapter 5 this volume) and PMT (Norman *et al.*, Chapter 3 this volume) suggest that motivation and self-efficacy are the proximal determinants of goal achievement. Thus, although implementation intentions are conceptualized as a post-intentional, volitional strategy, it is still possible that implementation intentions promote changes in behaviour because the if–then planning leads to increases in intention and/or self-efficacy. To investigate whether forming implementation intentions promotes goal attainment through motivational processes, Webb and Sheeran (2008) conducted a meta-analytic review. Across 13 studies, implementation intentions had little impact on intentions ($d_+ = 0.10$), and across nine studies, there was a similarly small effect on self-efficacy ($d_+ = 0.10$). Implementation intentions have also significantly affected the likelihood of goal achievement even when almost all of the participants scored at the top of the scale measuring goal intentions (i.e. already had very strong intentions prior to plan formation; Verplanken and Faes 1999; Sheeran and Orbell 2000). Finally, a re-analysis of data from Webb and Sheeran (2003, Study 1) indicated that participants who formed implementation intentions exhibited greater task persistence than ego-depleted participants even though both groups had equivalent low scores on the 'Reduced Motivation' subscale of the Multidimensional Fatigue Inventory (MFI-20; Smets *et al.* 1995). In summary, motivation appears not to be the mechanism by which implementation intentions promote goal achievement.

2.3.5 Summary of mechanisms

Evidence suggests that action initiation by implementation intentions is relatively immediate, efficient, and does not require conscious intent. Some researchers have asserted that the mechanisms underlying implementation intention effects may differ between health behaviours and behaviours studied in the laboratory (e.g. Sniehotta 2009; Hagger and Luszczynska 2014); however, to date, there is no evidence in support of alternative mechanisms for behaviours outside of the laboratory. Nonetheless, further research is needed to examine this issue.

3 Summary of research

3.1 Meta-analysis

Since implementation intentions facilitate identification of good opportunities to act, and initiate responses more automatically when those opportunities are encountered, forming an implementation intention should make it more likely that decisions become a reality compared with only forming a goal intention. The overall impact of forming implementation intentions on behavioural performance and goal achievement has been tested in several meta-analyses. Some of these meta-analyses have reviewed the effects of if–then planning on a range of behaviours (Koestner *et al.* 2002; Sheeran 2002; Gollwitzer and Sheeran 2006; Howard *et al.* 2009), while others have been domain-specific (diet: Adriaanse *et al.* 2011b; emotion control: Webb *et al.* 2012; physical activity: Bélanger-Gravel *et al.* 2013; Carraro and Gaudreau 2013), and yet others have focused on mechanisms (Webb and Sheeran 2008; Nyman and Yardley 2009). The effect size estimate used in most cases was d_+, which is the sample-weighted difference between means for an implementation intention condition versus a control condition divided by the within-group standard deviations. According to Cohen (1992), $d_+ = 0.20$ should be considered a 'small' effect size, $d_+ = 0.50$ is a 'medium' effect size, and $d_+ = 0.80$ is a 'large' effect size. Table 10.1 presents the effect sizes obtained in these reviews (note that effect sizes have been converted to d_+ where required).

In the largest review of the effects of forming implementation intentions conducted so far, Gollwitzer and Sheeran (2006) reported an effect size of medium-to-large magnitude ($d_+ = 0.65$) across 94 studies ($n = 8461$). In additional analyses, Gollwitzer and Sheeran (2006) reported effect sizes within different domains including health ($d_+ = 0.59$, $k = 23$, $n = 2861$). These findings are supported by reviews that focus specifically on health behaviours, such as diet and physical activity, although these suggest relatively smaller effects (Adriaanse *et al.* 2011b; Bélanger-Gravel *et al.* 2013; Carraro and Gaudreau 2013). Implementation intentions can also be used to modify emotional outcomes, where effect sizes tend to be large (Webb *et al.* 2012) or across a range of behaviours for clinical samples (Toli *et al.*, submitted). Thus, forming an implementation intention makes an important difference to whether or not desired outcomes are obtained, including when the outcomes are health-related, although the effects are somewhat smaller for physical activity and reducing unhealthy eating.

Table 10.1 Effect sizes in meta-analyses of the impact of implementation intentions on goal achievement and related outcomes

Research area	Researchers	Effect size d_+ (number of studies, k)
General	Koestner et al. (2002)	0.54 (k = 13)
	Sheeran (2002)	0.70 (k = 15)
	Gollwitzer and Sheeran (2006)	0.65 (k = 94)
	Howard et al. (2009)	0.54 (k = 9)
	Toli et al. (submitted)	0.63 (k = 27)
Emotion control	Webb et al. (2012)	0.91 (k = 21)
Diet	Adriaanse et al. (2011a)	0.43 (k = 24)
		Promoting healthy eating: 0.51 (k = 15)
		Reducing unhealthy eating: 0.29 (k = 9)
Physical activity	Carraro and Gaudreau (2013)	0.30 (k = 21): average post-intervention and follow-up
	Bélanger-Gravel et al. (2013)	0.24 (k = 19): follow-up

Several features of Gollwitzer and Sheeran's (2006) analysis serve to underline the efficacy of implementation intentions in promoting goal achievement. First, the review does not suffer from publication bias. Forty-nine per cent of the studies reviewed were unpublished; moreover, publication status had no impact on the effect size obtained for implementation intentions. Second, experimental designs (i.e. random assignment of participants to implementation intention vs. control conditions) yielded similar effect sizes to those obtained using correlational designs that assessed participants' use of implementation intentions using rating scales (d_+ = 0.65 and 0.70 respectively), which increases confidence in the findings. Finally, the efficacy of implementation intentions was not exaggerated by over-reliance on self-report measures of behaviour with similar sized effects when using self-report or objective outcome measures (d_+ = 0.63 and 0.67 respectively). In summary, implementation intentions benefited performance when assessed across a range of methods.

The efficacy of implementation intentions has also been noted in meta-analyses comparing the effect of a wide range of behaviour change techniques, including among internet-based interventions (Webb et al. 2010), on specific health behaviours such as smoking (Bartlett et al. 2014) or on the determinants of health behaviours such as self-efficacy (Olander et al. 2013; Williams and French 2011). These meta-analyses typically use taxonomies of behaviour change techniques and compare the effect sizes among studies that use a specific technique in the intervention condition with the effect sizes reported by studies that do not use the specific technique in the intervention condition. While these reviews are useful in comparing the effects of several techniques across a relatively broad range of literature, given the differences in several potentially important features across included studies, one should not ignore individual studies – particularly those using full-factorial designs. In the field of implementation intentions, studies have been conducted using this approach to identify the effect of implementation intentions alone and in conjunction with additional behaviour change techniques. For example, studies suggest that combining implementation intentions with motivational interventions (e.g. decisional balance sheets) produces stronger effects than using neither or either strategy alone (e.g. Prestwich et al. 2003, 2008; Sheeran et al. 2005).

3.2 Specific health behaviours

Implementation intentions have been used extensively to promote health behaviour change. Research to date has examined both health-protective behaviours (e.g. exercise, healthy food intake, vitamin intake, and cancer screening) and health-risk behaviours (e.g. unhealthy food intake, binge drinking, and smoking) and has used a variety of samples and measures of behaviour (see Table 10.2 for an overview of research to date).

3.2.1 Physical activity

Meta-analyses of the effects of forming implementation intentions on exercise (Bélanger-Gravel *et al.* 2013; Carraro and Gaudreau 2013) support the idea that forming implementation intentions can promote physical activity. Primary studies include interventions targeted at pregnant women (Gaston and Prapavessis 2014), prostate cancer survivors (although significant effects at one month disappeared at three months; McGowan *et al.* 2013), patients undergoing pulmonary rehabilitation (Rodgers *et al.* 2014), adults of low socio-economic status (Armitage and Arden 2010), and children (Armitage and Sprigg 2010). It should be noted that studies that have produced significant effects of implementation intentions on physical activity have tended to examine effects over relatively short periods (e.g. two weeks: Andersson and Moss 2011; four weeks/one month: Wiedemann *et al.* 2011; Gaston and Prapavessis 2014; two months: Rodrigues *et al.* 2013), while studies using longer-term follow-ups tend to report smaller effects on physical activity outcomes (three months: McGowan *et al.* 2013; six months: Prestwich *et al.* 2012; Rodgers *et al.* 2014). Formal meta-analytic tests of the length of follow-up suggested it did not impact on effect size (Bélanger-Gravel *et al.* 2013) or that the evidence was mixed (Carraro and Gaudreau 2013), but these reviews did not include several recent studies that incorporated long-term follow-ups producing small effects (e.g. Prestwich *et al.* 2012; Rodgers *et al.* 2014). Other studies have used implementation intentions successfully alongside other behaviour change techniques to promote physical activity but, by not adopting factorial designs, it is not possible to disentangle the unique effects of implementation intentions and the additional behaviour change techniques (Milne *et al.* 2002; Prestwich *et al.* 2010; Koring *et al.* 2012; Schwerdtfeger *et al.* 2012).

3.2.2 Diet

Since Adriaanse *et al.* (2011b) conducted their review of the effect of forming implementation intentions on dietary outcomes, the number of experimental studies published in the area has approximately doubled. A striking finding from Adriaanse and colleagues' review was that forming implementation intentions appeared to be more effective in promoting healthy dietary habits (e.g. promoting fruit and vegetable consumption) than in reducing unhealthy dietary habits (e.g. reducing dietary fat intake). Findings since then appear reasonably consistent with this pattern. Experimental studies focusing on promoting a healthy diet have reported significant effects of forming implementation intentions (Stadler *et al.* 2010; Zandstra *et al.* 2010; Knäuper *et al.* 2011; Guillaumie *et al.* 2012; Troop, 2013; Harris *et al.* 2014). In contrast, the pattern for reducing unhealthy snacking has been more mixed. While some studies have reported significant benefits of forming implementation intentions on reducing unhealthy food intake (Bukowska-Durawa *et al.* 2010; van Koningsbruggen *et al.* 2011; Karimi-Shahanjarini *et al.* 2013), some have reported more complex findings. For example, Verhoeven *et al.* (2013) found that forming one implementation intention was more effective than forming several implementation intentions.

Table 10.2   Applications of implementation intentions to health goals

Research area	Overview of empirical studies and reviews
Promoting health-protective behaviours	
Exercise	*Recent reviews*: Bélanger-Gravel *et al.* (2013), Carraro and Gaudreau (2013) *Additional studies not cited in these reviews*: Milne *et al.* (2002), Armitage and Arden (2010), Armitage and Sprigg (2010), Andersson and Moss (2011), Luszczynska *et al.* (2011), Wiedemann *et al.* (2011), Prestwich *et al.* (2012), Bélanger-Gravel *et al.* (2013), McGowan *et al.* (2013), Rodrigues *et al.* (2013), Epton *et al.* (2014), Gaston and Prapavessis (2014), Jessop *et al.* (2014), Rodgers *et al.* (2014)
Diet	*Recent review*: Adriaanse *et al.* (2011a) *Additional studies not cited in this review*: Adriaanse *et al.* (2010, 20011b), Bukowska-Durawa *et al.* (2010), Stadler *et al.* (2010), Tam *et al.* (2010), Zandstra *et al.* (2010), Knäuper *et al.* (2011), Kroese *et al.* (2011), Soureti *et al.* (2011), van Koningsbruggen *et al.* (2011), Guillaumie *et al.* (2012), Wiedemann *et al.* (2012), Benyamini *et al.* (2013), Karimi-Shahanjarini *et al.* (2013), Scholz *et al.* (2013), Troop (2013), Verhoeven *et al.* (2013), Epton *et al.* (2014), Harris *et al.* (2014), Prestwich *et al.* (2014a)
Cancer screening	
Breast self-examination	Orbell *et al.* (1997), Prestwich *et al.* (2005), Benyamini *et al.* (2011)
Testicular self-examination	Milne and Sheeran (2002), Steadman and Quine (2004), Heverin and Byrne (2011)
Breast screening	Rutter *et al.* (2006), Browne and Chan (2012)
Attendance for cervical screening	Sheeran and Orbell (2000), Walsh (2003)
Completing colorectal cancer screening	Lo *et al.* (2014), Neter *et al.* (2014)
Medication adherence	Sheeran and Orbell (1999), Steadman and Quine (2000), Liu and Park (2004), Jackson *et al.* (2006), Brown *et al.* (2009), Chatzisarantis *et al.* (2010), O'Carroll *et al.* (2013), Brom *et al.* (2014)
Reducing health-risk behaviours	
Smoking	Higgins and Conner (2003), Armitage (2007, 2008), Van Osch *et al.* (2008), Webb *et al.* (2009), Conner and Higgins (2010), Elfeddali *et al.* (2012), Epton *et al.* (2014)
Alcohol consumption	Murgraff *et al.* (1996, 2007), Fitzsimons *et al.* (2007), Gebhardt *et al.* (2008), Armitage (2009), Chatzisarantis and Hagger (2010), Armitage *et al.* (2011), Arden and Armitage (2012), Armitage and Arden (2012), Hagger *et al.* (2012a, 2012b), Epton *et al.* (2014)

Tam *et al.* (2010) found an interaction between implementation intention formation, regulatory fit, and habit strength. Specifically, when participants had weak unhealthy snacking habits, any related implementation intention formation was useful. However, when participants had strong unhealthy snacking habits, implementation intention formation required regulatory fit (promotion-focused individuals with promotion-focused implementation intentions; prevention-focused individuals with prevention-focused implementation intentions). Additional experimental studies have reported marginal (Kroese *et al.* 2011), mixed (i.e. a similar proportion of significant and null effects; Soureti *et al.* 2011) or non-significant effects of forming implementation intentions in reducing unhealthy food intake (Scholz *et al.* 2013; Prestwich *et al.* 2014a), with certain types of implementation intentions (e.g. negation implementation intentions: 'If [cue X] then not [habitual response Y]') being less effective than implementation intentions designed to replace the unhealthy snack with healthy snacks (Adriaanse *et al.* 2011a).

3.2.3 Cancer screening

Implementation intentions have been shown to be an effective behaviour change technique for increasing the likelihood of self-examinations. For example, in the first test of the efficacy of implementation intentions in promoting health-protective behaviour, Orbell *et al.* (1997) found that participants who formed implementation intentions were significantly more likely to perform a breast self-examination (BSE) than were control participants (64% and 14%, respectively). This group difference was similar when data from participants with strong goal intentions were analysed separately; here 100% of participants who formed implementation intentions conducted a BSE compared with just 53% of the control participants.

In a later study, Prestwich *et al.* (2005) examined the effect of involving partners in BSE using collaborative implementation intentions. While students were randomized to implementation intention or no implementation intention conditions, within each group they chose whether to involve their partner or not. Rates of BSE differed across groups at one-month follow-up (collaborative implementation intentions: 100%; partner/no implementation intention: 83%; implementation intention: 63%; control group: 26%). However, it should be noted that because the study did not fully randomize participants to conditions, it is difficult to draw clear conclusions about the impact of involving partners. In a related study, Benyamini *et al.* (2011) reported that participants who formed BSE plans individually versus participants who also involved their husbands in the BSE planning (but not the actual BSE behaviour) increased their rates of BSE to a similar extent.

Implementation intentions have also been used to successfully increase testicular self-examination (TSE) rates (Milne and Sheeran 2002; Steadman and Quine 2004). However, Heverin and Byrne (2011) reported that neither forming implementation intentions once or twice after watching a TSE demonstration video increased TSE rates compared with a demonstration video-only condition. It should be noted, however, that the demonstration video itself was highly effective, boosting TSE rates from 25% to above 80%, so perhaps there was no volitional problem for implementation intentions to address (see Section 2.2).

For other screening-related behaviours, the evidence regarding the benefits of implementation intentions is more mixed. Sheeran and Orbell (2000) used implementation intentions to increase cervical cancer screening rates (92% vs. 68% in the control group; see also Walsh 2003), while Browne and Chan (2012) used implementation intentions to increase the likelihood that young women would initiate a conversation with an older female family member concerning mammography (54% vs. 33% in the control group). Such interventions have been scaled-up to large populations with positive effects in relation to promoting adherence to colorectal cancer screening (Neter *et al.* 2014). However, another large-scale test of implementation intentions involving over 23,000 invitations (Lo *et al.* 2014) reported that asking participants to form three pre-formulated implementation intentions did not increase the likelihood that participants returned a screening test kit for colorectal cancer (39.7% uptake vs. 40.4% in the control condition; see also Rutter *et al.* 2006). The authors noted that the lack of an effect may have been attributable to the nature of the test kit, which may have reduced the motivation of individuals to take the test, which could, in turn, undermine the potential benefit of implementation intentions (see Section 4.2). Moreover, the manipulation was embedded in a leaflet (which requires no response from participants) rather than a questionnaire (where a response is required), which may have resulted in lower rates of implementation intention formation.

3.2.4 Medication adherence

Older adults who formed implementation intentions were five times more likely to take a blood pressure reading (Brom *et al.* 2014) and were more likely to monitor their blood glucose (Liu and Park 2004). Furthermore, there is evidence that people with epilepsy (Brown *et al.* 2009) and stroke survivors (O'Carroll *et al.* 2013) took their medication more regularly when they had formed implementation intentions, while students have been shown to be more likely to take vitamin C tablets (Sheeran and Orbell 1999; Steadman and Quine 2000) or multivitamin tablets (Chatzisarantis *et al.* 2010) when they had formed if–then plans, compared with control groups not forming implementation intentions. However, not all studies have reported positive effects of forming implementation intentions in relation to medication adherence. Jackson *et al.* (2006) reported that, in a sample of patients recruited through a pharmacist and taking a course of antibiotics, there was no difference in the proportion of individuals taking all of their medication between patients who formed their own implementation intentions, patients given an implementation intention, and one of two control groups (who differed only on whether they completed a questionnaire assessing constructs from the TPB; Ajzen 1991). Jackson *et al.* (2006) suggested that the implementation intention manipulations may not have promoted adherence, as the course of treatment was short (less than seven days on average) and the sample were highly motivated. Indeed, the studies demonstrating beneficial effects of forming implementation intentions on medication adherence have detected significant effects at longer follow-ups versus shorter follow-ups (e.g. Sheeran and Orbell 1999). On balance, the evidence across these studies suggests that implementation intentions represent a promising means of helping people to take their medication regularly and on time.

3.2.5 Alcohol intake

In the first test of the effect of forming implementation intentions on alcohol intake, Murgraff *et al.* (1996) reported that, compared with a control group, participants who were asked to form implementation intentions drank alcohol less frequently over a two-week period. More recently, Hagger *et al.* (2012a) found that combining implementation intentions with a motivational intervention (namely, a mental simulation task involving participants visualizing successful alcohol-related goal achievement and then reflecting on subsequent feelings arising from this achievement) was a particularly effective method to reduce drinking among a sub-sample of heavy drinking students. However, forming implementation intentions did not influence drinking when the full sample was considered, or within samples drawn from various countries reported elsewhere (Hagger *et al.* 2012b). Other successful applications have used implementation intentions to reduce the likelihood that students choose the offer of a free alcoholic drink (Chatzisarantis and Hagger 2010), to minimize binge drinking on Fridays but not Saturdays (Murgraff *et al.* 2007), and to reduce alcohol drinking in the general population using implementation intentions produced by the experimenter or by the participant themselves (Armitage 2009). Rivis and Sheeran (2013) found that implementation intentions attenuated the automatic influence of binge drinker stereotypes, and reduced binge drinking behaviour.

3.2.6 Smoking

Several studies have found that forming implementation intentions can help smokers to quit and prevent non-smokers from starting to smoke (but see van Osch *et al.* 2008). Armitage (2007) found that forming implementation intentions (specifying when and how to quit smoking in the following two months) significantly increased quit rates, compared with a control group, at two months in adult smokers (12% vs. 2%) and also reduced objectively measured levels of nicotine dependence. In adolescents, Conner and Higgins (2010) found that repeatedly forming implementation intentions every four months over a two-year period led to lower self-reported rates of smoking (26.3%) compared with three comparison groups (self-efficacy group: 34.0%; control 1: 30.5%; control 2: 34.5%). Conner and Higgins also found that implementation intentions led to lower rates of smoking on an objective measure of smoking (see also Higgins and Conner 2003). Using 12-month quit rates as their key outcome, Elfeddali *et al.* (2012) found that providing feedback on perceptions of smoking and quitting alongside implementation intention formation improved abstinence rates (33% in an observed case analysis) compared with a control group completing questionnaires only (22%). The implementation intention manipulation was delivered both before and after their quit date. Providing additional feedback on negative affect, self-efficacy, recovery self-efficacy and plans, in an augmented planning condition, did not improve quit rates further (31% in the observed case analysis). However, while implementation intentions may be useful in helping smokers to reduce the number of cigarettes smoked when their habit is weak or moderate, Webb *et al.* (2009) found that they may not be helpful for those with strong smoking habits. Whether implementation intentions are effective in breaking habits depends on the relative strength of implementation intentions. Breaking strong habits requires the formation of strong implementation intentions. Gollwitzer (2014) presents an overview of means through which the effects of implementation intentions can be strengthened to tackle habits including enriching implementation intention formation with imagery (e.g. Knäuper *et al.* 2011). Some sub-types or variants of implementation intentions (see Figure 10.1) may also prove more effective than others.

4 Developments

The first question that should be asked about the concept of implementation intentions is: 'Do implementation intentions facilitate the translation of intentions into action?' Findings from studies in social and health psychology and meta-analyses (see Section 3) indicate that the answer to this first question is 'yes'. A second question that should be asked in order to gain a more complete understanding of how implementation intentions can be used to promote health behaviours is *when* do implementation intentions facilitate translation of intentions into action?

An answer to this question can be gleaned from recent research on the moderators of implementation intention effects (Gollwitzer *et al.* 2010; Prestwich and Kellar 2014).

4.1 Presence of self-regulatory problems

Several factors are likely to determine how strongly implementation intentions affect goal achievement. The first key moderator of implementation intentions effects concerns the presence of a self-regulatory problem. If enacting a behaviour is easy and there are few obstacles to performance, then motivational factors (e.g. goal intentions, self-efficacy) should satisfactorily promote action; little additional benefit can be obtained from forming an implementation intention. A good example is Webb and Sheeran's (2003, Study 2) analysis of the impact of ego-depletion and implementation intention formation on Stroop performance. Webb and Sheeran found that implementation intentions had a strong effect on task speed and accuracy when participants were ego-depleted. However, when participants were not ego-depleted, implementation intentions did not benefit performance – presumably because participants possessed sufficient self-regulatory capacity to perform the task well (see also Lengfelder and Gollwitzer 2001). In addition, Gollwitzer and Brändstatter (1997, Study 1) used participants' ratings to divide goals into 'easy' versus 'difficult' categories and found that implementation intentions only promoted the achievement of difficult goals. Koestner *et al.* (2002) also showed that implementation intentions are more effective for difficult goals. These findings all seem to indicate that implementation intention effects are more likely to emerge when the focal behaviour presents a volitional challenge or when people have difficulty regulating their behaviour (but see Dewitte *et al.* [2003] for an alternative perspective that implementation intentions are effective also for easy goals as long as the baseline enactment rate is not too high, causing a 'ceiling effect').

4.2 Motivation and habits

Empirical findings indicate that the beneficial effects of forming implementation intentions are contingent upon the presence of strong superordinate goal intentions. For example, Sheeran *et al.* (2005) found a significant interaction between intention strength and the effect of forming implementation intentions, such that implementation intentions only affected the amount of independent study that students undertook when participants' goal intentions strongly favoured the behavioural performance. Similarly, the effect of forming implementation intentions has proved more pronounced among participants with strong (vs. weak) intentions in the context of various health behaviours, including physical activity (Prestwich *et al.*, 2003; Lippke *et al.* 2004; De Vet *et al.* 2009), diet (Prestwich *et al.* 2008), compliance with speed limits (Elliott and Armitage 2006), and sunscreen use (Van Osch *et al.* 2008); however, this finding does not always emerge (e.g. Sheeran and Silverman 2003; de Nooijer *et al.* 2006). There is evidence also that the effect of forming implementation intentions may be larger when *self-efficacy* is strong (Luszczynska and Haynes 2009; Luszczynska *et al.* 2011), particularly on tough tasks (Wieber *et al.* 2010), and that the effects of forming implementation intentions could be bolstered by self-efficacy-based interventions (Koestner *et al.* 2006). However, combining implementation intentions with self-efficacy-enhancing techniques failed to lead to more pronounced effects on fruit and vegetable intake (Guillaumie *et al.* 2012). Other moderators have been considered across multiple studies but have produced inconsistent results. For example, whereas Koestner *et al.* (2002) obtained evidence consistent with the idea that implementation intention effects were especially effective when participants' goal intentions were more *self-concordant* versus less self-concordant, Chatzisarantis *et al.* (2008) reported the opposite effect (i.e. implementation intention effects were strongest when motivation was self-discordant).

Habits constitute another potential moderator of the effect of forming implementation intentions on goal attainment. Specifically, evidence suggests that forming implementation intentions may be less effective when enacting the plan involves changing strong *habits*. In two studies, one conducted in the laboratory (a target detection task) and another in the field (smoking), Webb *et al.* (2009) showed that implementation intentions were more useful when habits were weak or moderate rather than when they were strong.

In summary, the strength of the respective superordinate goal intention, along with self-efficacy and habit, are likely to represent important moderators of action control by implementation intentions in many contexts.

4.3 Plan quality

A third potential moderator of implementation intention effects is the quality of implementation intention formation. Field studies have demonstrated that participants vary in the extent to which they follow instructions within implementation intention manipulations. For example, Michie *et al.* (2004) reported that only 63% of individuals who were asked to form a plan to attend an antenatal screening actually did so. Similarly, in a trial to promote physical activity, around 70% of participants in the experimental condition formed a specific implementation intention as directed (De Vet *et al.* 2011b), and rates were even lower (e.g. 18% of participants formed a specific implementation intention as directed for the target behaviour) in a trial designed to promote condom use (De Vet *et al.* 2011a). Studies have indicated that forming higher quality plans (as indexed by the extent to which individuals have followed directions to identify specific cues and responses) is related to higher levels of physical activity (Ziegelmann *et al.* 2006; De Vet *et al.* 2011b) and reduced levels of smoking (Van Osch *et al.* 2010) and alcohol intake (Armitage 2009). Relatedly, Allan *et al.* (2013) have demonstrated that forming implementation intentions is more effective when individuals are *poor planners*. Therefore, it is imperative that participants not only form plans, but form plans that specify an opportunity, an intended response, and link the two together. Poor planners may need even more assistance and could make use of volitional help sheets in this regard (see Section 6.2).

As well as examining the extent to which individuals follow the instructions to form implementation intentions and its impact on behaviour, the nature of the planning intervention itself is likely to influence the accessibility of cues and the strength of cue–response links. Certain procedures should, thereby, fortify implementation intention effects (for a detailed consideration of the effects of different types of implementation intentions, see Section 6.2). For example, Gollwitzer *et al.* (2002) manipulated the strength of participants' commitment to their implementation intention by providing feedback from extensive personality tests that supposedly indicated that participants would benefit from sticking closely to their plans (high commitment) or would benefit from not rigidly adhering to the plan (low commitment). Findings from a cued recall paradigm indicated that the high-commitment group had superior memory for selected opportunities compared with the low-commitment group. Prestwich *et al.* (2009) examined the efficacy of augmenting implementation intentions with text message reminders of their implementation intention designed to help strengthen the link between cue and response, finding that reminding individuals of their implementation intentions increased effects on physical activity (but see Schwerdtfeger *et al.* 2012). Thus, there is evidence that the degree of implementation intention formation, commitment, and plan reminders moderate the impact of if–then plans on goal achievement.

5 Operationalization of the model

5.1 Preliminary considerations

The paradigm adopted in most studies using implementation intentions to promote health goals has involved questionnaire measures followed by random assignment of participants to an experimental condition that contains questions designed to prompt implementation intention formation or to a control condition that does not contain these questions. Of course, random assignment should ensure that participants in both conditions have equivalent previous experience with, and motivation to achieve, the goal. However, an advantage of taking measures of experience and motivation is that randomization checks can be conducted and any differences on these variables can be controlled for in statistical analyses. Relatedly, if the behavioural follow-up involves further contact with participants, then measures of motivational variables could also be taken at the same time as the measure of behaviour. These procedures allow researchers to conduct statistical analyses to ensure that the impact of implementation intentions on goal attainment is not attributable to pre-intervention differences in motivation or past behaviour, or to potential differences in motivation accruing from the formation of the if–then plan.

Most studies of implementation intention effects in health psychology have involved passive control conditions – that is, participants in the control condition have not been asked to complete questionnaire items of similar content or duration as participants in the experimental group. Strictly speaking, this procedure confounds the impact of the experimental manipulation with potential differences in expectancies and attentional demands between conditions. However, studies that have employed active control conditions wherein participants formed implementation intentions about what to do after they had accomplished their goal (e.g. Aarts *et al.* 1999) or formed plans regarding an irrelevant goal (e.g. Sheeran *et al.* 2005) have obtained strong implementation intention effects as well. Nevertheless, it seems wise to employ an active control condition whenever possible in order to rule out alternative explanations of differences in behavioural performance or attained outcomes. Reviews have also found smaller effects of implementation intention formation on goal achievement when participants asked to form implementation intentions have been compared with participants in control conditions asked to form goal intentions, rather than control conditions where the goal is not specified or emphasized (Webb *et al.* 2012). This difference is understandable; the difference between implementation intention and goal intention instructions represents the effects of a volitional strategy, whereas the difference between implementation intention and no instructions likely represents the effects of both motivational and volitional processes because planning instructions typically also incorporate motivational instructions (e.g. participants are asked to increase the amount of exercise that they do, before being asked to form a plan to help them). Therefore, goal intention instructions represent the more stringent and specific comparison condition for evaluating the effect of forming implementation intentions.

Implementation intention manipulations can take many forms, although they each follow the format: 'if opportunity X, then response Y'. The variants of implementation intentions, and how they are manipulated, are described in Section 5.2 and illustrated in Figure 10.1. Because implementation intention inductions often ask participants to specify an appropriate opportunity and goal-directed response in an open-ended format, considerable care must be taken to ensure that participants do not skip relevant items. Answering open-ended questions can be perceived as onerous when participants have already completed a long questionnaire and have become used to ticking a box to indicate their response. Indeed, studies have reported that many participants may fail to formulate plans as instructed (e.g. Michie *et al.* 2004; De Vet *et al.* 2011a, 2011b). To alleviate this potential problem, some studies have hinted at the benefits of forming an implementation intention in order to encourage participants to complete the respective section of the questionnaire (e.g. Orbell *et al.* 1997; Sheeran and Orbell 1999; Milne *et al.* 2002). Even though this procedure seemed likely to generate expectancies about the impact of planning, none of these studies observed significant effects on subsequent motivation to perform the behaviour, and Chapman *et al.* (2009) have shown that such hints do not moderate the effects of forming implementation intentions on goal attainment. Other studies have used other techniques such as providing relevant examples and checklists to ensure that participants had formed implementation intentions accurately and sufficiently to meet the target goal (e.g. Prestwich *et al.* 2008). In summary, careful consideration needs be given to features of the overall questionnaire (e.g. length, order) and to the wording and layout of the implementation intention induction to ensure that participants engage with the process of forming an if–then plan.

5.2 Taxonomy of implementation intentions

Implementation intentions have the format 'If opportunity Y occurs, then I will initiate response Z.' The importance of using an if–then format in wording the plan was demonstrated by Oettingen *et al.* (2000, Study 3). All participants were asked to perform four concentration tasks on their computers each Wednesday morning for the next four weeks. Participants in the control condition were asked to indicate what time they would perform the task by responding to the statement, 'I will perform as many arithmetic tasks as possible each Wednesday at ____ (self-chosen time before noon)'. Participants in the implementation intention condition, on the other hand, indicated their chosen time by responding to the statement, 'If it is Wednesday at ____ (self-chosen time before noon), then I will perform as many arithmetic tasks as possible!' Despite the apparent similarity between the control and implementation intention instructions, the conditional structure of the implementation intention instructions had a dramatic impact on how closely participants performed the task to their intended time: the mean deviation from the intended start time was nearly five times higher in the control condition (8 hours) compared with the implementation intention condition (1.5 hours). These findings indicate that using the defining if–then format in implementation intention inductions is important to ensure strong implementation intention effects.

A number of variants on implementation intention interventions have emerged over recent years, such as collaborative implementation intentions, booster implementation intentions, and dyadic plans. Here, we present a taxonomy of implementation intention interventions in which we attempt to classify the different variants or sub-types of implementation intentions (see Figure 10.1). The taxonomy comprises seven questions or levels and the idea is that any if–then plan can be classified according to the different options under each level. Moreover, any option on one level can be paired with any option on another level. While certain combinations have been widely tested (e.g. questionnaire-manipulated implementation intentions, targeting individuals, without boosters, with single plans incorporating external cues to do more of a particular behaviour), other combinations have not been considered at all (e.g. mere-measurement implementation intention manipulations of dyadic planning).

5.2.1 Are implementation intentions formed spontaneously or prompted by an intervention?

Spontaneous implementation intentions, in which an individual forms an implementation intention without being prompted by an experimenter or researcher, have typically been assessed through correlational designs (e.g. Brickell *et al.* 2006) that measure the extent to which participants have specified when, where, and how they will perform goal-directed behaviours. In

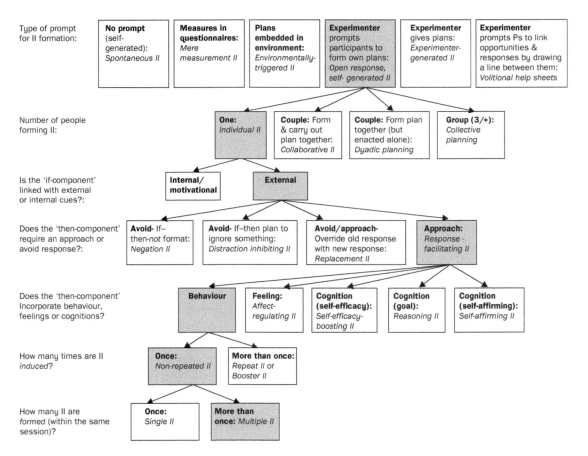

Figure 10.1 Taxonomy of implementation intentions (II) illustrating an II manipulation commonly used in field-based studies promoting health behaviours (shaded boxes reflect the II manipulation used by Prestwich *et al.* 2003)

contrast, there are a number of ways in which *prompted implementation intentions* can be generated and such studies typically adopt experimental designs where the effects of (prompted) planning are compared with an alternative or no intervention. For example, *mere measurement implementation intentions* involve simply embedding measures of implementation intentions within questionnaires (e.g. 'I have made a detailed plan regarding... when to exercise over the next 2 weeks, where to exercise over the next 2 weeks, how to exercise over the next 2 weeks, how often to exercise over the next 2 weeks', with anchors of 'not at all true' to 'exactly true') and have been used successfully to promote physical activity (e.g. Conner *et al.* 2010) and blood donation (e.g. Godin *et al.* 2010). *Volitional help sheets* list opportunities or temptations on one side of a page and possible responses on the other side. Participants are typically asked to choose an opportunity/temptation that is relevant to them, select a response from those provided, and then draw a line to link the relevant opportunity/temptation to the selected response. They have been used successfully to promote healthy behaviours such as physical activity (Armitage and Arden 2010), and to reduce unhealthy behaviours (alcohol intake: Armitage and Arden 2012; binge drinking: Arden and Armitage 2012; smoking: Armitage 2008).

Open-response, self-generated implementation intentions (the most commonly used type of implementation intention in field studies) directly ask participants to formulate their own plans. Examples of implementation intentions (e.g. '*If* it is the end of work on Mondays through to Fridays, *then* I will briskly walk home'; see Prestwich *et al.* 2012) are often provided alongside open-response, self-generated implementation intentions to illustrate how these plans should be formed. On the other hand, *experimenter-generated implementation intentions* (most often used in experimental, laboratory-based studies) provide participants with specific implementation intention(s) that they are required to use. In contrast to directly requesting implementation intention formation, the final type of prompted implementation intention formation relates to *environmentally triggered implementation intentions*. In this approach, if–then plans are induced indirectly by embedding them within features of the environment such as advertisements or product packaging. This approach has been utilized within a website advocating fair-trade products to increase purchasing of sustainable food items (see Fennis *et al.* 2011, Study 2). Environmentally triggered implementation intentions are distinguishable from spontaneous implementation intentions in that they are intentionally triggered by the interventionist.

5.2.2 How many people formulate the implementation intention? Individuals vs. pairs vs. groups

The vast majority of studies have focused on individuals forming if–then plans to support performance of their own health behaviour. However, Prestwich *et al.* (2005) developed *collaborative implementation intentions* that require pairs of individuals to identify critical opportunities and responses that they will enact together. Collaborative implementation intentions (e.g. '*If* it is the end of work on Mondays through to Fridays, *then we* will briskly walk home together') have been successfully used to promote physical activity (Prestwich *et al.* 2012) and breast self-examination (Prestwich *et al.* 2005), although they appear to be less effective in tackling risk behaviours such as unhealthy food intake (Prestwich *et al.* 2014a), possibly due to the difficulty in capturing all of the cues that can influence risk-related behaviour and ensuring that both individuals are together when these cues are encountered. A variant of collaborative implementation intentions, *dyadic planning* (Burkert *et al.* 2011), involves two people formulating if–then plans but with the target individual then enacting the target behaviour alone. For example, in the study by Burkert *et al.* (2011), participants in the dyadic planning condition completed, with the help of a partner, a planning sheet involving consideration of when, where, and how they alone would perform the target behaviour (regular pelvic floor exercises) while those in the individual condition completed the form alone. The idea of joint planning has also been extended to groups. *Collective planning* involves a group deciding when, where, and how to act towards their collective goal. This approach has been used to increase the likelihood of selecting the best choice on a decision-making task, to increase the probability that participants disengage from a failing course of action (investing in an unsuccessful, unpopular venture), and to increase cooperation in schoolchildren (for a review, see Wieber *et al.* 2012).

5.2.3 Cue component: is the 'if-component' linked with external or internal cues?

When formulating if–then plans, the cues can be external, such as an environmental feature (e.g. encountering an object, time of day, etc.) or internal, such as a feeling (e.g. boredom) or motivation (e.g. to be social). While the majority of studies have focused on the effects of if–then plans specifying external cues, there is some evidence in support of forming implementation intentions based on internal cues. For example, Adriaanse *et al.* (2009) demonstrated that forming implementation intentions based on motivational cues (e.g. feeling bored) but not situational cues (e.g. being at home) were significantly more effective than a control condition in promoting healthy snacking and reducing unhealthy snacking.

5.2.4 Response component 1: does the 'then-component' require an approach or avoidance response?

Implementation intentions have been used successfully to promote a variety of different responses. These successful applications include using implementation intentions to do more of a desired response or less of an undesired response, as well as being used to tackle a variety of behaviours, feelings or cognitions (see Section 5.2.5). Sub-types of implementation intentions may be delineated based on the different types of responses that are specified in the 'response' component of the plan. *Response facilitating implementation intentions* involve an individual planning how to initiate a response (e.g. planning to do an additional session of vigorous physical activity during the week). In contrast, *distraction-inhibiting implementation intentions* involve an individual formulating an if–then plan to ignore something (e.g. '*If* I see a person, *then* I will ignore his race'; Mendoza *et al.* 2010). Related to these concepts are *replacement implementation intentions* (that involve overriding an old response with a new one), or planning to not do something, termed *negation implementation intentions* (e.g. '*If* opportunity X, *then* not habitual response Y'), which have been shown to backfire (e.g. increase unhealthy snacking: Adriaanse *et al.* 2011a).

5.2.5 Response component 2: does the 'then-component' incorporate behaviour, feelings or cognitions?

While the majority of studies encourage implementation intention formation that specifies a behavioural response, others serve to activate other responses. *Reasoning implementation intentions* (Prestwich *et al.* 2008) involve an individual deciding what they will think at a specific opportunity in order that they will perform/not perform the target behaviour. Activating a higher-order goal within the risky situation in this fashion has been shown to enhance self-control in terms of reducing unhealthy food intake (Prestwich *et al.* 2008; van Koningsbruggen *et al.* 2011). Reasoning implementation intentions are distinct from activating a why mindset after forming an implementation intention, which has been shown to reduce implementation intention effects. For example, Wieber *et al.* (2014) asked all participants to form a goal intention (to hold a handgrip closed for as long as possible, Study 1; to respond to numbers quickly, Study 2) and then for some of these participants to supplement their goal intention with an if–then plan ('And if my muscles start hurting, then I will ignore the pain!'; 'And if the number 3 appears, then I will press the left mouse button particularly fast!'). Participants then either completed a second task to activate a *why* mindset (writing down *why* they would form and maintain personal relationships) or a *how* mindset (writing down *how* they would form and maintain personal relationships). While the why-mindset was shown to improve performance in the control (goal-intention) condition, it was shown to reduce the benefits of forming implementation intentions.

Bayer and Gollwitzer (2007) demonstrated that forming implementation intentions designed to boost self-efficacy (e.g. 'And if I start a new problem, then I will tell myself: I can solve it!') improved mathematical test performance in females (Study 1) and analytical reasoning test performance in males (Study 2). We term such plans *self-efficacy boosting implementation intentions*. In *self-affirming implementation intentions* (Armitage *et al.* 2011), means of affirming oneself are incorporated in the then-component of the plan (e.g. '*If* I feel threatened or anxious, *then* I will think about the things that I value about myself'). A final category of implementation intentions involves specifying a particular feeling in the then-component of the plan. For example, Azbel-Jackson (2012) investigated the effect of forming the plan: '*If* I see a weapon, *then* I will keep calm and relaxed!' on levels of arousal upon encountering the specified cue. We term such plans *affect-regulating implementation intentions*.

5.2.6 How many implementation intention inductions are used?

While most studies require participants to formulate implementation intentions once at the start of the study, some studies have encouraged participants to form new plans at some stage after the initial formulation of an if–then plan (*repeat implementation intentions*, de Vet *et al.* 2009; or *booster implementation intentions*, Luszczynska and Haynes 2009; Chapman and Armitage 2010). These plans could either be the same as the previous formed plan(s) or new. While de Vet *et al.* (2009) did not find a significant effect of implementation intentions (a repeated implementation intention vs. a non-repeated implementation intention condition) on physical activity, they did report that repeated implementation intentions were effective for strong intenders. Luszczynska and Haynes (2009) found that, compared with a control condition, a group who formed implementation intentions at baseline and then again at six weeks and nine weeks increased their fruit and vegetable intake more at four months. This study, however, did not include a condition in which implementation intentions were only formed once. Thus it is unclear how much benefit was gleaned from booster planning. Chapman and Armitage (2010) provide stronger evidence for the benefit of booster implementation intentions. They reported that participants who formed booster implementation intentions (booster at three months) consumed more fruit and vegetables at six months than participants who only formed a single plan. However, a study that manipulated the number of boosters observed no impact of the manipulation on dietary outcomes (Scholz *et al.* 2013).

5.2.7 How many implementation intentions are formed?

Studies have also compared the effect of forming different numbers of plans (multiple plans vs. single plans). For example, Wiedemann *et al.* (2012) asked participants to formulate one, two, three, four or five plans in relation to increasing their daily intake of fruit and vegetables (or none if they were assigned to the control condition). The number of plans formulated influenced effectiveness, with greater effects of planning on fruit and vegetable consumption being observed among participants who formed four or five plans. For physical activity, too, more plans seem to be associated with more success (Wiedemann *et al.* 2011). In contrast, Verhoeven *et al.* (2013) found that forming a single plan (in this case, to reduce unhealthy snacking) was more effective than forming multiple plans. The authors' explanation of this finding was that forming multiple plans could lead to interference at the moment of acting, especially if the plans are formed with respect to the same opportunity.

Variation in the number of plans could be restricted to the initial session or be manipulated across sessions (see booster/repeated implementation intentions). In a study that manipulated the number of boosters, the number of plans had no impact on dietary outcomes (Scholz *et al.* 2013). Rather than the number of plans, whether the plans are sufficient in order to reach the target goal may be the crucial factor. For example, if an individual had the goal to exercise five times per week but then planned only to go for a run in the evening every Saturday and Sunday, then their plan would likely be insufficient to reach the goal and forming more plans would most likely be beneficial.

6 Future directions

The concept of implementation intentions has shown clear promise for promoting health behaviour and hopefully continues to have a bright future in health psychology. Indeed, it is pleasing to note that since our original chapter on this topic (in the second edition of *Predicting Health Behaviour*, published in 2005), the number of primary studies has increased substantially. Accumulated evidence indicates that forming if–then plans makes an important difference to whether or not people realize their goals (e.g. Gollwitzer and Sheeran 2006) – both when goal attainment is contingent upon promoting wanted responses and controlling unwanted responses. In addition, a good deal of research indicates that implementation intentions promote goal achievement both by facilitating identification of specified opportunities to act and by automating goal-directed responses (e.g. Aarts *et al.* 1999; Webb and Sheeran 2008). Finally, there is evidence that a variety of factors moderate the impact of implementation intention formation on goal achievement, including difficulties in behaviour regulation, motivation-related variables and habits, and plan quality. In summary, substantial progress has been made in answering questions about *whether*, *when*, and *why* implementation intentions facilitate the enactment of goal intentions.

Despite this substantial progress, there remains considerable scope for future research to examine efficacy through rigorously conducted trials, to confirm mediating processes, and to identify additional moderating variables (see also Gollwitzer 2014). There have also been relatively few high-quality, pre-registered trials of implementation intentions using objective behavioural measures (see Hagger and Luszczynska 2014). While taking steps, for example, to blind key personnel to study condition and to protect the allocation sequence is rare in health behaviour interventions (e.g. Prestwich *et al.* 2014b, 2014c), such steps are important to ensure that estimates of the effects of forming implementation intentions on health behaviours are accurate. We would also point to the importance of pre-registering trials and publishing protocols, which can provide a number of benefits, including minimizing the risk of selective outcome reporting. (For examples of published protocols involving implementation intentions, see Conner *et al.* [2013] and Epton *et al.* [2014].)

As the body of empirical research on the effects of forming implementation intentions grows, there will likely be more opportunities to apply implementation intentions to population-level health behaviour change, especially as implementation intentions can be applied to large populations relatively easily (i.e. interventions are typically relatively short and cheap to implement). For example, Neter *et al.* (2014) successfully demonstrated, in an overall sample of nearly 30,000 adults aged 50–74, that forming implementation intentions can increase adherence to colorectal cancer screening.

While there has now been quite a lot of work on identifying when, and for whom, implementation intentions are most effective (for related reviews, see Gollwitzer *et al.* 2010; Prestwich and Kellar 2014), there is a need to conduct similar research on variants on implementation intentions (e.g. collaborative implementation intentions, dyadic plans). For these variants, the need for high-quality trials and for further work on mechanisms and to identify boundary conditions is particularly acute.

Some studies have assessed the impact of forming multiple implementation intentions. These have involved forming the same type of implementation intentions multiple times either at the start of the study period (i.e. *multiple plans*) and/or at a later stage (i.e. *booster/replacement implementation intentions*) or forming different types of implementation intentions (usually *coping plans* plus *action plans*). However, there remains considerable scope for examining whether combining different types of implementation intentions leads to stronger effects than using either type alone. For example, for behaviours that an individual sometimes performs alone and sometimes performs with a partner (e.g. dietary-related behaviours), combining individually formed implementation intentions with collaborative implementation intentions may yield stronger effects than forming either type of implementation intention alone. The ease with which implementation intentions can be applied within mobile- (e.g. Prestwich *et al.* 2010) and internet-based technologies (e.g. Hurling *et al.* 2006) also shows that there are opportunities to test whether implementation intentions augment the impact of technology-based interventions on behaviour change. Such studies should utilize full-factorial designs, whenever possible, to clearly identify the added benefit of if–then plans.

Finally, an exciting, recent development in research on if–then plans relates to interventions that combine mental contrasting with implementation intentions (MCII interventions; for reviews, see Oettingen and Gollwitzer 2010; Oettingen *et al.* 2013). Mental contrasting involves mentally elaborating the best outcome of a desired future and then elaborating the biggest obstacle to that future, and repeating this exercise for the second best outcome and second biggest obstacle. Mental contrasting energizes goal-striving and creates strong implicit links between future and reality and between obstacles and the means to overcome those obstacles; mental contrasting also changes rates of goal attainment in line with success expectancies (see Oettingen 2012 for a review). Mental contrasting aids implementation intention formation by helping participants to identify key volitional problems that stand in the way of their desired future – so that if–then plans can then be formulated to tackle those problems. MCII interventions have already proved effective in changing such health behaviours as fruit and vegetable consumption (Stadler *et al.* 2010), snacking habits (Adriaanse *et al.* 2010), and physical activity among chronic back pain sufferers (Christiansen *et al.* 2010).

While there is evidence that forming implementation intentions is effective in promoting health behaviour change, more work is needed to establish whether if–then plans promote long-lasting change through the mechanisms identified previously in laboratory work. When the effects of forming implementation intentions are examined in combination with other behaviour change techniques, it is important to adopt full-factorial designs to isolate both the independent and multiplicative effects of implementation intentions and the other techniques. Undertaking further research into the effects of forming implementation intentions on health behaviour represents a challenging, but important, step for health psychologists in order to advance both our theoretical understanding of the effects of implementation intentions on behaviour and their applied benefit.

References

Aarts, H., Dijksterhuis, A. and Midden, C. (1999) To plan or not to plan? Goal achievement or interrupting the performance of mundane behaviors, *European Journal of Social Psychology*, 29, 971–9.

Aarts, H., Gollwitzer, P.M. and Hassin, R. (2004) Goal contagion: perceiving is for pursuing, *Journal of Personality and Social Psychology*, 87, 23–37.

Abraham, C. and Sheeran, P. (2004) Implications of goal theories for the theories of reasoned action and planned behaviour, *Current Psychology*, 22, 218–33.

Abraham, C., Sheeran, P. and Johnson, M. (1998) From health beliefs to self-regulation: theoretical advances in the psychology of action control, *Psychology and Health*, 13, 569–92.

Abraham, C., Sheeran, P., Norman, P., Conner, M., Otten, W. and de Vries, N. (1999) When good intentions are not enough: modelling post-intention cognitive correlates of condom use, *Journal of Applied Social Psychology*, 29, 2591–612.

Achtziger, A., Bayer, U.C. and Gollwitzer, P.M. (2012) Committing to implementation intentions: attention and memory effects for selected situational cues, *Motivation and Emotion*, 36, 287–300.

Adriaanse, M.A., De Ridder, D.T.D. and De Wit, J.B.F. (2009) Finding the critical cue: implementation intentions to change one's diet work best when tailored to personally relevant reasons for unhealthy eating, Personality and Social Psychology Bulletin, 35, 60–71.

Adriaanse, M.A., Oettingen, G., Gollwitzer, P.M., Hennes, E.P., De Ridder, D.T.D. and De Wit, J.B.F. (2010) When planning is not enough: fighting unhealthy snacking habits by mental contrasting with implementation intentions (MCII), *European Journal of Social Psychology*, 40, 1277–93.

Adriaanse, M.A., van Oosten, J.M.F., de Ridder, D.T.D., de Wit, J.B.F. and Evers, C. (2011a) Planning what not to eat: ironic effects of implementation intentions negating unhealthy habits, *Personality and Social Psychology Bulletin*, 37, 69–81.

Adriaanse, M.A., Vinkers. C.D.W., De Ridder, D.T.D., Hox, J.J. and De Wit, J.B.F. (2011b) Do implementation intentions help to eat a healthy diet? A systematic review and meta-analysis of the empirical evidence, Appetite, 56, 183–93.

Ajzen, I. (1991) The theory of planned behavior, *Organizational Behavior and Human Decision Processes*, 50, 179–211.

Allan, J.L., Sniehotta, F.F. and Johnston, M. (2013) The best laid plans: planning skill determines the effectiveness of action plans and implementation intentions, Annals of Behavioral Medicine, 46, 114–20.

Andersson, E.K and Moss, T.P. (2011) Imagery and implementation intention: a randomised controlled trial of interventions to increase exercise behaviour in the general population, *Psychology of Sport and Exercise*, 12, 63–70.

Arden, M. and Armitage, C.J. (2012) A volitional help sheet to reduce binge drinking in students: a randomized exploratory trial, *Alcohol and Alcoholism*, 47, 156–9.

Armitage, C.J. (2007) Efficacy of a brief worksite intervention to reduce smoking: the roles of behavioral and implementation intentions, *Journal of Occupational Health Psychology*, 12, 376–90.

Armitage, C.J. (2008) A volitional help sheet to encourage smoking cessation: a randomized exploratory trial, *Health Psychology*, 27, 557–66.

Armitage, C.J. (2009) Effectiveness of experimenter-provided and self-generated implementation intentions to reduce alcohol consumption in a sample of the general population: a randomized exploratory trial, *Health Psychology*, 28, 545–53.

Armitage, C.J. and Arden, M.A. (2010) A volitional help sheet to increase physical activity in people with low socioeconomic status: a randomised exploratory trial, *Psychology and Health*, 25, 1129–45.

Armitage, C.J. and Arden, M.A. (2012) A volitional help sheet to reduce alcohol consumption in the general population: a field experiment, *Prevention Science*, 13, 635–43.

Armitage, C.J. and Sprigg, C.A. (2010) The roles of behavioral and implementation intentions in changing physical activity in young children with low socioeconomic status, *Journal of Sport and Exercise Psychology*, 32, 359–76.

Armitage, C.J., Harris, P.R. and Arden, M.A. (2011) Evidence that self-affirmation reduces alcohol consumption: randomized exploratory trial with a new, brief means of self-affirming, *Health Psychology*, 30, 633–41.

Azbel-Jackson, L. (2012) Regulation of arousal using implementation intentions. Unpublished doctoral thesis, University of Reading.

Bagozzi, R.P. and Kimmel, S.K. (1995) A comparison of leading theories for the prediction of goal-directed behaviour, *British Journal of Social Psychology*, 34, 437–61.

Bargh, J.A. (1992) The ecology of automaticity: towards establishing the conditions needed to produce automatic processing effects, *American Journal of Psychology*, 105, 181–99.

Bargh, J.A. (1994) The four horsemen of automaticity: awareness, efficiency, intention, and control in social interaction, in R.S. Wyer, Jr. and T.K. Srull (eds.) *Handbook of Social Cognition* (2nd edn., pp. 1–40). Hillsdale, NJ: Erlbaum.

Bargh, J.A., Gollwitzer, P.M., Lee-Chai, A., Barndollar, K. and Trötschel, R. (2001) The automated will: nonconscious activation and pursuit of behavioral goals, *Journal of Personality and Social Psychology*, 81, 1014–27.

Bartlett, Y.K., Sheeran, P. and Hawley, M.S. (2014) Effective behaviour change techniques in smoking cessation interventions for people with chronic obstructive pulmonary disease: a meta-analysis, *British Journal of Health Psychology*, 19, 181–203.

Baumeister, R.F., Bratlavsky, E., Muraven, M. and Tice, D.M. (1998) Egodepletion: is the active self a limited resource? *Journal of Personality and Social Psychology*, 74, 1252–65.

Bayer, U.C. and Gollwitzer, P.M. (2007) Boosting scholastic test scores by willpower: the role of implementation intentions, *Self and Identity*, 6, 1–19.

Bayer, U.C., Achtziger, A., Gollwitzer, P.M. and Moskowitz, G.B. (2009) Responding to subliminal cues: do if–then plans facilitate action preparation and initiation without conscious intent? *Social Cognition*, 27, 183–201.

Bélanger-Gravel, A., Godin, G., Bilodeau, A. and Poirier, P. (2013) The effect of implementation intentions on physical activity among obese older adults: a randomised control study, *Psychology and Health*, 28, 217–33.

Benyamini, Y., Ashery, L. and Shiloh, S. (2011) Involving husbands in their wives' health behaviour: does it work? *Applied Psychology: Health and Well-Being*, 3, 66–86.

Benyamini, Y., Geron, R., Steinberg, D.M., Medini, N., Valinsky, L. and Endevelt, R. (2013) A structured intentions and action-planning intervention improves weight loss outcomes in a group weight loss program, *American Journal of Health Promotion*, 28, 119–27.

Brandstätter, V., Lengfelder, A. and Gollwitzer, P.M. (2001) Implementation intentions and efficient action initiation, *Journal of Personality and Social Psychology*, 81, 946–60.

Brickell, T.A., Chatzisarantis, N.L.D. and Pretty, G.M. (2006) Using past behaviour and spontaneous implementation intentions to enhance the utility of the theory of planned behaviour in predicting exercise, *British Journal of Health Psychology*, 11, 249–62.

Brom, S.S., Schnitzspahn, K.M., Melzer, M., Hagner, F., Bernhard, A. and Kliegel, M. (2014) Fluid mechanics moderate the effect of implementation intentions on a health prospective memory task in older adults, *European Journal of Ageing*, 11, 89–98.

Brown, I., Sheeran, P. and Reuber, M. (2009) Enhancing antiepileptic drug adherence: a randomized controlled trial, *Epilepsy and Behavior*, 16, 634–9.

Browne, J.L. and Chan, A.Y.C. (2012) Using the theory of planned behaviour and implementation intentions to predict and facilitate upward family communication about mammography, *Psychology and Health*, 27, 655–73.

Bukowska-Durawa, A., Haynes, C. and Luszczynska, A. (2010) Plans not needed if you have high and stable self-efficacy: planning intervention and snack intake in the context of self-efficacy trajectories, *Polish Psychological Bulletin*, 41 (3), 91–7.

Burkert, S., Scholz, U., Gralla, O., Roigas, J. and Knoll, N. (2011) Dyadic planning of health-behavior change after prostatectomy: a randomized-controlled planning intervention, *Social Science and Medicine*, 73, 783–92.

Carraro, N. and Gaudreau, P. (2013) Spontaneous and experimentally induced action and coping planning for physical activity: a meta-analysis, *Psychology of Sport and Exercise*, 14, 228–48.

Chapman, J. and Armitage, C.J. (2010) Evidence that boosters augment the long-term impact of implementation intentions on fruit and vegetable intake, *Psychology and Health*, 25, 365–81.

Chapman, J., Armitage, C.J. and Norman, P. (2009) Comparing implementation intention interventions in relation to young adults' intake of fruit and vegetables, *Psychology and Health*, 24, 317–32.

Chatzisarantis, N.L.D. and Hagger, M.S. (2010) Effects of implementation intentions linking suppression of alcohol consumption to socializing goals on alcohol-related decisions, *Journal of Applied Social Psychology*, 40, 1618–34.

Chatzisarantis, N.L.D., Hagger, M.S. and Thórgersen-Ntoumani, C. (2008) The effects of self-discordance, self-concordance, and implementation intentions on health behaviour, *Journal of Applied Biobehavioral Research*, 13, 198–214.

Chatzisarantis, N.L.D., Hagger, M.S. and Wang, J.C.K. (2010) Evaluating the effects of implementation intention and self-concordance on behaviour, *British Journal of Psychology*, 101, 705–18.

Christiansen, S., Oettingen, G., Dahme, B. and Klinger, R. (2010) A short goal-pursuit intervention to improve physical capacity: a randomized clinical trial in chronic back pain patients, *Pain*, 149, 444–52.

Cohen, J. (1992) A power primer, *Psychological Bulletin*, 112, 155–9.

Conner, M. and Higgins, A.R. (2010) Long-term effects of implementation intentions on prevention of smoking uptake among adolescents: a cluster randomized controlled trial, *Health Psychology*, 29, 529–38.

Conner, M., Grogan, S., Lawton, R., Armitage, C., West, R., Siddiqi, K. *et al.* (2013) Study protocol: a cluster randomised controlled trial of implementation intentions to reduce smoking initiation in adolescents, *BMC Public Health*, 13, 54.

Conner, M., Sandberg, T. and Norman, P. (2010) Using action planning to promote exercise behaviour, *Annals of Behavioral Medicine*, 40, 65–76.

Cooke, R. and Sheeran, P. (2004) Moderation of cognition–intention and cognition–behaviour relations: a meta-analysis of properties of variables from the theory of planned behaviour, *British Journal of Social Psychology*, 43, 159–86.

Custers, R. and Aarts, H. (2010) The unconscious will: how the pursuit of goals operates outside of conscious awareness, *Science*, 329, 47–50.

De Nooijer, J., de Vet, E., Brug, J. and de Vries, N.K. (2006) Do implementation intentions help to turn good intentions into higher fruit intakes? *Journal of Nutrition Education and Behavior*, 38, 25–9.

De Vet, E., Gebhardt, W.A., Sinnige, J., Van Puffelen, A., Van Lettow, B. and De Wit, J.B.F. (2011a) Implementation intentions for buying, carrying, discussing and using condoms: the role of the quality of plans, *Health Education Research*, 26, 443–55.

De Vet, E., Oenema, A. and Brug, J. (2011b) More or better: do the number and specificity of implementation intentions matter in increasing physical activity? *Psychology of Sport and Exercise*, 12, 471–7.

De Vet, E., Oenema, A., Sheeran, P. and Brug, J. (2009) Should implementation intentions interventions be implemented in obesity prevention? The impact of if–then plans on daily physical activity in Dutch adults, International Journal of Behavioral Nutrition and Physical Activity, 6, 11.

Dewitte, S., Verguts, T. and Lens, W. (2003) Implementation intentions do not enhance all types of goals: the moderating role of goal difficulty, *Current Psychology*, 22, 73–89.

Elfeddali, I., Bolman, C., Candel, M.J.J.M., Wiers, R.W. and de Vries, H. (2012) Preventing smoking relapse via web-based computer-tailored feedback: a randomized controlled trial, *Journal of Medical Internet Research*, 14 (4), e109.

Elliott, M. and Armitage, C. (2006) Effects of implementation intentions on the self-reported frequency of drivers' compliance with speed limits, Journal of Experimental Psychology: Applied, 12, 108–17.

Epton, T., Norman, P., Dadzie, A.-S., Harris, P.R., Webb, T.L., Sheeran, P. *et al.* (2014) A theory-based online health behaviour intervention for new university students (U@Uni): results from a randomised controlled trial, *BMC Public Health*, 14, 563.

Fennis, B.M., Adriaanse, M.A., Stroebe, W. and Pol, B. (2011) Bridging the intention–behavior gap: inducing implementation intentions through persuasive appeals, *Journal of Consumer Psychology*, 21, 302–11.

Fitzsimons, G.J., Nunes, J.C. and Williams, P. (2007) License to sin: the liberating role of reporting expectations, *Journal of Consumer Research*, 34, 22–31.

Gaston, A. and Prapavessis, H. (2014) Using a combined protection motivation theory and health action process approach intervention to promote exercise during pregnancy, *Journal of Behavioral Medicine*, 37, 173–84.

Gebhardt, W.A., Van Empelen, P., Messchaert, E. and Kingma L. (2008) Implementation intentions and alcohol reduction among student association members, *Psychology and Health*, 23, 128.

Gilbert, S.J., Gollwitzer, P.M., Cohen, A.L., Oettingen, G. and Burgess, P.W. (2009) Separable brain systems supporting cued versus self-initiated realization of delayed intentions, *Journal of Experimental Psychology: Learning, Memory, and Cognition*, 35, 905–15.

Godin, G., Sheeran, P., Conner, M., Delage, G., Germain, M., Bélanger-Gravel, A. *et al.* (2010) Which survey questions change behavior? Randomized controlled trial of mere measurement interventions, *Health Psychology*, 29, 636–44.

Gollwitzer, P.M. (1990) Action phases and mindsets, in E.T. Higgins and J.R.M. Sorrentino (eds.) *The Handbook of Motivation and Cognition* (Vol. 2, pp. 53–92). New York: Guilford Press.

Gollwitzer, P.M. (1993) Goal achievement: the role of intentions, in W. Strobe and M. Hewstone (eds.) *European Review of Social Psychology* (Vol. 4, pp. 141–85). Chichester: Wiley.

Gollwitzer, P.M. (1996) The volitional benefits of planning, in P.M. Gollwitzer and J.A. Bargh (eds.) *The Psychology of Action: Linking Cognition and Motivation to Behavior* (pp. 287–312). New York: Guilford Press.

Gollwitzer, P.M. (1999) Implementation intentions: strong effects of simple plans, *American Psychologist*, 54, 493–503.

Gollwitzer, P.M. (2014) Weakness of the will: is a quick fix possible? *Motivation and Emotion*, 38, 305–22.

Gollwitzer, P.M. and Brandstätter, V. (1997) Implementation intentions and effective goal pursuit, *Journal of Personality and Social Psychology*, 73, 186–99.

Gollwitzer, P.M. and Schaal, B. (1998) Metacognition in action: the importance of implementation intentions, *Personality and Social Psychology Review*, 2, 124–36.

Gollwitzer, P.M. and Sheeran, P. (2006) Implementation intentions and goal achievement: a meta-analysis of effects and processes, *Advances in Experimental Social Psychology*, 38, 69–119

Gollwitzer, P.M., Achtziger, A., Schaal, B. and Hammelbeck, J.P. (2002) Intentional control of strereotypical beliefs and prejudicial feelings. Unpublished manuscript, University of Konstanz.

Gollwitzer, P.M., Bayer, U.C. and McCulluch, K.C. (2005) The control of the unwanted, in R.R. Hassin, J.S. Uleman and J.A. Bargh (eds.) *The New Unconscious* (pp. 485–515). New York: Oxford University Press.

Gollwitzer, P.M., Sheeran, P., Trötschel, R. and Webb, T. (2011) Self-regulation of behavioral priming effects, Psychological Science, 22, 901–7.

Gollwitzer, P.M., Wieber, F., Myers, A.L. and McCrea, S.M. (2010) How to maximize implementation intention effects, in C.R. Agnew, D.E. Carlston, W.G. Graziano and J.R. Kelly (eds.) Then a Miracle Occurs: Focusing on Behavior in Social Psychological Theory and Research (pp. 137–61). New York: Oxford University Press.

Guillaumie, L., Godin, G., Manderscheid, J., Spitz, E. and Muller, L. (2012) The impact of self-efficacy and implementation intentions-based interventions on fruit and vegetable intake among adults, *Psychology and Health*, 27, 30–50.

Hagger, M.S. and Luszczynska, A. (2014) Implementation intention and action planning interventions in health contexts: state of the research and proposals for the way forward, *Applied Psychology: Health and Well-Being*, 6, 1–47.

Hagger, M.S., Lonsdale, A. and Chatzisarantis, N.L.D. (2012a) A theory-based intervention to reduce alcohol drinking in excess of guideline limits among undergraduate students, *British Journal of Health Psychology*, 17, 18–43.

Hagger, M.S., Lonsdale, A., Koka, A., Hein, V., Pasi, H., Lintunen, T. *et al.* (2012b) An intervention to reduce alcohol consumption in undergraduate students using implementation intentions and mental simulations: a cross-national study, *International Journal of Behavioral Medicine*, 19, 82–96.

Hagger, M.S., Wood, C., Stiff, C. and Chatzisarantis, N.L. (2010) Ego depletion and the strength model of self-control: a meta-analysis, *Psychological Bulletin*, 136, 495–525.

Hallam, G.P., Webb, T.L., Sheeran, P., Miles, E., Wilkinson, I.D., Hunter, M.D. *et al.* (submitted) The neural correlates of emotion regulation by implementation intentions. Manuscript submitted for publication.

Harris, P.R., Brearley, I., Sheeran, P., Barker, M., Klein, W.M.P., Creswell, J.D. *et al.* (2014) Combining self-affirmation with implementation intentions to promote fruit and vegetable consumption, *Health Psychology*, 33, 729–36.

Heckhausen, H. and Gollwitzer, P.M. (1987) Thought contents and cognitive functioning in motivational versus volitional states of mind, *Motivation and Emotion*, 11, 101–20.

Heverin, M. and Byrne, M. (2011) The effect of implementation intentions on testicular self-examination using a demonstration video, *Irish Journal of Psychology*, 32, 40–8.

Higgins, A. and Conner, M. (2003) Understanding adolescent smoking: the role of the theory of planned behaviour and implementation intentions, *Psychology, Health and Medicine*, 8, 177–90.

Howard, G.S., Hill, T.L., Maxwell, S.E., Mourinho Baptista, T., Farias, M., Coelho, C. *et al.* (2009) What is wrong with research literatures? And how to make them right, *Review of General Psychology*, 13, 146–66.

Hurling, R., Fairley, B.W. and Dias, M.B. (2006) Internet-based exercise intervention systems: are more interactive designs better? *Psychology and Health*, 21, 757–72.

Jackson, C., Lawton, R.J., Raynor, D.K., Knapp, P.R., Conner, M.T., Lowe, C.J. *et al.* (2006) Promoting adherence to antibiotics: a test of implementation intentions, *Patient Education and Counseling*, 61, 212–18.

Jessop, D.C., Sparks, P., Buckland, N., Harris, P.R. and Churchill, S. (2014) Combining self-affirmation and implementation intentions: evidence of detrimental effects on behavioral outcomes, *Annals of Behavioral Medicine*, 47, 137–47.

Karimi-Shahanjarini, A., Rashidian, A., Omidvar, N. and Majdzadeh, R. (2013) Assessing and comparing the short-term effects of TPB only and TPB plus implementation intentions interventions on snacking behavior in Iranian adolescent girls: a cluster randomized trial, *American Journal of Health Promotion*, 27, 152–61.

Knäuper, B., McCollam, A., Rosen-Brown, A., Lacaille, J., Kelso, E. and Roseman, M. (2011) Fruitful plans: adding targeted mental imagery to implementation intentions increases fruit consumption, *Psychology and Health*, 26, 601–17.

Koestner, R., Horberg, E.J., Gaudreau, P., Powers, T., Di Dio, P., Bryan, C. *et al.* (2006) Bolstering implementation plans for the long haul: the benefits of simultaneously boosting self-concordance or self-efficacy, *Personality and Social Psychology Bulletin*, 32, 1547–58.

Koestner, R., Lekes, N., Powers, T.A. and Chicoine, E. (2002) Attaining personal goals: self-concordance plus implementation intentions equals success, *Journal of Personality and Social Psychology*, 83, 231–44.

Koring, M., Richert, J., Parschau, L., Ernsting, A., Lippke, S. and Schwarzer, R. (2012) A combined planning and self-efficacy intervention to promote physical activity: a multiple mediation analysis, *Psychology, Health and Medicine*, 17, 488–98.

Kroese, F.M., Adriaanse, M.A., Evers, C. and De Ridder, D.T.D. (2011) 'Instant success': turning temptations into cues for goal-directed behaviour, *Personality and Social Psychology Bulletin*, 37, 1389–97.

Lengfelder, A. and Gollwitzer, P.M. (2001) Reflective and reflexive action control in patients with frontal brain lesions, *Neuropsychology*, 15, 80–100.

Lippke, S., Ziegelmann, J.P. and Schwarzer, R. (2004) Initiation and maintenance of physical exercise: stage-specific effects of a planning intervention, *Research in Sports Medicine*, 12, 221–40.

Liu, L.L. and Park, D.C. (2004) Aging and medical adherence: the use of automatic processes to achieve effortful things, *Psychology and Aging*, 19, 318–25.

Lo, S.H., Good, A., Sheeran, P., Baio, G., Rainbow, S., Vart, G. *et al.* (2014) Preformulated implementation intentions to promote colorectal cancer screening: a cluster-randomized trial, *Health Psychology*, 33, 998–1002.

Luszczynska, A. and Haynes, C. (2009) Changing nutrition, physical activity and body weight among student nurses and midwives: effects of a planning intervention and self-efficacy beliefs, *Journal of Health Psychology*, 14, 1075–84.

Luszczynska, A., Schwarzer, R., Lippke, S. and Mazurkiewicz, M. (2011) Self-efficacy as a moderator of the planning–behaviour relationship in interventions designed to promote physical activity, *Psychology and Health*, 26, 151–66.

McBroom, W.H. and Reid, F.W. (1992) Towards a reconceptualization of attitude–behavior consistency, *Social Psychology Quarterly*, 55, 205–16.

McGowan, E.L., North, S. and Courneya, K.S. (2013) Randomized controlled trial of a behavior change intervention to increase physical activity and quality of life in prostate cancer survivors, *Annals of Behavioral Medicine*, 46, 382–93.

Mendoza, S.A., Gollwitzer, P.M. and Amodio, D.M. (2010) Reducing the expression of implicit stereotypes: reflexive control through implementation intentions, *Personality and Social Psychology Bulletin*, 36, 512–23.

Michie, S., Dormandy, E. and Marteau, T.M. (2004) Increasing screening uptake amongst those intending to be screened: the use of action plans, Patient Education and Counseling, 55, 218–22.

Milne, S. and Sheeran, P. (2002) Combining motivational and volitional interventions to prevent testicular cancer. Paper presented to the 13th General Meeting of the European Association of Experimental Social Psychology, San Sebastian, June.

Milne, S., Orbell, S. and Sheeran, P. (2002) Combining motivational and volitional interventions to promote exercise participation: protection motivation theory and implementation intentions, *British Journal of Health Psychology*, 7, 163–84.

Moors, A. and De Houwer, J. (2006) Automaticity: a theoretical and conceptual analysis, *Psychological Bulletin*, 132, 297–326.

Muraven, M. and Baumeister, R.F. (2000) Self-regulation and depletion of limited resources: does self-control resemble a muscle? *Psychological Bulletin*, 126, 247–59.

Murgraff, V., Abraham, C. and McDermott, M. (2007) Reducing Friday alcohol consumption among moderate, women drinkers: evaluation of a brief evidence-based intervention, *Alcohol and Alcoholism*, 42, 37–41.

Murgraff, V., White, D. and Phillips, K. (1996) Moderating binge drinking: it is possible to change behaviour if you plan it in advance, *Alcohol and Alcoholism*, 6, 577–82.

Neter, E., Stein, N., Barnett-Griness, O., Rennert, G. and Hagoel, L. (2014) From the bench to public health: population-level implementation intentions in colorectal cancer screening, *American Journal of Preventive Medicine*, 46, 273–80.

Nyman, S.R. and Yardley, L. (2009) Web-site-based tailored advice to promote strength and balance training: an experimental evaluation, *Journal of Aging and Physical Activity*, 17, 210–22.

O'Carroll, R.E., Chambers, J.A., Dennis, M., Sudlow, C. and Johnston, M. (2013) Improving adherence to medication in stroke survivors: a pilot randomised controlled trial, *Annals of Behavioral Medicine*, 46, 358–68.

Oettingen, G. (2012) Future thought and behavior change, *European Review of Social Psychology*, 23, 1–63.

Oettingen, G. and Gollwitzer, P.M. (2001) Goal setting and goal striving, in A. Tesser and N. Schwarz (eds.) *Blackwell Handbook in Social Psychology, Vol. 1: Intraindividual Processes* (pp. 329–47). Oxford: Blackwell.

Oettingen, G. and Gollwitzer, P.M. (2010) Strategies of setting and implementing goals: mental contrasting and implementation intentions, in J.E. Maddux and J.P. Tangney (eds.) *Social Psychological Foundations of Clinical Psychology* (pp. 114–35). New York: Guilford Press.

Oettingen, G., Hönig, G. and Gollwitzer, P.M. (2000) Effective self-regulation of goal attainment, *International Journal of Educational Research*, 33, 705–32.

Oettingen, G., Wittchen, M. and Gollwitzer, P.M. (2013) Regulating goal pursuit through mental contrasting with implementation intentions, in E.A. Locke and G.P. Latham (eds.) *New Developments in Goal Setting and Task Performance* (pp. 523–48). New York: Routledge.

Olander, E.K., Fletcher, H., Williams, S., Atkinson, L., Turner, A. and French, D.P. (2013) What are the most effective techniques in changing obese individuals' physical activity self-efficacy and behaviour: a systematic review and meta-analysis, International Journal of Behavioral Nutrition and Physical Activity, 10, 29.

Orbell, S. and Sheeran, P. (1998) 'Inclined abstainers': a problem for predicting health-related behavior, *British Journal of Social Psychology*, 37, 151–65.

Orbell, S. and Sheeran, P. (2000) Motivational and volitional processes in action initiation: a field study of the role of implementation intentions, *Journal of Applied Social Psychology*, 30, 780–97.

Orbell, S., Hodgkins, S. and Sheeran, P. (1997) Implementation intentions and the theory of planned behavior, *Personality and Social Psychology Bulletin*, 23, 945–54.

Papies, E.K., Aarts, H. and de Vries, N.K. (2009) Planning is for doing: implementation intentions go beyond the mere creation of goal-directed associations, *Journal of Experimental Social Psychology*, 45, 1148–51.

Parks-Stamm, E.J., Gollwitzer, P.M. and Oettingen, G. (2007) Action control by implementation intentions: effective cue detection and efficient response initiation, *Social Cognition*, 25, 248–66.

Prestwich, A. and Kellar, I. (2014) How can the impact of implementation intentions as a behaviour change intervention be improved, *European Review of Applied Psychology*, 64, 35–41.

Prestwich, A., Ayres, K. and Lawton, R. (2008) Crossing two types of implementation intentions with a protection motivation intervention for the reduction of saturated fat intake, *Social Science and Medicine*, 67, 1550–8.

Prestwich, A., Conner, M., Lawton, R., Bailey, W., Litman, J. and Molyneaux, V. (2005) Individual and collaborative implementation intentions and the promotion of breast self-examination, *Psychology and Health*, 20, 743–60

Prestwich, A., Conner, M., Lawton, R., Ward, J., Ayres, K. and McEachan, R. (2012) Randomized controlled trial of collaborative implementation intentions targeting working adults' physical activity, *Health Psychology*, 31, 486–95.

Prestwich, A., Conner, M.T., Lawton, R.J., Ward, J.K., Ayres, K. and McEachan, R.R.C. (2014a) Partner and planning-based interventions to reduce fat consumption: randomized controlled trial, *British Journal of Health Psychology*, 19, 132–48.

Prestwich, A., Kellar, I., Parker, R., MacRae, S., Learmonth, M., Sykes, B. *et al.* (2014b) How can self-efficacy be increased? Meta-analysis of dietary interventions, *Health Psychology Review*, 8, 270–85.

Prestwich, A., Lawton, R. and Conner, M. (2003) Use of implementation intentions and the decision balance sheet in promoting exercise behaviour, *Psychology and Health*, 18, 707–21.

Prestwich, A., Perugini, M. and Hurling, R. (2009) Can the effects of implementation intentions on exercise be enhanced using text messages? *Psychology and Health*, 24, 677–87.

Prestwich, A., Perugini, M. and Hurling, R. (2010) Can implementation intentions and text messages promote brisk walking? A randomized trial, *Health Psychology*, 29, 40–9.

Prestwich, A., Sniehotta, F.F., Whittington, C., Dombrowski, S.U., Rogers, L. and Michie, S. (2014c) Does theory influence the effectiveness of health behavior interventions? Meta-analysis, *Health Psychology*, 33, 465–74.

Rhodes, R. and De Bruijn, G.-J. (2013) How big is the physical activity intention–behaviour gap? A meta-analysis using the action control framework, *British Journal of Health Psychology*, 18, 296–309.

Rivis, A. and Sheeran, P. (2013) Automatic risk behavior: direct effects of drinker stereotypes on drinking behavior, *Health Psychology*, 32, 571–80.

Rodgers, W.M., Selzler, A.-M., Haennel, R.G., Holm, S., Wong, E.Y.L. and Stickland, M.K. (2014) An experimental assessment of the influence of exercise versus social implementation intentions on physical activity during and following pulmonary rehabilitation, *Journal of Behavioral Medicine*, 37, 480–90.

Rodrigues, R.C.M., Joao, T.M.S., Jayme Gallani, M.C.B., Cornelio, M.E. and Alexandre, N.M.C. (2013) The 'Moving Heart Program': an intervention to improve physical activity among patients with coronary heart disease, *Revista Latino-Americana de Enfermagem*, 21, 180–9.

Rogers, R.W. (1983) Cognitive and physiological processes in fear appeals and attitude change: a revised theory of protection motivation, in B.L. Cacioppo and L.L. Petty (eds.) *Social Psychophysiology: A Sourcebook* (pp. 153–76). London: Guildford Press.

Rutter, D.R., Steadman, L. and Quine, L. (2006) An implementation intentions intervention to increase uptake of mammography, *Annals of Behavioral Medicine*, 32, 127–34

Scholz, U., Ochsner, S. and Luszczynska, A. (2013) Comparing different boosters of planning interventions on changes in fat consumption in overweight and obese individuals: a randomized controlled trial, *International Journal of Psychology*, 48, 604–15.

Schwerdtfeger, A.R., Schmitz, C. and Warken, M. (2012) Using text messages to bridge the intention–behavior gap? A pilot study on the use of text message reminders to increase objectively assessed physical activity in daily life, *Frontiers in Psychology*, 3, article 270.

Sewacj, D., Ajzen, I. and Fishbein, M. (1980) Predicting and understanding weight loss: intentions, behaviors, and outcomes, in I. Ajzen and M. Fishbein (eds.) *Understanding Attitudes and Predicting Social Behavior* (pp. 101–12). Englewood Cliffs, NJ: Prentice-Hall.

Sheeran, P. (2002) Intention–behavior relations: a conceptual and empirical review, in W. Strobe and M. Hewstone (eds.) *European Review of Social Psychology* (Vol. 12, pp. 1–30). Chichester: Wiley.

Sheeran, P. and Orbell, S. (1999) Implementation intentions and repeated behavior: augmenting the predictive validity of the theory of planned behavior, *European Journal of Social Psychology*, 29, 349–69.

Sheeran, P. and Orbell, S. (2000) Using implementation intentions to increase attendance for cervical cancer screening, *Health Psychology*, 19, 283–9.

Sheeran, P. and Silverman, M. (2003) Evaluation of three interventions to promote workplace health and safety: evidence for the utility of implementation intentions, *Social Science and Medicine*, 56, 2153–63.

Sheeran, P., Abraham, C. and Orbell, S. (1999) Psychosocial correlates of heterosexual condom use: a meta-analysis, *Psychological Bulletin*, 125, 90–132.

Sheeran, P., Webb, T.L. and Gollwitzer, P.M. (2005) The interplay between goal intentions and implementation intentions, *Personality and Social Psychology Bulletin*, 31, 87–98.

Sheeran, P., White, D. and Phillips, K. (1991) Premarital contraceptive use: a review of the psychological literature, *Journal of Reproductive and Infant Psychology*, 9, 253–69.

Smets, E.M.A., Garssen, B., Bonke, B. and De Haes, J.C.J.M. (1995) The Multidimensional Fatigue Inventory (MFI): psychometric qualities of an instrument to assess fatigue, *Journal of Psychosomatic Research*, 39, 315–25.

Sniehotta, F.F. (2009) Towards a theory of intentional behaviour change: plans, planning and self-regulation, *British Journal of Health Psychology*, 14, 261–73.

Soureti, A., Murray, P., Cobain, M., Chinapaw, M., van Mechelen, W. and Hurling, R. (2011) Exploratory study of web-based planning and mobile text reminders in an overweight population, *Journal of Medical Internet Research*, 13, 232–42.

Stadler, G., Oettingen, G. and Gollwitzer, P.M. (2010) Intervention effects of information and self-regulation on eating fruits and vegetables over two years, *Health Psychology*, 29, 274–83.

Steadman, L. and Quine, L. (2000) Are implementation intentions useful for bridging the intention–behavior gap in adhering to long-term medication regimens? An attempt to replicate Sheeran and Orbell's (1999) intervention to enhance adherence to daily vitamin C intake. Paper presented to the British Psychological Society Division of Health Psychology Annual Conference, University of Kent at Canterbury, September.

Steadman, L. and Quine, L. (2004) Encouraging young males to perform testicular self-examination: a simple, but effective, implementation intention intervention, *British Journal of Health Psychology*, 9, 479–87.

Tam, L., Bagozzi, R.P. and Spanjol, J. (2010) When planning is not enough: the self-regulatory effect of implementation intentions on changing snacking habits, *Health Psychology*, 29, 284–92.

Toli, A., Webb, T.L. and Hardy, G.E. (submitted) Does forming implementation intentions help people with mental health problems to achieve goals? A meta-analysis of experimental studies with clinical and analogue samples. Manuscript submitted for publication.

Triandis, H.C. (1980) Values, attitudes, and interpersonal behaviour, in H. Howe and M. Page (eds.) *Nebraska Symposium on Motivation* (Vol. 27, pp. 195–259). Lincoln, NB: University of Nebraska Press.

Troop, N.A. (2013) Effect of dietary restraint on fruit and vegetable intake following implementation intentions, *Journal of Health Psychology*, 18, 861–5.

Van Koningsbruggen, G.M., Stroebe, W., Papies, E.K. and Aarts, H. (2011) Implementation intentions as goal primes: boosting self-control in tempting environments, *European Journal of Social Psychology*, 41, 551–7.

Van Osch, L., Lechner, L., Reubsaet, A. and De Vries, H. (2010) From theory to practice: an explorative study into the instrumentality and specificity of implementation intentions, *Psychology and Health*, 25, 351–64.

Van Osch, L., Lechner, L., Reubsaet, A., Wigger, S. and De Vries, H. (2008) Relapse prevention in a national smoking cessation contest: effects of coping planning, *British Journal of Health Psychology*, 13, 525–35.

Verhoeven, A.A.C., Adriaanse, M.A., De Ridder, D.T.D., De Vet, E. and Fennis, B.M. (2013) Less is more: the effect of multiple implementation intentions targeting unhealthy snacking habits, *European Journal of Social Psychology*, 43, 344–54.

Verplanken, B. and Faes, S. (1999) Good intentions, bad habits, and effects of forming implementation intentions on healthy eating, *European Journal of Social Psychology*, 29, 591–604.

Walsh, J.C. (2003) An evaluation of an intervention to improve attendance rates for cancer screening in the Irish Cervical Screening Programme (ICSP), *National Institute of Health Sciences Research Bulletin*, 2, 32–3.

Webb, T.L. and Sheeran, P. (2003) Can implementation intentions help to overcome ego-depletion? *Journal of Experimental Social Psychology*, 39, 279–86.

Webb, T.L. and Sheeran, P. (2004) Identifying good opportunities to act: implementation intentions and cue discrimination, *European Journal of Social Psychology*, 34, 407–19.

Webb, T.L. and Sheeran, P. (2006) Does changing behavioral intentions engender bahaviour change? A meta-analysis of the experimental evidence, *Psychological Bulletin*, 132, 249–68.

Webb, T.L. and Sheeran, P. (2007) How do implementation intentions promote goal attainment? A test of component processes, *Journal of Experimental Social Psychology*, 43, 295–302.

Webb, T.L. and Sheeran, P. (2008) Mechanisms of implementation intention effects: the role of goal intentions, self-efficacy, and accessibility of plan components, *British Journal of Social Psychology*, 47, 373–95.

Webb, T.L., Joseph, J., Yardley, L. and Michie, S. (2010) Using the internet to promote health behavior change: a systematic review and meta-analysis of the impact of theoretical basis, use of behavior change techniques, and mode of delivery on efficacy, *Journal of Medical Internet Research*, 12 (1), e4.

Webb, T.L., Sheeran, P., Gollwitzer, P.M. and Trötschel, R. (2012) Strategic control over the unhelpful effects of primed social categories and goals, *Journal of Psychology*, 220, 187–93.

Webb, T.L., Sheeran, P. and Luszczynska, A. (2009) Planning to break unwanted habits: habit strength moderates implementation intention effects on behavior change, *British Journal of Social Psychology*, 48, 507–23

Wieber, F. and Sassenberg, K. (2006) I can't take my eyes off it: attention attraction effects of implementation intentions, *Social Cognition*, 24, 723–52.

Wieber, F., Odenthal, G. and Gollwitzer, P. (2010) Self-efficacy feelings moderate implementation intention effects, *Self and Identity*, 9, 177–94.

Wieber, F., Sezer, L.A. and Gollwitzer, P.M. (2014) Asking 'why' helps action control by goals but not plans, *Motivation and Emotion*, 38, 65–78.

Wieber, F., Thürmer, J.L. and Gollwitzer, P.M. (2012) Collective action control by goals and plans: applying a self-regulation perspective to group performance, *American Journal of Psychology*, 125, 275–90.

Wieber, F., von Suchodoletz, A., Heikamp, T., Trommsdorff, G. and Gollwitzer, P.M. (2011) If–then planning helps school-aged children to ignore attractive distractions, Social Psychology, 42, 39–47.

Wiedemann, A.U., Lippke, S. and Schwarzer, R. (2012) Multiple plans and memory performance: results of a randomized controlled trial targeting fruit and vegetable intake, *Journal of Behavioral Medicine*, 35, 387–92.

Wiedemann, A.U., Lippke, S., Reuter, T., Ziegelmann, J.P. and Schuz, B. (2011) The more the better? The number of plans predicts health behaviour change, *Applied Psychology: Health and Well-Being*, 3, 87–106.

Williams, S.L. and French, D.P. (2011) What are the most effective intervention techniques for changing physical activity self-efficacy and physical activity behaviour – and are they the same? *Health Education Research*, 26, 308–22.

Zandstra, E.H., den Hoed, W., Van der Meer, N. and Van der Maas, A. (2010) Improving compliance to meal-replacement food regimens: forming implementation intentions (conscious IF–THEN plans) increases compliance, *Appetite*, 55, 666–70.

Ziegelmann, J., Lippke, S. and Schwarzer, R. (2006) Adoption and maintenance of physical activity: planning interventions in young, middle-aged, and older adults, *Psychology and Health*, 21, 145–63.

Chapter 11

Health behaviour change techniques

Susan Michie and Caroline E. Wood

1 Background

Preventable behaviours, such as smoking, physical inactivity, unhealthy eating habits, and excessive alcohol consumption have been identified as leading causes of morbidity and mortality in resource-rich countries (Mokdad *et al.* 2004; NICE 2007; Lozano *et al.* 2012; Murray *et al.* 2013). To decrease the prevalence of these behaviours, we need effective behaviour change interventions – that is, 'co-ordinated sets of activities assigned to change specified behaviour patterns' (Michie *et al.* 2011e). Thousands of studies have developed and evaluated interventions aimed at improving health behaviour across a range of populations and contexts, as evidenced in the Cochrane Collaboration's literature reviews. These interventions are usually complex and vary along several dimensions, including their content and mode of delivery. Content refers to the potentially active ingredients within an intervention, whereas mode of delivery refers to variables such as format, who delivered, to whom, for how long, and in what context (Davidson *et al.* 2003; Michie *et al.* 2009b).

Maximizing the efficiency of accumulating knowledge about behaviour change and developing more effective interventions requires clear reporting and an agreed standard for specifying the 'active ingredients' of interventions (Michie and Abraham 2004; Michie *et al.* 2009b, 2011e, 2013; Michie and Johnston 2012).

Building on previous work, a checklist for a general specification of interventions has been developed: the Template for Intervention Description and Replication (TIDieR) (Hoffman *et al.* 2013, 2014). The checklist aims to provide the minimum data required to report in interventions, including surgical, psychotherapeutic as well as behavioural interventions. The checklist was developed using consensus methods and advocates that those reporting interventions should specify at minimum: brief name of the intervention, why (i.e. the rationale), what materials, what procedure, who provided, how, where, when and how much, whether there was any tailoring, details of any changes that were made to the original intervention protocol, how well monitored, and how well delivered.

Good description of intervention content allows both replication in scientific investigation and implementation in practical applications. It also allows the possibility of evaluating the effectiveness of component behaviour change techniques, individually and in combination. Maximizing the efficient accumulation of evidence about interventions requires an understanding of *how* interventions work (i.e. their mechanisms of action and their theoretical explanations). To achieve this, interventions should be developed, evaluated, and implemented within theoretical frameworks (Rothman 2004; Michie and Johnston 2012). However, theoretical frameworks and detailed descriptions of interventions are often missing from published reports, meaning that we are left knowing little about their content, their functional components or why they have the effects they have.

In this chapter, we start by considering ways in which theory can be used to inform intervention design. Next, we present a methodology for specifying interventions in terms of their component behaviour change techniques (BCTs) and outline how this can improve intervention development, implementation, evaluation of intervention effectiveness, and investigation of mechanisms of action. We then consider how to take forward the identification of links between theory and BCTs and how to use this methodology to investigate the effectiveness of individual BCTs and combinations of BCTs in changing behaviour. We conclude with a discussion of implications of this approach and directions for future research.

2 What is theory?

The term 'theory' has been defined variably, for example: as an 'account of a process that is arrived at by a process of inference and that provides an explanation for observed phenomena and that generates predictions' (West and Brown 2013). It represents *a priori* assumptions about what human behaviour is and the influences on behaviour. In the context of behaviour change, theories seek to explain why, when, and how a behaviour does or does not occur and represent the accumulated knowledge of the mechanisms of action (mediators) and the influences that modify change (moderators). A consensus definition of theory has been developed by a multi-disciplinary group of researchers across psychology, sociology, anthropology, and economics, together with public health policy-makers: 'A set of concepts and/or statements which specify how phenomena relate to each other. Theory provides an organising description of a system that accounts for what is known, and explains and predicts phenomena' (Davis *et al.* 2014; Michie *et al.* 2014b). The terms 'theories' and 'models' are sometimes used interchangeably but are not the same. A scientific model is a descriptive representation of a system consisting of constructs and relationships between these that are used to describe relevant characteristics of a system, make predictions, and develop interventions. Theories are a subset of models that purport to explain a set of phenomena and are used to understand phenomena, guide observation, and develop interventions (West 2014; see www.ucl.ac.uk/behaviour-change/resources).

3 Use of theory for intervention design

In developing and evaluating interventions to change behaviour, the importance has been recognized of not just evaluating evidence of effectiveness but establishing *how* the intervention works. This is evident, for example, in guidance from the UK's Medical Research Council on developing and evaluating complex interventions (Craig *et al.* 2008). This includes understanding the target behaviour and drawing on theories of behaviour change to advance understanding of the likely processes of change before piloting and more formal testing is carried out (a process the guidance defines as 'modelling').

However, the practice of developing, evaluating, and reporting interventions without an explicit theoretical framework is widespread, as evidenced by many reviews. For example, a review of health behaviour interventions found that only a third of the 193 studies were based on theory (Painter *et al.* 2008). Of those using theory, 18% reported applying theory, 3.6% testing theory, and, 9.4% building theory. A similar review assessed theory use in 235 evaluations of interventions to increase guideline dissemination and implementation (Davies *et al.* 2010). Studies were classified using a descriptive framework that considered the *level* of theory use and the *stage* at which the theory was used. Studies that reported using theory were described as being 'explicitly theory-based'. Of the studies reviewed, only 6% reported having *explicitly* used theory and a further 22.5% were judged to be 'theory-inspired'. In a review of 190 studies of interventions to increase physical activity and healthy eating, 56% were found to explicitly report using theory, with only 10% reporting that theoretical constructs were used to guide selection of appropriate change techniques (Prestwich *et al.* 2014c).

There is a debate as to whether interventions are likely to be more effective when explicitly informed by a theoretical model of behaviour change than when not. There is some evidence of a positive association between use of theory and effectiveness (Swann *et al.* 2003; Albarracín *et al.* 2005; Noar *et al.* 2007; Albada *et al.* 2009; Glanz and Bishop 2010; Webb *et al.* 2010; Taylor *et al.* 2012), but other studies have found no association, or even a negative association (Stephenson *et al.* 2000; Roe *et al.* 2007; Gardner *et al.* 2011). Some literature reviews have reported mixed findings depending on the measure of effectiveness (Kim *et al.* 1997; Ammerman *et al.* 2002; Bhattarai *et al.* 2013).

There are several possible explanations for studies reporting null, negative or mixed findings. One is that the choice of theory may not have been appropriate. For example, if a behaviour is heavily influenced by habit or emotional states, then a theory that focuses on beliefs and reflective thought processes may not be appropriate when informing intervention design. A second explanation is that the theory may be appropriate but poorly applied to intervention development. In cases where theory has been applied to intervention design and evaluation, it is often only loosely referred to and/or only a few of the theoretical constructs have been targeted and/or the theoretical framework has not been used appropriately to tailor the intervention (i.e. selection of intervention recipients and selection of BCTs most appropriate for the recipients) (Painter *et al.* 2008; Davies *et al.* 2010; Prestwich *et al.* 2014c).

Methods have been developed to identify the extent to which behaviour change interventions have been informed by theory, have applied theory to intervention development and/or evaluation, have tested theory, and have developed theory (Painter *et al.* 2008; Prestwich *et al.* 2014c). One method developed to more precisely evaluate the extent to which theory has been applied to intervention development and evaluation is the 19-item Theory Coding Scheme (TCS) (Michie and Prestwich 2010).

The TCS enables researchers to ascertain: whether theory is mentioned, how theory has been used directly in intervention design, whether theory has influenced interventions indirectly (i.e. via the selection of participants and via the delivery to different groups of participants), how theory explains effects on behavioural outcomes, and whether the implications of the results for future development of the theory are addressed. The TCS has been found to demonstrate good inter-rater reliability for all items (all kappa values were 0.70 and above) except one sub-item, which had a lower, but still acceptable kappa ($\kappa = 0.64$). Since its development, the TCS has been applied to investigate the extent of theory use in interventions, including ones targeting physical activity and healthy eating (Prestwich *et al.* 2014a, 2014c), diabetes management for patients with Type-2 diabetes (Avery *et al.* 2012), and promotion of hand hygiene behaviours (Yardley *et al.* 2011).

If an appropriate theory is selected and applied well to intervention development, one would expect the resulting intervention to be more effective, since theory represents the accumulation of knowledge of how to change behaviour across different populations and contexts. Interventions developed without theory may fail to build on existing knowledge, may omit important processes needed for behaviour change to occur, and consequently may fail to optimize effectiveness. Another important reason for developing theoretically informed interventions is that it provides an opportunity to test and develop theory and therefore understanding of behaviour and behaviour change. In order to achieve this, theory should appropriately guide measurement, study design, and data analysis and interpretation (Lippke and Ziegelmann 2008; Michie 2008b; Prestwich *et al.* 2014c). To make use of theory in intervention design, and to learn about theoretical processes in evaluations of interventions, more thorough selection, application, and evaluation of theory by researchers working in the field of behavioural science is required. With these provisos, an appropriate and well-specified theory (i.e. one that describes a set of mechanisms that if targeted would have the potential to bring about behaviour change) should enable researchers to predict, explain, and bring about behaviour change.

3.1 Selecting behaviour change theories

Selecting the most appropriate theory to inform intervention development can be a challenging task because many theories address only a small sub-set of the relevant constructs (West and Brown 2013) or have the same or overlapping constructs (Michie *et al.* 2005). In addition, the same theoretical constructs may have different names, or the same labels may be used to describe somewhat different constructs, and constructs may be split into several sub-constructs and/or be part of higher-order constructs. To add to this, much of the published literature on health behaviour change is dominated by only a small number of theories, meaning that potentially useful theories are currently under-used (Painter *et al.* 2008; Prestwich *et al.* 2014c). In a systematic review of interventions to increase physical activity and healthy eating, for example, Prestwich *et al.* (2014a) found the literature was dominated by two theories: social cognitive theory and the transtheoretical model. Of the 107 studies reporting use of theory, 59 mentioned the former and 58 the latter.

3.1.1 Social cognition models

A widely used set of theoretical accounts of behaviour for predicting and/or changing health behaviours are social cognition models (SCMs) (Conner and Norman 1995, 2005; Armitage and Conner 2000; Rutter and Quine 2002; Glanz *et al.* 2008). They guide the identification of key cognitions that distinguish between those who do and do not perform health-related behaviours (Abraham *et al.* 2008). Social cognition models such as the health belief model (e.g. Janz and Becker 1984; see Abraham and Sheeran, Chapter 2 this volume), the theory of planned behaviour/

theory of reasoned action (Ajzen and Fishbein 1980; Ajzen 1991; see Conner and Sparks, Chapter 5 this volume), social cognitive theory (Bandura, 1991; see Luszczynska and Schwarzer, Chapter 7 this volume), protection motivation theory (Maddux and Rogers 1983; see Norman *et al.*, Chapter 3 this volume), and the transtheoretical model (Prochaska *et al.* 1992; Prochaska and Velicer 1997; see also stage theories: Sutton, Chapter 9 this volume; the health action process approach: Schwarzer and Luszczynska, Chapter 8 this volume; self-determination theory: Hagger and Chatzisarantis, Chapter 4 this volume; and the prototype/willingness model: Gibbons *et al.*, Chapter 6 this volume) propose that a number of motivational and volitional variables (e.g. threat, attitudes, behavioural intentions, action planning) predict health behaviours.

Although there is considerable evidence in support of SCMs as predictive models of behaviour across groups, several potential disadvantages to their application have been noted (Conner and Norman 1995, 2005; Armitage and Conner 2000; Norman *et al.* 2000; Ogden 2003). One argument against the usefulness of SCMs is that they provide an incomplete understanding of health behaviour change and, in some cases, over-simplify the behaviour change process (Armitage and Conner 2000). Interventions designed using SCMs tend to target factors relating to 'reflective' motivation involving goals, plans, and beliefs. Research on health behaviour over the last three decades has been dominated by SCMs with relatively little attention paid to theories involving more 'automatic' processes, such as drives, emotions, habits, and impulses (Glanz *et al.* 2008; West and Brown 2013; Michie *et al.* 2014b). Social cognition models also pay relatively little attention to capability and opportunity that are necessary factors for behaviour to occur. This may be one reason that a significant proportion of the variance in behavioural outcomes remains unaccounted for by SCMs (Sutton 1998; Ogden 2003). Second, ascertaining the importance of constructs within these models is often confounded, as constructs often overlap and measurement is usually based on self-report (Conner and Norman 1995, 2005; Schwarzer 2001; Ogden 2003). Third, SCMs have been developed to explain differences between groups rather than change within individuals over time; this limits their usefulness in informing interventions to change. Another limitation is that SCMs focus on intra-individual, and to some extent interpersonal, constructs rather than the broader social, cultural, and environmental context which provides the 'opportunity' for people to engage with an activity and influences how we think and feel about particular activities, and therefore how we behave (Glanz and Bishop 2010).

Syntheses of the evidence for effectiveness of behaviour change interventions have identified a set of principles associated with effective interventions (Abraham *et al.* 2009) and concluded that the most effective interventions are those that simultaneously target change mechanisms at different levels (i.e. individual, community, and population) (NICE 2007). This suggests that, when designing and evaluating behaviour change interventions, there is likely to be benefit from drawing on a broader range of theories of behaviour change than those falling under the SCM umbrella. A number of useful compendia have been produced of theories related to health behaviour (e.g. Glanz *et al.* 2002; Conner and Norman 2005; Michie *et al.* 2008b; Nutbeam *et al.* 2010; Davis *et al.* 2014).

One of these (Davis *et al.* 2014; Michie *et al.* 2014b) resulted from a cross-disciplinary review of theories of behaviour and behaviour change, led by a team of psychologists, sociologists, anthropologists, and economists. It identified 83 theories that together included a total of 1659 constructs. These showed a considerable range of constructs beyond the intra-psychic constructs most commonly associated with SCMs, and also a considerable overlap between them.

The published compendium, 'The ABC of Behaviour Change' (Michie *et al.* 2014b), consists of summaries of the primary source of each theory, a list of the component constructs of each theory, and a network analysis to identify reported connections and influences between theories. It is accompanied by a searchable database so that all theories with a particular construct, or combination of constructs, can be identified (www.behaviourchangetheories.com).

3.1.2 The COM-B model of behaviour

One of the models identified by the review (the 'COM-B model of behaviour'; see Figure 11.1) seeks to provide a comprehensive and parsimonious summary of the general drivers of behaviour: the factors that need to be in place for behaviour change to occur (Michie *et al.* 2011e, 2014a). These are capability, opportunity, and/or motivation, which also feature in two of the other theories identified in the review: the 'Needs-Opportunities-Abilities Model' (Gatersleben and Vlek 1998) and the 'Motivation-Opportunities-Abilities Model' (Olander and Thorgersen 1995). Furthermore, these are also consistent with the three necessary and sufficient conditions for behaviour as identified by the 'grand theorists' at a US consensus meeting to consider the integration of theory, held in the 1990s (Fishbein *et al.* 2001). In COM-B, capability, opportunity, and motivation are conceptualized as being part of a mutually influencing system, rather than as a list of factors, with a variety of entry points to promote behaviour change.

The model elaborates motivation into reflective and automatic processes, capability into psychological and physical aspects, and opportunity into physical and social aspects. This model seeks to be simple but comprehensive and to provide a framework within which other theories can be considered. For example, the constructs of SCMs fall mainly into the reflective motivation segment of COM-B, and minimally or not at all in the other five components. The COM-B has been used to provide a method of analysing behaviour in context to formulate a 'behavioural diagnosis' of what needs to shift to change behaviour. This can be linked with the intervention functions that are likely to be effective, given the diagnosis, and the policy categories that are likely to provide appropriate support for the identified intervention.

A framework for moving from diagnosis by COM-B to intervention design has been developed: the 'Behaviour Change Wheel' (BCW), which will be discussed in detail below (Michie *et al.* 2014a). Possibly because of their simplicity, COM-B and the BCW have been used by disciplines

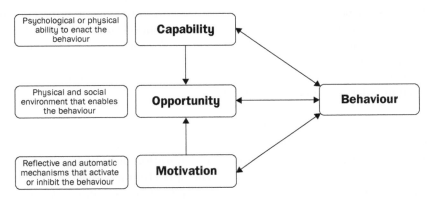

Figure 11.1 The COM-B model of behaviour (Michie *et al.* 2011e)

beyond psychology and by professional groups beyond researchers, such as policy-makers and intervention designers (e.g. Sallis *et al.* 2010; Charani *et al.* 2013; Jackson *et al.* 2014). Policy-makers have used this method both for intervention and policy design and to retrofit existing policies to identify whether there are important omissions and intervention functions or policy categories that could be added.

Social cognition models differ from COM-B/BCW as a method for intervention development in several ways. For example, SCMs are predictive models that can be used to identify constructs that have been found in particular contexts to be associated with the target behaviour. These are often referred to as 'determinants' that can be targeted by an intervention with the aim of changing behaviour. 'Determinants' are a subset of maintaining factors, those that account for any variance in behaviour between individuals. By limiting interventions to targeting such determinants, there is a danger of missing out three types of potential levers of change:

1. Maintaining factors that are not identified as determinants of individual behaviour, either because there is insufficient variation between individuals, or too much;
2. Factors that are not currently maintaining the behaviour but have changed the behaviour in the past;
3. Specific factors that may never have influenced behaviour but potentially could (e.g. novel incentives).

COM-B, on the other hand, is a system within which to consider where change within that system is most likely to bring about change in behaviour. This is informed by a comprehensive assessment, preferably drawing on more than one source and type of information, to construct a formulation about its original causation, development, and maintenance. Information about a behaviour's development is of special importance, as one can track how the behaviour has changed in intensity and frequency over time and identify the antecedents, correlates, and consequences of these changes. One can also ascertain the change strategies the person, group or population has tried in different contexts and the effects of those strategies, which provides valuable information for designing interventions. Current maintaining factors also provide information, although this information tends to be less rich as it does not capture influences on variation over time. Information about the causes of, and responses to, natural variation and interventions over time, and about current maintaining factors, is used to develop a formulation of the target behaviour in its context. By considering what has influenced behaviour in the past and the current potential and limitations of the individual(s) and the context, interventions most likely to be effective can be developed. This is a holistic, dialectical assessment, formulation, and planning process for behaviour change, developed on the basis of a dynamic model of an individual rather than a mechanistic process of identifying determinants of behaviour based on factors accounting for variation in current behaviour between individuals.

3.1.3 The theoretical domains framework

A second general framework that has been widely used across disciplines is the Theoretical Domains Framework (TDF), which represents an elaboration of COM-B's six components into 14 domains (Michie *et al.* 2005; Cane *et al.* 2012). The opportunity and capability components of COM-B map fairly directly to TDF domains (e.g. psychological capability having the domains of 'Knowledge' and 'Skills'). The motivational components incorporate several domains. Automatic motivation is reflected in the domains of 'Reinforcement' and 'Emotion' and reflective motivation in the domains of 'Professional/social role and identity', 'Beliefs about capabilities', 'Optimism', 'Beliefs about consequences', 'Intentions', and 'Goals'. The TDF was developed in response to non-psychologists who wished to draw on theory in developing and evaluating interventions but did not know how to evaluate or select among the large number of theories, many of which overlapped. The TDF was developed by psychologists and implementation researchers, starting with 128 constructs from 33 theories of behaviour and behaviour change. It has been used in many contexts to understand why desired behaviours are not occurring, for example, why evidence-based health care is not being practised. This understanding provides a theoretical basis for intervention design (Francis *et al.* 2012; French *et al.* 2012).

The TDF has been used by research teams across many countries and health care systems to investigate implementation problems and inform interventions to change professional practice (e.g. McKenzie *et al.* 2008; Francis *et al.* 2009; Bussieres *et al.* 2012; Patey *et al.* 2012). Research using the TDF to improve the implementation of guidelines, for example, has covered a variety of health settings and target behaviours, including: smoking cessation by midwives (Beenstock *et al.* 2012) and by dental providers (Amemori *et al.* 2011), transfusion prescribing (Francis *et al.* 2009), hand hygiene (Dyson *et al.* 2011), acute lower back pain in primary care (French *et al.* 2012), mental health (Michie *et al.* 2007a), and GP prescribing for upper-respiratory tract infections (Treweek *et al.* 2011).

The TDF has been used as a basis for designing interventions, using a matrix linking domains to BCTs (Michie *et al.* 2008b; French *et al.* 2012). The matrix was the result of a consensus exercise that identified the BCTs judged to be likely to be effective for changing each domain. Thus, a TDF assessment of a problem requiring behaviour change identifies the domains judged to explain the target behaviour either occurring or not occurring (depending on what the problem is). Guided by the particular application of the intervention, the BCTs likely to change those domains are then selected and form the basis of the intervention. A good report of the steps taken to apply this approach to intervention design is a study by French *et al.* (2012), who developed a theory-based intervention to increase GPs' implementation of guidelines for managing lower back pain.

French *et al.* (2012) used a four-step, systematic approach to help guide their intervention design process. First, they identified the behavioural problem based on gaps between evidence and practice documented in the literature. They specified these target behaviours in detail, clarifying what behaviour (or series of linked behaviours) would be targeted for change, who would perform the behaviour(s), and where and when the behaviour(s) would be performed. Second, they assessed the problem using qualitative methods underpinned by their chosen theoretical framework. The authors used the TDF on the basis of being the most likely to inform the pathways of behaviour change. Third, they selected techniques to overcome the barriers and enhance enablers. Their selection was informed by the chosen theoretical framework and by what was considered to be acceptable and likely to be supported within the local context, feasible to deliver, and could be implemented as part of an integrated intervention. Fourth, they determined which mediators of change could be measured to evaluate the pathways of change. Their selection of outcome measures was guided by considerations of validity, reliability, and feasibility of use in the local context. The intervention led to small changes in GP intentions to practise in a manner that is consistent with evidence-based guidelines. The changes to actual behaviour were not statistically significant; however, the conclusions from this study were flagged as limited due to recruitment problems.

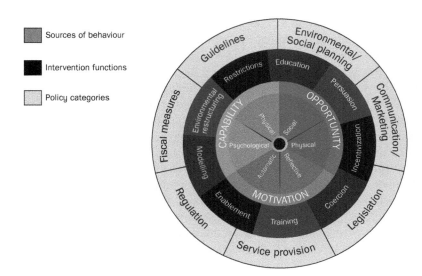

Figure 11.2 The Behaviour Change Wheel (BCW; Michie *et al.* 2011e)

French *et al.* (2012) suggest that although iterative adjustment and refinement is needed to suit specific contexts and settings, the four-step process is a useful guide for those developing complex implementation interventions. This approach has since been developed and is outlined in the 'Behaviour Change Wheel Guide to Designing Interventions' (Michie *et al.* 2011e, 2014a).

3.1.4 The Behaviour Change Wheel

The Behaviour Change Wheel (BCW) (see Figure 11.2; Michie *et al.* 2011e) is a framework of nine intervention functions and seven policy categories, linked to the COM-B model. It is the result of a synthesis of 19 behaviour change frameworks identified in a systematic literature review of frameworks of behaviour change (Geller *et al.* 1990; Goel *et al.* 1996; Cohen and Scribner 2000; Vlek 2000; Walter *et al.* 2003; Population Services International 2004; Perdue *et al.* 2005; West 2006; Leeman *et al.* 2007; Maibach *et al.* 2007; Nuffield Council 2007; DEFRA 2008; Knott *et al.* 2008; Abraham *et al.* 2010; Cochrane Effective Practice and Organisation of Care Group 2010; Dolan *et al.* 2010 Dunton *et al.* 2010; White 2010; Bartholomew *et al.* 2011). These frameworks were evaluated against three criteria: comprehensiveness (i.e. the framework should cover every intervention that has been or could be developed), coherence (i.e. categories are all exemplars of the same type and specificity of entity), and linked to a model of behaviour. Since there was considerable overlap between the 19 frameworks and none met all three criteria, they were synthesized. The steps taken to do this can be seen in the electronic supplements accompanying Michie *et al.* (2011e).

The Behaviour Change Wheel can be used as a tool to guide intervention design (see www. behaviourchangewheel.com). To summarize, an assessment of the target behaviour in context is made using COM-B (or TDF) to make a 'behavioural diagnosis' of what needs to shift in order for behaviour change to occur. The judgement of which of the COM-B components or TDF domains are likely to be important to change informs which of the intervention functions are likely to be effective, which, in turn, has implications for which policy categories and specific BCTs are likely to be effective and therefore should be considered when designing the intervention.

The Behaviour Change Wheel and COM-B model have been applied to understand and develop interventions for a range of behaviours and behavioural outcomes, including medication adherence (Jackson *et al.* 2014), reducing childhood obesity (Hendriks *et al.* 2012), and increasing attentive eating (Robinson *et al.* 2013). The COM-B model has also been used to inform the improvement of existing interventions, for example, the 'Clean Your Hands Campaign', an intervention to improve hand hygiene in health workers in all acute National Health Service (NHS) hospital trusts in England and Wales (Stone *et al.* 2012). The intervention involved installation of bedside alcohol hand rub, posters, and other materials promoting hand hygiene and engagement with the campaign. Regular hand hygiene audits were carried out to evaluate adherence. Evaluation of interview, observational, and documentary data using the COM-B model revealed that the intervention was targeting 'opportunity' (e.g. alcohol hand rub installed beside each bed) and 'motivation' (e.g. persuasive posters displayed in the ward) to carry out the behaviour. However, no intervention was in place to increase their 'capability'. While nurses had the capability to clean their hands, there was room for improvement in the capability to pay attention to this behaviour over other competing behaviours, to develop routines for noticing when the behaviour did not happen, and to put in place action plans for acting in the future. These findings informed the development of a programme to train staff to set goals, observe their own behaviour, and to develop action plans on the basis of feedback. The addition and implementation of goal-setting, one-to-one feedback, and action planning led to staff being 13–18% more likely to clean their hands (Fuller *et al.* 2012) and decreased infection rates of methicillin-resistant (MRSA), methicillin-sensitive (MSSA), and *Clostridium difficile* (Stone *et al.* 2012). (For detailed guidance and more examples of this method, see Michie *et al.* [2014a].)

The word 'functions' rather than 'categories' is used, as the functions are not mutually exclusive in that the same BCT may have more than one function. There was considerable overlap between the 19 frameworks of behaviour change. A synthesis of intervention functions was conducted, resulting in nine intervention functions (Michie *et al.* 2011e): 'Education', 'Persuasion', 'Incentivization', 'Coercion', 'Training', 'Restriction', 'Environmental restructuring', 'Modelling', and 'Enablement'. Seven policy categories were identified: 'Communication and marketing', 'Guidelines', 'Fiscal', 'Regulation', 'Legislation', 'Environmental/social planning', and 'Service provision'. These terms are defined in the published article and in the guide (Michie *et al.* 2011e, 2014a). While some level of judgement may inevitably be needed, there are matrices to guide the process of moving from behavioural diagnoses using COM-B (or TDF) to selecting intervention functions, policy categories, and BCTs. The choice of BCTs will depend on the local context, and this is helped by considering six criteria, with the acronym 'APEASE': 'Affordability', 'Practicability', 'Effectiveness', 'Acceptability', 'Safety', and 'Equitability' (Michie *et al.* 2014a).

4 Behaviour change techniques

Over the past decade, several guidance documents have been published advocating the importance of clear and precise reporting of interventions in behavioural science. For example, CONSORT guidelines for reporting randomized controlled trails recommend the reporting of the 'precise details' of interventions as 'actually administered' (Moher *et al.* 2003). Similarly, the TREND statement for reporting non-randomized trials recommends that authors should report in full the content and context of their intervention as well as full details of the control conditions (Des Jarlais *et al.* 2004). The UK's Medical Research Council (MRC) guidance for developing and evaluating complex interventions also calls for a full specification of the 'active ingredients' (i.e. the BCTs) within interventions as a necessary step for investigating how they exert their effect and for designing more effective interventions (Craig *et al.* 2008). A shared and standardized method of classifying intervention content is required and is necessary if interventions are to be successfully replicated across different behaviours and populations, and understood across a range of research groups, disciplines, and countries (Michie *et al.* 2011a).

Behaviour change techniques provide a means of characterizing intervention content to facilitate the implementation, delivery, and evaluation of behaviour change interventions. They are defined as the observable, replicable components of behaviour change interventions with the aim of being the smallest components that in optimal circumstances can bring about change. They can be used individually but are more commonly used in combination with other BCTs (Michie and Johnston 2013). Specifying intervention content by BCTs: (1) promotes accurate replication of intervention content in comparative efficacy research; (2) facilitates faithful implementation of intervention protocols in research and in practical applications; (3) enables systematic reviewers to extract and synthesize information about intervention content; (4) enables intervention designers to draw on a more comprehensive list of BCTs (other than those that are familiar to them or those can be brought to mind); and (5) prompts investigation of mechanisms of action by linking BCTs with theoretical constructs.

4.1 The Behaviour Change Technique Taxonomy v1

Drawing on published lists of BCTs (e.g. Prochaska *et al.* 1992; Hardeman *et al.* 2000; Conn *et al.* 2002; Albarracín *et al.* 2005), researchers have started to develop 'taxonomies' of BCTs that can be used to specify the potentially active ingredients of interventions. A taxonomy is, strictly speaking, a hierarchical structure (Stavri and Michie 2012). Sets of BCTs have been identified in relation to particular behavioural domains, including: physical activity and healthy eating, 40 BCTs (Abraham and Michie 2008; Michie *et al.* 2011b); smoking cessation, 53 BCTs (Michie *et al.* 2011d); reducing excessive alcohol consumption, 42 BCTs (Michie *et al.* 2012b); and increasing condom use, 47 BCTs (Abraham *et al.* 2012).

While these taxonomies represented a significant step forward compared with previous vague or inconsistent terminology used for intervention descriptions, they were developed somewhat in parallel and using slightly different methods for different behaviours. Recognizing that these varied methods may encourage silos of research rather than a shared language that could be used across behavioural domains, Michie and colleagues built on the published taxonomies to generate a more extensive and advanced cross-domain taxonomy (Michie *et al.* 2011a, submitted b). This was conducted in collaboration with a wide number of international experts across domains, disciplines, and countries: 30 serving on an international advisory board, 37 taking part in consensus exercises, 40 taking part in coding studies, and 327 giving feedback in workshops and training tutorials. In all, more than 400 experts from 12 countries were involved in developing the Behaviour Change Technique Taxonomy version 1 (BCTTv1; see Table 11.1; Michie *et al.* 2011a, 2013; Cane *et al.* 2015), a hierarchically structured taxonomy comprising 93 distinctive, non-overlapping BCTs clustered into 16 groupings, each with a clear label and

Table 11.1 The Behaviour Change Technique Taxonomy v1 (BCTTv1): 93 BCTs and 16 groupings (Michie *et al.* 2013)

1. Goals and planning
1.1 Goal-setting (behaviour)
1.2 Problem-solving
1.3 Goal-setting (outcome)
1.4 Action planning
1.5 Review behaviour goal(s)
1.6 Discrepancy between current behaviour and goal
1.7 Review outcome goal(s)
1.8 Behavioural contract
1.9 Commitment

2. Feedback and monitoring
2.1. Monitoring of behaviour by others without feedback
2.2. Feedback on behaviour
2.3. Self-monitoring of behaviour
2.4. Self-monitoring of outcome(s) of behaviour
2.5. Monitoring of outcome(s) of behaviour without feedback
2.6. Biofeedback
2.7. Feedback on outcome(s) of behaviour

3. Social support
3.1. Social support (unspecified)
3.2. Social support (practical)
3.3. Social support (emotional)

4. Shaping knowledge
4.1. Instruction on how to perform the behaviour
4.2. Information about antecedents
4.3. Re-attribution
4.4. Behavioural experiments

5. Natural consequences
5.1. Information about health consequences
5.2. Salience of consequences
5.3. Information about social and environmental consequences
5.4. Monitoring of emotional consequences
5.5. Anticipated regret
5.6. Information about emotional consequences

6. Comparison of behaviour
6.1. Demonstration of the behaviour
6.2. Social comparison
6.3. Information about others' approval

7. Associations
7.1. Prompts/cues
7.2. Cue signalling reward
7.3. Reduce prompts/cues
7.4. Remove access to the reward
7.5. Remove aversive stimulus
7.6. Satiation
7.7. Exposure
7.8. Associative learning

8. Repetition and substitution
8.1. Behavioural practice/rehearsal
8.2. Behaviour substitution
8.3. Habit formation
8.4. Habit reversal
8.5. Over-correction
8.6. Generalization of target behaviour
8.7. Graded tasks

9. Comparison of outcomes
9.1. Credible source
9.2. Pros and cons
9.3. Comparative imagining of future outcomes

10. Reward and threat
10.1. Material incentive (behaviour)
10.2. Material reward (behaviour)
10.3. Non-specific reward
10.4. Social reward
10.5. Social incentive
10.6. Non-specific incentive
10.7. Self-incentive
10.8. Incentive (outcome)
10.9. Self-reward
10.10. Reward (outcome)
10.11. Future punishment

11. Regulation
11.1. Pharmacological support
11.2. Reduce negative emotions
11.3. Conserving mental resources
11.4. Paradoxical instructions

12. Antecedents
12.1. Restructuring the physical environment
12.2. Restructuring the social environment
12.3. Avoidance/reducing exposure to cues for the behaviour
12.4. Distraction
12.5. Adding objects to the environment
12.6. Body changes

13. Identity
13.1. Identification of self as role model
13.2. Framing/reframing
13.3. Incompatible beliefs
13.4. Valued self-identify
13.5. Identity associated with changed behaviour

14. Scheduled consequences
14.1. Behaviour cost
14.2. Punishment
14.3. Remove reward
14.4. Reward approximation
14.5. Rewarding completion
14.6. Situation-specific reward
14.7. Reward incompatible behaviour
14.8. Reward alternative behaviour
14.9. Reduce reward frequency
14.10. Remove punishment

15. Self-belief
15.1. Verbal persuasion about capability
15.2. Mental rehearsal of successful performance
15.3. Focus on past success
15.4. Self-talk

16. Covert learning
16.1. Imaginary punishment
16.2. Imaginary reward
16.3. Vicarious consequences

definition, and examples. The grouping structure was introduced as it was recognized that 93 BCTs are too many to be able to easily recall without being conceptually grouped.

4.1.1 Training for users of BCTTv1

The process of specifying behaviour change interventions by BCTs requires a certain level of skill and familiarity with BCT labels, definitions, and examples in the taxonomy. It also requires the coder specifying the content to make a series of complex interpretative judgements to ascertain the presence or absence of a BCT. An effective programme of coder training is required to build a sufficient level of skill for identification of BCTs to be reliable and valid. Reliability refers to the extent to which coders agree with one another and validity refers to the extent to which coders agree with consensus reached by expert BCT coders. As part of the BCTTv1 project (for more information, see www.ucl.ac.uk/health-psychology/bcttaxonomy), two methods of coder training were developed: one-day workshops and distance group-based tutorials. Training effectiveness was evaluated in terms of increased: (1) agreement between trainees; (2) trainee agreement with expert consensus about the presence of BCTs; (3) trainee confidence in BCT identification; and (4) numbers of trainees achieving coding competence (i.e. agreement with expert consensus) (Wood *et al.* 2014).

A self-directed online training resource has also been launched (www.bct-taxonomy.com). The resource is based on the tutorial training programme model and is aimed at both those new to the taxonomy and trained users to give them the opportunity to refresh their knowledge and skills. It trains users on all 93 BCTs from BCTTv1. To further facilitate accuracy and ease and speed of applying BCTTv1 to characterizing intervention content, a smartphone app version of the taxonomy has been developed that can be used alongside the BCTTv1 online training resource.

4.2 Applications of the BCT approach

The BCT approach has been used to describe intervention content and to identify effective BCTs within complex interventions. An example of the former is seen in Michie and colleagues' characterization of the smoking cessation text messaging intervention, 'TxT2Stop' (Michie *et al.* 2012a). The SMS programme had previously been shown to double smokers' chances of quitting (Free *et al.* 2011). To enable development of similar interventions in other countries and improve the existing programme, the BCT content of the intervention was specified using an adapted version of a taxonomy previously used to specify BCTs in face-to-face behavioural support for smoking cessation (Michie *et al.* 2011d). Thirty-four BCTs were identified across the messages used in the Txt2Stop programme. Systematic identification of BCTs provides a basis for experimental manipulation of the content to ascertain which BCTs are the active components of the intervention.

A second example of the approach is seen in the characterization of interventions aiming to reduce the decline of physical activity during pregnancy (Currie *et al.* 2013). A systematic literature review identified 14 relevant BCTS, which showed that participants in intervention groups were more physically active post-intervention than participants in the control group. Two reviewers, working independently, used BCTTv1 to specify intervention content into component BCTs. Common BCTs employed were related to 'Goals and planning', 'Feedback', 'Repetition and substitution', 'Shaping knowledge', and 'Comparison of behaviour'. Currie *et al.* (2013) concluded that a range of BCTs from these groupings can be implemented to reduce the decline in physical activity throughout pregnancy.

Other applications of the BCT approach have included examining the effectiveness of specific BCTs, for example, within motivational interviewing interventions (Morton *et al.* 2014), evaluating a national sexual health and relationships educational package (Dale *et al.* 2014), improving oral hygiene behaviours (Schwarzer *et al.* 2015), increasing young adults' condom use intentions and behaviour (Newby *et al.* 2013), and prevention of childhood obesity among pre-school-aged children (Po'e *et al.* 2013).

To understand not only what works but how an intervention works, we need to understand the causal mechanisms explaining intervention effects (Michie and Abraham 2004; Michie *et al.* 2008b, 2009a). This includes understanding which BCTs are driving effectiveness. Some studies have used meta-regression to assess whether the absence or presence of particular BCTs is associated with effectiveness e.g. (Albarracín *et al.* 2005; Michie *et al.* 2009a; Webb *et al.* 2010; Ivers *et al.* 2012). Others have investigated theoretically based BCT combinations in terms of effectiveness and their interactions, such as whether they are working additively or synergistically with one another (Peters *et al.* 2013; Johnson and Michie 2014; Michie *et al.* 2014c). Recent work has sought to explore these relationships by applying 'classification and regression trees' (CART) to meta-analytic data ('meta-CART') (Dusseldorp *et al.* 2013). Application of this approach is discussed in Section 4.3.2.

4.2.1 Defining and assessing professional competence

In addition to intervention development and evaluation, BCTs can be an important method for defining and assessing professional competence. A number of competency frameworks have been developed to help ensure quality of intervention delivery. The Health Behaviour Change Competency Framework (HBCC; Dixon and Johnston 2012) is a hierarchical framework of competencies for those delivering health behaviour change interventions. The BCTs are grouped according to 'Motivation development', 'Action on motivation', and 'Prompted or cued behaviour'. The HBCC framework has informed the basis of a training programme delivered by NHS Health Scotland. The competences for behavioural support for smoking cessation interventions have also been defined by BCTs, grouped according to functions of motivation, self-regulation, adjuvant activities (e.g. social support, medication), and general aspects of the interaction (delivery of the intervention, information gathering, and general communication) and professionalism (Michie *et al.* 2011c). This forms the basis for a national smoking cessation training programme for stop smoking specialists in England and Wales that has been shown to be effective (see www.ncsct.co.uk) (Brose *et al.* 2013; West and Michie 2013).

4.2.2 Assessing the quality and quantity of intervention delivery

Behavioural change techniques can be used to investigate the translation of evidence into practice and to assess the quality and quantity of intervention delivery (e.g. Michie *et al.* 2011c; Dixon and Johnston 2012; Lorencatto *et al.* 2012, 2013, 2014). For example, specifying behavioural support interventions by BCTs has also enabled the development of evidence-based treatment manuals for smoking cessation interventions (Brose *et al.* 2011) and development of a method to assess the fidelity of the delivery for smoking cessation behavioural support (Lorencatto *et al.* 2013).

In a study by Lorencatto *et al.* (2013), treatment manuals and transcripts of 34 audio-recorded individual behaviour support sessions for smoking cessation were coded into component BCTs. Fidelity was assessed by comparing the proportion of BCTs specified in the manuals with the proportion of BCTs delivered in the sessions. Fidelity was assessed according to session type (i.e. session prior to or after quitting), practitioner, duration, and by BCT. Fidelity was markedly low, with a mean of just 41% of BCTs specified in the treatment manual being delivered per session by stop smoking practitioners. Fidelity varied by practitioner from 32% to 49%. The authors recommended that there should be more routine monitoring in the English Stop Smoking Services to increase fidelity to treatment manuals.

4.2.3 Using BCTs to investigate intervention effectiveness

Behavioural change techniques can have a number of different impacts, such as initiation or termination of a behaviour or change in the frequency, duration or intensity of the behaviour (Michie and Johnston 2013). Evaluating the effectiveness of behaviour change interventions is challenging, since they are nearly always complex in one or more of the following ways: consisting of several interacting components, having a wide scope for variation in the way that interventions are delivered or engaged with (Herbert and Bo 2005), targeting a number of population groups and/or organizational levels and resulting in different kinds of outcome (Craig *et al.* 2008). The BCT methodology is a starting point for investigating the effectiveness of component BCTs. It also allows the study of how modifying factors, such as mode of delivery, intervention intensity, target behaviour, target population, and context, may make BCTs more or less effective (Peters *et al.* 2013; Johnson and Michie 2014; Michie *et al.* 2014c).

Evidence synthesis using traditional meta-analysis in which complex interventions are treated as 'lumps' is not able to move beyond reporting average effect sizes (usually modest) and measures of heterogeneity (usually large). This is not very informative for intervention designers. Other methods of evidence synthesis based on BCT analyses of intervention content are emerging. A recent scoping of the behaviour change literature identified 57 studies testing the effectiveness of BCTs (Michie *et al.* submitted a). Five methods for evaluating BCT effectiveness were identified: 10 used meta-analysis (Knittle *et al.* 2010; Webb *et al.* 2010; Avery *et al.* 2012; Taylor *et al.* 2012; Bull *et al.* 2013; Hill *et al.* 2013; Johnson *et al.* 2013; Olander *et al.* 2013; Bartlett *et al.* 2014; French *et al.* 2014), nine used meta-regression (Michie *et al.* 2009a; Stavri and Beard 2009; Dombrowski *et al.* 2010; Abraham *et al.* 2012; Michie *et al.* 2012b; Prestwich *et al.* 2014b; Denford *et al.* 2014; Hartmann-Boyce *et al.* 2014; Lara *et al.* 2014), nine were experimental studies (Sather *et al.* 2011; Brown *et al.* 2012; Dombrowski *et al.* 2012; Sniehotta *et al.* 2012; Suresh *et al.* 2012; Fletcher *et al.* 2013; Robinson *et al.* 2014), four were correlational studies (West *et al.* 2010, 2011; Murray *et al.* 2013; Hankonen *et al.* 2014), and one study reported the use of meta-CART methods (Dusseldorp *et al.* 2013). The remaining 24 studies were systematic reviews in which effective interventions were compared with non-effective interventions in terms of component BCTs. Articles not included in the review were 14 reviews that had used BCTs to characterize interventions regardless of their effectiveness and 27 study protocols or intervention development articles using a BCT taxonomy.

Several studies have used meta-regression guided by theory to investigate the effectiveness of both individual BCTs and combinations of BCTs that theory predicts would work synergistically together to bring about behaviour change (Smoak *et al.* 2006; Michie *et al.* 2009b; Gardner *et al.* 2010; Dombrowski *et al.* 2012; Ivers *et al.* 2012). Two reviews of interventions to increase physical activity and healthy eating investigated a combination of BCTs predicted by control theory (Carver and Scheier 1982) to be effective (Michie *et al.* 2009b; Dombrowski *et al.* 2010). Interventions combining the BCTs self-monitoring, goal-setting, and action planning were twice as effective as those that did not. Similar methods have been applied in a recent Cochrane review of audit and feedback interventions, finding that interventions were more effective if they included goal-setting and action planning in addition to feedback (Ivers *et al.* 2012). Drawing on a different theory, the Information-Motivation-Behavioural Skills Model (Fisher and Fisher 1992), a review of interventions to reduce risky sexual behaviours found that the theoretically based combination of BCTs associated with the provision of information, motivation, and enhancement of behaviour skills was more effective than other interventions. More recently, meta-analyses using classification and regression trees, referred to as 'meta-CART' (Dusseldorp *et al.* 2013), have been used to explore BCT effectiveness. A re-analysis of the data collected by Michie *et al.* (2009a) found that providing information about the links between behaviour and health was effective if combined with *either* goal-setting *or* with providing information on the consequences of the behaviour *and* using follow-up prompts.

The BCT methodology also has the potential to support the investigation of effective components of complex interventions in primary research. Traditional approaches to intervention development (i.e. constructing an intervention *a priori* before evaluating it in an RCT) evaluate the intervention as a whole rather than isolating the effects of individual BCTs. However, the use of some BCTs may reduce overall effectiveness, some may have a positive effect while others may have no effect. An experimental paradigm to test the effectiveness of BCTs and their interactions is the fractional factorial design, such as used in the Multiphase Optimization Strategy (MOST; Collins *et al.* 2007, 2011). The method starts with a 'screening phase' in which cells from a factorial design of all BCTs are selected to test in a 'fractional factorial' design. Selection is guided by theory and empirical evidence.

The 'refining phase' builds on the first draft of the intervention and seeks to establish the optimal dose of the tested BCTs and whether dose differs according to individual or group characteristics. Decisions about dose are again based on results from RCTs. At the end of this phase, the developers have an optimized 'final draft' intervention consisting of active BCTs at the optimised dosages. In the final phase of the MOST approach, the 'confirming' phase, the intervention is evaluated in a standard RCT. This phase prompts consideration of whether the intervention is efficacious and whether the effects of the intervention are large enough to warrant implementation of the intervention.

Strecher *et al.* (2008) provide an example of this approach as part of their development of a tailored web-based programme for smoking cessation. Strecher *et al.* based the content of their programme on cognitive-behavioural theory and methods of smoking cessation and relapse prevention (e.g. stimulus control, self-efficacy enhancement, and suggestions for coping with tempting situations, events, and emotions). The BCTs selected for testing within this theory included those concerning outcome expectancies, message personalization, timing of message exposure, and efficacy expectations. For some of these, the depth of tailoring was manipulated. A fractional factorial design with 16 arms was implemented, which allowed testing of all main effects and several interactions. The systematic selection procedure within the MOST approach enabled identification of effective intervention components (i.e. engagement, message source, degree of message tailoring, and timing of message exposure) that could be generalized to other computerized smoking cessation interventions. The fractional factorial design also enabled efficient examination of the study aims, including the effect of different depths of tailoring.

A second paradigm is *N*-of-1 studies, in which BCTs can be sequentially introduced within individuals over time in planned or randomized sequences. *N*-of-1 studies serve two main functions: they can be used to evaluate the impact of an intervention of proven effectiveness on individuals, and build the evidence surrounding intervention effectiveness (Craig *et al.* 2008). Experimental *N*-of-1 studies enable the testing of intervention effectiveness in terms of individual or combinations of BCTs; correlational *N*-of-1 studies can be used to investigate change processes and test theoretically specified mechanisms of action. Using series of *N*-of-1 studies, it is possible to assess effectiveness across individuals as well as across several points in time, using time-series analyses. One can investigate how change over time varies across individuals by additionally using multi-level modelling (Quinn *et al.* 2013).

An example of using this approach is a study testing the suitability of *N*-of-1 studies as a means of testing the effectiveness of BCTs based on self-regulation theory (goal-setting and self-monitoring) for promoting walking in healthy adult volunteers (Sniehotta *et al.* 2012). Ten normal or overweight adults were provided with pedometers and were sent daily text messages prompting them to set a step count and/or to monitor their number of steps taken. Participants took part in the intervention for 60 days. Single cases were analysed individually and the primary outcome was the number of steps taken over the 60 days. Mean step counts were higher on days that participants received goal-setting text messages and also higher on days they were prompted to self-monitor. Four participants significantly increased their walking, two on self-monitoring days and two on goal-setting days, compared with the control condition. The remaining six participants did not benefit from the intervention. The authors suggest in their conclusion that *N*-of-1 designs are suitable for testing the effectiveness of interventions at the individual level.

The effectiveness of BCTs can also be assessed using large observational datasets including demographic data, intervention content coded by BCT, contextual factors and outcomes. An example of this is identifying effective BCTs for behavioural support for smoking cessation in a national dataset (West *et al.* 2010, 2011). The first study carried out by West *et al.* (2010) assessed the associations between inclusion of specific BCTs in behavioural support for smoking cessation and the success rates of English Stop Smoking Services. Treatment manuals were obtained from 43 Stop Smoking Services and coded by BCTs using a 43-item smoking behaviour taxonomy (Michie *et al.* 2011d). The manuals contained an average of 22 BCTs. Nine BCTs were associated with both self-reported and carbon-monoxide (CO) verified 4-week quit rates (e.g. advise on medication, measure CO, provide rewards contingent on abstinence, and strengthen ex-smoker identity), and five were associated with CO verified but not self-reported quit rates (e.g. advise on/facilitate use of social support, provide reassurance). The second study (West *et al.* 2011) investigated whether there were any group-based BCTs that added to effectiveness over and above the BCTs used for individual behavioural support in the English Stop Smoking Services. Of the 14 group-based BCTs identified in treatment manuals, two (i.e. 'communicating group membership' and a 'betting game') were associated with increased one-month quit rates.

4.3 Establishing links between BCTs and theory

In this chapter, we have reviewed some of the advances in methods for understanding behaviour and designing interventions. These include frameworks for the systematic development of interventions, informed by a theoretical understanding of behaviour (e.g. the TDF [Michie *et al.* 2005; Cane *et al.* 2012] and the BCW [Michie *et al.* 2011e, 2014a]), and for specifying intervention content using consensus-based methods (e.g. BCTTv1 [Michie *et al.* 2011a, 2013]). Such advances have provided tools to use across disciplines and beyond academia for conceptualizing and changing behaviour (Michie *et al.* 2007b; Michie and Johnston 2012). Theory-based intervention design and evaluation have also been strengthened by the development of methods to assess the extent to which interventions have been informed by formal theories (e.g. the TCS; Prestwich *et al.* 2014c). Although BCTs change behaviour on the basis of a wide variety of mechanisms of action, these are seldom made explicit. Bandura has outlined some links between social cognitive theory (Bandura 1991) and BCTs, although no systematic method for this has been reported. In this section, we describe how work is advancing in establishing systematic methods for linking theory and BCTs.

Fishbein and colleagues reported the work of a small group of world-leading behaviour change theorists who identified key constructs that would enable the prediction and understanding of behaviour drawn from five of the most widely used theories of behaviour change: the health belief model (Janz and Becker 1984), social cognitive theory (Bandura 1991), the theory of reasoned action (Ajzen and Fishbein 1980), self-regulation theory (Kanfer and Gaelick 1991), and self-control theory (Fishbein *et al.* 2001; Mischel 2011). The group agreed that intentions, environmental barriers/facilitators, and skills were necessary for behaviour to occur. The theorists reached a consensus about linkages between theoretical models, constructs, and intentions; however, consensus was not reached about the causal model linking constructs to behaviour. The theorists concluded that (a) if strong intention to perform the behaviour has not yet been formed, then the focus of the intervention should be on constructs that increase motivation, and (b) if strong intention has been formed but has not yet been acted upon, then the focus should be on improving skills needed in order to perform the behaviour or removing barriers to facilitate the behaviour. They agreed, therefore, that effective interventions were likely to be those that focused on strengthening intentions, removing environmental barriers to change, and increasing skills required to perform the behaviour.

There have been some efforts to link theoretical constructs and domains to BCTs (Fishbein *et al.* 2001; Albarracín *et al.* 2005; Abraham and Michie 2008; Michie *et al.* 2008a, 2008b, 2011c). For example, Abraham and Michie (2008) linked BCTs from their 26-item taxonomy onto a variety of theoretical accounts of behaviour change (e.g. control theory; Carver and Scheier 1982), social comparison theory (Festinger 1954), and social cognitive theory (Bandura 1991). For example, the BCTs 'Provide information on consequences' and 'Provide information about others' approval' were linked to constructs relating to personal beliefs about the behaviour reflected in the theory of planned behaviour (Ajzen 1991) and social cognitive theory (Bandura 1991).

Michie *et al.* (2008a) adopted small-group consensus methods to link BCTs used by facilitators delivering a physical activity intervention for adults at risk of Type 2 diabetes to four theories: the theory of planned behaviour (Ajzen 1991), self-regulation theory (Kanfer and Gaelick 1991), operant learning theory (Skinner 1938), and relapse prevention theory (Marlatt and George, 1984). This was part of a study investigating the extent to which BCTs and their theoretical base were delivered by facilitators according to protocol (Hardeman *et al.* 2007), and the extent to which those receiving the intervention engaged with the BCTs. Using this method, the authors were able to show that the theoretical basis of the intervention protocol was reflected in delivery (although on average only 42% of BCTs are delivered), whereas the theoretical basis of the intervention was not reflected in participant engagement. The way that participants talked about changing behaviour suggested they were drawing on BCTs associated with operant learning theory more heavily than would be suggested by the emphasis placed on it within the protocol.

Building on this research, Michie *et al.* sought to link BCTs to theoretical domains in the TDF (Michie *et al.* 2008b). They identified BCTs from textbooks and two published systematic reviews with definitions then being developed via a process of brainstorming. A total of 35 BCTs were identified from the two systematic reviews (Hardeman *et al.* 2000; Abraham and Michie 2008). Nine textbooks, covering a range of behavioural therapies and approaches were then consulted (Gambrill 1977; Stern 1978; Kanfer and Goldstein 1986; Sherman 1990; Bergin and Garfield 1994; Leslie and O'Reilly 1999; Kazdin 2001; Sarafino 2001; Leslie 2002). Michie *et al.* systematically identified 53 BCTs from these textbooks. Having identified 88 BCTs in total, the study team members individually rated the extent to which they considered each of the 35 BCTs identified from the reviews would be effective in changing each behaviour (as identified by Fishbein *et al.* 2001; Michie and Abraham 2004). Reasonable agreement (>70%) was reached among the study team and these data were used to build a matrix of BCT–theoretical domain linkages.

Another approach, 'intervention mapping' (Kok *et al.* 2004; Bartholomew *et al.* 2011), outlines six systematic steps to aid planning and development of behaviour change interventions:

1. The needs assessment: involving a scientific, epidemiological, behavioural, and social analysis of the population and their problem.
2. Definition of proximal programme objectives: involving explication of who and what will change as a result of the intervention.
3. Selection of theoretical methods and practical strategies: the goal of this step is to generate a list of intervention methods and techniques informed by the analysis performed in steps 1 and 2 and to develop practical and appropriate ways of delivering them.
4. Production of the programme components and production: involving the design of the intervention programme with careful reconsideration of the intended participants and context, and piloting the programme strategies and materials.
5. Consideration of the programme's adoption, implementation, and sustainability: involving the identification of performance objectives. Objectives are operationalized using theory-informed strategies and methods. Detailed plans are drawn up for accomplishing programme adoption and evaluation.
6. Generating an evaluation plan to assess change in health and quality-of-life problems, behaviour and environment, and determinants of performance objectives: all variables have been defined in a measurable way throughout the programme development process.

The intervention mapping approach has been widely implemented to develop interventions targeting a range of behaviours, including healthy eating in children (Weber Cullen *et al.* 1998; Pérez-Rodrigo *et al.* 2005), preventing transmission of sexually transmitted diseases in high-risk minority adolescents (Tortolero *et al.* 2005), and decreasing lower-back pain in the workplace (Ammendolia *et al.* 2009). It provides intervention designers with a systematic process to follow; however, it does not cover the full range of intervention components available that could be important. Step 3 in the intervention mapping process also requires intervention designers to base their selection of specific BCTs on a theoretical model. The successful selection of techniques appropriate to the model is dependent on the designer having a good knowledge and understanding of the possible theories and models to use, being aware of the full range of BCTs available, and having the understanding and skills to link theoretical constructs and BCTs.

The ABC of Behaviour Change Theories provides a resource for designers to consider a wide range of theories (Davis *et al.* 2014; Michie *et al.* 2014b) (see www.behaviourchangetheories.com) but further work is required to help designers evaluate and choose between them. Some initial work has been carried out to assess the quality of theories and to develop quality criteria to guide intervention designers in selecting the most appropriate theory (Michie and Prestwich 2010; Davis *et al.* 2014). Having reviewed the health behaviour change literature as to what makes a theory scientifically useful (e.g. West 2006; Glanz *et al.* 2008), Davis *et al.* (2014) consulted an advisory board of 24 UK experts from across psychology, anthropology, sociology, economics, and epidemiology, and identified nine criteria as being conceptually important for a good theory. They were: (1) clarity of constructs (e.g. 'has the case been made for the independence of constructs from each other?'); (2) clarity of relationships between constructs (e.g. 'are the relationships between constructs clearly specified?'); (3) measurability (e.g. 'is an explicit methodology for measuring the constructs given?'); (4) testability (e.g. 'has the theory been specified in such a way that it can be tested?'); (5) being explanatory (e.g. 'has the theory been used to explain/account for a set of observations? Either statistically or logically'); (6) describing causality (e.g. 'has the theory been used to describe mechanisms of change?'); (7) achieving parsimony (e.g. 'has the case for parsimony been made?'); (8) generalizability (e.g. 'have generalizations been investigated across (i) behaviours?, (ii) populations?, (iii) contexts?'); and (9) having an evidence base.

Work is currently underway by Michie and colleagues to explore the relationships among constructs within theory and to map constructs across theories and to develop and test a methodology for linking theoretical constructs and domains to BCTs (Michie *et al.* 2014d). A set of criteria for assessing the quality of theories have been developed by a multidisciplinary expert group (Davis *et al.* 2014; Michie *et al.* 2014b). Future work includes developing a method to apply the criteria to examine the quality of behaviour change theories for use in designing and evaluating interventions.

An example of a study explicitly linking BCTs to theoretical mechanisms is a randomized controlled trial to test the impact of partner-based interventions on changes to physical activity and healthy eating (Prestwich *et al.* 2014a). Previous research had shown that partner-based interventions had the potential to encourage greater levels of motivation and intrinsic motivation (Prestwich *et al.* 2005) and increase social influence and self-efficacy by processes such as 'modelling' (Bandura 1977). Such BCTs as the provision of structured support, encouraging the person to involve family members and/or friends as forms of social support, and setting implementation intentions were all positively associated with intervention effectiveness across a range of different behaviours (e.g. van Osch *et al.* 2009). Prestwich *et al.* noted that the effectiveness of specific BCTs or constructs was being driven by theories such as the theory of planned behaviour (Ajzen 1991) and social cognitive theory (Bandura 1986), and thus changes to these BCTs and/or constructs had potential to mediate intervention effectiveness. In most of this work, judgement of which BCTs are associated with which mechanisms of action has been done using small-group consensus methods among members of the research team. Establishing a methodology for linking BCTs to their mechanisms of action is a much-needed next step for advancing the science of behaviour change and its applications.

4.3.1 Developing a methodology for linking BCTs and theory

Achieving a consensus about BCT–theory links will enable the translation of theory into intervention design (Michie *et al.*, 2008b, 2011e, 2014a) and enable effective interventions to be explained in terms of their theoretical mechanisms (Michie *et al.* 2009b; McEachan *et al.* 2011;

Dombrowski *et al.* 2012; Ivers *et al.* 2012). It will also become possible to more rigorously test theory and ascertain BCT effectiveness. Developing a consensus about how theories link to BCTs requires intensive work informed both by systematic reviews of the literature and by consensus exercises among cross-disciplinary behaviour change experts. This is the focus of a current project (Michie *et al.* 2014d) that aims to connect three methodologies: BCTTv1 (Michie *et al.* 2011a, 2013), the TDF (Cane *et al.* 2012), and the 83 theories identified by the interdisciplinary behaviour change theory project (Davis *et al.* 2014; Michie *et al.* 2014b). The aim is to begin to develop a 'Behaviour Change Ontology', specifying the concepts within, and relationships between, the five domains of BCTs, modes of delivery, mechanisms of action, context, and behaviour. Ontologies refer to taxonomic descriptions of the concepts applied in a specific domain and of the relationships between them (Bickmore *et al.* 2011).

5 Conclusion and the future

The work and ideas discussed in this chapter are presented as small steps along the path of developing a systematic, theory-based, and usable methodology for developing, evaluating, and reporting behaviour change interventions. Continued development of this methodology alongside increasingly sophisticated designs and experimental methods will enable behavioural science to begin to more effectively unpack the 'black boxes' of complex interventions to change behaviour.

Social cognition models have been widely implemented in the health behaviour change literature and continue to be popular choices for intervention designers building theory-based interventions. We have suggested that there is likely to be value in broadening the conceptualization of influences on behaviour beyond social cognition to automatic processes in motivation such as emotions, impulses, desires, and to the influences of capability and opportunity on behaviour (see Norman and Conner, Chapter 12 this volume). Integrative theories of behaviour and behaviour change (e.g. COM-B [Michie 2011e, 2014a], PRIME theory [West and Brown 2013], and the CEOS model [Borland 2014]) encapsulate both automatic and reflective processes of motivation and aid systematic identification of factors that may need to 'shift' in order for behaviour change to occur. However, a study of the 83 theories identified in our review, of which COM-B, PRIME, and CEOS are three, show that many bring different and potentially important constructs, and relationships between constructs, to the understanding, prediction, and change of behaviour. Broad frameworks (such as the BCW and TDF) include a wide range of factors influencing the behaviour that may be missed by a simpler, less comprehensive model. However, they do not include directional relationships between variables that are key to understanding behaviour in order to change it. An initial assessment using a broad framework can be combined with specific formal theories relevant to a particular theoretical domain. Developing methods for testing theory (which require a reliable method for linking theoretical constructs and BCTs, among other things) is a necessary requisite for the advance of behavioural science and its application.

For translating theory into interventions and for testing theory, we have highlighted the need for a shared terminology accessible across research groups, disciplines, and countries that can be used to describe how theoretical constructs can be operationalized. The Behaviour Change Technique Taxonomy v1 (BCTTv1) (Michie *et al.* 2011a, 2013) provides a means of characterizing the active content of complex behaviour change interventions to facilitate intervention replication, delivery, evaluation, and reporting. Researchers have already sought to explore links between theoretical constructs and BCTs; work is now under way to provide a more rigorous methodology for this process, agreed across a range of disciplines, work areas, and countries, and to build a resource for use by intervention designers (Michie *et al.* 2014d).

Evidence about the effectiveness of individual BCTs and combinations of BCTs is accumulating as intervention evaluations are being published at a rapid and accelerating rate. To enable the rapid integration of these data within a structure so that they can be easily accessed and used, we require a more comprehensive Behaviour Change Ontology – that is, a structure that systematically represents and organizes the essential elements of behaviour change interventions, codifies our collective knowledge, provides a consensus on concepts, terms, and relationships, and specifies and formalizes them. We are collaborating with computational and informational scientists to begin the work of developing taxonomies for elements in the ontology where they do not exist and constructing links between them. The elements in our Behaviour Change Ontology are: BCTs, mechanisms of action (i.e. theory), types of behaviour, modes of delivery, and context (situation and population). The vision is to develop methods and create an integrated human–computer expert network for the efficient and rapid synthesis of scientific findings that would continuously advance and update knowledge. These data would be classifiable into, and retrievable from, the ontological structure. The result would be a systematized 'clearinghouse' of continuously updated evidence-based intervention components and an open-access, searchable database for intervention designers to identify the intervention characteristics most likely to be effective for their behavioural targets and contexts. This would form a step change towards the more rapid development and optimization of real-world behaviour change interventions.

References

Abraham, C. and Michie, S. (2008) A taxonomy of behavior change techniques used in interventions, *Health Psychology*, 27, 379–87.

Abraham, C., Conner, M., Jones, F. and O'Connor, D. (2008) *Health Psychology: Topics in Applied Psychology*. London: Hodder Education.

Abraham, C., Good, A., Huedo-Medina, T., Warren, M. and Johnson, B. (2012) Reliability and utility of the SHARP taxonomy of behaviour change techniques, *Psychology and Health*, 27, 1–2.

Abraham, C., Kelly, M., West, R. and Michie, S. (2009) The UK National Institute for Health and Clinical Excellence public health guidance on behaviour change: a brief introduction, *Psychology, Health and Medicine*, 14 (1), 1–8.

Abraham, C., Kok, G., Schaalma, H. and Luszczynska, A. (2010) Health promotion, in P. Martin, F. Cheung, M. Kyrios, L. Littlefield, L. Knowles and M. Overmier (eds.) *The International Association of Applied Psychology Handbook of Applied Psychology* (pp. 83–111). Oxford: Wiley-Blackwell.

Ajzen, I. (1991) The theory of planned behaviour, *Organizational Behavior and Human Decision Processes*, 50, 179–211.

Ajzen, I. and Fishbein, M. (1980) *Understanding Attitudes and Predicting Social Behaviour*. London: Pearson.

Albada, A., Ausems, M., Bensing, J. and van Dulmen, S. (2009) Tailored information about cancer risk and screening: a systematic review, *Patient Education and Counseling*, 77, 155–71.

Albarracín, D., Gillette, J.C., Earl, A.N., Glasman, L.R., Durantini, M.R. and Ho, M.-H. (2005) A test of major assumptions about behavior change: a comprehensive look at the effects of passive and active HIV-prevention interventions since the beginning of the epidemic, *Psychological Bulletin*, 131, 856–97.

Amemori, M., Michie, S., Korhonen, T., Murtomaa, H. and Kinnunen, T.H. (2011) Assessing implementation difficulties in tobacco use prevention and cessation counselling among dental providers, *Implementation Science*, 6, 50.

Ammendolia, C., Cassidy, D., Steenstra, I., Soklaridis, S., Boyle, E., Eng, S. *et al.* (2009) Designing a workplace return-to-work program for occupational low back pain: an intervention mapping approach, *BMC Musculoskeletal Disorders*, 10, 65.

Ammerman, A., Lindquist, C., Lohr, K. and Hersey, J. (2002) The efficacy of behavioral interventions to modify dietary fat and fruit and vegetable intake: a review of the evidence, *Preventive Medicine*, 35, 25–41.

Armitage, C. and Conner, M. (2000) Social cognition models and health behaviour: a structured review, *Psychology and Health*, 15, 173–89.

Avery, L., Flynn, D., van Wersch, A., Sniehotta, F. and Trenell, M. (2012) Changing physical activity behavior in Type 2 diabetes: a systematic review and meta-analysis of behavioral interventions, *Diabetes Care*, 35, 2681–9.

Bandura A. (1977) Self-efficacy: toward a unifying theory of behavioral change, *Psychological Review*, 84, 191–215.

Bandura, A. (1991) Social cogntiive theory of moral thought and action, in W.J. Kurtines and L. Gewirtz (eds.) *Handbook of Moral Behavior and Development* (Vol. 1, pp. 45–103). Hillsdale, NJ: Erlbaum.

Bartholomew, L., Parcel, G., Kok, G., Gottlieb, N. and Fernandez, M. (eds.) (2011) *Planning Health Promotion Programs: An Intervention Mapping Approach* (3rd edn.). San Francisco, CA: Jossey-Bass.

Bartlett, Y., Sheeran, P. and Hawley, M. (2014) Effective behaviour change techniques in smoking cessation interventions for people with chronic obstructive pulmonary disease: a meta-analysis, *British Journal of Health Psychology*, 19, 181–203.

Beenstock, J., Sniehotta, F.F., White, M., Bell, R., Milne, E.M. and Araujo-Soares, V. (2012) What helps and hinders midwives in engaging with pregnant women about stopping smoking? A cross-sectional survey of perceived implementation difficulties among midwives in the North East of England, *Implementation Science*, 7, 36.

Bergin, A.E. and Garfield, S. (1994) *Handbook of Psychotherapy and Behaviour Change* (4th edn.). Chichester: Wiley.

Bhattarai, N., Prevost, A., Wright, A., Charlton, J., Rudisill, C. and Gulliford, M. (2013) Effectiveness of interventions to promote healthy diet in primary care: systematic review and meta-analysis of randomised controlled trials, *BMC Public Health*, 13, 1203.

Bickmore, T., Schulman, D. and Sidner, C. (2011) A reusable framework for health counseling dialogue systems based on a behavioral medicine ontology, *Journal of Biomedical Informatics*, 44, 183–97

Borland, R. (2014) *Understanding Hard to Maintain Behaviour Change: A Dual Process Approach*. Oxford: Wiley-Blackwell.

Brose, L., West, R., McDermott, M., Fidler, J., Croghan, E. and McEwen, A. (2011) What makes for an effective stop-smoking service? *Thorax*, 66, 924–6.

Brose, L., West, R., Michie, S. and McEwen, A. (2013) Validation of content of an online knowledge training program, *Nicotine and Tobacco Research*, 15, 997–8.

Brown, J., Michie, S., Geraghty, A., Miller, S., Yardley, L., Gardner, B. *et al.* (2012) A pilot study of StopAdvisor: a theory-based interactive internet-based smoking cessation intervention aimed across the social spectrum, *Addictive Behaviors*, 37, 1365–70.

Bull, E., Dombrowski, S. and Johnston, M. (2013) Behaviour change techniques within diet, activity and smoking interventions for low-income groups: a systematic review, *Psychology and Health*, 28, 70–5.

Bussieres, A.E., Patey, A.M., Francis, J.J., Sales, A.E., Grimshaw, J.M., Brouwers, M. *et al.* (2012) Identifying factors likely to influence compliance with diagnostic imaging guideline recommendations for spine disorders among chiropractors in North America: a focus group study using the Theoretical Domains Framework, *Implementation Science*, 7, 82.

Cane, J., O'Connor, D. and Michie, S. (2012) Validation of the theoretical domains framework for use in behaviour change and implementation research, *Implementation Science*, 7, 37.

Cane, J., Richardson, M., Johnston, M., Lahda, R. and Michie, S. (2015) From lists of behaviour change techniques (BCTs) to structured hierarchies: comparison of two methods of developing a hierarchy of BCTs, *Health Psychology*, 20. 130–50.

Carver, C.S. and Scheier, M.F. (1982) Control theory: a useful conceptual framework for personality–social, clinical, and health psychology, *Psychological Bulletin*, 92, 111–35.

Charani, E., Castro-Sanchez, E., Sevdalis, N., Kyratsis, Y., Drumright, L., Shah, N. *et al.* (2013) Understanding the determinants of antimicrobial prescribing within hospitals: the role of 'prescribing etiquette', *Clinical Infectious Diseases*, 57, 188–96.

Cochrane Effective Practice and Organisation of Care Group (EPOC) (2010) Cochrane Effective Practice and Organisation of Care Group: EPOC-specific resources for review authors [http://epoc.cochrane.org/epoc-specific-resources-review-authors].

Cohen, D. and Scribner, R. (2000) An STD/HIV prevention intervention framework, *AIDS Patient Care and STDS*, 14, 37–45.

Collins, L., Baker, T., Mermelstein, R., Piper, M., Jorenby, D., Smith, S. *et al.* (2011) The multiphase optimization strategy for engineering effective tobacco use interventions, *Annals of Behavioral Medicine*, 41, 208–26.

Collins, L., Murphy, S. and Strecher, V. (2007) The multiphase optimization strategy (MOST) and the sequential multiple assignment randomized trial (SMART): new methods for more potent eHealth interventions, *American Journal of Preventive Medicine*, 32 (5 suppl.), S112–S118.

Conn, V., Valentine, J. and Cooper, H. (2002) Interventions to increase physical activity among aging adults: a meta-analysis, *Annals of Behavioral Medicine*, 24, 190–200.

Conner, M. and Norman, P. (1995) Predicting health check attendance among prior attenders and non-attenders: the role of prior behaviour in the theory of planned behaviour, *Journal of Applied Social Psychology*, 26, 1010–26.

Conner, M. and Norman, P. (2005) *Predicting Health Behaviour*. Buckingham: Open University Press.

Craig, P., Dieppe, P., Macintyre, S., Michie, S., Nazareth, I. and Petticrew, M. (2008) Developing and evaluating complex interventions: the new Medical Research Council guidance, *British Medical Journal*, 337, 979–83.

Currie, S., Sinclair, M., Murphy, M., Madden, E., Dunwoody, L. and Liddle, D. (2013) Reducing the decline in physical activity during pregnancy: a systematic review of behaviour change interventions, *PLoS One*, 8 (6), e66385.

Dale, H., Raftery, B. and Locke, H. (2014) Behaviour change and sexual health: SHARE programme evaluation, *Health Education*, 114, 2–19.

Davidson, K.W., Goldstein, M., Kaplan, R.M., Kaufmann, P.G., Knatterud, G.L., Orleans, C.T. *et al.* (2003) Evidence-based behavioral medicine: what is it and how do we achieve it? *Annals of Behavioral Medicine*, 26, 161–71.

Davies, P., Walker, A.E. and Grimshaw, J.M. (2010) A systematic review of the use of theory in the design of guideline dissemination and implementation strategies and interpretation of the results of rigorous evaluations, *Implementation Science*, 5, 14.

Davis, R., Campbell, R., Hildon, Z. and Michie, S. (2014) Theories of behaviour and behaviour change across disciplines: a systematic review, *Health Psychology Review*.

DEFRA (2008) *A Framework for Pro-Environmental Behaviours: Report*. London: DEFRA.

Denford, S., Taylor, R., Campbell, J. and Greaves, C. (2014) Effective behavior change techniques in asthma self-care interventions: systematic review and meta-regression, *Health Psychology*, 33, 577–87.

Des Jarlais, D., Lyles, C. and Crepaz, N. (2004) Improving the reporting quality of nonrandomized evaluations of behavioral and public health interventions: the TREND statement, *American Journal of Public Health*, 94, 361–6.

Dixon, D. and Johnston, M. (2012) *Health Behavior Change Competency Framework: Competences to Deliver Interventions to Change Lifestyle Behaviors that Affect Health* [http://www.phorcast.org.uk/document_store/1318587875_wBBR_health_behaviour_change_competency_framework.pdf].

Dolan, P., Halpern, D., King, D., Vlaev, I. and Hallsworth, M. (2010) *MINDSPACE: Influencing Behaviour through Public Policy*. London: Institute for Government.

Dombrowski, S.U., Sniehotta, F.F., Avenell, A., Johnston, M., MacLennan, G. and Araújo-Soares, V. (2010) Identifying active ingredients in complex behavioural interventions for obese adults with obesity-related co-morbidities or additional risk factors for co-morbidities: a systematic review, *Health Psychology Review*, 6, 7–32.

Dombrowski, S.U., Sniehotta, F.F., Johnston, M., Broom, I., Kulkarni, U., Brown, J. *et al.* (2012) Optimizing acceptability and feasibility of an evidence-based behavioral intervention for obese adults with obesity-related co-morbidities or additional risk factors for co-morbidities: an open-pilot intervention study in secondary care, *Patient Education and Counseling*, 87, 108–19.

Dunton, G., Cousineau, M. and Reynolds, K. (2010) The intersection of public policy and health behaviour theory in the physical activity arena, *Journal of Physical Activity and Health*, 7 (suppl.), S91–S98.

Dusseldorp, E., van Genugten, L., van Buuren, S., Verheijden, M.W. and van Empelen, P. (2013) Combinations of techniques that effectively change health behavior: evidence from Meta-CART analysis, *Health Psychology* [DOI: 10.1037/hea0000018].

Dyson, J., Lawton, R., Jackson, C. and Cheater, F. (2011) Does the use of a theoretical approach tell us more about hand hygiene behaviour? The barriers and levers to hand hygiene, *Journal of Infection Prevention*, 12, 17–24.

Festinger, L. (1954) A theory of social comparison processes, *Human Relations*, 7, 117–40.

Fishbein, M., Triandis, H., Kanfer, F., Becker, M., Middlestadt, S. and Eichler, A. (2001) Factors influencing behaviour and behaviour change, in A. Baum, T. Revenson, J. Singer and N. Imahwah (eds.) *Handbook of Health Psychology* (pp. 3–17). Hillsdale, NJ: Erlbaum.

Fisher, J.D. and Fisher, W.A. (1992) Changing AIDS-risk behavior, *Psychological Bulletin*, 111, 455–74.

Fletcher, A., Wolfenden, L., Wyse, R., Bowman, J., McElduff, P. and Duncan, S. (2013) A randomised controlled trial and mediation analysis of the 'Healthy Habits', telephone-based dietary intervention for preschool children, *International Journal of Behavioral Nutrition and Physical Activity*, 10, 43.

Francis, J., O'Connor, D. and Curran, J. (2012) Theories of behaviour change synthesised into a set of theoretical groupings: introducing a thematic series on the theoretical domains framework, *Implement Science*, 7, 35 [DOI: 10.1186/1748-5908-7-35].

Francis, J., Stockton, C., Eccles, M., Johnston, M., Cuthbertson, B., Grimshaw, J. *et al.* (2009) Evidence based selection of theories for designing behaviour change interventions: using methods based on theoretical construct domains to understand clinicians' blood transfusion behaviour. *British Journal of Health Psychology*, 14 (4), 625-46.

Francis, J., Tinmouth, A., Stanworth, S., Grimshaw, J., Johnston, M., Hyde, C. *et al.* (2009) Using theories of behaviour to understand transfusion prescribing in three clinical contexts in two countries: development work for an implementation trial, *Implementation Science*, 4, 70.

Free, C., Knight, R., Robertson, S., Whittaker, R., Edwards, P., Zhou, W. *et al.* (2011) Smoking cessation support delivered via mobile phone text messaging (txt2stop): a single-blind, randomised trial, *Lancet*, 378, 49–55.

French, D., Olander, E., Chisholm, A. and McSharry, J. (2014) Which behaviour change techniques are most effective at increasing older adults' self-efficacy and physical activity behaviour? A systematic review, *Annals of Behavioral Medicine*, 48, 225–34.

French, S., Green, S., O'Connor, D., McKenzie, J., Francis, J., Michie, S. *et al.* (2012) Developing theory-informed behaviour change interventions to implement evidence into practice: a systematic approach using the Theoretical Domains Framework, *Implementation Science*, 7, 38.

Fuller, C., Michie, S., Savage, J., McAteer, J., Besser, S., Charlett, A. *et al.* (2012) The Feedback Intervention Trial (FIT) – improving hand hygiene compliance in UK healthcare workers: a stepped wedge cluster randomised controlled trial, *PLoS One*, 7 (10), e41617.

Gambrill, E.D. (1977) *Behaviour Modification: Handbook of Assessment, Intervention and Evaluation*. San Francisco, CA: Jossey Boss.

Gardner, B., Wardle, J., Poston, L. and Croker, H. (2011) Changing diet and physical activity to reduce gestational weight gain: a meta-analysis, *Obesity Reviews*, 12, e602–20.

Gardner, B., Whittington, C., McAteer, J., Eccles, M. and Michie, S. (2010) Using theory to synthesise evidence from behaviour change interventions: the example of audit and feedback, *Social Science and Medicine*, 70, 1618–25.

Gatersleben, B. and Vlek, C. (1998) Household consumption, quality of life, and environmental impacts: a psychological perspective and empirical study, in K.J. Noorman and T.S. Uiterkamp (eds.) *Green Households? Domestic Consumers, Environment and Sustainability* (pp. 141–83). London: Earthscan.

Geller, S., Berry, T., Ludwig, T., Evans, R., Gilmore, M. and Clarke, S. (1990) A conceptual framework for developing and evaluating behavior change interventions for injury control, *Health Education Research*, 5, 125–37.

Glanz, K. and Bishop, D.B. (2010) The role of behavioral science theory in development and implementation of public health interventions, *Annual Review of Public Health*, 31, 399–418.

Glanz, K., Rimer, B. and Lewis, F. (2002) *Health Behavior and Health Education: Theory, Research and Practice*. San Francisco, CA: Wiley.

Glanz, K., Rimer, B. and Viswanath, K. (eds.) (2008) *Health Behaviour and Health Education: Theory, Research and Practice* (4th edn.). San Francisco, CA: Jossey-Bass.

Goel, P., Ross-Degnan, D., Berman, P. and Soumerai, S. (1996) Retail pharmacies in developing countries: a behavior and intervention framework, *Social Science and Medicine*, 42, 1155–61.

Hankonen, N., Sutton, S., Prevost, A., Simmons, R., Griffin, S., Kinmonth, A. *et al.* (2014) Which behavior change techniques are associated with changes in physical activity, diet and body mass index in people with recently diagnosed diabetes? *Annals of Behavioral Medicine* [DOI: 10.1007/s12160-014-9624-9].

Hardeman, W., Griffin, S., Johnston, M., Kinmonth, A. and Wareham, N. (2000) Interventions to prevent weight gain: a systematic review of psychological models and behaviour change methods, *International Journal of Obesity and Related Metabolic Disorders*, 24, 131–43.

Hardeman, W., Michie, S., Fanshawe, T., Prevost, T., McLoughlin, K. and Kinmonth, A. (2007) Fidelity of delivery of a physical activity intervention: predictors and consequences, *Psychology and Health*, 23, 11–24.

Hartmann-Boyce, J., Johns, D., Jebb, S. and Aveyard, P. (2014) Effect of behavioural techniques and delivery mode on effectiveness of weight management: systematic review, meta-analysis and meta-regression, *Obesity Reviews*, 15, 598–609.

Hendriks, A., Gubbels, J., De Vries, N., Seidell, J., Kremers, S. and Jansen, M. (2012) Interventions to promote an integrated approach to public health problems: an application to childhood obesity, *Journal of Environmental and Public Health* [DOI: 10.1155/2012/913236].

Herbert, H. and Bo, K. (2005) Analysis of quality of interventions in systematic reviews, *British Medical Journal*, 331, 507–9.

Hill, B., Skouteris, H. and Fuller-Tyszkiewicz, M. (2013) Interventions designed to limit gestational weight gain: a systematic review of theory and meta-analysis of intervention components, *Obesity Reviews*, 14, 435–50.

Hoffmann, T., Erueti, C. and Glasziou, P. (2013) Poor description of non-pharmacological interventions: analysis of consecutive sample of randomised trials, *British Medical Journal*, 347, f3755.

Hoffmann, T.C., Glasziou, P.P., Boutron, I., Milne, R., Perera, R., Moher, D. *et al.* (2014) Better reporting of interventions: template for intervention description and replication (TIDieR) checklist and guide, *British Medical Journal*, 348.

Ivers, N., Jamtvedt, G., Flottorp, S., Young, J.M., Odgaard-Jensen, J., French, S.D. *et al.* (2012) Audit and feedback: effects on professional practice and healthcare outcomes, *Cochrane Database Systematic Reviews*, 6, Cd000259.

Jackson, C., Eliasson, L., Barber, N. and Weinman, J. (2014) Applying COM-B to medication adherence: a suggested framework for research and interventions, *European Health Psychologist*, 16 (1), 7–17.

Janz, N. and Becker, M. (1984) The Health Belief Model: a decade later, *Health Education Quarterly*, 11, 1–47.

Johnson, B., Lennon, C., Huedo-Medina, T., Spina, M., Sagherian, M. and Ballester, E. (2013) Behaviour change techniques succeed best under optimal circumstances, *Psychology and Health*, 28 (suppl. 1), 15.

Johnson, B.T. and Michie, S. (2014) Towards healthy theorizing about health behaviours in the maze of messy reality: a reaction to Peters, de Bruin, and Crutzen (2013), *Health Psychology Review* [DOI: 10.1080/17437199.2014.900722].

Kanfer, F. and Gaelick, L. (1991) Self-management methods, in F. Kanfer and A. Goldstein (eds.) *Helping People Change: A Textbook of Methods* (pp. 305–60). New York: Pergamon Press..

Kanfer, F.H. and Goldstein, AP. (1986) *Helping People Change: A Textbook of Methods*. New York: Pergamon Press.

Kazdin, A.E. (2001) *Behavior Modification in Applied Settings* (6th edn.). Belmont, CA: Wadsworth/Thomson.

Kim, N., Stanton, B., Li, X., Dickersin, K. and Galbraith, J. (1997) Effectiveness of the 40 adolescent AIDS-risk reduction interventions: a quantitative review, *Journal of Adolescent Health*, 20, 204–15.

Knittle, K., Maes, S. and de Gucht, V. (2010) Psychological interventions for rheumatoid arthritis: examining the role of self-regulation with a systematic review and meta-analysis of randomized controlled trials, *Arthritis Care and Research (Hoboken)*, 62, 1460–72.

Knott, D., Muers, S. and Aldridge, S. (2008) *Achieving Culture Change: A Policy Framework*. London: Strategy Unit.

Kok, G., Schaalma, H., Ruiter, R.A.C., Van Empelen, P. and Brug, J. (2004) Intervention mapping: protocol for applying health psychology theory to prevention programmes, *Journal of Health Psychology*, 9, 85–98.

Lara, J., Hobbs, N., Moynihan, P., Meyer, T., Adamson, A., Errington, L. *et al.* (2014) Effectiveness of dietary interventions among adults of retirement age: a systematic review and meta-analysis of randomized controlled trials, *BMC Medicine*, 12, 60.

Leeman, J., Baernholdt, M. and Sandelowski, M. (2007) Developing a thoery-based taxonomy of methods for implementing change in practice, *Journal of Advanced Nursing*, 58, 191–200.

Leslie, J.C. (2002) *Essential Behavior Analysis*. London: Arnold.

Leslie, J.C. and O'Reilly, M.F. (1999) *Behavior Analysis: Foundations and Applications to Psychology*. Amsterdam: Harwood Academic.

Lippke, S. and Ziegelmann, J. (2008) Theory-based health behavior change: developing, testing, and applying theories for evidence-based interventions, *Applied Psychology*, 57, 698–716.

Lorencatto, F., West, R., Bruguera, C. and Michie, S. (2014) A method for assessing fidelity of delivery of telephone behavioral support for smoking ceessation, *Journal of Consulting and Clinical Psychology*, 82, 482–91.

Lorencatto, F., West, R., Christopherson, C. and Michie, S. (2013) Assessing fidelity of delivery of smoking cessation behavioural support in practice, *Implementation Science*, 8, 40.

Lorencatto, F., West, R., Stavri, Z. and Michie, S. (2012) How well is intervention content described in published reports of smoking cessation interventions? *Nicotine and Tobacco Research*, 14, 1019–26.

Lozano, R., Naghavi, M., Foreman, K., Lim, S., Shibuya, K., Aboyans, V. *et al.* (2012) Global and regional mortality from 235 causes of death for 20 age groups in 1990 and 2010: a systematic analysis for the Global Burden of Disease Study 2010, *Lancet*, 380, 2095–128.

Maddux, J. and Rogers, R. (1983) Protection motivation and self-efficacy: a revised theory of fear appeals and attitude change, *Journal of Experimental Social Psychology*, 19, 469–79.

Maibach, E., Abroms, L. and Marosits, M. (2007) Communication and marketing as tools to cultivate the public's health: a proposed 'people and places' framework, *BMC Public Health*, 7, 88.

Marlatt, G. and George, W. (1984) Relapse prevention: introduction and overview of the model, *British Journal of Addiction*, 79, 261–73.

McEachan, R.R.C., Conner, M., Taylor, N.J. and Lawton, R.J. (2011) Prospective prediction of health-related behaviours with the Theory of Planned Behaviour: a meta-analysis, *Health Psychology Review*, 5, 97–144.

McKenzie, J.E., French, S.D., O'Connor, D.A., Grimshaw, J.M., Mortimer, D., Michie, S. *et al.* (2008) IMPLEmenting a clinical practice guideline for acute low back pain evidence-based manageMENT in general practice (IMPLEMENT): cluster randomised controlled trial study protocol, *Implementation Science*, 3, 11.

Michie, S. and Abraham, C. (2004) Interventions to change health behaviours: evidence-based or evidence-inspired? *Psychology and Health*, 19, 29–49.

Michie, S. and Johnston, M. (2012) Theories and techniques of behaviour change: developing a cumulative science of behaviour change, *Health Psychology Review*, 6, 1–6.

Michie, S. and Johnston, M. (2013) Behaviour change techniques, in M. Gellman and R.J. Turner (eds.) *Encyclopeadia of Behavioural Medicine* (pp. 182–7). London: Springer.

Michie, S. and Prestwich, A. (2010) Are interventions theory-based? Development of a theory coding scheme, *Health Psychology*, 29, 1–8.

Michie, S., Abraham, C., Eccles, M., Francis, J., Hardeman, W. and Johnston, M. (2011a) Strengthening evaluation and implementation by specifying components of behaviour change interventions: a study protocol, *Implementation Science*, 6, 10.

Michie, S., Abraham, C., Whittington, C., McAteer, J. and Gupta, S. (2009a) Effective techniques in healthy eating and physical activity interventions: a meta-regression, *Health Psychology*, 28, 690–701.

Michie, S., Ashford, S., Sniehotta, F., Dombrowski, S., Bishop, A. and French, D. (2011b) A refined taxonomy of behaviour change techniques to help people change their physical activity and healthy eating behaviours: the CALO-RE taxonomy, *Psychology and Health*, 26, 1479–98.

Michie, S., Atkins, L. and West, R. (2014a) *The Behaviour Change Wheel: A Guide to Designing Interventions*. London: Silverback Publishing.

Michie, S., Campbell, R., Brown, J., West, R. and Gainforth, H. (2014b) *ABC of Theories of Behaviour Change*. London: Silverback Publishing.

Michie, S., Churchill, S. and West, R. (2011c) Identifying evidence-based competences required to deliver behavioural support for smoking cessation, *Annals of Behavioral Medicine*, 41, 59–70.

Michie, S., Fixsen, D., Grimshaw, J. and Eccles, M. (2009b) Specifying and reporting complex behaviour change interventions: the need for a scientific method, *Implementation Science*, 4, 40.

Michie, S., Free, C. and West, R. (2012a) Characterising the 'Txt2Stop' smoking cessation text messaging intervention in terms of behaviour change techniques, *Journal of Smoking Cessation*, 7, 55–60.

Michie, S., Hardeman, W., Fanshawe, T., Toby Prevost, A., Taylor, L. and Kinmonth, A. (2008a) Investigating theoretical explanations for behaviour change: the case study of ProActive, *Psychology and Health*, 23, 25–39.

Michie, S., Hyder, N., Walia, A. and West, R. (2011d) Development of a taxonomy of behaviour change techniques used in individual behavioural support for smoking cessation, *Addictive Behaviors*, 36, 315–19.

Michie, S., Jochelson, K., Markham, W. and Bridle, C. (2009c) Low-income groups and behaviour change interventions: a review of intervention content, effectiveness and theoretical frameworks, *Journal of Epidemiology and Community Health*, 63, 610–22.

Michie, S., Johnson, B. and Johnston, M. (2014c) Advancing cumulative evidence on behaviour change techniques and interventions, *Health Psychology Review* [DOI: 10.1080/17437199.2014.912538].

Michie, S., Johnston, M., Abraham, C., Lawton, R., Parker, D. and Walker, A. (2005) Making psychological theory useful for implementing evidence based practice: a consensus approach, *Quality and Safety in Health Care*, 14, 26–33.

Michie, S., Johnston, M., Francis, J., Hardeman, W. and Eccles, M. (2008b) From theory to intervention: mapping theoretically derived behavioural determinants to behaviour change techniques, *Applied Psychology*, 57, 660–80.

Michie, S., Johnston, M., Rothman, A., Kelly, M. and de Bruin, M. (2014d) *Developing Methodology for Designing and Evaluating Theory-based Complex Interventions: An Ontology for Linking Behaviour Change Techniques to Theory*. Cambridge: Medical Research Council.

Michie, S., Pilling, S., Garety, P., Whitty, P., Eccles, M., Johnston, M. *et al.* (2007a) Difficulties implementing a mental health guideline: an exploratory investigation using psychological theory, *Implementation Science*, 2, 1–8.

Michie, S., Richardson, M., Johnston, M., Abraham, C., Francis, J., Hardeman, W. *et al.* (2013) The behavior change technique taxonomy (v1) of 93 hierarchically clustered techniques: building an international consensus for the reporting of behavior change interventions, *Annals of Behavioral Medicine*, 46, 81–95.

Michie, S., Rothman, A. and Sheeran, P. (2007b) Advancing the science of behaviour change, *Psychology and Health*, 22, 249–53.

Michie, S., Sheals, K. and West, R. (submitted a) Assessing the effectiveness of behaviour change techniques: proposed methods of evidence synthesis. Manuscript submitted for publication.

Michie, S., van Stralen, M. and West, R. (2011e) The behaviour change wheel: a new method for characterising and designing behaviour change interventions, *Implementation Science*, 6, 42.

Michie, S., Whittington, C., Hamoudi, S., Zarnani, F., Tober, G. and West, R. (2012b) Identification of behaviour change techniques to reduce excessive alcohol consumption, *Addiction*, 107, 1431–40.

Michie, S., Wood, C., Johnston, M., Abraham, C., Francis, J. and Hardeman, W. (submitted b) Behaviour change techniques: the devlelopment and evaluation of a taxonomic method for reporting and describing behaviour change interventions, *Health Technology Assessment*.

Mischel, W. (2011) Self-control theory, in P.A.M. Van Lange, A.W. Kruglanski and E.T. Higgins (eds.) *Handbook of Theories of Social Psychology* (pp. 1–22). Thousand Oaks, CA: Sage.

Moher, D., Schulz, K. and Altman, D. (2003) The CONSORT statement: revised recommendations for improving the quality of reports of parallel-group randomised trials, *Clinical Oral Investigations*, 7, 2–7.

Mokdad, A.H., Marks, J.S., Stroup, D.F. and Gerberding, J.L. (2004) Actual causes of death in the United States, 2000, *Journal of the American Medical Association*, 291, 1238–45.

Morton, K., Beauchamp, M., Prothero, A., Joyce, L., Saunders, L., Spencer-Bowdage, S. *et al.* (2014) The effectiveness of motivational interviewing for health behaviour change in primary care settings: a systematic review, *Health Psychology Review* [DOI: 10.1080/17437199.2014.882006].

Murray, C., Richards, M., Newton, J., Fenton, K., Anderson, H., Atkinson, C. *et al.* (2013) UK health performance: findings of the Global Burden of Disease Study 2010, *Lancet*, 381, 997–1020.

Murray, R., Szatkowski, L. and Ussher, M. (2013) Evaluation of a refined, nationally disseminated self-help intervention for smoking cessation ('quit kit-2'), *Nicotine and Tobacco Research*, 15, 1365–71.

Newby, K., French, D., Brown, K. and Lecky, D. (2013) Increasing young adults' condom use intentions and behaviour through changing chlamydia risk and coping appraisals: study protocol for a cluster randomised controlled trial of efficacy, *BMC Public Health*, 13, 528.

NICE (2007) *Behaviour Change: The Principles for Effective Interventions* (PH6) [http://www.nice.org.uk/guidance/ph6/resources/guidance-behaviour-change-the-principles-for-effective-interventions-pdf].

Noar, S., Benac, C. and Harris, M. (2007) Does tailoring matter? Meta-analytic review of tailored print health behavior change interventions, *Psychological Bulletin*, 133, 673–93.

Norman, P., Conner, M. and Bell, R. (2000) The theory of planned behaviour and exercise: evidence for the moderating role of past behaviour, *British Journal of Health Psychology*, 5, 249–61.

Nuffield Council (2007) *Public Health: Ethical Issues – A Guide to the Report* [http://nuffieldbioethics.org/wp-content/uploads/2014/07/Public-Health-short-guide.pdf].

Nutbeam, D., Harris, E. and Wise, W. (2010) *Theory in a Nutshell: A Practical Guide to Health Promotion Theories*. Maidenhead: McGraw-Hill.

Ogden, J. (2003) Some problems with social cognition models: a pragmatic and conceptual analysis, *Health Psychology*, 22, 424–8.

Olander, F. and Thorgersen, J. (1995) Understanding of consumer behaviour as a prerequisute for environmental protection, *Journal of Consumer Policy*, 18, 345–85.

Olander, E., Fletcher, H., Williams, S., Atkinson, L., Turner, A. and French, D. (2013) What are the most effective techniques in changing obese individuals' physical activity self-efficacy and behaviour: a systematic review and meta-analysis, *International Journal of Behavioral Nutrition and Physical Activity*, 10, 29.

Painter, J., Borba, C., Hynes, M., Mays, D. and Glanz, K. (2008) The use of theory in health behavior research from 2000 to 2005: a systematic review, *Annals of Behavioral Medicine*, 35, 358–62.

Patey, A., Islam, R., Francis, J., Bryson, G. and Grimshaw, J. (2012) Anesthesiologists' and surgeons' perceptions about routine pre-operative testing in low-risk patients: application of the Theoretical Domains Framework (TDF) to identify factors that influence physicians' decisions to order pre-operative tests, *Implementation Science*, 7, 52.

Perdue, W., Mensah, G., Goodman, R. and Moulton, A. (2005) A legal framework for preventing cardiovascular diseases, *American Journal of Preventive Medicine*, 29, 139–45.

Pérez-Rodrigo, C., Wind, M., Hildonen, C., Bjelland, M., Aranceta, J., Klepp, K. *et al.* (2005) The Pro Children intervention: applying the intervention mapping protocol to develop a school-based fruit and vegetable promotion programme, *Annals of Nutrition and Metabolism*, 49, 267–77.

Peters, G.-J.Y., de Bruin, M. and Crutzen, R. (2013) Everything should be as simple as possible, but no simpler: towards a protocol for accumulating evidence regarding the active content of health behaviour change interventions, *Health Psychology Review* [DOI: 10.1080/17437199.2013.848409].

Po'e, E., Heerman, W., Mistry, R. and Barkin, S. (2013) Growing Right Onto Wellness (GROW): a family-centered, community-based obesity prevention randomized controlled trial for preschool child–parent pairs, *Contemporary Clinical Trials*, 36, 436–49.

Population Services International (2004) *PSI Behaviour Change Framework 'Bubbles'*. Washinton, DC: PSI.

Prestwich, A., Conner, M., Lawton, R., Bailey, W., Litman, J. and Molyneaux, V. (2005) Individual and collaborative implementation intentions and the promotion of breast self-examination, *Psychology and Health*, 20, 743–60.

Prestwich, A., Conner, M., Lawton, R., Ward, J., Ayres, K. and McEachan, R. (2014a) Partner- and planning-based interventions to reduce fat consumption: randomized controlled trial, *British Journal of Health Psychology*, 19, 132–48.

Prestwich, A., Kellar, I., Parker, R., MacRae, S., Learmonth, M., Sykes, B. *et al.* (2014b) How can self-efficacy be increased? Meta-analysis of dietary interventions, *Health Psychology Review*, 8, 270–85.

Prestwich, A., Sniehotta, F., Whittington, C., Dombrowski, S., Rogers, L. and Michie, S. (2014c) Does theory influence the effectiveness of health behavior interventions? Meta-analysis, *Health Psychology*, 35, 465–74.

Prochaska, J. and Velicer, W. (1997) The transtheoretical model of health behavior change, *American Journal of Health Promotion*, 12, 38–48.

Prochaska, J., DiClemente, C. and Norcross, J. (1992) In search of how people change: applications to addictive behaviors, *American Psychologist*, 47, 1102–14.

Quinn, F., Johnston, M. and Johnston, D.W. (2013) Testing an integrated behavioural and biomedical model of disability in *N*-of-1 studies with chronic pain, *Psychology and Health*, 28, 1391–1406.

Robinson, E., Higgs, S., Daley, A., Jolly, K., Lycett, D., Lewis, A. *et al.* (2013) Development and feasibility testing of a smart phone based attentive eating intervention, *BMC Public Health*, 13, 639.

Robinson, J., Gaber, R., Hultgren, B., Eilers, S., Blatt, H., Stapleton, J. *et al.* (2014) Skin self-examination education for early detection of melanoma: a randomized controlled trial of Internet, workbook, and in-person interventions, *Journal of Medical Internet Research*, 16 (1), e7.

Roe, L., Hunt, P., Bradshaw, H. and Rayner, M. (2007) *Health Promotion Interventions to Promote Healthy Eating in the General Population: A Review*. Abingdon-on-Thames: Health Education Authority.

Rothman, A.J. (2004) 'Is there nothing more practical than a good theory?' Why innovations and advances in health behavior change will arise if interventions are used to test and refine theory, *International Journal of Behavioral Nutrition and Physical Activity*, 1, 11.

Rutter, D. and Quine, L. (2002) Social cognition models and changing health behaviours, in D. Rutter and L. Quine (eds.) *Changing Health Behaviour: Intervention and Research with Social Cognition Models* (pp. 1–27). Buckingham: Open University Press.

Sallis, A., Birkin, R. and Munir, F. (2010) Working towards a 'fit note': an experimental vignette survey of GPs, *British Journal of General Practice*, 60, 245–50.

Sarafino, E.P. (2001) *Behavior Modification: Principles of Behaviour Change* (2nd edn.). Boston, MA: McGraw Hill.

Sather, C., Lagges, A., Cupp, H., Brubaker, J., LaMothe, V., Marshall, A. *et al.* (2011) BMI screening starting between ages 2–5 years impacts obesity and related morbidity better than current recommendations, *Gastroenterology*, 140 (suppl. 1), S-618.

Schwarzer, R. (2001) Social-cognitive factors in changing health-related behaviors, *Current Directions in Psychological Science*, 10, 47–51.

Schwarzer, R., Antoniuk, A. and Gholami, M. (2015) A brief intervention changing oral self-care, self-efficacy, and self-monitoring, *British Journal of Health Psychology*, 20: 56–67.

Sherman, W.M. (1990) *Behavior Modification*. New York: Harper.

Skinner, B.F. (1938) *Behavior of Organisms*. New York: Appleton-Century-Croft.

Smoak, N.D., Scott-Sheldon, L.A.J., Johnson, BT; Carey, M.P. and the SHARP Research Team (2006) Sexual risk reduction interventions do not inadvertently increase the overall frequency of sexual behavior: a meta-analysis of 174 studies with 116,735 participants, *Journal of Acquired Immune Deficiency Syndromes*, 41, 374–84.

Sniehotta, F., Presseau, J., Hobbs, N. and Araujo-Soares, V. (2012) Testing self-regulation interventions to increase walking using factorial randomized *N*-of-1 trials, *Health Psychology*, 31, 733–7.

Stavri, Z. and Beard, E. (2009) Applying a taxonomy of behaviour change techniques to smoking cessation: are published descriptions adequate? *Psychology and Health*, 24, 370–5.

Stavri, Z. and Michie, S. (2012) Classification systems in behavioural science: current systems and lessons from the natural, medical and social sciences, *Health Psychology Review*, 6, 113–40.

Stephenson, J., Imrie, J. and Sutton, S. (2000) Rigorous trials of sexual behaviour interventions in STD/HIV prevention: what can we learn from them? *Aids*, 14 (suppl. 3), S115–S124.

Stern, R. (1978) *Behavioural Techniques*. London: Academic Press.

Stone, S., Fuller, C., Savage, J., Cookson, B., Hayward, A., Cooper, B. *et al.* (2012) Evaluation of the national Cleanyourhands campaign to reduce *Staphylococcus aureus* bacteraemia and *Clostridium difficile* infection in hospitals in England and Wales by improved hand hygiene: four year, prospective, ecological, interrupted time series study, *British Medical Journal*, 344, e3005.

Strecher, V.J., McClure, J.B., Alexander, G.L., Chakraborty, B., Nair, V.N., Konkel, J.M. *et al.* (2008) Web-based smoking-cessation programs: results of a randomized trial, *American Journal of Preventive Medicine*, 34, 373–81.

Suresh, R., Jones, K., Newton, J. and Asimakopoulou, K. (2012) An exploratory study into whether self-monitoring improves adherence to daily flossing among dental patients, *Journal of Public Health Dentistry*, 72, 1–7.

Sutton, S. (1998) Predicting and explaining intentions and behavior: how well are we doing? *Journal of Applied Social Psychology*, 28, 1317–38.

Swann, C., Bowe, K., McCormick, G. and Kosmin, M. (2003) *Teenage Pregnancy and Parenthood: A Review of Reviews*. London: Health Development Agency.

Taylor, N., Conner, M. and Lawton, R. (2012) The impact of theory on the effectiveness of worksite physical activity interventions: a meta-analysis and meta-regression, *Health Psychology Review*, 6, 33–73.

Tortolero, S., Markham, C., Parcel, G., Peters, R., Escobar-Chaves, S., Basen-Engquist, K. *et al.* (2005) Using intervention mapping to adapt an effective HIV, sexually transmitted disease, and pregnancy prevention program for high-risk minority youth, *Health Promotion Practice*, 6, 286–98.

Treweek, S., Ricketts, I., Francis, J., Eccles, M., Bonetti, D., Pitts, N. *et al.* (2011) Developing and evaluating interventions to reduce inappropriate prescribing by general practitioners of antibiotics for upper respiratory tract infections: a randomised controlled trial to compare paper-based and web-based modelling experiments, *Implementation Science*, 6, 16.

Van Osch, L., Beenackers, M., Reubsaet, A., Lechner, L., Candel, M. and De Vries, H. (2009) Action planning as predictor of health protective and health risk behavior: an investigation of fruit and snack consumption, *International Journal of Behavioral Nutrition and Physical Activity*, 6, 69.

Vlek, C. (2000) Essential psychology for environmental policy making, *International Journal of Psychology*, 35, 153–67.

Walter, I., Nutley, S. and Davies, H. (2003) Developing a taxonomy of interventions used to increase the impact of research. Unpublished discussion paper, Research Unit for Research Utilisation, Department of Management, University of St. Andrews.

Webb, T., Joseph, J., Yardley, L. and Michie, S. (2010) Using the internet to promote health behavior change: a systematic review and meta-analysis of the impact of theoretical basis, use of behavior change techniques, and mode of delivery on efficacy, *Journal of Medical Internet Research*, 12 (1), e4.

Weber Cullen, K., Bartholomew, K., Parcel, G. and Kok, G. (1998) Intervention mapping: use of theory and data in the development of a fruit and vegetable nutrition program for girl scouts, *Journal of Nutrition Education*, 30, 188–95.

West, R. (2006) Tobacco control: present and future, *British Medical Bulletin*, 77/78, 123–36.

West, R. and Brown, J. (2013) *Theory of Addiction* (2nd edn.). London: Wiley-Blackwell.

West, R. and Michie, S. (2013) Carbon monoxide verified 4-week quit rates in the English Stop Smoking Services before versus after establishment of the National Centre for Smoking Cessation and Training, *Smoking in Britain*, 1, 3.

West, R., Evans, A. and Michie, S. (2011) Behavior change techniques used in group-based behavioral support by the English stop-smoking services and preliminary assessment of association with short-term quit outcomes, *Nicotine and Tobacco Research*, 13, 1316–20.

West, R., Walia, A., Hyder, N., Shahab, L. and Michie, S. (2010) Behavior change techniques used by the English Stop Smoking Services and their associations with short-term quit outcomes, *Nicotine and Tobacco Research*, 12, 742–47.

White, P. (2010) PETeR: A universal model for health interventions.

Wood, C.E., Richardson, M., Johnston, M., Abraham, C., Francis, J., Hardeman, W. *et al.* (2014) Applying the behaviour change technique (BCT) taxonomy v1: a study of coder training, *Translational Behavioral Medicine: Research, Policy and Practice* [DOI: 10.1007/s13142-014-0290-z].

Yardley, L., Miller, S., Schlotz, W. and Little, P. (2011) Evaluation of a web-based intervention to promote hand hygiene: exploratory randomized controlled trial, *Journal of Medical Internet Research*, 13 (4), e107.

Chapter 12

Predicting and changing health behaviour: future directions

Paul Norman and Mark Conner

1 Introduction

Despite an extensive research base on the application of social cognition models (SCMs) to the prediction of health behaviour, there are a range of issues for future work to address. In Section 2, we highlight seven issues focusing on: (1) the impact of personality traits on health behaviour, (2) the assessment of risk perceptions, (3) the utility of other SCMs, (4) the impact of past behaviour/habit, (5) automatic influences on health behaviour, (6) the maintenance of health behaviour, and (7) critiques of the use of SCMs to predict health behaviour. Recently, there has also been a growing interest in the development of interventions based on the main SCMs to change health behaviour (see Rutter and Quine 2002). In Section 3, we consider six issues relating to: (1) the practicality of SCMs for developing health behaviour interventions, (2) the impact of changes in cognitions on changes in health behaviour, (3) habit-based interventions, (4) self-affirmation interventions, (5) integrating work on behaviour change techniques and theory-based interventions, and (6) evaluating theory-based health behaviour interventions.

2 Predicting health behaviour: future directions

2.1 The impact of personality traits on health behaviour

There is a growing literature linking various individual difference variables to health behaviours, including executive control function (Hall and Fong 2007), action versus state orientation (Kuhl 1985), and assessment versus locomotion aspects of self-regulation (Kruglanski *et al.* 2000). This section focuses on the category of individual difference variables receiving the most attention in the literature, namely, personality traits. Research demonstrating mediated, direct, and moderating effects of personality traits in predicting health behaviour is reviewed.

The extensive literature linking personality traits to health outcomes (see Marshall *et al.* 1994) has recently been expanded to examine the impact of these traits on health behaviour (Hampson 2012). To date, most of this research has focused on the influence of the 'big five' personality traits (i.e. neuroticism, extraversion, conscientiousness, openness, and agreeableness) on health behaviour (e.g. Siegler *et al.* 1995; Schwartz *et al.* 1999; Conner and Abraham 2001). Such personality traits are considered as distal predictors in the main SCMs that shape beliefs about the behaviour in question, which, in turn, determine intention and behaviour. Thus, the impact of personality traits should be mediated by social cognitive variables, and a number of studies support this. For example, Siegler *et al.* (1995) found that the effect of conscientiousness on mammography attendance was mediated by knowledge of breast cancer and the perceived costs of seeking mammography. Other research has reported mediated and direct effects for personality traits when predicting health behaviour. For example, extraversion has been shown to explain additional variance in exercise behaviour, over and above that explained by the theory of planned behaviour (e.g. Courneya *et al.* 1999). Similarly, Conner and Abraham (2001) reported that conscientiousness had a direct effect on exercise behaviour, whereas extraversion and neuroticism only had indirect effects, and openness and agreeableness had no effects.

Conscientiousness and extraversion have been a particular focus of research in this area. Conscientiousness refers to the ability to control one's behaviour and to complete tasks. Those with high conscientiousness scores are seen to be more organized, careful, dependable, self-disciplined, and achievement-oriented than those low in conscientiousness (McCrae and Costa 1987). Friedman *et al.* (1995) showed that conscientious children were less likely to become heavy smokers and drinkers and this partly accounted for them living longer. Conscientious individuals tend to engage in greater physical activity, less excessive alcohol use, less drug use, less unhealthy eating, less risky sex (Hagger-Johnson and Shickle 2010), less tobacco use (Hampson *et al.* 2000, 2006), and show better adherence to medical regimens (O'Cleirigh *et al.* 2007). A comprehensive meta-analysis conducted by Bogg and Roberts (2004) showed conscientiousness to be positively related to a range of protective health behaviours (e.g. exercise) and negatively related to a range of risky health behaviours (e.g. smoking).

High conscientiousness scores have also been associated with greater use of problem-focused, positive reappraisal, and support-seeking coping strategies (Watson and Hubbard 1996), and less frequent use of escape avoidance and self-blame coping strategies (O'Brien and DeLongis 1996). Such characteristics and activities are likely to facilitate the performance of aversive or difficult health behaviours that individuals are motivated to perform. Conscientiousness should therefore moderate the relationship between health beliefs and health behaviour. For example, in a retrospective study, Schwartz *et al.* (1999) found that conscientiousness moderated the relationship between breast cancer-related distress and mammography uptake such that under high levels of distress, those with high conscientiousness scores were more likely to have attended mammography screening than those with low conscientiousness scores. Conscientiousness scores had no differential impact under low levels of distress. In relation to exercise, Rhodes *et al.* (2002, 2005) reported conscientiousness to significantly moderate the intention–exercise behaviour relationship, with higher levels of conscientiousness associated with stronger intention–behaviour relationships. Conner *et al.* (2007b) reported a similar moderation effect, but only for exercise completed in non-usual weeks. In relation to smoking initiation, Conner *et al.* (2009) showed intentions to be stronger predictors of resisting smoking for an adolescent sample with higher versus lower levels of conscientiousness.

The moderating role of extraversion on intention–behaviour relations has also been examined in a number of studies on exercise behaviour. Extraverts are seen to have an increased tendency to seek out situations in which opportunities to be active present themselves (Eysenck 1981). Individuals with high extraversion scores may be more likely to encounter opportunities to act on their intentions to exercise, which will therefore increase the strength of intention–behaviour relations. Consistent with this position, extraversion has been found to moderate the relationship between exercise intentions and behaviour (e.g. Rhodes *et al.* 2003). Interestingly, other studies have shown that the direct effect of extraversion on exercise behaviour is primarily due to the activity facet of extraversion, rather than the positive affect or sociability facets (e.g. Rhodes and Courneya 2003). According to McCrae and Costa (1990), the activity facet describes an individual's tendency to be energetic, busy, and forceful. With respect to exercise behaviour, it is possible that this facet may also be responsible for the moderating role of extraversion on intention–behaviour relations.

In conclusion, Abraham *et al.* (2000) have noted that the literatures on the links between personality and health behaviour, and between SCMs and health behaviour have developed in parallel with little cross-referencing. Personality and social cognitive influences may therefore be usefully integrated into a single account of health behaviour (see also Bermudez 1999; Ferguson 2013). In such an account, personality traits are likely to be distal predictors of health behaviour, their impact being mediated by the variables contained in current SCMs. However, given the direct effects of conscientiousness and extraversion on health behaviour reported in some studies, it is possible that individual differences may add to the prediction of health behaviour. In addition, personality traits may also be important moderators of intention–behaviour relations for certain health behaviours and populations.

2.2 The assessment of risk perceptions

Risk perceptions are central to most SCMs that have been applied to the prediction of health behaviour. For example, models that have been developed specifically to predict health behaviour – the health action process approach (HAPA), health belief model (HBM), and protection motivation theory (PMT) – all contain constructs that explicitly focus on risk perceptions. In addition, other models such as the theory of planned behaviour (TPB) and social cognitive theory (SCT) focus on perceptions of risk, indirectly, via other constructs, such as behavioural beliefs in the TPB and outcome expectancies in SCT. However, despite the central role afforded to risk perceptions in many SCMs, research evidence for a link between risk perceptions and health behaviour is weak. For example, in a meta-analysis of PMT studies, Milne *et al.* (2000) reported that perceived vulnerability had relatively weak correlations with intention ($r = 0.16$), concurrent behaviour ($r = 0.13$), and future behaviour ($r = 0.12$).

There are a number of potential reasons for these weak effects. First, in cross-sectional studies, it is not possible to determine whether risk perceptions drive behaviour in line with SCMs (e.g. individuals who believe they are at risk of HIV infection are more likely to use condoms), or whether risk perceptions are inferred from current behaviour (e.g. individuals who use condoms infer that they are at low risk of HIV infection) (Weinstein and Nicolich 1993). In the former case, a positive correlation is expected between perceived risk and behaviour, whereas in the latter case, a negative correlation is expected. Teasing apart these two rival positions in cross-sectional studies is difficult. The obtained correlation between perceived risk and concurrent behaviour is a function of the relative sizes of these two sub-samples and is therefore likely to be attenuated. A similar argument can be made when considering the relationship between perceived risk and intention.

Second, the weak effects typically found for perceived risk may also be due to the way in which risk perceptions are measured. Studies typically ask respondents to estimate the likelihood that an event will occur in the future (e.g. 'How likely is it that you will become infected with the AIDS virus in the next two years?'). As Van der Velde and Hooykaas (1996) note, such questions provide unconditional risk estimates as respondents can take into account an unspecified range of factors, including their current behaviour, when providing a risk estimate. In contrast, conditional risk items ask respondents to estimate the likelihood that an event will occur in the future if no preventive action is taken (e.g. 'How likely is it that you will become infected with the AIDS virus in the next two years, if you don't use condoms?'). Van der Velde and Hooykaas (1996) reported that an unconditional measure of perceived risk resulted in stronger, and theoretically consistent, correlations with condom use intentions.

Third, the typically weak relationship between perceived risk and health-protective behaviour might be due to some people underestimating their risk status. In particular, research has shown that most people tend to believe that they are at less risk than their peers. This tendency is referred to as 'unrealistic optimism' (Weinstein and Klein 1996; Shepperd *et al.* 2013) and has been found in relation to a wide range of health problems, including diabetes (Weinstein 1984), high blood pressure (Weinstein 1987), HIV (Gold and Aucote 2003), breast cancer (Skinner *et al.* 1998), liver disease, heart disease, and stroke (Harris and Middleton 1994). Weinstein (1983) explains the existence of such optimistic biases by arguing that individuals show selective focus when making comparative risk judgements, for example focusing primarily on their risk-reducing rather than their risk-increasing behaviour. In addition, this selective focus is compounded by egocentrism such that individuals tend to ignore others' risk-reducing behaviour when making comparative risk judgements. Moreover, there is some evidence that unrealistic optimism may inhibit the performance of precautionary behaviours (see Helweg-Larsen and Shepperd 2001). For example, Dillard *et al.* (2006) found that smokers with higher levels of unrealistic optimism had lower intentions to quit smoking.

As the above discussion highlights, there are various reasons for the weak relationship between perceived risk and health behaviour. Risk perceptions are unlikely to have a strong, proximal impact on behaviour. Instead, perceived risk may be considered to be a distal predictor that influences behaviour through other social cognitive variables. For example, Schwarzer (1992) argues that perceptions of risk may stimulate people to start thinking about the benefits of engaging in a health-protective behaviour and their ability to perform the behaviour, which, in turn, determine goal intentions. Relatedly, in the precaution adoption process model (PAPM; Weinstein 1988), risk perceptions are held to have their most important effects in the early stages of the precaution adoption process.

2.3 Other social cognition models

2.3.1 The theory of interpersonal behaviour

According to the theory of interpersonal behaviour (TIB; Triandis 1977, 1980), behaviour is a function of four factors: (a) intentions, (b) habits, (c) facilitating conditions, and (d) physiological arousal. Intentions here are defined as the self-instructions that individuals give themselves to behave in certain ways and are operationalized in a similar manner as in the theory of planned behaviour (TPB; Ajzen 1988). Triandis (1980: 204) also affords a predictive role to habits, which are 'situation–behavior sequences that are or have become automatic, so that they occur without self-instruction'. Triandis emphasizes the importance of a close correspondence between the situation, response (i.e. behaviour), and reinforcement in the development of habits. However, even when people have formed strong intentions or have developed strong habits, environmental constraints may be encountered that impede performance of the behaviour. As a result, facilitating conditions (low vs. high) are likely to have a strong influence on the likelihood of behaviour. Finally, the likelihood of performance of a behaviour is also dependent on the physiological arousal/state of the individual, which may vary from zero (i.e. asleep) to 1.00 (i.e. extremely aroused). In general, increasing levels of physiological arousal are likely to facilitate performance of a behaviour, although under very high levels of arousal behaviour may be impeded. Triandis (1980) proposes that probability of action is a function of intentions plus habits multiplied by physiological arousal and facilitating conditions. Most applications of the model do not assess physiological arousal (or assume it to be optimum) and simply test the additive effects of the remaining three factors (i.e. intention, habit, and facilitating conditions) on behaviour. Triandis further proposes that repeated behaviours are likely to be determined by habit, whereas novel behaviours are likely to be determined by intention. Thus, an interaction is hypothesized between intention and habit, such that intention should become a weaker predictor of behaviour as habit strength increases.

Intention is seen to be a linear function of three factors. The first is the consequences component, which focuses on the perceived consequences of performing the behaviour weighted by the value attached to these consequences. The second is the affective component, which focuses on the affective reactions that the individual associates with performing the behaviour (e.g. joy, displeasure, etc.). Third are social factors, which refer to the individual's internalization of his or her reference group's subjective culture as well as specific interpersonal agreements made with other group members. These factors determine the extent to which an individual perceives a behaviour to be appropriate, desirable, and morally correct.

The TIB has been successfully applied to a range of health behaviours, including exercise (e.g. Godin and Gionet 1991), mammography screening (e.g. Lauver *et al.* 2003a), cervical cancer screening (e.g. Seibold and Roper 1979), influenza vaccinations (e.g. Nowalk *et al.* 2004), and HIV-risk-related behaviours (e.g. Apostolopoulos *et al.* 2003). For example, Apostolopoulos *et al.* (2003) used the TIB to predict the sexual behaviour of American undergraduates on their spring-break vacation. Variables from the TIB were able to explain 75% of the variance in engaging in casual sex with social influences (i.e. having made a 'pact' to have causal sex), prior experience of casual sex, and facilitating factors (i.e. drinking prior to sexual activity and impulsivity) emerging as significant predictors. The TIB variables also explained 69% of the variance in engaging in unprotected sex with two facilitating factors (i.e. the (un)availability of condoms and impulsivity) emerging as significant predictors. A number of studies have tested the hypothesis, derived from the TIB, that habit should moderate intention–behaviour relations. Gardner (2014) reviewed 24 studies that had tested this hypothesis and found that 18 reported evidence that intention became a weaker predictor of behaviour as habit strength increased.

The TIB has been found to provide strong predictions of health behaviour and, as a result, should provide a sound basis for the development of effective interventions. However, to date, there have been few TIB-based intervention studies. Caron *et al.* (2004) reported an evaluation of the 'Protection Express Program' to encourage safer sexual behaviour among high school students in Canada. The programme draws upon the TIB (and TPB) and a teaching model based on the principles of social cognitive theory (Bandura 1986). The intervention was found to have significant impacts on all TIB and TPB variables at nine-month follow-up, although no differences were found between intervention and control schools in postponing sexual intercourse and consistent condom use. Lauver et al. (2003b) used the TIB to develop an intervention to increase mammography uptake in women who had not been screened in the previous 13 months. A tailored discussion with a nurse that focused on the women's beliefs, feelings, and perceived barriers about screening, as specified by the TIB, led to increased mammography uptake at (15–22 months) follow-up.

The TIB has a number of similarities with the TPB, which may explain its strong predictive validity. For example, the cognitive component, social norm component, and facilitating/impeding conditions parallel the attitude, subjective norm, and perceived behavioural control components of the TPB. In addition, both the TIB and the TPB (a) posit intention to be a key mediating variable between more distal predictor variables and behaviour, (b) state that external variables (e.g. age, gender, personality) should have their influence through the variables contained in the models, (c) emphasize the importance of measuring the predictor variables and behaviour at the same level of specificity in terms of action, target, context, and time, and (d) suggest that the relative weights of the predictor variables for both intention and behaviour should vary as a function of the population and behaviour under study.

The TIB also has a number of positive features. First, it explicitly distinguishes between cognitive and affective reactions towards performing a behaviour. Second, by focusing on group norms, roles, and interpersonal agreements, the social factors component of the TIB considers a wider range of normative influences than the subjective norm component of the TPB. Third, the TIB also focuses on moral considerations within the social factors component, which, again, some researchers have suggested should be added to the TPB (e.g. Manstead 2000). Fourth, and most importantly, the TIB includes habit as a predictor of future behaviour along with intention and facilitating conditions. Triandis (1977) equates habit with the frequency of past behaviour and this, in part, may explain the strong predictive validity of the model reported in many applications, given that past behaviour is often found to be the best predictor of future behaviour (Ouellette and Wood 1998). However, Gardner (2014) has questioned whether the frequency of past behaviour should be used as a measure of habit strength (see Section 2.4 for a fuller discussion).

A number of additional comments are worth making on the TIB as a model of health behaviour. First, intention is proposed to mediate the influence of more distal TIB predictors on behaviour. However, few TIB studies have tested this mediation hypothesis, instead either considering the impact of all the TIB variables on behaviour in a single regression equation (e.g. Apostolopoulos et al. 2003) or only examining the predictors of intention (e.g. Gagnon and Godin 2000). Second, many tests of the TIB have been performed in conjunction with other SCMs, including the theories of reasoned action (e.g. Boyd and Wandersman 1991) and planned behaviour (e.g. Belanger et al. 2002) and the transtheoretical model of change (e.g. Lauver et al. 2003). The TIB variables are typically found to explain additional variance in intention and behaviour. Third, there is a lack of consistency in the description and operationalization of the model in the literature. Thus, studies may list different constructs as being part of the TIB, employ different labels to describe the same constructs, and operationalize specific TIB variables in different ways. Fourth, the TIB does not explicitly include self-efficacy as a predictor.

Instead, Triandis (1980) argues that perceptions of the ease/difficultly of performing a behaviour are covered by the consequences component. However, this is an important omission given that self-efficacy is widely recognized as being one of the most powerful predictors of health behaviour (see Luszczynska and Schwarzer, Chapter 7 this volume). Finally, further experimental/intervention work is required both to test the structure of the model and to aid the design of effective health behaviour interventions.

2.3.2 Temporal self-regulation theory

Hall and Fong (2007) proposed temporal self-regulation theory (TST) as a new, comprehensive model of the biological, cognitive, and social influences on health behaviour. According to TST, intention to engage in a health behaviour is determined by the perceived probability that performing the behaviour will lead to certain outcomes (i.e. connectedness beliefs) weighted by both the value of the outcomes and their perceived closeness in time (i.e. temporal valuations). Intention, in turn, predicts future behaviour. However, the strength of this relationship is moderated by behavioural pre-potency and self-regulatory capacity. Behavioural pre-potency encompasses the influence of internal biological drives (e.g. hunger, thirst), salient environmental cues, and the frequency of past behaviour. As behavioural pre-potency increases, the intention–behaviour relationship should become weaker. Self-regulatory capacity encompasses state- and trait-like factors (e.g. executive function, self-control) that influence an individual's ability to regulate their behaviour. As self-regulatory capacity increases, the intention–behaviour relationship should become stronger. Both behavioural pre-potency and self-regulatory capacity are also hypothesized to have direct, positive effects on behaviour. According to TST, the predictive strength of intention, behavioural pre-potency, and self-regulatory capacity may vary according to temporal contingencies in the social and physical environment. For example, repeated health behaviours performed in supportive contexts should be primarily predicted by behavioural pre-potency and secondarily by intention and self-regulatory capacity, whereas repeated health behaviours performed in non-supportive contexts should be jointly determined by intention, behavioural pre-potency, and self-regulatory capacity. Finally, TST proposes feedback loops between behavioural performance and connectedness beliefs, temporal valuations, behavioural pre-potency, and self-regulatory capacity. Thus, prior performance of a behaviour may provide information relating perceived links between the behaviour and various outcomes as well as the perceived closeness of the outcomes in time; repeated performance of a behaviour may also lead to habitual responses that will increase behavioural pre-potency; and some health behaviours, such as exercise, may have positive effects on cognitive function, thereby increasing self-regulatory capacity (Hillman *et al.* 2006).

To date, there have been few applications of TST, although extensive evidence exists for specific hypotheses derived from TST (see Hall and Fong 2007). For example, Booker and Mullan (2013) assessed intentions to pursue a healthy lifestyle, past performance of health behaviours (i.e. behavioural pre-potency), and three measures of self-regulatory capacity. Both intention and behavioural pre-potency, but not the measures of self-regulatory capacity, were significantly correlated with the number of health behaviours performed at one-week follow-up. Booker and Mullan (2013) also assessed perceived environmental triggers to determine whether participants considered their environments to be supportive or non-supportive. For those experiencing supportive environments, only behavioural pre-potency was a significant predictor of health behaviour at follow-up, in line with predictions. For those experiencing non-supportive environments, intention and self-regulatory capacity (i.e. planning and response inhibition) were predictive of health behaviour.

Several studies have focused specifically on whether measures of executive function explain additional variance in future behaviour, over and above that explained by intention, and moderate the strength of the intention–behaviour relationship. Various aspects of executive function have been assessed, including planning (Tower of London/Hanoi), inhibition control (Go/NoGo, Stroop), cognitive flexibility (Winconsin Card Sorting Task), and decision-making (Iowa Gambling Task). For example, Hall *et al.* (2008) found that scores on the Go/NoGo task (i.e. inhibition control) explained additional variance in both physical activity and dietary behaviour at one-week follow-up. Moreover, the Go/NoGo task moderated the strength of the intention–behaviour relationship for both behaviours such that stronger relationships were found as executive functioning increased in strength. However, subsequent research has failed to replicate these findings in relation to hygienic food handling (Fulham and Mullan 2011). Non-significant findings have also been reported for the Winconsin Card Sorting Task (Mullan *et al.* 2011; Allom *et al.* 2013) and for the Iowa Gambling Task (Allom *et al.* 2013). In contrast, measures of planning (Tower of London/Hanoi) have been found to explain addition variance in, and moderate intention–behaviour relations for, binge drinking and breakfast consumption (Wong and Mullan 2009; Mullan *et al.* 2011). However, non-significant results have been reported in relation to sunscreen use and sun-protection behaviour (Allom *et al.* 2013).

Temporal self-regulation theory has a number of novel features that point to its potential as a comprehensive SCM of health behaviour. First, TST acknowledges the importance of time perspective. As noted by Hall and Fong (2007), many health behaviours are characterized by long-term positive health benefits but short-term costs. In contrast, for many health-risk behaviours, the positive short-term benefits outweigh the long-term negative health consequences. Weighting outcome expectancies by temporal evaluations helps to explain why health-risk behaviours are often chosen over health-promoting behaviours. Second, TST acknowledges the intention–behaviour gap and identities two key factors that may serve to strengthen (i.e. self-regulatory capacity) or weaken (i.e. behavioural pre-potency) the intention–behaviour relationship. Third, by including past behaviour and environmental cues as factors that increase behavioural pre-potency, TST taps into recent work that has shown that behaviours performed frequently in stable contexts may lead to the development of habitual responses (see Section 2.4). Fourth, TST also draws on recent neuroscience work that highlights the importance of the prefrontal cortex and anterior cingulate for executive functioning, including behavioural self-regulation.

Despite the potential of TST, further methodological work is needed on the measurement of key components of the model (Hall and Fong 2010). Considering self-regulatory capacity, most tests of TST to date have employed measures that assess the output of the executive system (e.g. Go/NoGo task, Winconsin Card Sorting Task, Iowa Gambling Task). These tasks measure different facets of executive function (e.g. behavioural inhibition, planning, cognitive flexibility). Thus, more work is needed to identify which of these facets are most important for the prediction of different health behaviours. In addition, it is possible to assess the neurophysiological correlates of the operation of the executive system using a range of non-invasive brain imaging techniques. Functional magnetic resonance imaging (fMRI) provides high-resolution measurement of the blood flow correlates of brain activity changes but is relatively expensive and there are limitations on the types of experimental tasks that can be practically implemented in the MRI environment. Other techniques, such as electroencephalography (EEG) and functional near infrared spectroscopy (fNIRS), monitor changes in electrical activity and blood oxygenation respectively. These both provide less expensive and more practical solutions, although measurements are limited to cortical structures and spatial resolution is lower than for fMRI. Considering behavioural pre-potency, self-reported past behaviour is typically used as a proxy measure. However, methodological work is needed on the measurement of other facets of behavioural pre-potency, including the nature, quality, and salience of environmental cues as well as internal biological drives. Finally, further empirical work is needed to test the predictive utility of TST. In particular, studies that assess all components of the model (i.e. the predictors of intention as well as of behaviour) are required.

2.3.3 Control theory

The main SCMs covered in this book consider goal intentions as the key proximal determinant of behaviour. Aside from the health action process approach, these theories do not specify the processes that intervene between intention formation (i.e. goal-setting) and goal attainment (de Bruin *et al.* 2012). An important exception is control theory (Carver and Scheier 1982), which focuses on the processes intervening between goal-setting and goal attainment (for a review, see Inzlicht *et al.* 2014). Two key processes are distinguished: goal-monitoring and goal-striving. Monitoring of goal progress involves periodic evaluation of one's ongoing performance relative to a desired standard. Monitoring progress should promote goal attainment because it serves to identify discrepancies between the current state and the desired state, and thus enables individuals to recognize when goal-striving is required. Goal-striving is expending effort or exerting self-control in order to help bring behaviour or outcomes in line with the desired standard. For example, through monitoring their intake of calories, dieters can better decide whether they should avoid having an extra helping in order to meet their weight control goal. According to control theory, monitoring goal progress and then acting on discrepancies are the processes through which individuals move from goal-setting to goal attainment.

The majority of studies using control theory in relation to health behaviours focus on the impact of self-monitoring of goal progress and goal-striving on goal attainment. For example, de Bruin *et al.* (2012) reported that a self-report measure tapping both progress monitoring and responding to discrepancies was strongly associated with medication adherence ($r = 0.63$) and vigorous exercise ($r = 0.43$). This measure added to predictions of behaviour over and above measures of goal intentions and partially mediated the effect of intentions on behaviour.

Prompting the self-monitoring of goal progress and goal-striving has also been used to promote behaviour change in a number of studies. For example, in a review of interventions designed to promote healthy eating and physical activity, Michie *et al.* (2009) reported that 38% of studies used self-monitoring. Michie *et al.* (2009) reported that interventions combining progress monitoring with one of four other behaviour change techniques consistent with control theory (intention formation, specific goal-setting, feedback on performance, review of behavioural goals) was associated with larger effects on physical activity and dietary behaviour. Similar findings were reported in a systematic review of behavioural interventions for obese adults (Dombrowski *et al.* 2012). Harkin *et al.* (submitted), in the most comprehensive review of progress monitoring to date, reported progress monitoring to have a medium-sized effect on goal attainment.

The above findings emphasize the importance of progress monitoring as a key behavioural mechanism by which people strive to achieve goals. At the conceptual level, these findings suggest that models of behaviour positing a direct relationship between intentions and behaviour neglect a key volitional process – progress monitoring – that intervenes between goal-setting and goal attainment. It is notable that progress monitoring has a bigger impact on performance (Harkins *et al.* submitted) than do goal intentions (Webb and Sheeran 2006), suggesting that effective goal-striving requires that one not only decide upon an appropriate goal but also compare the relevant behaviour/outcomes to that standard on an ongoing basis. Monitoring goal progress serves to identify the discrepancy between the current and desired state and enables the person to decide how best to allocate effort among salient goals (Carver and Scheier 1982) and to decide when and how to exercise restraint or initiate corrective action. Many of the SCMs considered in this book might usefully add constructs such as monitoring goal progress and goal-striving.

2.4 The role of past behaviour and habit

A major shortcoming of the main SCMs is their inability to account fully for the influence of past behaviour on future behaviour. Past behaviour is often found to have a strong relationship with future behaviour that is not mediated by social cognitive variables. For example, the meta-analysis of McEachan *et al.* (2011) included 86 health-related TPB studies that reported past behaviour–behaviour relationships. Past behaviour was found to explain, on average, an additional 5.3% of the variance in future behaviour, after taking account of TPB variables. Similar findings have been noted in relation to other SCMs, although tests of the impact of past behaviour on future behaviour are less common than in TPB studies. For example, the HBM has been found to be unable to fully mediate the effect of past behaviour in relation to the uptake of flu immunizations (Cummings *et al.* 1979) and the performance of breast self-examination (Norman and Brain 2005). Direct effects for past behaviour have also been reported in PMT studies on binge drinking (Murgraff *et al.* 1999), exercise (Plotnikoff *et al.* 2009), safe sex behaviours (Aspinwall *et al.* 1991), breast self-examination (Hodgkins and Orbell 1998), and treatment adherence (Norman *et al.* 2003). Such findings have led to a call for past behaviour to be included in SCMs as an additional predictor variable (e.g. Bentler and Speckhart 1979). However, Ajzen (1987) has cautioned against such a move, pointing out that past behaviour has no explanatory value – one is unlikely to exercise tomorrow *because* one exercised yesterday. Instead, it is necessary to offer a theoretical account of the ways in which past behaviour may influence future behaviour, as has been provided by Ouellette and Wood (1998) in their review of past behaviour–future behaviour relations. They proposed that past behaviour may impact on future behaviour through one of two routes, depending on the frequency of the opportunity to perform the behaviour and the stability of the context in which the behaviour is performed.

First, for behaviours that are performed relatively infrequently in unstable contexts, past behaviour may provide individuals with information that shapes their beliefs about the behaviour, which, in turn, determine intention and future behaviour (i.e. a conscious response). For such behaviours, past behaviour affects future behaviour indirectly through its influence on beliefs and intention. Such an account is consistent with the structure of major SCMs. For example, Rogers (1983) sees prior experience (i.e. past behaviour) as an intrapersonal source of information that may initiate the cognitive processes outlined in PMT, while Bandura (1986) contends that personal (mastery) experience is an important source of self-efficacy.

The second way in which past behaviour may impact on future behaviour is through the formation of a habitual response. Thus, for behaviours that are performed relatively frequently in stable contexts, the impact of past behaviour may reflect the operation of habitual responses that do not require the mediation of intention. For such behaviours, intentions (and other social cognitive variables) may lose their predictive validity and past behaviour will have a direct effect on future behaviour. The idea behind this proposition is that the repeated execution of the same behaviour (i.e. response) in the same context is likely to lead to formation of a habitual response. As a result, the behaviour is performed automatically and efficiently with little effort or conscious awareness in response to relevant stimulus cues. The direct effect of past behaviour on future behaviour can therefore be interpreted in terms of the operation of habits that have been defined as 'learned sequences of acts that have become automatic responses to specific cues' (Verplanken and Aarts 1999: 104). (See also Gardner [2014] for a fuller discussion of the definition of habits in which automaticity is highlighted as the key component.)

Ouellette and Wood's (1998) analysis of past behaviour–future behaviour relations is important for two main reasons. First, it allows for the direct effect of past behaviour on future behaviour found in many studies to be interpreted in terms of the operation of habits, and second, it delineates the circumstances under which intention and past behaviour are expected to predict behaviour (i.e. frequency of opportunity/stability of context). In particular, for behaviours that are performed relatively infrequently in unstable contexts, intention should be the primary predictor of future behaviour (reflecting the operation of conscious responses), whereas for behaviours that are performed relatively frequently in stable contexts, past behaviour is expected to be the primary predictor of future behaviour (reflecting the operation of habitual responses). Ouellette and Wood (1998) conducted a meta-analysis to test these predictions in which behaviours were classified according to whether they had the opportunity to be performed frequently in stable environmental contexts or infrequently in unstable environmental contexts. When the joint effects of past behaviour and intention were assessed, past behaviour ($\beta = 0.45$) was found to be a stronger predictor than intention ($\beta = 0.27$) of frequent/stable behaviours, whereas intention ($\beta = 0.62$) was a stronger predictor than past behaviour ($\beta = 0.12$) of infrequent/unstable behaviours. These results are consistent with the idea that infrequent/unstable behaviours are primarily under the control of intentional processes, whereas frequent/stable behaviours are primarily under the control of habitual processes. However, as noted by Sheeran (2002), these findings should be treated with some caution given that the regression analyses were based on only eight studies of frequent/stable behaviours and six studies of infrequent/unstable behaviours.

In addition, care needs to taken when attributing residual variance to habit, even for frequent/stable behaviours, as the direct effect of past behaviour on future behaviour may simply indicate that a model is not sufficient and that additional, social cognitive predictors need to be considered. As Ajzen (1991) argues, assuming that the determinants of behaviour remain stable over time, the past behaviour–future behaviour correlation can be taken as an indication of the ceiling of a model's predictive validity. If a model contains all the important proximal determinants of a behaviour (i.e. is sufficient), then the addition of past behaviour in a regression analysis should not explain additional variance in future behaviour. Thus, when a direct effect is found between past behaviour and future behaviour, this may indicate that the model is not sufficient rather than the operation of habitual responses. Moreover, even when past behaviour is found to explain additional variance in future behaviour, part of this effect may be the result of shared method variance inasmuch as measures of past behaviour and future behaviour are likely to be more similar than measures of intention and future behaviour.

Ajzen (2002) has provided a more fundamental critique of Ouellette and Wood (1998). Ajzen (2002) notes that the habitual account of the direct effect of past behaviour on future behaviour is based on the premise that habitual responses are likely to form when behaviours are performed repeatedly in stable contexts. However, this explanation does not account for the residual impact of past behaviour that is often found for low-frequency behaviours such as attendance at health checks (e.g. Norman and Conner 1996). Furthermore, it is clear from Ouellette and Wood's (1998) study that intention is a significant predictor of both infrequent/unstable and frequent/stable behaviours, even in conjunction with past behaviour. Ajzen (2002) argues that for behaviours that are performed frequently, intentions themselves might be automatically activated by situational cues and used to guide behaviour without the need for conscious awareness or control. As Heckhausen and Beckmann (1990: 38) propose, 'intents resemble plans about how to act when predetermined cues or conditions occur. Once formed, however, the intents no longer require much conscious control. Instead, they are triggered as automatic or quasi-automatic operations.' In many ways, this conceptualization of well-formed intentions has parallels with the concept of implementation intentions (Gollwitzer 1993), which are seen to mimic habitual responses by linking an intended action to an environmental cue. Finally, Ajzen (2002) notes that inferring the existence of a habit from a strong past behaviour–future behaviour correlation and then using the concept to explain the existence of the strong correlation involves a circular argument. Instead, an independent measure of habit is required to be able to use habit as an explanation for the existence of strong past behaviour–future behaviour correlations. Using frequency of past behaviour as a measure of habit strength fails to capture all of the defining features of a habitual response. Habitual behaviours are performed frequently (i.e. have a history of repetition), but they are also performed automatically, efficiently, and with little effort or conscious awareness in response to stable environmental cues. In short, it is necessary to develop measures of habit strength that show discriminant validity with respect to frequency of past behaviour when attempting to provide an explanation for the strength of past behaviour–future behaviour relations. A number of measures of habit strength have been reported in the literature.

In line with Ouellette and Wood (1998), some studies have sought to measure habit strength by assessing behavioural frequency and the stability of the context in which the behaviour is performed. For example, Danner et al. (2008) assessed the frequency with which three behaviours (snacking, drinking milk, and drinking alcohol) had been performed in the past four weeks (on 9-point response scales) and the extent to which the time (of day), place (physical location), and situation (circumstances) were similar each time the behaviour was performed (on 9-point response scales). The behavioural frequency and context stability items were multiplied together to provide a measure of habit strength, which was found to predict subsequent behaviour and moderate intention–behaviour relations for two of the three behaviours in line with predictions. However, a key limitation of this measure of habit strength is that it assesses the factors that are likely to lead to the formation of habits, rather than habit strength itself.

Verplanken et al. (1994) developed a script-based, or response-frequency, measure of habit strength in which participants are presented with a series of habit-related situations and instructed to respond as quickly as possible with their behavioural choice. The number of times a participant responds with the same behavioural choice over different situations is taken as a measure of habit strength. This measure has been shown to moderate the intention–future behaviour relationship in relation to travel mode choice in line with predictions (Verplanken et al. 1998). However, such script-based measures of habit strength have a number of limitations. First, it is possible to question the extent to which habits are akin to behavioural scripts, which are knowledge structures that contain 'a standard sequence of events characterizing typical activities' (Abelson 1981: 715). Second, Ajzen (2002) has argued that it may be more appropriate to interpret the response-frequency measure of habit strength as a generalized measure of intention. Third, the measure is restricted to choice behaviours that are executed in different contexts, which goes against the importance that is afforded to the stability of the environmental context in the formation of habits. Fourth, the development of such a measure requires extensive pilot work to identify key situations and, finally, its administration requires a controlled research environment, which is not always available when conducting applied research.

Various self-report measures of habit strength have been used that ask participants to indicate how often they perform a behaviour 'by force of habit' or 'without awareness' (e.g. Kahle and Beatty 1987; Conner and McMillan 1999). Such measures have been found to be predictive of future behaviour, although they have not been shown to moderate intention–future behaviour relations (e.g. Conner and McMillan 1999). In addition, they have three common shortcomings: (1) they ask for simultaneous estimates of behavioural frequency and the extent to which the behaviour is habitual in nature; (2) they tend to be single-item measures; and (3) they do not assess all of the defining features of habitual responses.

In response to these criticisms, Verplanken and Orbell (2003) developed a 12-item self-report index of habit strength that is based on the key features of habitual responses – that is, a history of repetition (e.g. 'X is something I do frequently'), automaticity (e.g. 'X is something I do without having to consciously remember'), and expression of one's identity (cf. Trafimow and Wyer 1993) (e.g. 'X is something that's typically "me"'). Verplanken and Orbell (2003) reported that the self-report habit index (SRHI) was a reliable measure that correlated with the response-frequency measure of habit and with frequency of past behaviour. In addition, it discriminated successfully between three behaviours differing in average behavioural frequency and between behaviours performed weekly versus daily. Subsequent research with the SRHI has found it to correlate significantly, and prospectively, with a range of health behaviours, including car and bicycle use (Gardner 2009), physical activity (de Bruijn et al. 2012; van Bree et al. 2013), unhealthy snacking behaviour (Aukje et al. 2012), fruit consumption (de Bruijn et al. 2007), binge drinking (Norman 2011; Gardner et al. 2012b), and breast self-examination (Norman and Cooper 2011). In a meta-analysis of 22 studies, Gardner et al. (2011) reported an average weighted correlation of 0.44 between the SRHI and measures of nutrition behaviour and physical activity. Gardner et al. (2011) also reported that the SRHI moderated intention–behaviour relations in eight of nine tests, such that intention became a weaker predictor of behaviour with increasing level of habit strength. However, it should be noted that many of these tests used cross-sectional designs. In addition, intention typically remained a significant predictor of behaviour even under high levels of habit strength. Some more recent studies have reported positive moderation effects (de Bruijn et al. 2012; Gardner et al. 2012b) such that intention becomes a stronger predictor of behaviour with increasing level of habit strength. Thus, intentional and habitual processes may complement each other, such that those with strong intentions may seek out opportunities, or develop conducive environments, to engage in the behaviour, and those who have strong habits may be more likely to respond to these opportunities and environmental cues (Norman 2011). Moreover, on a theoretical level, it is not clear why intentions should lose their predictive validity as habit strength increases (Ajzen 2002); people are likely to continue to hold positive intentions even if the behaviour is under the control of habitual processes. As noted by Gardner et al. (2011), measures of intention and habit strength are often strongly, and positively, correlated.

The SRHI is the most popular measure of habit strength. However, the conceptual validity of the measure has been questioned (Gardner *et al.* 2012a; Sniehotta and Presseau 2012; Gardner 2014). The SRHI assess three components of habit, namely, automaticity, behavioural frequency, and identity. As argued by Gardner (2014), identity is not a defining feature of habits. Moreover, the identity items of the SRHI have been found to load on to a separate factor with other identity measures (Gardner *et al.* 2012b). In addition, behavioural frequency cannot be used to distinguish between habitual and intentional influences on future behaviour. As a result, the inclusion of items assessing behavioural frequency in the SRHI is likely to inflate its correlation with future behaviour. In contrast, automaticity is a key defining feature of habits that can distinguish between habitual and intentional behaviour. Gardner *et al.* (2012a) therefore developed a sub-scale of the SRHI consisting of four automaticity items: the self-report behavioural automaticity index (SRBAI). An analysis of 34 published datasets and four primary datasets indicated that the SRBAI had strong correlations with behaviour (though slightly weaker than for the SRHI) and moderated intention–behaviour relations in the same way as, and typically stronger than, the SRHI. Given the increased parsimony and conceptual clarity offered by the SRBAI, it is likely to become the measure of choice when assessing habit strength in future studies. Nonetheless, as acknowledged by Gardner *et al.* (2012a), it has a number of limitations. First, the SRBAI does not assess cues to habits. However, given the idiosyncratic nature of the cues that trigger automatic responses, this is likely to be difficult to incorporate into a measure of habit strength. Second, as with other self-report measures of habit strength, it is possible to question the extent to which people are able to accurately report on the non-conscious (e.g. automatic) processes that guide behaviour (cf. Nisbett and Wilson 1977). Third, the SRBAI requires validation against 'gold standard' experimental tests of the strength of cue–response associations (Danner *et al.* 2011).

2.5 Dual-process models

The research reviewed in this volume predominantly focuses on reflective influences on health behaviour. This work emphasizes the role of key variables such as outcome expectancies, self-efficacy, and the formation of strong and stable goal intentions in determining health behaviour. In the last few years, the development of 'dual-process' models has drawn attention to the role of non-reflective influences on behaviour. The reflective–impulsive model (RIM) developed by Strack and Deutsch (2004) represents an important dual-process model in relation to furthering our understanding of the different influences on health behaviours. The RIM distinguishes two separate but interacting systems that together guide behaviour: the reflective and the impulsive. The reflective system is seen as reasoned, conscious, and intentional and many of the models outlined in this book attempt to describe the key constructs that influence behaviour in this system. In contrast, the impulsive system consists of associative clusters that have been created by temporal or spatial co-activation of external stimuli, affective reactions, and associated behavioural tendencies (Hofmann *et al.* 2008). Once a valence-laden association is established in the impulsive system, a simple perceptual input can automatically trigger an affective evaluation and associated behaviour. Sheeran *et al.* (2013) provide a useful review of impulsive processes and health behaviours and distinguish three areas of research: implicit cognition, implicit affect, and implicit motivation (see also Hofmann *et al.* 2008).

Implicit cognition refers to knowledge or processes that remain outside of awareness. The most prominent focus for work on health behaviours has been in relation to attentional bias. This is typically measured using a modified Stroop task. For example, Calitri *et al.* (2010) reported that greater attentional bias for healthy food words and less attentional bias for unhealthy food words both predicted reductions in body mass index over a period of a year. Training to reduce attentional bias has been shown to promote reduction in alcohol consumption and delayed relapse over a three-month period among people with alcohol dependence (Schoenmakers *et al.* 2010). The formation of implementation intentions (if–then plans) has also been shown to reduce attentional bias and impact on habitual behaviours like consumption of high-fat foods (Achtziger *et al.* 2008).

Implicit affect is usually tapped by implicit attitudes. The most widely used implicit attitude measure is the Implicit Association Test (IAT; Greenwald *et al.* 1998). The IAT is a computerized method for measuring indirectly the strength of the association between pairs of concepts via a discrimination task. It relies on the assumption that if two concepts are highly associated (congruent), the discrimination task will be easier, and therefore quicker, when the associated concepts share the same response key than when they require different response keys (for more details about the procedure, see Greenwald *et al.* 1998). Implicit attitudes have been found to be associated with intentions to use (Czopp *et al.* 2004) and use of condoms (Stacy *et al.* 2006), smoking (Payne *et al.* 2007), snack consumption (Conner *et al.* 2007b), and physical activity (Calitri *et al.* 2009). Various reviews also suggest that implicit attitudes are predictive of behaviour even after taking account of explicit attitude measures (Hofmann *et al.* 2008; Rooke *et al.* 2008) or other explicit cognitions such as outcomes expectancies, self-efficacy, and intention (Conroy *et al.* 2010; Cheval *et al.* 2015). However, there is continuing debate about the power of implicit attitudes to predict behaviour after controlling for affective attitudes (Conner *et al.* 2011; Ayres *et al.* 2012), suggesting that some explicit measures may also tap these impulsive influences. Interventions to change implicit attitudes have used evaluative conditioning, which attempts to change the valance of the evaluation by pairing the stimulus with another positive or negative stimulus. In one of the few studies on health behaviours, Hollands *et al.* (2011) measured implicit and explicit attitudes to snacks and then paired images of snacks with aversive images of obesity and heart disease. Evaluative conditioning reduced the favourability of implicit attitudes to snack without changing explicit attitudes and also reduced the likelihood of choosing a snack as a reward. Mediation analyses showed the change in implicit attitude partially explained the impact of evaluative conditioning on behaviour. Wiers *et al.* (2011) used a computer task to train alcohol-dependent patients to make an avoidance movement (i.e. push) to pictures of alcohol and an approach movement (i.e. pull) to non-alcoholic drinks and showed this reduced relapse rates, compared with a control condition, from 59% to 43% over a one-year period.

Implicit motivation refers to goal pursuit that is not guided by an agentic self and that operates outside of conscious intention and awareness (Sheeran *et al.* 2013). Research on goal-priming has shown that mental representations of goals can be activated without the individual knowing about or intending it. This can be achieved through subliminal presentation of goal-relevant stimuli or through subtle and unobtrusive supraliminal presentation. Stroebe *et al.* (2008) showed that subliminally priming the goal of eating enjoyment inhibited the goal of controlling one's weight in restrained eaters. Albarracin *et al.* (2009) showed that participants primed with exercise words consumed more food in a taste test than controls. Fishbach *et al.* (2003) showed that participants exposed to magazines about food or slimming in a room while they waited to participate in an experiment were more likely to activate a slimming goal and to subsequently choose an apple over a chocolate bar compared with controls. In a field study, Papies and Hamstra (2010) showed that priming the goal of dieting via a subtle exposure to a poster led to a reduced number of snacks being consumed by restrained eaters.

Further research on the individual and combined effects of reflective and impulsive influences on health behaviours is required to address a number of outstanding questions. First, what is the relative predictive power of reflective and impulsive influences? Second, when might we expect reflective and impulsive influences to act independently or interact in producing behaviour? Third, what conditions promote or inhibit the relative power of reflective and impulsive influences to determine behaviour and how can this be harnessed to produce behaviour change? The answers to these questions are likely to provide us with a fuller understanding of the relative impact of reflective and impulsive influences on health behaviour.

2.6 Maintenance of health behaviour

Research with SCMs has tended to focus on the initiation of health behaviour. This is appropriate for behaviours where health benefits are associated with one-off performance (e.g. immunization). However, other health behaviours (e.g. healthy eating, exercise) provide little or no health benefit unless maintained over prolonged periods of time. A greater understanding is required of the factors determining maintenance of health behaviour; it is likely that these will be different from the factors important in the initiation of health behaviour. In addition, although health benefits of maintenance behaviours may be most strongly associated with consistent performance over prolonged periods of time, interruptions or lapses may be common for these behaviours (e.g. healthy eating; Conner and Armitage 2002). Hence, an appropriate focus may be on performance over prolonged periods of time that minimizes lapses (Shankar *et al.* 2004).

Distinguishing initiation and maintenance is a key component of various stage models (see Sutton, Chapter 9 this volume) and has been specifically noted in relation to physical activity (Sherwood and Jeffery 2000), weight control (Jeffery *et al.* 1999), and recovery from addictions (Marlatt and Gordon 1985). A complex but key issue is how initiation versus maintenance is defined. Stage models such as the transtheoretical model of change (TTM; Prochaska *et al.* 1992) suggest distinguishing the two based on a fixed period of time: initiation is the first six months following behaviour change; maintenance is beyond six months. However, this period of time is essentially arbitrary and appears to be based on when most relapses occur (Orleans 2000). Others have argued that maintenance occurs when the behaviour is performed effortlessly and efficiently, without the need to specify a timeframe (e.g. Bargh 1992). However, this definition equates the maintenance of behaviour with habitual control (and is therefore restricted to behaviours that can be performed frequently in stable contexts). Moreover, it does not allow for the possibility that behaviours can be maintained through intentional control. A more useful distinction between initiation and maintenance might focus on variations in the factors that determine the decision to initiate or maintain the behaviour.

Various theories of the factors important for the maintenance of behaviour have been developed, including the relapse prevention model (Marlatt and Gordon 1985) and the TTM (Prochaska *et al.* 1992). Basic to these theories is the idea that different factors are important in the decision to initiate and maintain a behaviour. This is distinct from other SCMs that assume the same factors underlie initiation and maintenance. The evidence here is mixed. For example, in their meta-analysis of the PMT, Floyd *et al.* (2000) reported that response efficacy and self-efficacy had similar effect sizes for both initiation and maintenance behaviours. Conner *et al.*

(2002) reported the TPB to be predictive of long-term healthy eating over a six-year period, although Sheeran *et al.* (2001) showed the TPB to predict attendance at individual screening appointments, but not repeated attendance.

Here we highlight six theories that outline different factors that are important in the decision to initiate a behaviour compared with the decision to maintain a behaviour. These theories propose that either different factors or the same factors acting via different processes are important in determining the decision to initiate or maintain a behaviour.

First, Rothman (2000) focuses on the role of outcome expectancies and satisfaction with outcomes in the initiation and maintenance of behaviour. The decision to initiate a behaviour is held to be based on a consideration of the potential benefits afforded by the new pattern of behaviour compared with the current situation (i.e. outcome expectancies). Initiating a new behaviour thus depends on holding favourable expectancies regarding future outcomes. Because the process of behavioural initiation can be conceptualized as the attempt to reduce the discrepancy between a current state and a desired reference state, it is viewed as an approach-based self-regulatory system (Carver and Scheier 1990). In contrast, decisions to maintain a behaviour involve decisions about whether the outcomes associated with the new pattern of behaviour are sufficiently desirable to warrant continued action (King *et al.* 2002). Thus, the decision to maintain a behaviour depends principally on perceived satisfaction with received outcomes (e.g. Kassovou *et al.* 2014). Because the process of behavioural maintenance can be conceptualized as the attempt to maintain the discrepancy between a current state and an undesired reference state, it is viewed as an avoidance-based self-regulatory system (Carver and Scheier 1990). Another implication of this view is that while high expectations may be an important facilitator to initiating a behaviour, these expectations must be realistic in order that dissatisfaction with the received outcomes does not inhibit maintenance (see also Sears and Stanton 2001). Rothman (2000) suggests that satisfaction will depend upon comparisons of received outcomes with expectations about what rewards a new pattern of behaviour will provide. Thus, interventions that heighten expectations may be useful in initiating behaviour change but be detrimental to the maintenance of a behaviour. More recently, Rothman *et al.* (2011) have proposed that, in addition to satisfaction with perceived outcomes, automatic influences are important for behaviours that are maintained over extended periods of time.

Second, self-efficacy has been found to be a key predictor of initiation and maintenance across a variety of behavioural domains, including physical activity (e.g. Dzewaltowski *et al.* 1990), oral health behaviours (e.g. Syrjala *et al.* 2001), cardiac rehabilitation (e.g. Oldridge 1988), and AIDS-preventive behaviours (e.g. Kok *et al.* 1991). It is also a variable that distinguishes action and maintenance stages from earlier stages in the TTM (e.g. Marcus and Simkin 1994). In the HAPA, action self-efficacy is a key predictor of intention and initial performance of health behaviour, whereas coping and recovery self-efficacy are important for the maintenance of health behaviour and recovering from lapses, respectively (see Schwarzer and Luszczynska, Chapter 8 this volume). Similarly, in relapse prevention theory (Marlatt and Gordon 1985), the importance of self-efficacy is highlighted in relation to recovering from slips and relapses.

Third, social support, though only tangentially included in the major SCMs, may also be important in relation to initiation and maintenance. In relation to weight loss, for example, social support appears to be an important predictor of initial weight loss attempts and longer-term maintenance (Wing *et al.* 1991). In terms of initiation, social support may need to take the form of encouragement from others to try weight loss behaviours, while in terms of maintenance, social support may need to take the form of knowing others with whom to perform the behaviour. Social support has also been found to have small-to-moderate effects on maintenance of exercise behaviours (Sherwood and Jeffery 2000). Such effects are sometimes direct and at other times mediated by changes in self-efficacy. Social support may be just one important part of a supportive environment that is key to the maintenance of behaviours (Orleans 2000).

Fourth, self-determination theory (SDT; Deci and Ryan 1985) specifies the different motivational determinants that might be relevant to initiation versus maintenance of behaviour. In particular, SDT views successful maintenance as based on the internalization of motivation to act. So while successful initiation of a health behaviour may be possible even where the motivation is external (e.g. a health professional's recommendation), such motivation is not likely to be sufficient to maintain the behaviour. Internalization here refers to the process whereby the individual comes fully to accept the regulation of the behaviour as internally determined. Such internalized motivation has been reported to be related to the maintenance of physical activity (Laitakari *et al.* 1996), diabetic dietary self-care (Senécal *et al.* 2000), smoking cessation (Williams *et al.* 2002), and medication adherence (Williams *et al.* 1998). However, it is unclear whether these impacts of internalized motivation are independent of self-efficacy.

Fifth, the relapse prevention model (RPM; Marlatt and Gordon 1985) provides an account of the factors important to maintenance and relapse from maintenance (for a comprehensive review, see Larimer *et al.* 1999). The RPM focuses on those situations that place an individual at risk from relapse and the coping strategies an individual might use to prevent relapse via increasing self-efficacy. High-risk situations might include emotional states and social pressure. Relapse can be tackled through the avoidance of high-risk situations, increasing self-efficacy, and changing the interpretation of minor lapses. The latter is particularly important. Individuals who make internal, stable, and global attributions for a lapse and experience negative emotions such as guilt are more likely to relapse. For example, Stetson *et al.* (2005) reported that, among male exercisers, weaker perceptions of control and higher levels of guilt over lapses in high-risk situations were associated with reduced levels of exercise at three-month follow-up. Relapse prevention training has been applied to marijuana dependence (Stephens *et al.* 1994), physical activity (Knapp 1988), weight management (Perri *et al.* 2001), and smoking cessation (Curry and McBride 1994). The RPM has usefully focused attention on the importance of successfully managing lapses as a means to increase maintenance of a health behaviour.

Finally, in attempting to integrate theory and research in this area, Voils *et al.* (2014) outline five cognitive and behavioural process that have different effects for the initiation and maintenance of health behaviour. First, in terms of self-regulatory focus, during initiation the focus is on approaching a favoured state (e.g. weight loss), whereas during maintenance the focus is on avoiding an unfavoured state (e.g. weight gain). Second, in relation to outcome beliefs, in line with most SCMs, initiation of health behaviour is dependent on the anticipation of positive outcomes, whereas its maintenance is dependent on satisfaction with the obtained outcomes (Rothman 2000). Third, in terms of planning and associated self-efficacy, having formed an intention, individuals need to develop action plans (e.g. implementation intentions; see Prestwich *et al.*, Chapter 10 this volume) detailing when, where, and how they will initiate the behaviour, whereas they need to develop plans to deal with high-risk situations (i.e. relapse prevention; Marlatt and Gordon 1985) to maintain the behaviour. In line with the HAPA (Schwarzer and Luszczynska, Chapter 8 this volume), individuals also need to be confident in their ability to perform a behaviour (i.e. action self-efficacy) in order to initiate it, whereas they need to be confident in their ability to overcome barriers (i.e. maintenance self-efficacy) and to get back on track after relapses (i.e. recovery self-efficacy) to maintain it. Fourth, in relation to self-monitoring, during initiation self-monitoring is typically guided by others (e.g. the interventionist), whereas during maintenance it is more likely to be self-guided. Thus, the locus of control shifts from external to internal consistent with SDT that proposes that initiation of behaviour can be based on extrinsic motivation but maintenance is based on intrinsic motivation (Deci and Ryan 1985). Fifth, in terms of social support, during initiation it may be provided by the intervention context (e.g. weight loss group), whereas during maintenance it may be provided by the individual's existing social network.

Voils *et al.* (2014) put forward a conceptual model of behaviour initiation and maintenance (CMBIM) that outlines a number of key motivational and volitional variables that are important in the initiation and maintenance of health behaviour. According to this model, (favourable) outcomes expectations and action self-efficacy determine intention to initiate a behaviour. In order to translate this intention into behaviour, the individual needs to form action plans. Having initiated the behaviour, satisfaction with outcomes, together with maintenance and recovery self-efficacy determine intention to maintain a behaviour. This intention then requires relapse prevention planning to ensure that the behaviour is maintained. This model has a number of positive features. First, it incorporates the distinction between motivational and volitional (i.e. post-intentional) phases of health behaviour that is lacking in many SCMs (the HAPA is an exception to this). As a result, it contains both motivational (e.g. outcome expectancies) and volitional (e.g. action planning) variables. Second, it also incorporates the distinction between the initiation of health behaviour (that most SCMs focus on) and its maintenance, outlining different variables for each phase. However, despite its potential, there have been no formal tests of the model to date. In addition, there is scope to question some of the proposed relationships in the model. In particular, it may be useful to outline direct links between self-efficacy and behaviour (initiation and maintenance) as included in other SCMs, such as SCT. Similarly, it may be more appropriate to consider relapse self-efficacy as a volitional variable. In addition, the model may benefit from a greater emphasis on, and integration of, social influences on behaviour.

In summary, the above theories provide useful insights into the factors that are important for the maintenance of health behaviour. A number of conclusions and issues for further research can be drawn. First, the key role of self-efficacy is evident in a number of the above theories. In particular, high levels of self-efficacy appear to be important for maintenance and for dealing with temporary lapses. Second, motivation appears as a central construct in a number of the models. For example, in SDT the importance of intrinsic motivation is emphasized, particularly in relation to maintaining health behaviours. Third, the need for integration of these different models of maintenance is apparent. The conceptual model of behaviour initiation and maintenance presented by Voils *et al.* (2014) represents a promising first step in this direction.

2.7 Critiques of the social cognition approach

The use of SCMs to predict health behaviour has a number of advantages, as outlined by Conner and Norman (Chapter 1 this volume). In this section, we consider critiques of specific SCMs (e.g. Sarver 1983; Liska 1984; Eagly and Chaiken 1993; Trafimow 2009; Head and Noar 2014; Sniehotta *et al.* 2014) and the general SCM approach (Greve 2001; Ogden 2003; Noar and Zimmerman 2005;

Johnston and Johnston 2013) that have raised a number of important issues. These are grouped under the headings of *falsification, rationality, methodological issues*, and *sufficiency*.

A first important criticism of SCMs is that they are not falsifiable (Smedslund 2000; Greve 2001; Ogden 2003; Trafimow 2009). For example, Ogden (2003) argues that SCMs cannot be disconfirmed. Ogden supports this conclusion by arguing that researchers do not conclude they have disconfirmed the theory under test when they find that one or more of the theory's antecedent variables do not predict the outcome measure or that the findings do not explain all or most of the variance in intentions or behaviour. Ajzen and Fishbein (2004) highlight that the logic of this argument is unsound; to conclude that a theory has been disconfirmed under such circumstances would not be consistent with the theories being tested. Taking the example of the TRA/TPB, numerous descriptions of the theory make clear that the extent to which each of the antecedent variables predicts intentions or behaviour is a function of the population and behaviour under study. For a specific behaviour and population, one or more antecedents may indeed not be predictive without disproving the theory. However, evidence disproving the theory would be obtained if none of the antecedent variables were predictive of intentions or behaviour. In this way, the TRA/TPB could be disconfirmed. A similar argument to Ogden's is made by Greve (2001), who argues that models like the TPB fail the Smedslund test. The test requires us to imagine the reverse empirical relation and ask if true, would we then discard the theory. If the answer is no, then the test is failed, and this failure suggests that the theory is not falsifiable. Consider the study by Armitage and Conner (1999). According to Greve, if Armitage and Conner had found that as people's intention to eat a low-fat diet increased they actually were less likely to do so, we would not believe the finding. According to Greve, this study fails the Smedslund test – no matter what was found, we would still believe the theory. However, closer examination suggests that this criticism is not well founded. In particular, Greve neglects the possibility that no correlation could have been found, in which case we would have less confidence in the TPB. If that finding had been replicated using a variety of operationalizations of the variables, we might be quite confident in rejecting the theory. Even in the extreme case described by Greve, if replicated in a sufficient variety of ways, the scientific community would come to agree that increasing intentions might decrease the probability of following a low-fat diet. Subsequent research attention would then be directed towards identifying the circumstances under which such counter-intentional behaviour occurs. On this basis, it appears incorrect to characterize the TPB as failing the Smedslund test. Trafimow (2009) makes a similar argument in relation to the TRA, and argues that a number of falsification tests have been successfully conducted and in some cases have even contributed to the further development of the theory.

A second important criticism of SCMs is that they are too rational and deliberative and fail to take account of other affective/emotional, non-conscious or irrational determinants of human behaviour (Sheeran *et al.* 2013; Sniehotta *et al.* 2014). As we noted in Section 2.5 on dual-process models, the SCMs considered in this volume do indeed focus on the reflective as opposed to the impulsive influences on behaviour and there is reason to believe that taking account of both sets of influences may provide a more complete and more predictive account of health behaviours. In addition, a number of studies have begun to consider the role of affective influences on health behaviours within SCMs such as the TPB (e.g. Conner *et al.* 2014). Nevertheless, Fishbein and Ajzen (2010) and Ajzen (2011, 2014) make the point that the TRA/TPB does not propose that people are rational or behave in a rational manner. The TPB makes no assumptions about the objectivity or veridicality of behavioural, normative or control beliefs. It is assumed that various non-cognitive, non-conscious or irrational factors may influence the formation of these beliefs. The TPB only assumes that people's attitudes, subjective norms, and perceptions of control follow reasonably and consistently from these beliefs, and in this way influence their intentions and behaviour. Fishbein and Ajzen (2010) also make the point that SCMs like the TRA/TPB still do a reasonable job of predicting behaviours that are associated with significant risk, are addictive or habitual, or are performed when aroused or intoxicated with legal or illegal drugs, despite the supposed greater influence of various affective/emotional determinants in such cases. Moreover, this is despite a potential problem with the way in which SCM studies are typically conducted. In particular, differences may exist between the contemplation of a behaviour (e.g. when filling in an SCM questionnaire) and its performance in a real-life context. It may be that the health cognitions activated when completing the questionnaire are different from the ones accessible at the point of performing the behaviour (Ajzen and Sexton 1999), leading to the health cognitions being poor representations of those which exist in the behavioural situation and thus being poor predictors of action. It may be particularly difficult for individuals to correctly anticipate the strong emotions that drive their behaviour in real life (Ajzen and Fishbein 2005). This would lead to problems with incorporating emotional factors within typical SCM applications. Nevertheless, it should be noted that there is usually considerable consistency between intentions and behaviours where one might expect marked differences in emotional state between the context in which the questionnaire is completed and the one in which the behaviour is performed (for example, regarding condom use, Albarracin *et al.* [2001] report intention–behaviour $r_+ = 0.45$ across 96 data sets, although mainly based on self-reported behaviour).

A third important criticism of SCMs is based on methodological grounds. There are a number of strands to these methodological critiques. For example, Ogden (2003) has claimed that SCMs contain only analytic truths (as opposed to synthetic truths that can be known through testing) because the correlations observed between measured cognitions are likely to be attributable to overlap in the way the constructs are measured. She claims that this argument extends to measures of behaviour because these are often based on self-report. We would dispute this interpretation of the literature for two main reasons: (1) it is not at all apparent that Ogden's explanation would account for the observed patterns of correlations among cognitions that are reported in the literature; and (2) high levels of prediction of behaviour are also found with objective measures of behaviour that do not rely on self-report and thus cannot be biased in the way Ogden describes. For example, in their meta-analysis of the TPB, Armitage and Conner (2001) showed that intention and perceived behavioural control still accounted for 21% of variance in behaviour when objectively measured. Ogden (2003) makes the related argument that the application of SCMs leads to the creation of cognitions rather than the measurement of such cognitions, which, in turn, influences behaviour. As Ajzen and Fishbein (2004) point out, this is a common concern in questionnaire and interview studies and has become referred to as the 'question–behaviour effect' (Dholakia 2010). A number of studies have shown that measuring components of SCMs can have an impact on behaviour. For example, Godin *et al.* (2008) showed that measuring components of the TPB in relation to blood donation produced a 6–9% increase in blood donation compared with not measuring these components. A meta-analysis by Rodrigues *et al.* (2015) indicated that measuring health cognitions is consistently associated with a small effect on health behaviours (see also Wood *et al.* submitted). Although Fishbein and Ajzen (2010) argue that this does not invalidate models like the TRA/TPB, we may need to remain aware of such effects when examining behaviour change using SCMs and employ more sophisticated designs (e.g. Soloman four-group designs).

A further methodological criticism has been the over-reliance on correlational tests of SCMs (Sniehotta *et al.* 2014). Although models such as the PMT have received more experimental tests, there are fewer such tests for models such as the TPB. Nevertheless, a growing number of meta-analyses have examined studies that have successfully manipulated individual health cognitions in SCMs and reported the effects on intentions and behaviour. For example, Webb and Sheeran (2006) meta-analysed 46 studies that had successfully changed intentions and reported they were associated with a small-to-medium-sized effect on behaviour. More recently, Sheeran *et al.* (submitted) reported that studies that successfully changed attitudes, norms, and self-efficacy were associated with medium-sized changes in intentions and small-to-medium-sized changes in behaviour. Further research that uses experimental designs to manipulate components of SCMs and observes effects on intentions and behaviour would represent useful contributions to this area.

A final and related methodological criticism has been the fact that SCMs have tended to be tested in between-subject designs when they are assumed to be theories that apply to individuals (Johnston and Johnston 2013). The majority of tests of SCMs do indeed employ between-subject correlational designs that assess the extent to which individuals with stronger intentions, self-efficacy, outcome expectancies or other health cognitions are also the ones most likely to perform the behaviour. However, within-subject correlational tests do exist. A number of such tests use within-subject correlations to examine if individuals are indeed most likely to perform those behaviours that they have the most positive health cognitions towards (e.g. Conner *et al.* 2003). A more recent and sophisticated approach to this question has been to use multi-level modelling to examine both the within-subject and between-subject relationships in a single analysis. Conner *et al.* (2014) provide one example of this in relation to testing extensions of the TPB across multiple behaviours. These studies have generally confirmed the findings using between-subject analyses.

A fourth and final important criticism of SCMs is based on sufficiency (Head and Noar 2014; Sniehotta *et al.* 2014). A number of commentators have lamented the large proportion of variance left unexplained in both intentions and behaviour by SCMs. In part, this reflects limits on the predictive validity of health cognitions due to their imperfect measurement. Reliability of measures of intentions, self-efficacy, and other health cognitions rarely exceed 0.80, meaning they contain less than 64% meaningful variance, attenuating the variance in intentions and behaviour they could theoretically explain. One response to the lack of variance explained in intentions and behaviour has been the search for additional variables. A strength of most SCMs is that they predict intentions and action across a broad range of behaviours and populations using a limited number of health cognitions (i.e. they are parsimonious). Although an additional variable might add to the predictive power of SCMs in one domain, that same variable may not be predictive in other domains. Head and Noar (2014) comment on this tension between generalizability and utility in using SCMs and come down in favour of the latter for the health behaviour field given the applied focus. There is some merit in this view when the focus is on changing behaviour (see Conner and Norman, Chapter 1 this volume) because we want to identify all the key determinants of behaviour within a domain in order to target them in an intervention. This links to a related criticism of SCMs that they are not models of behaviour change (Ajzen 2014; Sniehotta *et al.* 2014) in that they help identify targets of interventions (i.e. different health cognitions) designed to change behaviour rather than necessarily saying how to change these health cognitions. Nevertheless, as we noted earlier, a growing body of literature is identifying the impacts of changing the relevant health cognitions on changes in intentions and behaviour and also identifying the interventions that can be used to change these health cognitions (Webb and Sheeran 2006; Sheeran *et al.* submitted).

In summary, critiques have raised a number of concerns over the application of SCMs to the prediction of health behaviour. In particular, these critiques have focused on falsification, rationality, methodological issues, and sufficiency of SCMs. We believe that such debate can be useful in identifying the general strengths and weaknesses of this approach. In addition, the individual models have been subjected to considerable critical analysis in the literature and many unresolved issues are detailed in other chapters in this book. We believe that such critiques are crucial for the continuing development of the models. Despite the success of the social cognition approach to the prediction of health behaviour, there are still many issues for future work to address.

3 Changing health behaviour: future directions

3.1 The practicality of social cognition models

Social cognition models can be used to inform the development of interventions to change health behaviour. Brawley (1993) argues that it is possible to assess the extent to which a model provides a sound framework for intervention design on the basis of its *practicality*. To have a high level of practicality, a model must (a) have predictive utility, (b) describe the relationships between key constructs, (c) offer guidelines for the assessment of these constructs, (d) allow the translation of these constructs into operational manipulations, and (e) provide the basis for detecting the reasons why an intervention succeeds or fails. Each of these factors will be considered in turn in relation to the major SCMs.

First, it is clear that many of the SCMs have good predictive utility and, as such, provide a sound basis for developing interventions. For example, the meta-analysis conducted by McEachan *et al.* (2011) indicated that the TPB explained 44.3% of the variance in intentions and 19.3% of the variance in health behaviour in prospective tests. Similar meta-analytic results have been reported in relation to PMT (Milne *et al.* 2000) and the PWM (Todd *et al.* 2014). In contrast, the HBM (Harrison *et al.* 1992; Carpenter 2010) and TTM (Herzog *et al.* 1999) have received less empirical support.

Second, models should describe the relationships between key constructs. This requirement is easily satisfied by many SCMs. For example, in the HAPA, risk perception, outcome expectancies, and action self-efficacy predict intention, which, in turn, is predictive of behaviour along with planning (action and coping), self-efficacy (coping and recovery), and action control. In contrast, the HBM has been criticized for failing to detail the links between the model's variables (Abraham and Sheeran, Chapter 2 this volume), and Bridle *et al.* (2005) have argued that the TTM also requires greater model specification (see also Sutton, Chapter 9 this volume).

Third, a model should provide guidelines for the assessment of key constructs. For example, recommendations exist for the construction of both direct and indirect measures of attitude, subjective norm, and perceived behavioural control within the TPB (Ajzen 1988; Conner and Sparks, Chapter 5 this volume). In addition, there are clear guidelines for the measurement of self-efficacy (Bandura 1986; Luszczynska and Schwarzer, Chapter 7 this volume). The TTM has also benefited from considerable work that has developed measures of stages of change, pros and cons, confidence and temptation, and the processes of change (Prochaska *et al.* 1992). In contrast, the psychometric rigour of many applications of the HBM has been questioned (Harrison *et al.* 1992).

Fourth, it should be possible to translate a model's key constructs into operational manipulations – that is, it should be possible to design interventions to change these variables. However, a common critique of the major SCMs is that while they can be used to identify the key variables for interventions to target, they provide few guidelines on how to change these variables. An exception to this critique is SCT. Thus, Bandura (1986) outlines various sources of self-efficacy that can be targeted to enhance self-efficacy through the use of personal mastery experience, vicarious experience, persuasive communications, and physiological feedback. In addition, PMT has its roots in the fear-drive model (Hovland *et al.* 1953), which revealed that presenting a fear-inducing message followed by an action plan detailing how to deal with the threat increased the likelihood of performance of the recommended action (e.g. Leventhal *et al.* 1965). This work on action plans has since been incorporated into the model of action phases (Heckhausen 1991). In particular, the formation of implementation intentions has been found to be a powerful technique for ensuring that goal intentions are translated into behaviour (Prestwich *et al.*, Chapter 10 this volume).

Fifth, a model should provide a basis for detecting the reasons why an intervention succeeds or fails. It is clear that the major SCMs have the potential to provide such an account. For example, HBM-based interventions should produce changes in HBM cognitions, which, in turn, should lead to changes in behaviour. In other words, if an HBM-based intervention is successful in changing health behaviour, this effect should occur through (i.e. be mediated by) the beliefs that were targeted in the intervention. However, there is a need for greater reporting of mediation analyses in the literature (Michie and Abraham 2004).

3.2 The impact of changes in cognitions on changes in behaviour

To the extent that SCMs are able to predict health behaviour, they should provide a sound basis for developing interventions. As detailed in this volume, there is considerable evidence that SCMs provide strong predictions of intentions and, to a lesser extent, health behaviour. Moreover, there is a growing literature that suggests that theory-based interventions can have significant, and typically stronger, effects on health behaviour (Webb *et al.* 2010). However, the strongest evidence for the SCM approach comes from experimental work that shows that changing variables outlined in SCMs leads to changes in health behaviour. A series of meta-analyses have addressed this issue.

Sheeran *et al.* (2014) examined whether interventions that successfully heightened threat appraisals (i.e. perceived risk, perceived severity, anticipatory emotions, anticipated emotions) also produced changes in intentions and behaviour. Across 239 studies that produced a significant difference in threat appraisals between the intervention and control conditions, the overall effect on threat appraisals was $d_+ = 0.50$, which constitutes a medium-to-large effect. In turn, heightened threat appraisals had a small-to-medium effect on intentions ($d_+ = 0.37$) and a small effect on subsequent behaviour ($d_+ = 0.23$). Encouragingly, interventions that also produced changes in coping appraisals (e.g. response-efficacy, self-efficacy) produced larger effect sizes.

Sheeran *et al.* (submitted) further examined the impact of changing attitudes, norms, and self-efficacy on intentions and behaviour. Interventions that produced significant effects on these variables ($d_+ = 0.46$; $d_+ = 0.54$; $d_+ = 0.60$ respectively) led to medium-sized changes in intentions ($d_+ = 0.50$; $d_+ = 0.41$; $d_+ = 0.50$ respectively) and small-to-medium-sized changes in behaviour ($d_+ = 0.37$; $d_+ = 0.20$; $d_+ = 0.46$ respectively).

The above meta-analyses indicate that successfully changing cognitions produces changes in health-related intentions and behaviour, thereby providing strong experimental evidence for the SCM approach to changing health behaviour. It is noteworthy that the effects of changing cognitions are stronger on intentions than on behaviour, consistent with correlational evidence indicating that SCMs provide stronger predictions of intentions than behaviour. Moreover, Webb and Sheeran (2006) reported that interventions that had medium-to-large effects on intentions ($d_+ = 0.66$) only had small- to medium-sized effects on behaviour ($d_+ = 0.36$). Together, these sources of evidence point to the existence of an intention–behaviour gap and highlight the need to identify variables and interventions that help people translate their intentions into behaviour. Additional volitional strategies, such as forming implementation intentions (Prestwich *et al.*, Chapter 10 this volume), may be needed to bridge the intention-behaviour gap.

3.3 Habit-based interventions

In their meta-analysis, Sheeran *et al.* (submitted) reported that changes in attitudes and self-efficacy produced larger changes in infrequently performed (e.g. cancer screening, self-examination) than frequently performed (e.g. exercise, alcohol use) preventive behaviours ($d_+ = 0.53$ vs. 0.34; $d_+ = 0.67$ vs. 0.40 respectively), suggesting that it may be more difficult to change behaviours that are performed frequently. As argued by Ouellette and Wood (1998), behaviours that are performed frequently (in stable contexts) are likely to come under habitual, rather than intentional, control. As a result, they may be more resistant to change, especially in response to interventions based on the major SCMs that are likely to focus on more deliberative, rather than automatic, influences on health behaviour. Rothman *et al.* (2009) suggest two possibilities for changing habitual behaviour. First, deliberate self-control strategies, such as vigilant monitoring, may be used to overcome unwanted habits (Quinn *et al.* 2010). Second, the environmental cues that trigger habitual behaviour may be altered. This could be achieved either through public health policy initiatives (e.g. curbing advertising, reducing the availability of alcohol through licensing laws) (Toomey *et al.* 2007) or through individuals making changes to the structure of their own environments. Accordingly, a small number of individual-focused habit-based interventions have been developed and tested in exploratory trials in recent years.

For example, Lally *et al.* (2008) tested a brief habit-based weight loss intervention. Participants were given a 'Ten Top Tips for Weight Loss' leaflet that listed 10 everyday eating and exercise behaviours that are associated with successful weight loss (e.g. reduced consumption of fatty foods, 10,000 steps per day) along with tips of how to incorporate the behaviours into their daily routines. The intervention resulted in increased weight loss at eight weeks compared with the waiting-list control condition. In addition, the intervention group also had higher automaticity scores (on items from the SRHI; Verplanken and Orbell 2003) at eight-week follow-up. Moreover, changes in automaticity scores were correlated with the amount of weight loss in the intervention condition over a 32-week follow-up period.

The weight-loss intervention developed by Carels *et al.* (2014) focused on promoting healthy habits and disrupting unhealthy habits in relation to dietary behaviours and physical activity. To form new healthy habits, participants were encouraged to (a) develop predictable and sustainable routines, (b) anticipate and minimize potential disruptions to these routines, (c) ensure that new healthy behaviours are reinforced immediately, and (d) form implementation intentions to support the initiation of new behaviours. To disrupt unwanted unhealthy habits, participants were encouraged to (a) change their current routines, (b) not reinforce unhealthy behaviours, (c) remove environmental triggers for unhealthy behaviours, and (d) form implementation intentions to perform healthy behaviours in response to old cues. The habit-based intervention produced significant weight loss at the end of the 12-week programme, as did an educational programme focusing on relationships with food, body image, and stereotypes/myths. However, the habit-based intervention led to greater maintenance of weight loss at six-month follow-up than did the educational programme.

Taken together, the results of these trials highlight the potential of interventions that focus on the formation of new habits and the disruption of old habits through an analysis of environmental cues and associated responses. Such habit-based interventions may be particularly useful for targeting those health behaviours that are performed frequently and are resistant to change via deliberative pathways. In addition, such interventions may also be useful to supporting the maintenance of newly acquired health behaviours. However, tests of these interventions to date have been small-scale and there have been some null findings (Carels *et al.* 2010). Further tests are warranted before strong conclusions can be made.

3.4 Self-affirmation interventions

Attempts to change health behaviour through targeting social cognitive variables may fail because people engage in defensive processing and therefore reject the health message. Leffingwell *et al.* (2007) reported that alcohol-using students were more critical of a health message about the dangers of alcohol use and rated the problem as less important than non-drinking students. Moreover, these effects were more pronounced for frequent and heavy drinkers (i.e. those at greater risk). According to self-affirmation theory (Steele 1988), health messages may not only threaten people's physical integrity (i.e. by outlining risks to their health), but also their self-integrity (i.e. their sense of being sensible, rational, and morally adequate people). As a result, people may resist health messages (e.g. through message derogation) in order to reduce the threat to their self-integrity.

Self-affirmation – the process of reflecting on one's cherished values, actions or values in an unrelated domain – provides a simple technique for bolstering self-integrity and reducing the need to engage in defensive processing. As a result, self-affirmed individuals should engage in more open-minded and balanced processing of health messages, which should lead to more positive intentions and greater changes in health behaviour. For example, Cooke *et al.* (2014) randomly allocated participants to a self-affirmed condition, in which they were asked to list their most important value and write why it was important to them, or a non-affirmed control condition, before reading a health message about physical activity. Self-affirmed participants were found to have more positive attitudes, stronger intentions, and higher levels of physical activity at one-week follow-up. Similar effects have been reported across a range of health behaviours, and have been summarized in two meta-analytic reviews.

Sweeney and Moyer (2015) included 16 studies in their meta-analysis and reported that self-affirmation manipulations (SAMs) had small, but significant, effects on intentions (d_+ = 0.26) and behaviour (d_+ = 0.27). These effects were not moderated by type of self-affirmation manipulation, health message or health behaviour. A more extensive meta-analysis conducted by Epton *et al.* (2015) included 52 studies, but reported similar findings. Self-affirmation manipulations had small, but significant, effects on message derogation (d_+ = 0.17), intentions (d_+ = 0.14), and behaviour (d_+ = 0.32). Few moderation effects were found, although SAMs were found to have stronger effects on behaviour when the timing of the health threat was proximal, when writing a values essay was used as the manipulation, and when samples had smaller proportions of white participants.

A striking feature of the results reported by Epton *et al.* (2015) was the larger effect size found on behaviour than intention. According to self-affirmation theory, self-affirmed individuals should engage in less defensive processing, which should result in more positive intentions, which, in turn, should lead to changes in health behaviour. The larger effect size for behaviour is not consistent with this account and suggests that SAMs may have direct effects on behaviour that operate via non-deliberative/reflective routes. For example, Logel and Cohen (2012) reported that self-affirmed women lost more weight over 10 weeks than non-affirmed women in the absence of a health message. Logel and Cohen (2012) suggest that SAMs may bolster self-control by ensuring that people are focused on higher values rather than more immediate impulses, or by buffering people against stressors that deplete self-regulatory resources. An alternative interpretation is that the positive intentions that are engendered by SAMs are not always translated into behaviour. For example, Cooke *et al.* (2014) reported that the positive effect of their SAM on behaviour was not mediated by intention. In addition, in the meta-analysis reported by Sweeney (2015), the size of the effect on intentions did not predict the size of the effect on behaviour. These findings suggest that SAMs may need to be combined with volitional techniques, such as implementation intentions, to translate positive intentions into behaviour. Two studies have tested this possibility, with mixed results. Harris *et al.* (2014) found that fruit and vegetable consumption was highest among self-affirmed participants who also formed an implementation intention. In contrast, Jessop *et al.* (2014) found that forming an implementation intention had a detrimental effect on exercise behaviour in self-affirmed participants. As noted by Jessop *et al.* (2014), the mechanisms through which SAMs and implementation intentions operate may be incompatible given that SAMs orient individuals towards high-level construals (e.g. superordinate goals) whereas implementation intentions orient people towards low-level construals (e.g. the processes important to goal attainment).

Despite some promising findings and its intuitive appeal, there are a number of issues for future work on self-affirmation to consider. First, more work is needed on the processes through which self-affirmation works, including attentional bias, temporal construal, judgemental confidence, and self-regulatory resources (Epton *et al.* 2015). Second, more attention is needed on the quality of the health messages. Self-affirmation manipulations should only produce positive effects on intentions and behaviour when health messages are strong. If they are weak, SAMs should lead to greater message rejection due to increased message scrutiny. Klein *et al.* (2011) reported that self-affirmed participants only reported increased feelings of vulnerability and intentions to reduce caffeine consumption after reading health messages containing strong versus weak arguments. Third, more work is needed to develop SAMs that are suitable for use in non-laboratory settings and with non-student samples so that they can be more easily incorporated into health behaviour interventions. This may be particularly challenging given awareness of the goal of the SAM may reduce its impact (Sherman *et al.* 2009).

3.5 Behaviour change techniques in theory-based interventions

As detailed in the preceding chapters, the last 10 years have witnessed a marked increase in the development and evaluation of interventions based on SCMs. This work is important as it seeks to both develop effective interventions to change key health behaviours, and provide the strong tests of the proposed causal relationships within SCMs. Thus, to the extent that the SCMs identify the key proximal determinants of health behaviour, developing interventions to change these determinants should produce changes in health behaviour. There is good evidence to support the argument that changes in cognitions lead to changes in behaviour (Sheeran *et al.* 2014, submitted). As detailed in Chapter 11, there has been a parallel strand of work that has sought to identify the key techniques for changing health behaviour. This has resulted in a taxonomy of (health) behaviour change techniques (BCTs; Michie *et al.* 2013) that can be used to describe interventions and to identify the most effective techniques, either in isolation or combination, for changing health behaviour. To date, there has been little cross-fertilization between these two strands of work. Work on theory-based interventions has focused on testing the effectiveness of interventions that target social cognitive variables with little attention to the BCTs being employed, whereas work on BCTs has focused on categorizing different techniques that have been used in interventions to change health behaviour with little attention to underlying theory. Few intervention studies have made explicit links between intervention techniques and targeted cognitions. For example, in their review of physical activity and diet interventions, Prestwich *et al.* (2014) noted that only 9.3% of theory-based intervention studies indicated that every theoretical construct in the underlying theory had been specifically targeted by at least one intervention technique. This suggests that interventions rarely target all theoretical constructs from the underlying theory. Similarly, only 10.7% of studies indicated that every intervention technique targeted at least one theoretical construct in the underlying theory. This suggests that intervention techniques are often utilized without considering how they target a theoretical construct from the underlying theory.

Michie and Wood (Chapter 11 this volume) outline some initial work that has sought to integrate work on theory-based interventions and BCTs. We believe that this represents a key development in the field both in terms of maximizing intervention effectiveness and providing stronger tests of theory. This is likely to be of mutual, and synergistic, benefit. Thus, SCMs identify what to target in health behaviour interventions, but most are silent on how to change targeted variables. Theory-based interventions are therefore likely to benefit from a consideration of specific techniques that can be used to change targeted cognitions and, in turn, behaviour. An analysis of BCTs helps to identify those techniques that can be used to change behaviour, but SCMs are needed to understand how they produce change (i.e. mediation). Integrating these two strands of work may require the development of a taxonomy of cognition change techniques (i.e. CCTs) that can be used to change specific cognitions outlined in SCMs as predictive of health behaviour. Thus, the effectiveness of interventions is likely to be maximized when they target key cognitions using techniques that are able to produce changes in these cognitions. Moreover, such interventions can then be tested not only in terms of their effects on health behaviour, but also whether they produce changes in the targeted cognitions and whether changes in these cognitions mediate intervention effects on behaviour (thereby providing stronger tests of theory).

3.6 Evaluating theory-based interventions

A number of reviews have noted that many theory-based intervention studies are poorly designed (Hardeman *et al.* 2002; Michie and Abraham 2004; Bridle *et al.* 2005). The literature reveals a range of limitations both in the design (i.e. a lack of randomized controlled trials, appropriate control groups, blinding of participants, intervention details, measurement of potential mediators, long-term follow-ups) and analysis (i.e. a lack of 'intention to treat' and mediation analyses) of theory-based interventions. These factors undermine the quality of research evaluating the effectiveness of theory-based interventions. Michie and Abraham (2004) called for increased theoretical and methodological rigour in the design and evaluation of interventions in order to accelerate the development of effective theory-based interventions. In particular, they highlight the recommendations made by Oakley *et al.* (1995) that evaluations of interventions should (a) include randomly allocated or matched control groups, (b) report pre- and post-test intervention data, (c) report 'intention to treat' analyses or control for differential attrition in the intervention and control groups, and (d) report analyses for all outcome variables targeted by the intervention. Michie and Abraham (2004) further recommend that (e) the description of interventions should be sufficiently detailed to enable replication, (f) experimental examinations of specific intervention techniques, both in isolation and combination, should be conducted to identify those techniques that are critical to intervention effectiveness, and (g) measures of the theory-based determinants of behaviour should be taken to allow (h) mediation analyses to identify the underlying mechanisms responsible for any behaviour change.

Rothman (2004) has noted that reports of health behaviour interventions typically fail to describe the extent to which theory has been used to inform the development and evaluation of the intervention. This represents an important barrier to assessing the effectiveness of theory-based interventions. Moreover, many theory-based interventions are only loosely based on theory – that is, theory-inspired rather than theory-based (Michie and Abraham 2004). As a result, Michie and Prestwich (2010) developed a 19-item Theory Coding Scheme (TCS) to provide a reliable means for assessing the use of theory in development and evaluation of health behaviour interventions. The TCS covers the full range of ways that theory can be used in the development and evaluation of health behaviour interventions, including the design of the intervention, the variables targeted, the choice of intervention techniques, the use of tailoring, the (secondary outcome) measures assessed, and the use of mediation analyses. Use of the coding scheme has two main potential benefits. First, it is likely to lead to the more appropriate use of theory in the development and evaluation of health behaviour interventions as researchers may use the coding scheme as a checklist to ensure that their intervention is, in fact, theory-based. Second, it is likely to lead to a more rigorous and systematic examination of the effectiveness of theory-based interventions through reviews and meta-analyses by providing a means to assess the extent of theory use and whether this is related to intervention effectiveness. Both these benefits are likely to aid the scientific development of theory-based interventions.

Finally, many health behaviour interventions are poorly reported. This represents a significant barrier to replication by other researchers and adoption by health professionals. For example, Glasziou *et al.* (2014) noted that only 29% of reports of non-pharmacological interventions provided an adequate description of the intervention. Against this backdrop, an international group of experts developed a list of minimum requirements for the reporting of interventions through a series of Delphi surveys, expert meetings, and pilot work. The TIDieR (Template for Intervention Description and Replication) checklist comprises 12 items (Hoffmann *et al.* 2014) that should be reported/described for all interventions, including health behaviour change interventions:

1. *Brief Name* – a title that describes the intervention.
2. *Why* – the underlying theory or rationale for essential elements of the intervention.
3. *What: Materials* – the intervention materials (full details can be supplied through the use of online supplementary material).
4. *What: Procedures* – the procedures, activities, and processes used in the intervention.
5. *Who Provided* – the background/expertise of those delivering the intervention.
6. *How* – the mode of delivery of the intervention and whether it was delivered to individuals or a group.
7. *Where* – the types of location where the intervention was delivered.
8. *When and How Much* – the duration, timing, and frequency of the intervention.
9. *Tailoring* – whether/how the intervention was tailored.
10. *Modification* – whether/how the intervention was modified during the course of the study.
11. *How Well: Planned* – whether/how intervention fidelity and adherence was assessed and/or encouraged.
12. *How Well: Actual* – the extent to which intervention fidelity and adherence was achieved.

4 Concluding comments

An adequate social cognitive account of health behaviour should be able to predict health behaviour *and* account for, and promote, health behaviour change (Fishbein 1997). The main SCMs of health behaviour have been found to provide strong predictions of health-related intentions and, to a lesser extent, behaviour. Recent years have witnessed increased theoretical and empirical work on the variables that are important in the volitional (i.e. post-intentional) phases of health behaviour. A parallel strand of work has focused on non-intentional (i.e. automatic, non-conscious) influences on health behaviour, which has led to the development of dual-process models. There is a clear need for these two strands of work on post-intentional and non-intentional influences to be formally incorporated into SCMs of health behaviour. Hall and Fong's (2007) theory of temporal self-regulation provides a good example of such an endeavour. In addition, more theoretical and empirical work is needed to identify the key predictors of the maintenance of health behaviour. The conceptual model of behaviour initiation and maintenance presented by Voils *et al.* (2014) represents an important development that awaits further testing and refinement. Social cognition models are being increasingly used to inform the development of interventions to change health behaviour. These interventions have produced some important effects on health cognitions, intentions, and behaviour. However, there is a need for more stringent evaluations and better reporting of theory-based interventions. In addition, there is great potential in formally integrating work on SCMs and behaviour change techniques (BCTs). Thus, work on SCMs can identity the key proximal variables to target in interventions, whereas work on BCTs can identify the best techniques to change these variables in order to produces changes in health behaviour.

As highlighted throughout this book, there are many important questions still to be addressed before the full potential of a social cognition approach to the prediction, and promotion, of health behaviour is realized. These questions represent a challenging, and exciting, agenda for future research on SCMs and health behaviour.

References

Abelson, R.P. (1981) Psychological status of the script concept, *American Psychologist*, 36, 715–29.

Abraham, C., Norman, P. and Conner, M. (2000) Towards a psychology of health-related behaviour change, in P. Norman, C. Abraham and M. Conner (eds.) *Understanding and Changing Health Behaviour: From Health Beliefs to Self-Regulation* (pp. 242–369). Amsterdam: Harwood Academic.

Achtziger, A., Gollwitzer, P.M. and Sheeran, P. (2008) Implementation intentions and shielding goal striving from unwanted thoughts and feelings, *Personality and Social Psychology Bulletin*, 34, 381–93.

Ajzen, I. (1987) Attitudes, traits and actions: dispositional prediction of behavior in personality and social psychology, in L. Berkowitz (ed.) *Advances in Experimental Social Psychology* (Vol. 20, pp. 1–64). New York: Academic Press.

Ajzen, I. (1988) *Attitudes, Personality and Behavior*. Buckingham: Open University Press.

Ajzen, I. (1991) The theory of planned behavior, *Organizational Behavior and Human Decision Processes*, 50, 179–211.

Ajzen, I. (2002) Residual effects of past on later behavior: habituation and reasoned action perspectives, *Personality and Social Psychology Review*, 6, 107–22.

Ajzen, I. (2011) The theory of planned behaviour: reactions and reflections, *Psychology and Health*, 26, 1113–27.

Ajzen, I. (2014) The theory of planned behaviour is alive and well, and not ready to retire: a commentary on Sniehotta, Presseau, and Araujo-Soares, *Health Psychology Review* [DOI: 10.1080/17437199.2014.883474].

Ajzen, I. and Fishbein, M. (2004) Questions raised by a reasoned action approach: reply on Ogden (2003), *Health Psychology*, 23, 431–4.

Ajzen, I. and Fishbein, M. (2005) The influence of attitudes on behavior, in D. Albarracin, B.T. Johnson and M.P. Zanna (eds.) *Handbook of Attitudes and Attitude Change: Basic Principles* (pp. 173–221). Mahwah, NJ: Erlbaum.

Ajzen, I. and Sexton, J. (1999) Depth of processing, belief congruence, and attitude–behavior correspondence, in S. Chaiken and Y. Trope (eds.) *Dual-process Theories in Social Psychology* (pp. 117–38). New York: Guilford Press.

Albarracin, D., Johnson, B.T., Fishbein, M. and Muellerleile, P.A. (2001) Theories of reasoned action and planned behavior as models of condom use: a meta-analysis, *Psychological Bulletin*, 127, 142–61.

Albarracin, D., Leeper, J. and Wang, W. (2009) Immediate increases in eating after exercise promotion messages, *Obesity*, 17, 1451–2.

Allom, V., Mullan, B. and Sebastian, J. (2013) Closing the intention–behaviour gap for sunscreen use and sun protection behaviours, *Psychology and Health*, 28, 477–94.

Apostolopoulos, Y., Sonmez, S. and Yu, C.H. (2003) HIV-risk behaviours of American spring break vacationers: a case of situational disinhibition? *International Journal of STD and AIDS*, 13, 733–43.

Armitage, C.J. and Conner, M. (1999) The theory of planned behaviour: assessment of predictive validity and 'perceived control', *British Journal of Social Psychology*, 38, 35–54.

Armitage, C.J. and Conner, M. (2001) Efficacy of the theory of planned behaviour: a meta-analytic review, *British Journal of Social Psychology*, 40, 471–99.

Aspinwall, L.G., Kemeny, M.E., Taylor, S.E., Schneider, S.G. and Dudley, J.P. (1991) Psychosocial predictors of gay men's AIDS risk-reduction behavior, *Health Psychology*, 10, 432–44.

Aukje, A.C., Verhoeven, M.A., Adriaanse, C.E. and de Ridder, D.T.D. (2012) The power of habits: unhealthy snacking behaviour is primarily predicted by habit strength, *British Journal of Health Psychology*, 17, 758–70.

Ayres, K., Conner, M.T., Prestwich, A. and Smith, P. (2012) Do implicit measures of attitudes incrementally predict snacking behaviour over explicit affect-related measures? *Appetite*, 58, 835–41.

Bandura, A. (1986) *Social Foundations of Thought and Action: A Cognitive Social Theory*. Englewood Cliffs, NJ: Prentice-Hall.

Bargh, J.A. (1992) The ecology of automaticity: toward establishing the conditions needed to produce automatic processing effects, *American Journal of Psychology*, 105, 181–99.

Belanger, D., Godin, G., Alary, M. and Bernard, P.M. (2002) Factors explaining the intention to use condoms among injecting drug users participating in a needle exchange program, *Journal of Applied Social Psychology*, 32, 1047–63.

Bentler, P. and Speckhart, G. (1979) Models of attitude–behavior relations, *Psychological Review*, 86, 542–6.

Bermudez, J. (1999) Personality and health protective behavior, *European Journal of Personality*, 13, 83–103.

Bogg, T. and Roberts, B.W. (2004) Conscientiousness and health-related behaviors: a meta-analysis of the leading behavioral contributors to mortality, *Psychological Bulletin*, 130, 887–919.

Booker, L. and Mullan, B. (2013) Using the temporal self-regulation theory to examine the influence of environmental cues on maintaining a healthy lifestyle, *British Journal of Health Psychology*, 18, 745–62.

Boyd, B. and Wandersman, A. (1991) Predicting undergraduate condom use with the Fishbein and Ajzen and the Triandis attitude–behavior models: implications for public health interventions, *Journal of Applied Social Psychology*, 21, 1810–30.

Brawley, L.R. (1993) The practicality of using social psychological theories for exercise and health research and intervention, *Journal of Applied Sport Psychology*, 5, 99–115.

Bridle, C., Riemsma, R.P., Pattenden, J., Sowden, A.J., Mather, L., Watt, I.S. *et al.* (2005) Systematic review of the effectiveness of health interventions based on the transtheoretical model, *Psychology and Health*, 20, 283–301.

Calitri, R., Lowe, R., Eves, F.F. and Bennett, P. (2009) Associations between visual attention, implicit and explicit attitude and behaviour for physical activity, *Psychology and Health*, 24, 1105–23.

Calitri, R., Pothos, E.M., Tapper, K., Brunstrom, J.M. and Rogers, P.J. (2010) Cognitive biases to healthy and unhealthy food words predict change in BMI, *Obesity*, 18, 2282–7.

Carels, R.A., Burmeister, J.M., Koball, A., Oehlhof, M.W., Hinman, N., LeRoy, M. *et al.* (2014) A randomized trial comparing two approaches to weight loss: differences in weight loss maintenance, *Journal of Health Psychology*, 19, 296–311.

Carels, R.A., Young, K.M., Koball, A., Gumble, A., Darby, L.A., Wagner Oehlhof, M. *et al.* (2010) Transforming your life: an environmental modification approach to weight loss, *Journal of Health Psychology*, 16, 430–8.

Caron, F., Godin, G., Otis, J. and Lambert, L.D. (2004) Evaluation of a theoretically based AIDS/STD peer education program on postponing sexual intercourse and on condom use among adolescents attending high school, *Health Education Research*, 19, 185–97.

Carpenter, C.J. (2010) A meta-analysis of the effectiveness of health belief model variables in predicting behaviour, *Health Communication*, 25, 661–9.

Carver, C.S. and Scheier, M.F. (1982) Control theory: a useful conceptual framework for personality, social, clinical and health psychology, *Psychological Bulletin*, 92, 111–35.

Carver, C.S. and Scheier, M. (1990) Principles of self-regulation: action and emotion, in E.T. Higgins and R. Sorrentino (eds.) *Handbook of Motivation and Cognition: Foundations of Social Behavior* (Vol. 2, pp. 645–72). New York: Guilford Press.

Cheval, B., Sarrazin, P., Isoard-Gauther, S., Radel, R. and Friese, M. (2015) Reflective and impulsive processes explain (in)effectiveness of messages promoting physical activity: a randomized controlled trial, *Health Psychology*, 34, 10–19.

Conner, M. and Abraham, C. (2001) Conscientiousness and the theory of planned behavior: toward a more complete model of the antecedents of intentions and behavior, *Personality and Social Psychology Bulletin*, 27, 1547–61.

Conner, M. and Armitage, C.J. (2002) *The Social Psychology of Food.* Buckingham: Open University Press.

Conner, M. and McMillan, B. (1999) Interaction effects in the theory of planned behaviour: studying cannabis use, *British Journal of Social Psychology*, 38, 195–222.

Conner, M., Grogan, S., Fry, G., Gough, B. and Higgins, A.R. (2009) Direct, mediated and moderated impacts of personality variables on smoking initiation in adolescents, *Psychology and Health*, 24, 1085–1104.

Conner, M., McEachan, R., Taylor, N., O'Hara, J. and Lawton, J. (2014) Role of affective attitudes and anticipated affective reactions in predicting health behaviors, *Health Psychology* [DOI: 10.1037/hea0000143].

Conner, M., Norman, P. and Bell, R. (2002) The theory of planned behavior and healthy eating, *Health Psychology*, 21, 194–201.

Conner, M., Perugini, M., O'Gorman, R., Ayres, K. and Prestwich, A. (2007a) Relations between implicit and explicit measures of attitudes and measures of behavior: evidence of moderation by individual difference variables, *Personality and Social Psychology Bulletin*, 33, 1727–40.

Conner, M., Povey, R., Sparks, P., James, R. and Shepherd, R. (2003) Moderating role of attitudinal ambivalence within the theory of planned behaviour, *British Journal of Social Psychology*, 42, 75–94.

Conner, M., Prestwich, A. and Ayres, K. (2011) Using explicit affective attitudes to tap impulsive influences on health behavior: a commentary on Hofmann et al. (2008), *Health Psychology Review*, 5, 145–9.

Conner, M., Rodgers, W. and Murray, T. (2007b) Conscientiousness and the intention–behavior relationship: predicting exercise behaviour, *Journal of Sports and Exercise Psychology*, 29, 518–33.

Conroy, D.E., Hyde, A.L., Doerksen, S.E. and Ribiero, N.F. (2010) Implicit attitudes and explicit motivation prospectively predict physical activity, *Annals of Behavioral Medicine*, 39, 112–18.

Cooke, R., Trebaczyk, H., Harris, P. and Wright, A.J. (2014) Self-affirmation promotes physical activity, *Journal of Sport and Exercise Psychology*, 36, 217–23.

Courneya, K.S., Bobick, T.M. and Schinke, R.J. (1999) Does the theory of planned behavior mediate the relation between personality and exercise behavior? *Basic and Applied Social Psychology*, 21, 317–24.

Cummings, K.M., Jette, A.M. and Brock, B.M. (1979) Psychological determinants of immunization behaviour in a Swine Influenza campaign, *Medical Care*, 17, 639–49.

Curry, S.J. and McBride, C.M. (1994) Relapse prevention for smoking cessations: review and evaluation of concepts and interventions, *Annual Review of Public Health*, 15, 345–66.

Czopp, A.M., Montieth, M.J., Zimmerman, R.S. and Lynam, D.R. (2004) Implicit attitudes as potential protection from risky sex: predicting condom use with the IAT, *Basic and Applied Social Psychology*, 26, 227–36.

Danner, U.N., Aarts, H. and de Vries, N.K. (2008) Habit vs. intention in the prediction of future behaviour: the role of frequency, context stability and mental accessibility of past behaviour, *British Journal of Social Psychology*, 47, 245–65.

Danner, U.N., Aarts, H., Papies, E.K. and de Vries, N.K. (2011) Paving the path for habit change: cognitive shielding of intentions against habit intrusion, *British Journal of Health Psychology*, 16, 189–200.

De Bruijn, G.-J., Kremers, S.P.J., de Vet, E., de Nooijer, J., van Mechelen, W. and Brug, J. (2007) Does habit strength moderate the intention–behaviour relationship in the theory of planned behaviour? The case of fruit consumption, *Psychology and Health*, 22, 899–916.

De Bruijn, G.-J., Rhodes, R. and van Osch, L. (2012) Does action planning moderate the intention–habit interaction in the exercise domain? A three-way interaction analysis investigation, *Journal of Behavioral Medicine*, 35, 509–19.

De Bruin, M., Sheeran, P., Kok, G., Hiemstra, A., Prins, J.M., Hospers, H.J. *et al.* (2012) Self-regulatory processes mediate the intention–behavior relation for adherence and exercise behaviors, *Health Psychology*, 31, 695–703.

Deci, E.L. and Ryan, R.M. (1985) *Intrinsic Motivation and Self-determination in Human Behavior.* New York: Plenum Press.

Dholakia, U.M. (2010) A critical review of question-behavior effect research, *Review of Marketing Research*, 7, 147–99.

Dillard, A.J., McCaul, K.D. and Klein, W.M.P. (2006) Unrealistic optimism in smokers: implications for smoking myth endorsement and self-protective motivation, *Journal of Health Motivation*, 11, 93–102.

Dombrowski, S.U., Sniehotta, F.F., Avenell, A., Johnston, M., MacLennan, G. and Araújo-Soares, V. (2012) Identifying active ingredients in complex behavioural interventions for obese adults with obesity-related co-morbidities or additional risk factors for co-morbidities: a systematic review, *Health Psychology Review*, 6, 7–32.

Dzewaltowski, D.A., Noble, J.M. and Shaw, J.M. (1990) Physical activity participation: social cognitive theory versus the theories of reasoned action and planned behavior, *Journal of Sport and Exercise Psychology*, 12, 388–405.

Eagly, A.H. and Chaiken, S. (1993) *The Psychology of Attitudes*. Fort Worth, TX: Harcourt Brace Jovanovich.

Epton, T., Harris, P.R., Kane, R., van Koningsbruggen, G.M. and Sheeran, P. (2015) The impact of self-affirmation on health behavior change: a meta-analysis, *Health Psychology*, 34, 187–96.

Eysenck, H.J. (ed.) (1981) *A Model for Personality*. Berlin: Springer.

Ferguson, E. (2013) Personality is of central concern to understand health: towards a theoretical model for health psychology, *Health Psychology Review*, 7, S32–S70.

Fishbach, A., Friedman, R.S. and Kruglanski, A.W. (2003) Leading us not unto temptation: momentary allurements elicit overriding goal activation, *Journal of Personality and Social Psychology*, 84, 296–309.

Fishbein, M. (1997) Predicting, understanding, and changing socially relevant behaviors: lessons learned, in C. McGarty and A.S. Haslam (eds.) *The Message of Social Psychology* (pp. 77–101). Oxford: Blackwell.

Fishbein, M. and Ajzen, I. (2010) *Predicting and Changing Behavior: The Reasoned Action Approach*. New York: Psychology Press.

Floyd, D.L., Prentice-Dunn, S. and Rogers, R.W. (2000) A meta-analysis of research on protection motivation theory, *Journal of Applied Social Psychology*, 30, 407–29.

Friedman, H.S., Tucker, J.S., Schwartz, J.E., Martin, L.R., Tomlinson-Keasay, C., Wingard, D.L. *et al.* (1995) Childhood conscientiousness and longevity: health behaviors and cause of death, *Journal of Personality and Social Psychology*, 68, 696–703.

Fulham, E. and Mullan, B. (2011) Hygienic food handling behaviors: attempting to bridge the intention–behavior gap using aspects from temporal self-regulation theory, *Journal of Food Protection*, 74, 925–32.

Gagnon, M.P. and Godin, G. (2000) The impact of new antiretroviral treatments on college students' intention to use a condom with a new sexual partner, *AIDS Education and Prevention*, 12, 239–51.

Gardner, B. (2009) Modelling motivation and habit in stable travel mode contexts, *Transportation Research Part F: Traffic Psychology and Behaviour*, 12, 68–76.

Gardner, B. (2014) A review and analysis of the use of 'habit' in understanding, predicting and influencing health-related behaviour, *Health Psychology Review* [DOI: 10.1080/17437199.2013.876238].

Gardner, B., Abraham, C., Lally, P. and de Bruijn, G.-J. (2012a) Towards parsimony in habit measurement: testing the convergent and predictive validity of an automaticity subscale of the Self-Report Habit Index, *International Journal of Behavioral Nutrition and Physical Activity*, 9, 102.

Gardner, B., de Bruijn, G.J. and Lally, P. (2011) A systematic review and meta-analysis of applications of the self-report habit index to nutrition and physical activity behaviours, *Annals of Behavioral Medicine*, 42, 174–87.

Gardner, B., de Bruijn, G.-J. and Lally, P. (2012b) Habit, identity, and repetitive action: a prospective study of binge-drinking in UK students, *British Journal of Health Psychology*, 17, 565–81.

Glasziou, P.P., Meats, E., Heneghan, C. and Shepperd, S. (2014) What is missing from descriptions of treatment in trials and reviews? *British Medical Journal*, 336, 1472–4.

Godin, G. and Gionet, N.J. (1991) Determinants of an intention to exercise of electric power commissions' employees, *Ergonomics*, 34, 1221–30.

Godin, G., Sheeran, P., Conner, M. and Germain, M. (2008) Asking questions changes behavior: mere measurement effects on frequency of blood donation, *Health Psychology*, 27, 179–84.

Gold, R.S. and Aucote, H.M. (2003) 'I'm less at risk than most guys': gay men's unrealistic optimism about becoming infected with HIV, *International Journal of STD and AIDS*, 14, 18–23.

Gollwitzer, P.M. (1993) Goal achievement: the role of intentions, in W. Stroebe and M. Hewstone (eds.) *European Review of Social Psychology* (Vol. 4, pp. 141–85). Chichester: Wiley.

Greenwald, A.G., McGhee, D.E. and Schwartz, J.K.L. (1998) Measuring individual differences in implicit cognition: the implicit association test, *Journal of Personality and Social Psychology*, 74, 1464–80.

Greve, W. (2001) Traps and gaps in action explanation: theoretical problems of a psychology of human action, *Psychological Bulletin*, 108, 435–51.

Hagger-Johnson, G. and Shickle, D. (2010) Conscientiousness, perceived control over HIV and condom use in gay/bisexual men, *Psychology and Sexuality*, 1, 62–74.

Hall, P.A. and Fong, G.T. (2007) Temporal self-regulation theory: a model for individual health behavior, *Health Psychology Review*, 1, 6–52.

Hall, P.A. and Fong, G.T. (2010) Temporal self-regulation theory: looking forward, *Health Psychology Review*, 4, 83–92.

Hall, P.A., Fong, G.T., Epp, L.J. and Elias, L. (2008) Executive function moderates the intention–behavior link for physical activity and dietary behavior, *Psychology and Health*, 23, 309–26.

Hampson, S.E. (2012) Personality processes: mechanisms by which personality traits 'get outside the skin', *Annual Review of Psychology*, 63, 315–39.

Hampson, S.E., Andrews, J.A., Barckley, M., Lichtenstein, E. and Lee, M.E. (2000) Conscientiousness, perceived risk, and risk-reduction behaviors: a preliminary study, *Health Psychology*, 19, 496–500.

Hampson, S.E., Goldberg, L.R., Vogt, T.M. and Dubanoski, J.P. (2006) Forty years on: assessments of children's personality traits predict self-reported health behaviors and outcomes at midlife, *Health Psychology*, 25, 57–64.

Hardeman, W., Johnston, M., Johnston, D., Bonetti, D., Wareham, N.J. and Kinmouth, A.L. (2002) Application of the theory of planned behaviour in behaviour change interventions: a systematic review, *Psychology and Health*, 17, 123–58.

Harkin, B., Webb, T.L., Chang, B.P.I., Prestwich, A., Conner, M., Kellar, I. *et al.* (submitted) Does monitoring goal progress promote goal attainment? A meta-analysis of the experimental evidence. Manuscript submitted for publication.

Harris, P. and Middleton, W. (1994) The illusion of control and optimism about health: on being less at risk but no more in control than others, *British Journal of Social Psychology*, 33, 369–86.

Harris, P.H., Brearley, I., Sheeran, P., Barker, M., Klein, W.M.P., Creswell, J.D. *et al.* (2014) Combining self-affirmation with implementation intentions to promote fruit and vegetable consumption, *Health Psychology*, 33, 729–36.

Harrison, J.A., Mullen, P.D. and Green, L.W. (1992) A meta-analysis of studies of the health belief model with adults, *Health Education Research*, 7, 107–16.

Head, K.J. and Noar, S.M. (2014) Facilitating progress in health behaviour theory development and modification: the reasoned action approach as a case study, *Health Psychology Review*, 8, 34–52.

Heckhausen, H. (1991) *Motivation and Action*. Berlin: Springer.

Heckhausen, H. and Beckmann, J. (1990) Intentional action and action slips, *Psychological Review*, 97, 36–48.

Helweg-Larsen, M. and Shepperd, J.A. (2001) Do moderators of the optimistic bias affect personal or target risk estimates: a review of the literature, *Personality and Social Psychology Review*, 1, 74–95.

Herzog, T.A., Abrams, D.B., Emmons, K.M., Linnan, L. and Shadel, W.G. (1999) Do processes of change predict smoking stage movements? A prospective analysis of the transtheoretical model, *Health Psychology*, 18, 369–75.

Hillman, C.H., Motl, R.W., Pontifex, M.B., Posthuma, D., Stubbe, J.H., Boomsma, D.I. *et al.* (2006) Physical activity and cognitive function in a cross-section of younger and older community-dwelling individuals, *Health Psychology*, 25, 678–87.

Hodgkins, S. and Orbell, S. (1998) Can protection motivation theory predict behaviour? A longitudinal study exploring the role of previous behaviour, *Psychology and Health*, 13, 237–50.

Hoffmann T.C., Glasziou, P.P., Boutron, I., Milne, R., Perera, R., Moher, D. *et al.* (2014) Better reporting of interventions: template for intervention description and replication (TIDieR) checklist and guide, *British Medical Journal*, 348, g1687.

Hofmann, W., Friese, M. and Wiers, R.W. (2008) Impulsive versus reflective influences on health behavior: a theoretical framework and empirical review, *Health Psychology Review*, 2, 111–37.

Hollands, G.J., Prestwich, A. and Marteau, T.M. (2011) Using aversive images to enhance healthy eating food choices and implicit attitudes: an experimental test of evaluative conditioning, *Health Psychology*, 30, 195–203.

Hovland, C., Janis, I.L. and Kelley, H. (1953) *Communication and Persuasion*. New Haven, CT: Yale University Press.

Inzlicht, M., Legault, L. and Teper, R. (2014) Exploring the mechanisms of self-control improvement, *Current Directions in Psychological Science*, 23, 302–7.

Jeffery, R.W., French, S.A. and Rothman, A.J. (1999) Stages of change as a predictor of success in weight control in adult women, *Health Psychology*, 18, 543–6.

Jessop, D.C., Sparks, P., Buckland, N., Harris, P.R. and Churchill, S. (2014) Combining self-affirmation and implementation intentions: evidence of detrimental effects on behavioral outcomes, *Annals of Behavioral Medicine*, 47, 137–47.

Johnston, D.W. and Johnston, M. (2013) Useful theories should apply to individuals, *British Journal of Health Psychology*, 18, 469–73.

Kahle, L.R. and Beatty, S.E. (1987) The task situation and habit in the attitude–behavior relationship: a social adaptation view, *Journal of Social Behavior and Personality*, 2, 218–32.

Kassovou, A., Turner, A., Hamborg, T. and French, D.P. (2014) Predicting maintenance of attendance at walking groups: testing constructs from three leading maintenance theories, *Health Psychology*, 33, 752–6.

King, C.M., Rothman, A.J. and Jeffery, R.W. (2002) The challenge study: theory-based interventions for smoking and weight-loss, *Health Education Research*, 17, 522–30.

Klein, W.M., Harris, P.R., Ferrer, R.A. and Zajac, L.E. (2011) Feelings of vulnerability in response to threatening messages: effects of self-affirmation, *Journal of Experimental Social Psychology*, 47, 1237–42.

Knapp, D.N. (1988) Behavioral management techniques and exercise promotion, in R.K. Dishman (ed.) *Exercise Promotion: Its Impact on Public Health* (pp. 203–55). Champaign, IL: Human Kinetics.

Kok, G.J., De Vries, H., Mudde, A.N. and Strecher, V.J. (1991) Planned health education and the role of self-efficacy: Dutch research, *Health Education Research*, 6, 231–8.

Kruglanski, A.W., Thompson, E.P., Higgins, E.T., Atash, M.N., Pierro, A., Shah, J.H. *et al.* (2000) To 'do the right thing' or to 'just do it': locomotion and assessment as distinct self-regulatory imperatives, *Journal of Personality and Social Psychology*, 79, 793–815.

Kuhl, J. (1985) Volitional mediators of cognition–behavior consistency: self-regulatory processes and action versus state orientation, in J. Kuhl and J. Beckman (eds.) *Action Control: From Cognition to Behavior* (pp. 101–28). New York: Springer.

Laitakari, J., Vuori, I. and Oja, P. (1996) Is long-term maintenance of health-related physical activity possible? An analysis of concepts and evidence, *Health Education Research*, 11, 463–77.

Lally, P., Chipperfield, A. and Wardle, J. (2008) Healthy habits: efficacy of simple advice on weight control based on a habit-formation model, *International Journal of Obesity*, 32, 700–7.

Larimer, M.E., Palmer, R.S. and Marlatt, G.A. (1999) Relapse prevention: an overview of Marlatt's cognitive-behavioral model, *Alcohol Research and Health*, 23, 151–60.

Lauver, D.R., Henriques, J.B., Settersten, L. and Bumann, M.C. (2003a) Psychosocial variables, external barriers, and stage of mammography adoption, *Health Psychology*, 22, 649–53.

Lauver, D.R., Settersten, L., Kane, J.H. and Henriques, J.B. (2003b) Tailored messages, external barriers, and women's utilization of professional breast cancer screening over time, *Cancer*, 97, 2724–35.

Leffingwell, T.R., Neumann, C., Leedy, M.J. and Babitzke, A.C. (2007) Defensively biased responding to risk information among alcohol-using college students, *Addictive Behaviors*, 32, 158–65.

Leventhal, H., Singer, R. and Jones, S. (1965) Effects of fear and specificity of recommendation upon attitudes and behaviour, *Journal of Personality and Social Psychology*, 2, 313–21.

Liska, A.E. (1984) A critical examination of the causal structure of the Fishbein/Ajzen attitude–behavior model, *Social Psychology Quarterly*, 47, 61–74.

Logel, C. and Cohen, G.L. (2012) The role of the self in physical health: testing the effect of a values-affirmation intervention on weight loss, *Psychological Science*, 23, 53–5.

Manstead, A.S.R. (2000) The role of moral norm in the attitude–behavior relation, in D.J. Terry and M.A. Hogg (eds.) *Attitudes, Behavior, and Social Context* (pp. 11–30). Mahwah, NJ: Erlbaum.

Marcus, B.H. and Simkin, L.R. (1994) The transtheoretical model: applications to exercise behaviour, *Medical Science in Sport and Exercise*, 26, 1400–4.

Marlatt, G.A. and Gordon, J. (eds.) (1985) *Relapse Prevention: Maintenance Strategies in Addictive Behavior Change*. New York: Guilford Press.

Marshall, G.N., Wortman, C.B., Vickers, R.R., Kusulas, J.W. and Hervig, L.K. (1994) The five-factor model of personality as a framework for personality-health research, *Journal of Personality and Social Psychology*, 67, 278–86.

McCrae, R.R. and Costa, P.T., Jr. (1987) Validation of the five-factor model of personality across instruments and observers, *Journal of Personality and Social Psychology*, 54, 81–90.

McCrae, R.R. and Costa, P.T., Jr. (1990) *Personality in Adulthood* (2nd edn.). New York: Guilford Press.

McEachan, R.R.C., Conner, M., Taylor, N.J. and Lawton, R.J. (2011) Prospective prediction of health-related behaviors with the theory of planned behavior: a meta-analysis, *Health Psychology Review*, 5, 97–144.

Michie, S. and Abraham, C. (2004) Interventions to change health behaviours: evidence-based or evidence-inspired? *Psychology and Health*, 19, 29–49.

Michie, S. and Prestwich, A. (2010) Are interventions theory-based? Development of a theory coding scheme, *Health Psychology*, 29, 1–8.

Michie, S., Abraham, C., Whittington, C., McAteer, J. and Gupta, S. (2009) Effective techniques in healthy eating and physical activity interventions: a meta-regression, *Health Psychology*, 28, 690–701.

Michie, S., Richardson, M., Johnston, M., Abraham, C., Francis, J., Hardeman, W. *et al.* (2013) The behavior change technique taxonomy (v1) of 93 hierarchically clustered techniques: building an international consensus for the reporting of behavior change interventions, *Annals of Behavioral Medicine*, 46, 81–95.

Milne, S., Sheeran, P. and Orbell, S. (2000) Prediction and intervention in health-related behavior: a meta-analytic review of protection motivation theory, *Journal of Applied Social Psychology*, 30, 106–43.

Mullan, B.C., Wong, C., Allom, V. and Pack, S. (2011) The role of executive function in bridging the intention–behaviour gap for binge-drinking in university students, *Addictive Behaviors*, 36, 1023–6.

Murgraff, V., White, D. and Phillips, K. (1999) An application of protection motivation theory to riskier single-occasion drinking, *Psychology and Health*, 14, 339–50.

Nisbett, R.E. and Wilson, T.D. (1977) Telling more than we can know: verbal reports on mental processes, *Psychological Review*, 84, 231–59.

Noar, S.M. and Zimmerman, R.S. (2005) Health behavior theory and cumulative knowledge regarding health behaviors: are we moving in the right direction? *Health Education Research*, 20, 275–90.

Norman, P. (2011) The theory of planned behavior and binge drinking among undergraduate students: assessing the impact of habit strength, *Addictive Behaviors*, 36, 502–7.

Norman, P. and Brain, K. (2005) An application of an extended health belief model to the prediction of breast self-examination among women with a family history of breast cancer, *British Journal of Health Psychology*, 10, 1–16.

Norman, P. and Conner, M. (1996) Predicting health check attendance among prior attenders and non-attenders: the role of prior behaviour in the theory of planned behaviour, *Journal of Applied Social Psychology*, 26, 1010–26.

Norman, P. and Cooper, Y. (2011) The theory of planned behaviour and breast self-examination: assessing the impact of past behaviour, context stability and habit strength, *Psychology and Health*, 26, 1156–72.

Norman, P., Searle, A., Harrad, R. and Vedhara, K. (2003) Predicting adherence to eye patching in children with amblyopia: an application of protection motivation theory, *British Journal of Health Psychology*, 8, 67–82.

Nowalk, M.P., Zimmerman, R.K., Shen, S.H., Jewell, I.K. and Raymund, M. (2004) Barriers to pneumococcal and influenza vaccination in older community-dwelling adults (2000–2001), *Journal of the American Geriatrics Society*, 52, 25–30.

O'Brien, T.B. and DeLongis, A. (1996) The interactional context of problem-, emotion-, and relationship-focused coping: the role of the big five personality factors, *Journal of Personality*, 64, 775–813.

O'Cleirigh, C., Ironson, G., Weiss, A. and Costa, P.T. (2007) Conscientiousness predicts disease progression (CD4 number and viral load) in people living with HIV, *Health Psychology*, 26, 473–80.

Oakley, A., Fullerton, D., Holland, J., Arnold, S., Francedawson, M., Kelly, P. *et al.* (1995) Sexual health education interventions for young people: a methodological review, *British Medical Journal*, 310, 158–62.

Ogden, J. (2003) Some problems with social cognition models: a pragmatic and conceptual analysis, *Health Psychology*, 22, 424–8.

Oldridge, N. (1988) Cardiac rehabilitation exercise program: compliance and compliance enhancing strategies, *Sports Medicine*, 6, 42–55.

Orleans, C.T. (2000) Promoting maintenance of health behaviour change: recommendations for the next generation of research and practice, *Health Psychology*, 19, 76–83.

Ouellette, J. and Wood, W. (1998) Habit and intention in everyday life: the multiple processes by which past behavior predicts future behavior, *Psychological Bulletin*, 124, 54–74.

Papies, E.K. and Hamstra, P. (2010) Goal priming and eating behavior: enhancing self-regulation by environmental cues, *Health Psychology*, 29, 384–8.

Payne, B.K., McClernon, F.J. and Dobbins, I.G. (2007) Automatic affective responses to smoking cues, *Experimental and Clinical Psychopharmacology*, 15, 400–9.

Perri, M.G., Nezu, A.M., McKelvey, W.F., Shermer, R.L., Renjilian, D.A. and Viegener, B.J. (2001) Relapse prevention training and problem solving therapy in the long-term management of obesity, *Journal of Consulting and Clinical Psychology*, 69, 722–6.

Plotnikoff, R.C., Trinh, L., Courneya, K.S., Karunamuni, N. and Sigal, R.J. (2009) Predictors of aerobic physical activity and resistance training among Canadian adults with type 2 diabetes: an application of the protection motivation theory, *Psychology of Sport and Exercise*, 10, 320–8.

Prestwich, A., Sniehotta, F.F., Whittington, C., Dombrowski, S.U., Rogers, L. and Michie, S. (2014) Does theory influence the effectiveness of health behavior interventions? Meta-analysis, *Health Psychology*, 33, 465–74.

Prochaska, J.O., DiClemente, C.C. and Norcross, J.C. (1992) In search of how people change: applications to addictive behaviors, *American Psychologist*, 47, 1102–14.

Quinn, J.M., Pascoe, A.T., Wood, W. and Neal, D.T. (2010) Can't control yourself? Monitor those bad habits, *Personality and Social Psychology Bulletin*, 36, 499–511.

Rhodes, R.E. and Courneya, K.S. (2003) Relationships between personality, an extended theory of planned behaviour model and exercise behaviour, *British Journal of Health Psychology*, 8, 19–36.

Rhodes, R.E., Courneya, K.S. and Hayduk, L.A. (2002) Does personality moderate the theory of planned behavior in the exercise domain? *Journal of Sport and Exercise Psychology*, 24, 120–32.

Rhodes, R.E., Courneya, K.S. and Jones, L.W. (2003) Translating exercise intentions into behavior: personality and social cognitive correlates, *Journal of Health Psychology*, 8, 447–58.

Rhodes, R.E., Courneya, K.S. and Jones, L.W. (2005) The theory of planned behavior and lower-order personality traits: interaction effects in the exercise domain, *Personality and Individual Differences*, 38, 251–65.

Rodrigues, A.M., O'Brien, N., French, D.P., Glidewell, L. and Sniehotta, F.F. (2015) The question–behavior effect: genuine effect or spurious phenomenon? A systematic review of randomized controlled trials with meta-analyses, *Health Psychology*, 34, 61–78.

Rogers, R.W. (1983) Cognitive and physiological processes in fear appeals and attitude change: a revised theory of protection motivation, in J.T. Cacioppo and R.E. Petty (eds.) *Social Psychophysiology: A Source Book* (pp. 153–76). New York: Guilford Press.

Rooke, S.E., Hine, D.W. and Thorsteinsson, E.B. (2008) Implicit cognition and substance use: a meta analysis, *Addictive Behaviors*, 33, 1314–28.

Rothman, A.J. (2000) Toward a theory-based analysis of behavioral maintenance, *Health Psychology*, 19, 64–9.

Rothman, A.J. (2004) 'Is there nothing more practical than a good theory?' Why innovations and advances in health behavior change will arise if interventions are used to test and refine theory, *International Journal of Behavioral Nutrition and Physical Activity*, 11, 1–7.

Rothman, A.J., Baldwin, A.S., Hertel, A.W. and Fuglestad, P.T. (2011) Self-regulation and behavior change: disentangling behavioral initiation and behavioral maintenance, in K.D. Vohs and R.F. Baumeister (eds.) *Handbook of Self-regulation: Research, Theory, and Applications* (pp. 106–22). New York: Guilford Press.

Rothman, A.J., Sheeran, P. and Wood, W. (2009) Reflective and automatic processes in the initiation and maintenance of food choices, *Annals of Behavioral Medicine*, 28 (suppl.), 4–17.

Rutter, D.R. and Quine, L. (eds.) (2002) *Changing Health Behaviour*. Buckingham: Open University Press.

Sarver, V.T., Jr. (1983) Ajzen and Fishbein's 'theory of reasoned action': a critical assessment, *Journal for the Theory of Social Behaviour*, 13, 155–63.

Schoenmakers, T.M., de Bruin, M., Lux, I.F., Goertz, A.G., van Kerkhof, D.H. and Wiers, R.W. (2010) Clinical effectiveness of attentional bias modification training in abstinent alcoholic patients, *Drug and Alcohol Dependence*, 109, 30–6.

Schwartz, M.D., Taylor, K.L., Willard, K.S., Siegel, J.E., Lamdan, R.M. and Moran, K. (1999) Distress, personality, and mammography utilization among women with a family history of breast cancer, *Health Psychology*, 18, 327–32.

Schwarzer, R. (1992) Self-efficacy in the adoption and maintenance of health behaviors: theoretical approaches and a new model, in R. Schwarzer (ed.) *Self-efficacy: Thought Control of Action* (pp. 217–43). London: Hemisphere.

Sears, S.R. and Stanton, A.L. (2001) Expectancy-value constructs and expectance violation as predictors of exercise adherence in previously sedentary women, *Health Psychology*, 20, 326–33.

Seibold, D.R. and Roper, R.E. (1979) Psychosocial determinants of health care intentions: test of the Triandis and Fishbein models, in D. Nimmo (ed.) *Communication Yearbook 3* (pp. 625–43). New Brunswick, NJ: Transaction Books.

Senécal, C., Nouwen, A. and White, D. (2000) Motivation and dietary self-care in adults with diabetes: are self-efficacy and autonomous self-regulation complementary to competing constructs? *Health Psychology*, 19, 452–7.

Shankar, A., Conner, M. and Jones, F. (2004) Psychosocial predictors of maintenance of health behaviours. Unpublished manuscript, School of Psychology, University of Leeds.

Sheeran, P. (2002) Intention–behavior relations: a conceptual and empirical review, in W. Stroebe and M. Hewstone (eds.) *European Review of Social Psychology* (Vol. 12, pp. 1–36). Chichester: Wiley.

Sheeran, P., Conner, M. and Norman, P. (2001) Can the theory of planned behavior explain patterns of behavior change? *Health Psychology*, 20, 12–19.

Sheeran, P., Gollwitzer, P.M. and Bargh, J.A. (2013) Nonconscious processes and health, *Health Psychology*, 32, 460–73.

Sheeran, P., Harris, P.R. and Epton, T. (2014) Does heightening risk appraisals change people's intentions and behavior? A meta-analysis of experimental studies, *Psychological Bulletin*, 140, 511–43.

Sheeran, P., Maki, A., Montanaro, E., Bryan, A., Klein, W.M.P., Miles, E. *et al.* (submitted) The impact of changing attitudes, norms, and self-efficacy on health-related intentions and behavior: a meta-analysis. Manuscript submitted for publication.

Shepperd, J.A., Klein, W.M.P., Waters, E.A. and Weinstein, N.D. (2013) Taking stock of unrealistic optimism, *Perspectives on Psychological Science*, 8, 395–411.

Sherman, D.K., Cohen, G.L., Nelson, L.D., Nussbaum, A.D., Bunyan, D.P. and Garcia, J. (2009) Affirmed yet unaware: exploring the role of awareness in the process of self-affirmation, *Journal of Personality and Social Psychology*, 97, 745–64.

Sherwood, N.E. and Jeffery, R.W. (2000) The behavioral determinants of exercise: implications for physical activity interventions, *Annual Review of Nutrition*, 20, 21–44.

Siegler, I.C., Feaganes, J.R. and Rimer, B.K. (1995) Predictors of adoption of mammography in women under age 50, *Health Psychology*, 14, 274–8.

Skinner, C.S., Kreuter, M.W., Kobrin, S.C. and Strecher, V.J. (1998) Perceived and actual breast cancer risk: optimistic and pessimistic biases, *Journal of Health Psychology*, 3, 181–93.

Smedslund, J. (2000) A pragmatic basis for judging models and theories in health psychology: the axiomatic method, *Journal of Health Psychology*, 5, 133–49.

Sniehotta, F.F. and Presseau, J. (2012) The habitual use of the self-report habit index, *Annals of Behavioral Medicine*, 43, 139–40.

Sniehotta, F.F., Presseau, J. and Araujo-Soares, V. (2014) Time to retire the theory of planned behaviour, *Health Psychology Review*, 8, 1–7.

Stacy, A.W., Ames, S.L., Ullman, J.B., Zogg, J.B. and Leigh, B.C. (2006) Spontaneous cognition and HIV risk behaviour, *Psychology of Addictive Behaviors*, 20, 196–206.

Steele, C.M. (1988) The psychology of self-affirmation: sustaining the integrity of the self, *Advances in Experimental Social Psychology*, 21, 261–302.

Stephens, R.S., Roffman, R.A. and Simpson, E.E. (1994) Treating adult marijuana dependence: a test of the relapse prevention model, *Journal of Consulting and Clinical Psychology*, 62, 92–9.

Stetson, B.A., Beacham, A.O., Frommelt, S.J., Boutelle, K.N., Colem J.D., Ziegler, C.H. *et al.* (2005) Exercise slips in high-risk situations and activity patterns in long-terms exercisers: an application of the relapse prevention model, *Annals of Behavioral Medicine*, 30, 25–35.

Strack, F. and Deutsch, R. (2004) Reflective and impulsive determinants of social behaviour, *Personality and Social Psychology Review*, 8, 220–47.

Stroebe, W., Mensink, W., Aarts, H., Schut, H. and Kruglanski, A.W. (2008) Why dieters fail: testing the goal conflict model of eating, *Journal of Experimental Social Psychology*, 44, 26–36.

Sweeney, A.M. and Moyer, A. (2015) Self-affirmation and responses to health messages: a meta-analysis on intentions and behavior, *Health Psychology*, 34, 149–59.

Syrjala, A.M., Knuuttila, M.L. and Syrjala, L.K. (2001) Self-efficacy perceptions in oral health behaviour, *Acta Odontologica Scandinavica*, 59, 1–6.

Todd, J., Kothe, E., Mullan, B. and Monds, L. (2014) Reasoned versus reactive prediction of behavior: a meta-analysis of the prototype willingness model, *Health Psychology Review*, 8, 1–24.

Toomey, T., Lenk, K.M. and Wagenaar, A.C. (2007) Environmental policies to reduce college drinking: an update of research findings, *Journal of Studies on Alcohol and Drugs*, 68, 208–19.

Trafimow, D. (2009) The theory of reasoned action: a case study of falsification in psychology, *Theory and Psychology*, 19, 501–18.

Trafimow, D. and Wyer, R.S. (1993) Cognitive representation of mundane social events, *Journal of Personality and Social Psychology*, 64, 365–76.

Triandis, H.C. (1977) *Interpersonal Behavior*. Monterey, CA: Brooks-Cole.

Triandis, H.C. (1980) Values, attitudes and interpersonal behavior, in M.M. Page (ed.) *Nebraska Symposium on Motivation 1979* (pp. 195–259). Lincoln, NB: University of Nebraska Press.

Van Bree, R.J.H., van Stralen, M.M., Bolman, C., Mudde, A.N., de Vries, H. and Lechner, L. (2013) Habit as moderator of the intention–physical activity relationship in older adults: a longitudinal study, *Psychology and Health*, 28, 514–32.

Van der Velde, W. and Hooykaas, C. (1996) Conditional versus unconditional risk estimates in models of AIDS-related risk behaviour, *Psychology and Health*, 12, 87–100.

Verplanken, B. and Aarts, H. (1999) Habit, attitude and planned behaviour: is habit an empty construct or an interesting case of automaticity? *European Review of Social Psychology*, 10, 101–34.

Verplanken, B. and Orbell, S. (2003) Reflections on past behavior: a self-report index of habit strength, *Journal of Applied Social Psychology*, 33, 1313–30.

Verplanken, B., Aarts, H., van Knippenberg, A. and Moonen, A. (1998) Habit versus planned behaviour: a field experiment, *British Journal of Social Psychology*, 37, 111–28.

Verplanken, B., Aarts, H., van Knippenberg, A. and van Knippenberg, C. (1994) Attitude versus general habit: antecedents of travel mode choice, *Journal of Applied Social Psychology*, 24, 285–300.

Voils, C.I., Gierisch, J.M., Yancy, W.S., Sandelowski, M., Smith, R., Bolton, J. *et al.* (2014) Differentiating behavior initiation and maintenance: theoretical framework and proof of concept, *Health Education and Behavior*, 41, 325–36.

Watson, D. and Hubbard, B. (1996) Adaptational style and dispositional structure: coping in the context of the five-factor model, *Journal of Personality*, 64, 737–74.

Webb, T.L. and Sheeran, P. (2006) Does changing behavioural intentions engender behavior change? A meta-analysis of experimental evidence, *Psychological Bulletin*, 132, 249–68.

Webb, T.L., Joseph, J., Yardley, L. and Michie, S. (2010) Using the internet to promote health behavior change: a systematic review and meta-analysis of the impact of theoretical basis, use of behavior change techniques, and mode of delivery on efficacy, *Journal of Medical Internet Research*, 12, e4.

Weinstein, N.D. (1983) Reducing unrealistic optimism about illness susceptibility, *Health Psychology*, 2, 11–20.

Weinstein, N.D. (1984) Why it won't happen to me: perceptions of risk factors and illness susceptibility, *Health Psychology*, 3, 431–57.

Weinstein, N.D. (1987) Unrealistic optimism about susceptibility to health problems: conclusions from a community-wide sample, *Journal of Behavioural Medicine*, 10, 481–99.

Weinstein, N.D. (1988) The precaution adoption process, *Health Psychology*, 7, 355–86.

Weinstein, N.D. and Klein, W. (1996) Unrealistic optimism: present and future, *Journal of Social and Clinical Psychology*, 15, 1–8.

Weinstein, N.D. and Nicolich, M. (1993) Correct and incorrect interpretations of correlations between risk perceptions and risk behaviors, *Health Psychology*, 12, 235–45.

Wiers, R.W., Eberl, C., Rinck, M., Becker, E. and Lindenmeyer, J. (2011) Retraining automatic action tendencies changes alcoholic patients' approach bias for alcohol and improves treatment outcome, *Psychological Science*, 22, 290–7.

Williams, G.C., Gagné, M., Ryan, R.M. and Deci, E.L. (2002) Facilitating autonomous motivation for smoking cessation, *Health Psychology*, 21, 40–50.

Williams, G.C., Rodin, G.C., Ryan, R.M., Grolnick, W.S. and Deci, E.L. (1998) Autonomous regulation and long-term medication adherence in medical outpatients, *Health Psychology*, 17, 269–76.

Wing, R.R., Marcus, M.D., Epstein, L.H. and Jawad, A. (1991) A 'family-based' approach to the treatment of obese Type II diabetic patients, *Journal of Consulting and Clinical Psychology*, 59, 156–62.

Wong, C. and Mullan, B. (2009) Predicting breakfast consumption: an application of the theory of planned behaviour and the investigation of past behaviour and executive function, *British Journal of Health Psychology*, 14, 489–504.

Wood, C., Conner, M., Sandberg, T., Taylor, N., Godin, G., Miles, E. *et al.* (submitted) A meta-analysis of the question–behavior effect: mechanisms and moderators. Manuscript submitted for publication.

Index

Page numbers in *italics* indicate figures and tables.

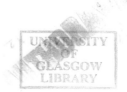

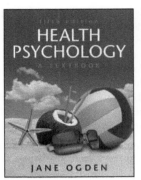

HEALTH PSYCHOLOGY
A Textbook
Fifth Edition

Jane Ogden

9780335243839 (Paperback)
eBook: 9780335243846
2012

The market leading textbook in the field, *Health Psychology* by Jane Ogden
is essential reading for all students and researchers of health psychology. It
will also be invaluable to students of medicine, nursing and allied health.
Retaining the breadth of coverage, clarity and relevance that has made it a
favourite with students and lecturers, this fourth edition has been thoroughly
revised and updated.

Key features:

- New chapter on women's health issues, exploring recent research into
  pregnancy, miscarriage, birth, menopause and related areas
- Updated "Focus on Research" examples to introduce contemporary
  topics and emerging areas for research in health psychology, including
  exercise, smoking and pain
- Includes new data, graphs and further reading plus suggestions about
  where to access the most recent publications and other data

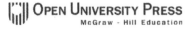

www.openup.co.uk